Critical Care Nursing

Caring for the critically ill adult

For Jane, Benjamin and Claire
and for Sally, Aaron and Rebecca

Critical Care Nursing

Caring for the critically ill adult

Edited by

Brian Millar and Philip Burnard
*University of Wales College of Medicine
Cardiff*

Baillière Tindall

LONDON PHILADELPHIA TORONTO SYDNEY TOKYO

Baillière Tindall 24–28 Oval Road
W. B. Saunders London NW1 7DX

The Curtis Center
Independence Square West
Philadelphia, PA 19106-3399, USA

Harcourt Brace & Company
55 Horner Avenue
Toronto, Ontario, M8Z 4X6, Canada

Harcourt Brace & Company, Australia
30–52 Smidmore Street
Marrickville
NSW 2204, Australia

Harcourt Brace & Company, Japan
Ichibancho Central Building
22-1 Ichibancho
Chiyoda-ku, Tokyo 102, Japan

A catalogue record for this book is available from the British Library
ISBN 0-7020-1549-0

Typeset by Paston Press Ltd, Loddon, Norfolk
Printed and bound in Great Britain by Bath Press, Avon

Contents

Foreword: Carol Ball

It is interesting to reflect on the diversity of issues which currently impact on the practice of nursing in Critical Care Areas. Whereas, in the past, the major focus was purely physiological, it is now self evident that critical care nursing should be placed in a broader context. This is necessary from a political, professional and personal standpoint.

Millar and Burnard are to be commended for the inception of this text, which provides a breadth of information related to critical care, rather than a narrow perspective. All the authors included have extensive knowledge of their subject area, evidenced by their erudition and the reference material provided. Areas of particular interest are quality of care and the often neglected issue of the impact of critical illness on the family.

None of the usual problems which beset multi-author works, namely overlap and repetition, are evident in this text. Each chapter stands as an entity in itself and presents a particular area, pertinent to critical care, for consideration. Uniformity of presentation is achieved through the use of a specific format. Case studies are provided, which aid the novice in critical care to understand some of the complex issues discussed and a list of key terms is available for reference. Areas for further study are also identified.

Those involved in higher education will also find the text of value, as it provides a definitive focus for many of the concepts addressed during postgraduate study, which frequently appear divorced from the nurse's everyday experience of critical care. Of equal importance to all nurses is the clear and concise prose style of all the authors. Every effort is made to engender understanding of the sometimes complex issues under discussion. The result is an excellent text relevant to all nurses currently practising in the arena of Critical Care Nursing.

Carol Ball MSc, DipNE, RN
Course Director MSc in Nursing, City University, St Bartholomew's, Princess Alexandra and Newham College of Nursing and Midwifery, St Bartholomew's Hospital, London

Preface

Caring for the Critically Ill Adult provides a foundation upon which the general concepts of critical care nursing practice, including knowledge and skills, are built. The rapid developments in science and technology, combined with advances in nursing practice and education, have provided a stimulus for collecting the contributors to this book. The purpose of the book is to provide a research-based resource for those intending to nurse, or indeed currently nursing in critical care units. Our intention is to illustrate the value of reflective practice for developing not only the knowledge and skills of critical care nursing but also the 'holistic' care which critically ill patients and their families deserve.

GENERAL COMMENTS

This text is specifically geared to the student in the field of critical care nursing who is working towards a career as a critical care nurse. The student will find its content applicable from classroom through clinical practice, and later as a registered practitioner. For those already registered the text will provide a valuable resource tool; it is also useful for those students on postgraduate courses. The authors have drawn upon the expertise and abilities of critical care managers, practitioners, researchers and educators, eliminating the need for supplemental textbooks.

Throughout the book the authors have tried to minimize gender specific language whenever possible. We recognize the influence that language has on how we think and behave. This book is a tribute to all those who have dedicated their professional career to the care of the critically ill, wherever it is required.

ORGANIZATION

Caring for the Critically Ill Adult is divided into five units, with all of the authors following a similar format for the presentation of their chapter(s).

Section one describes the important concepts for caring for the critically ill adult. It begins by introducing the reader to the world of critical care nursing, the role and responsibilities of the critical care nurse in providing individualized patient care. Topics covered include the impact of technology, delivering care through the application of nursing theory/models, primary nursing in the critical care unit, and the use and application of complementary therapies in caring for the critically ill individual.

Section two provides knowledge of fundamental issues in the institution which influence the care of the critically ill adult. Individual chapters explore the contribution of management and education to the development of quality critical care nursing practice, the impact of stress and burnout, and the increasing importance of quality assurance in the care of the critically ill adult. Practical skills are emphasized.

The major focus for **Section three** is the family of the critically ill person. Specific chapters focus upon caring for families, as well as examining the increasing importance of ethical issues for the critical care nurse practitioner. In this section the authors also acknowledge the importance of more than one source of knowledge; a chapter examines the importance of spirituality for the client and the family, and the sensitive issue of death and dying in critical care is reviewed with practical examples and skills being provided throughout.

Section four emphasizes the contributions to both our knowledge and understanding of the care of the critically ill person form other disciplines. Chapters address the importance of concepts from disciplines such as psychology and sociology. Communication knowledge and skills are explored, as are the use of counselling skills in the critical care unit.

Finally, though by no means less important, we offer a brief glimpse into the future. Futurists such as Toffler and Ferguson have been predicting the challenges facing us for some two decades. In their vision a key challenge will be harnessing the explosion in information technology which is gradually invading all aspects of our professional and personal lives. We are delighted that a colleague of ours, and a personal friend and mentor, Nancy Gantz, a Vice President of Nursing in the USA, has been able to contribute to this book. Nancy has extensive experience in working within critical care and has been involved in the introduction and development of information technology systems in critical care in the USA. Her experience and vision are a tremendous asset to this book. In some respects, her chapter may be familiar to some, and new ground for others. We believe, however, that the impact of information technology in critical care here in the UK has yet to be fulfilled. This important chapter concludes our book by providing an insightful and stimulating vision for a future critical care where the human skills of critical care nurses are combined with the latest available technology to provide the highest quality nursing care possible for patients and their families.

SPECIAL FEATURES

Throughout the planning and development of this book our primary purpose has been to aid the reader. The following special features have been incorporated:

☐   **Chapter format:** Each chapter begins by outlining its content, allowing the reader quick reference to each topic.

☐   **Aims:** All of the contributors have provided a set of aims/objectives to help the reader quickly identify what they can learn from the chapter.

☐   **Glossary of terms:** A list of key terms have been identified and defined by the contributors and are emphasized in the chapter itself.

☐   **Self learning:** Clinical examples are provided where appropriate for self-assessment and reflection. A short list of guiding questions are provided to help you assess your learning outcomes from reading the chapter or consider the relevance to your own practice.

☐   Finally, all of the chapters include a brief Further Reading list for those who want to develop their knowledge and skills about a topic further.

Our intention to provide comprehensive coverage of the fundamental principles of caring for the critically ill is evident in the choice of the contributors. Each is an expert in his or her field, and we believe that they have provided a wholly new and exciting foundation text for critical care nursing in the United Kingdom. We hope that the reader will find this book refreshing and applicable to their practice, and a stimulus to continue the process of developing and learning about the field of critical care nursing. As editors we would welcome the comments, criticisms and ideas of the reader for the improvement of future editions.

List of Contributors

Rachel Ashcroft BSc(Hons), RN, ENB 998, ENB 100 is currently travelling around the world. Previously she was based at Southampton General Hospital where she was a staff nurse in ITU. She has a degree in Nursing Studies from the University of Surrey, and qualifications in chiropractic, aromatherapy, and anatomy, physiology and massage. She is a member of the Institute of Professional Therapists.

Belinda L Atkinson BSc(Hons), RGN, RSCN, Dip N(Lond) currently holds the post of Clinical Services Manager, Intensive Care Units for Southampton University Hospitals. She was a founder member of the British Association of Critical Care Nurses, and held the office of President between 1989–1991. She currently represents the United Kingdom and Europe as the liaison member for the World Federation of Societies of Intensive and Critical Care Medicine.

Philip Burnard PhD MSc, RGN, RMN, DipN, Cert Ed, RNT is Director of Postgraduate Nursing Studies at the University of Wales College of Medicine in Cardiff. He has written a variety of books about communication, counselling, education and ethics. He has contributed to nursing and health care journals in the UK, USA, Italy, Finland and the Czech State. His research interests include counselling skills, AIDS counselling, experiential learning and forensic psychiatric nursing.

Rebecca Carter BN(Hons), RGN, Dip HV, RHV gained a Bachelor of Nursing Upper Second Class Honours Degree from the University of Wales College of Medicine, Cardiff, graduating in 1990. Her final year dissertation was a study researching qualified nurses' perceptions of the spiritual care of patients. At the time of writing she is working in the Community in West Sussex as Health Visitor for Mid-Downs Health Authority.

Helen Ellis RGN, Dip N, BSc, MSc (Manchester), ENB 100, ENB 920 is based in the Lancashire College of Nursing and Health Studies, Preston as ENB 100 course teacher, and is responsible for development of Critical Care Pathways for Framework and Higher National Award. She is currently Chairperson for Education Forum and Chairperson for Education Forum BACCN 1990.

Nancy Rollins Gantz PhD, MBA, RN, CNA is Assistant Vice President, Patient Care Services, Executive Director, Regional Heart Center, Deaconess Medical Center, Spokane, Washington, USA.

Penny Irwin BA(Hons), RGN, SCM, ENB 100, MSc is Senior Nurse, Quality Assurance and Nurse Manager for Clinical Nurse Specialists, the Barts NHS Group, London. In 1983–1985 she undertook a hyperbaric oxygen research trial funded by the Multiple Sclerosis Society at St Thomas' Hospital, and in 1988–1989 completed a MSc at Manchester University.

Netta Lloyd-Jones RGN, Dip N (Dist) is a Nurse Teacher in the Continuing Education Department of the South Wales Institute of Nursing and Midwifery Education, responsible initially for the W.N.B. courses 100 and 115, and both Certificate and Diploma level modules in general intensive and critical care nursing. She is an active member of the British Association of Critical Care Nurses (BACCN), acting as Chairman from 1982–1992, and is currently National Representative for Wales and National Membership Secretary. She is undertaking a Masters in Nursing at the University of Wales College of Medicine.

Kim Manley RN, Dip N(Lond), RCNT, BA, MN (Wales), PGCE(A) is currently Clinical Nurse Specialist on the Chelsea and Westminster Nursing Development Unit/ITU and also lecturer in nursing one day a week to the Masters in Nursing Course at the Institute of Advanced Nursing Education of the RCN. She has a Masters degree in nursing from the University of Wales, specializing in the implementation and evaluation of Primary Care in Intensive Care.

Brian Millar RGN, DN (Lond), MN (Wales), PGCE(A) is currently a lecturer in Nursing Studies at the School of Nursing Studies, University of Wales College of Medicine in Cardiff. Since coming to Cardiff he has helped to start the Welsh Intensive Care Group (Now the Welsh Branch of BACCN) and has undertaken research into family needs and family nursing in ITU. Currently he is working on a PhD on the subject of promoting family-nursing interventions.

Paul Morrison BA, PhD, RMN, RGN, PGCE, CPsychol, AFBPsS is a lecturer in the School of Nursing Studies, University of Wales College of Medicine in Cardiff, where he teaches psychology. He trained in psychiatric and general nursing and worked as a staff nurse, charge nurse and research nurse before taking up his present post. He studied psychology at University College of North Wales in Bangor, and completed a PhD in applied psychology at Sheffield Hallam University.

Evelyn P. Parsons BSc, PhD, DIA, MIPM (Sociology/Social Policy), a medical sociologist, is a lecturer in the School of Nursing Studies at the University of Wales College of Medicine Cardiff and a Research Fellow in the Institute of Medical Genetics. She is currently responsible for the psychosocial evaluation of the newborn screening programme for Duchenne muscular dystrophy in Wales.

Jim Richardson BA, RGN, RSCN, PGCE is currently Lecturer in Nursing Studies (Care of the Child), School of Nursing Studies, University of Wales College of Medicine. He has been involved in child health nursing both here in the United Kingdom and abroad in Finland, and has undertaken visits to Latvia as a consultant through the World Health Organisation. His interests include cultural aspects of child health care and adaptation of families to chronic childhood illnesses.

Christopher Turnock RGN, DPSN, DANS, MSc, NT is currently a nurse teacher in the Continuing Nurse Education and Research Unit of Newcastle and Northumbria College of Health Studies, where he has been the course teacher to the ENB Intensive Care Nursing course. He previously worked as a staff nurse on the intensive care unit at Newcastle General Hospital and has undertaken research into the views of intensive care nurses on the psychological needs of their patients.

David Thompson BSc, MA, PhD, RGN, RMN, ONC, FRCN is Reader in Cardiac Nursing at the Institute of Nursing in Oxford. He has spent 15 years of his professional life specialising in cardiac nursing, holding a variety of clinical and academic posts. He is actively engaged in research, and has published widely in the scientific and popular press.

Ann Ceinwen Tuxill BA(Hons) (Philosophy) is presently Principal Lecturer, School of Health and Community Studies, Sheffield Hallam University, where she teaches Ethics and Social Responsibility on a range of degree courses. She has published widely in this area, and in 1989 presented a paper on Ethics in Critical Care to the Annual Conference of the British Association of Critical Care Nurses.

Section 1
CARING FOR THE
CRITICALLY ILL INDIVIDUAL

This section identifies and explores the key role of the nurse in critical care. It describes the important concepts of caring for the critically ill adult and introduces the crucial responsibilities of the nurse to provide individualized patient care.

1
CRITICAL CARE TODAY
Belinda L. Atkinson

CHAPTER AIMS

This chapter will outline several issues concerning the provision of critical care services today. Many of these, and others, will be discussed in greater detail by the authors of subsequent chapters. In some respects, it is difficult to be totally comprehensive because critical care is a dynamic, expanding and rapidly changing speciality – features which, in themselves, make it an exciting and rewarding specialist area to be involved with. Specifically, this chapter aims to set the scene by considering the following issues:

☐ The history of critical care;

☐ Current issues;

☐ Applications to clinical practice.

INTRODUCTION

Throughout the world, health-care remains high on the political agenda; and it can be suggested that there are two main reasons for this – firstly, that health-care consumes large quantities of financial resources; and secondly, that it affects mankind universally (but not necessarily equally) – regardless of race, creed, class or background. In addition, efforts by various countries to rationalize health care services have, in many cases, led to explicit rationing in an effort to promote cost-effectiveness.

Critical care is central to this debate, because although it is costly, it can – by virtue of limited resources – be only applied selectively to a small section of the population. It is this very need to be selective that gives rise to many of the debates and dilemmas surrounding the provision of critical care services. Many of the resulting issues are complex, but few can be discussed in isolation,

and each needs to be taken in the context of critical care as a whole. In essence, the Gestalt theory applies – the whole is indeed greater than the sum of the parts.

In addition, we now live in an age of rapid communication and travel – both also products of developing technology. The result produces a sense of geographical proximity – so that we are able to feel more intimately concerned with problems and events that might previously have seemed rather remote.

However, one of the advantages of this new apparent closeness is that one now has the opportunity to share issues and concerns relating to health care – and, of course, in this case in particular, critical care – between nurses and other health care professionals worldwide.

It would seem that both reassurance and concerns have resulted. Reassurance because it has been found that others are experiencing similar problems, but concerns because it has been found that some problems occur on a larger scale than had previously been envisaged. However, the way to develop critical care practice, and, in particular, critical care nursing is surely to analyse the experience of others on a large scale and extract and develop the very best. In turn, this requires the development of certain skills by critical care nurses, which have implications in their own right in terms of the provision of education, research opportunities, management development, and so on. Critical care nursing can be said to have long been an art, but the time has come to substantiate the practice and develop the science.

Firstly, though, it is necessary to start by going back to the beginning, because the genesis of modern critical care, and indeed, of some of today's issues, occurs in a former decade.

THE HISTORY OF CRITICAL CARE

Critical care has a long history, although the main phases of development have perhaps been concentrated at certain specific time points. It would seem that the earliest reference to this type of care appears in Florence Nightingale's *Notes on Hospitals*, written in 1859, where she stated:

> "It is not uncommon, in small country hospitals to have a recess or small room leading from the operating theatre; in which patients remain until they have recovered, or at least recovered from the immediate effects of the operation."

Lenihan, writing in 1979, described how the origins of modern intensive care can be seen in the efforts made during the Second World War to develop facilities for the treatment of shock. He further describes how "as army surgical units moved nearer the battle fronts, between 1943 and 1945, specialised teams were assembled to provide pre-operative and post-operative intensive care with good results."

Later, the 1950s saw the advent of units for assisted ventilation, as the result of a polio epidemic, which was affecting most of the western world. These units occurred first in Denmark, at the Rigshospital in Copenhagen; and then spread throughout Europe, North America and elsewhere.

Hillman (1990) suggests that one of the features of intensive care, then as now, was the cooperation between different specialities, in this case anaesthetists and physicians, to solve old problems in a new way. It was also soon realized that these patients were best treated in a common area, thus optimizing medical, nursing and technological resources – and so the concept of an intensive care unit was born.

The 1960s and 1970s saw the development of intensive care units on a relatively rapid scale, with a gradual increase in size and sophistication. Units were present in almost all teaching hospitals and in many district general hospitals. The level of facility which should be provided in each type of centre remains contentious today, and will be referred to again subsequently in the chapter concerned with management of the critical care unit.

The 1980s, however, saw something of a change in this pattern. Several intensivists, including Tinker (1978), have previously referred to the soundness, economic and otherwise, of grouping critically ill patients together in the same area. However, with the emergence of developing specialities, and the latter present-day need for specialities to 'market' themselves in a cost-effective manner in the new health service financing arrangements, there has begun to be fragmentation of intensive care services. Whether this is a good thing or not probably remains to be seen. In itself, though, it has led to the adaption of the term 'critical care' to embrace all high-tech, specialist services, e.g. intensive care, cardiothoracic intensive care, coronary care, neurosciences intensive care, and so on.

The way in which critical care has developed has given rise to some specific issues which will now be examined in greater detail.

CURRENT ISSUES – EXTRACTS FROM THE LITERATURE

"Thirty years ago, when intensive care was young, so were our patients – usually under forty, and suffering from well defined diseases with a known course. We knew that if our efforts were successful then the patient would be able to resume life as it had been prior to the illness; there was nothing to lose and everything to gain . . . we accepted virtually all the patients referred to us and, for all of them, we did everything in our power to help. We could perceive no external forces restricting our action: financial resources covered our needs, we were never criticised for abusing our power; we seemed to have the publics' blessing for all we did."

So wrote the French physician Maurice Rapin, in 1987, shortly before his somewhat premature death – and this extract would seem to be a good starting point from which to examine some of the current issues in critical care today. During the last 30 years, the care of seriously ill patients has, as has already been suggested, developed very rapidly – and the practice of critical care today is very different to that of 30 years ago outlined by Maurice Rapin.

Therapeutic techniques have become increasingly complex, and, together with advances in technology and new practices, have resulted in the ability to care for increasingly sick and complex patients – patients who would probably have had little or no chance of surviving, only a few years ago.

Speaking of current practice in 1987 Rapin stated that "patients are older, suffer from more serious disorders, and usually have more than one failing vital organ, and we are now capable of supporting the failing vital functions almost indefinitely . . . new medical techniques are now available which yield results before unimaginable . . . physicians have become more and more aggressive in their approach to disease."

Rapin is not the only writer to have alluded to the complexities that have emerged in modern-day critical care practice. Tinker (1978) stated that "the high costs of intensive care have inevitably invited questions on the ethics of concentrating so much of the resources on a relatively small number of patients."

Jacobs (1988) suggests that "treatment of critically ill patients in high technology intensive care units has become rather complex, and very expensive."

Sprung (1990) states that "critical care medicine is currently being practised in difficult times. Great technological advances have been curtailed by limited resources, and have led to frustrating ethical dilemmas".

And finally, the King's Fund Panel (1989) stated that "at a time when resources for health services are tightly constrained, it is important to ensure that the money available is used effectively and efficiently."

We are concerned here with current issues and how they affect the state of critical care today – and in particular, critical care nursing. However, it has already been suggested that the practice of critical care is complex and multi-faceted, and it is therefore difficult to separate out specific areas as the whole concept of critical care needs to be taken as a complete entity, and the relevant components put in appropriate context.

Knaus (1989), again writing of the early days of intensive care as compared with today, states:

"Only a few intensivists practising today remember those times, and none of us expect to relive them. The world of intensive care today presents different challenges. We can no longer accept all patients referred to us, we realise our ability to help patients with multiple as opposed to single organ system failure is limited, and we feel increasingly restricted by reduced budgets; but increased demands for professional and public accountability."

This sentiment was echoed by Edwards (1992) in a television documentary. He suggests that "intensive care has been a victim of its own success. Ten years ago, complex patients would not have had the same chance of survival – but in many cases we are still treating them with the same resources."

What are the main issues?

In searching for a concise overview of the main problems encountered in the clinical practice of critical care, the author returned to the work of Maurice Rapin (1987). Here, he categorizes the most controversial intensive care situations into three groups – because these require physicians and the multidisciplinary team to make decisions regarding treatment. Discussions with critical care personnel in other countries would, additionally, suggest that these do not appear to differ much around the world. They are:

"1. Irreversible deterioration of higher cerebral functions.
2. The indefinite need for artificial ventilation.
3. Irreversible failure of the left ventricle." (Rapin 1987).

In addition, technology itself can perhaps be viewed as a double edged sword, because better information can now generally be obtained regarding the patient's diagnosis and condition, and there is a wider range of therapeutic possibilities at the physician's disposal, having made the decision to treat. However, and conversely, the ability of such technology to sustain life almost indefinitely has produced dilemmas of its own – largely revolving around how far to proceed, and when to withdraw. In recent years, there is little doubt that the issues surrounding this area have risen to the forefront frequently in many different contexts.

In April 1991, Professor William Knaus from the United States of America, addressed the annual Intensive Care Society (UK) meeting. In a paper discussing the prediction of outcome from critical care, Professor Knaus made the following general points:

☐ We care for the most 'expensive' people in our society; and these are also some of the most vulnerable.

☐ We (the critical care team) are required to make frequent decisions which influence the time and circumstances of a person's death.

☐ We have to consider quality of life – is it, indeed possible, to create an outcome which is worse for the patient than death?

☐ And finally, we must find ways of rationally distributing the greatly increased variety of medical services. (Knaus 1991, unpublished).

This implies the need to make rational decisions about who should receive critical care, based upon the probability of being able to benefit the patient rather than on pure bed availability. This is an important issue because, at the time of writing, the provision and number of critical care beds in the United Kingdom is a highly political issue, and has gained media coverage on an increasing number of occasions. In essence, it is necessary to develop efficient systems of audit and cost containment, and to consider issues relating to the quality of life, and to enhance skills for rational ethical decision making.

"Successful treatment" states Harris, in the *Journal of Medical Ethics* (1987), "removes the danger to life, or at least postpones it, and so survival rates of treatment have been regarded as a good indicator of success. However, equally clearly, it is also of crucial importance to those treated, that the health offered them not only removes the threat to life, but also leaves them able to enjoy the remission granted. In short, gives them reasonable quality, as well as extended quantity of life."

To take the discussion of critical care as it is today further, it is necessary to return again momentarily to the beginning, and consider what critical care is – and, perhaps, what it is not.

Many questions have been raised concerning the delivery of critical care, and those posed by the American National Institute of Health in 1984 probably still represent the most common questions asked internationally. These include:

☐ Is there empirical evidence that intensive care units cause a decrease in patient morbidity or mortality? Which patients are most likely to benefit from intensive care?

☐ What skills are essential for personnel in a critical care unit? How should this personnel be trained and organized to ensure the best care for patients most in need?

☐ What special technology and therapeutic intervention should be routinely available for the most effective ICU function?

☐ How is a hospital's critical care delivery system best structured: one large multi-specialty unit or multiple small sub-specialty units?

☐ How has the development of critical care units affected the traditional functions of a hospital?

☐ What direction should critical care research follow?

The answers to many of these questions are still being sought, and some suggestions will be made as to the type of discussion points frequently encountered. As a starting point, it is becoming increasingly apparent when global concerns relating to critical care are examined, that there are one or two that occur time and time again. In essence, it will have by now become apparent that these revolve around the cost of such care; the justification for its expense, and the equitable distribution of critical care resources amongst the population.

If (as it appears to be increasingly assumed) critical care is a costly service to provide, then there has to be something said about its audit and cost benefit analysis. One of the problems with the way in which the National Health Service is funded is that if funding for intensive care units is not appropriate it tends to impinge upon the resources of other departments – often leading to inter-departmental friction, and increased scrutiny of local, and in many cases, global intensive care practice. Therefore, it is necessary that the question is asked – does intensive care work, and what are the benefits to patients, to the health care system and to society generally?

Many efforts have been made in recent years to produce empirical data to substantiate the use of intensive care units, and some aspects of the evaluation of critical care practice will be covered in more depth in subsequent chapters, so comments here will be of a more general nature, and perhaps more specifically related to intensive care.

In 1988, the Kings Fund College in London staged a consensus conference on intensive care. It is interesting to note that the questions raised were, in essence, similar to those that have already been referred to from the USA:

- [ ] Is there scientific evidence that ICU's cause a decrease in mortality and morbidity?
- [ ] What criteria should be set for admission and discharge to ICUs?
- [ ] Which classes of patients are likely to benefit most from which procedures that are carried out in an ICU?
- [ ] For what extra cost is therapeutic benefit gained by using intensive care?

- [ ] What scale of provision is needed in the NHS? What are the pros and cons of a large multi-specialty unit or small sub-speciality units? (King's Fund, 1989).

These questions will be referred to in more detail in the chapter concerned with management of the critical care unit. It is, however, interesting to note that the areas causing concern have changed little in the last decade.

The second point of interest regarding the Kings Fund conference was that the consensus conference, as such, failed – and the main reason given for this was the fact that the panel had insufficient data with which to arrive at a consensus opinion, and provide answers to the questions posed.

It was therefore decided not to hold the conference, but instead to produce a report summarizing the current state of knowledge about intensive care, highlighting the absence of evidence, and calling for a substantial programme of research (Kings Fund, 1989).

This, of course, raises questions about the efficiency of audit of intensive and critical care practice at present, and there are many studies currently underway in various countries looking to redress this matter.

Indeed, Christine Hancock, General Secretary of the Royal College of Nursing of the United Kingdom, stated in 1990 that "Doctors and nurses have been trying for decades to develop effective systems for auditing professional activity in health care."

Scoring systems of various types have become a commonplace activity in critical care practice. Much of this work has originated from the United States, and, in particular, from the work of Professor William Knaus and his colleagues in Washington. Professor Knaus is noted for devising the Acute Physiology and Chronic Health Evaluation (APACHE) scoring system (Knaus, 1988).

The United Kingdom APACHE scoring system trial is but one example of a current study of critical care audit (Rowan/ICS), and there are, at the time of writing, others in the data collection and planning stages in other European centres – some under the auspices of the European Society of Intensive Care Medicine. This particular study attempts to validate the APACHE 2 scoring system for use in the United Kingdom. Ledingham (1985) suggested that the use of methods such as APACHE 2 allows assessment of performance between different intensive care units, and should prove helpful in evaluating new treatment and determining which patients will derive most benefits from intensive care.

It has been suggested already that the cost implications of critical care are significant, and may give rise to many controversies regarding the use and abuse of the service. It is perhaps unclear exactly what critical care costs, and it is difficult to make meaningful comparisons between different monetary systems.

Furthermore, the cost of health care is currently leading most countries in Europe to reorganize their health care systems in an effort to reduce costs. Health expenditure in Britain has grown, but the rate of growth is slow; and our overall expenditure is still one of the smallest in Europe (Smith, 1991).

In respect of critical care we know, for instance, that in the UK, the cost of keeping a patient in the intensive care unit is roughly three to four times that of keeping a patient in a general ward per day. Limited, unpublished studies in the UK have also shown that a patient costs more during the first 24 hours after admission, and that this as a general rule tends to decrease subsequently. It is also known that certain drugs and therapeutic treatments are expensive.

Currently, attempts are being made by various groups to study the cost of intensive care from a management aspect.

There are two levels of audit – local unit audit and national audit. The first deals with results in specific units, and the second helps researchers to compare their own results with others. To do this, the data sets used must be compatible in terms of comparison. It is also often difficult to determine the fine line between collecting too much and too little data.

In May 1990, the Intensive Care Society of the United Kingdom published guidelines for audit in intensive care, as the results of a working party. The following general recommendations were made:

☐ Basic intensive care audit must be standardized, so that results can be compared between units.

☐ Data sets must be appropriately structured and limited so that collection is possible in the maximum number of units. This may, of course, mean that individual units need to add to the basic data set for their own purposes.

☐ The data collected should also include information on nurse staffing and patient dependency levels.

☐ Examination of costs is probably considered too complex to include as part of the basic data set.

☐ The use of diagnostic coding and diagnostic related groups is particularly difficult in critical care, and this problem needs to be addressed.

☐ Outcome must be recorded at unit discharge, and at hospital discharge.

☐ Withdrawal of treatment should be recorded, with reasons.

☐ And finally, long-term follow-up of patients discharged from ICU should be considered.

Evaluation of critical care in the long term is important, because we need to consider quality of life in our deliberations on the effectiveness of treatment.

Loirat et al. (1990), from Paris, state that "intensive care medicine is very costly. Rationalization of health expenditure begins to affect hospital budgets and can lead to explicit rationing – intensive care is not exempt from this process and the only way to justify our expenses will be to make a proper evaluation of intensive care activities."

However, increasing attention to justification of the purposes of critical care and examination of the results leads the health care professional into the debate of who and for how long? That is to say, in terms of patient benefit, how do we rationalize the use of critical care – who do we treat and when do we stop? For a more detailed discussion of the ethical aspects surrounding this debate, the reader is referred to the appropriate chapter, but again, some organizational comments are made here.

The Kings Fund panel suggested that "Primarily intensive care should be given in the expectations of beneficial consequences, when such benefits can be achieved at acceptable cost. It should not be provided in situations where possible harm outweighs the prospective benefit" (King's Fund, 1989).

Perhaps this sounds simple, but in reality it is never so clear cut. The same panel suggested that a simple scale should be used:

- [ ] expected to survive: potentially recoverable;
- [ ] prognosis uncertain;
- [ ] death probable shortly whatever is done;
- [ ] and death apparently imminent;

and that in the UK, intensive care should be considered for the first two of these categories, if the costs are not prohibitive.

These recommendations are controversial – everyone can quote the patient who survived despite the odds being highly unlikely. But it is predictable that the time will come where clinicians and others may well be forced into making decisions as to who gets critical care, based on some similar type of scale or scoring system.

"Selection for intensive care", stated the Kings Fund Panel, "should be based on broad concepts of prognosis, derived from statistical analysis of comparable cohorts of patients, backed up by sound clinical trials." It is such data that is currently deficient in the field of critical care in the UK and probably in other countries as well.

Having made the decision to treat, it has also to be considered that in some cases, it may later become appropriate to withdraw therapy and allow the patient a dignified death. Decision making in this respect is also often problematic in critical care, and increasingly so today, when the ability exists to prolong life with sophisticated technology.

Indeed, Knaus (1987) stated that "the complexity of modern intensive care and the amount of information currently available, frequently makes it impossible for one individual to use personal intuitive judgement to decide on the course of treatment. Often, the best course of action will only

become apparent through a careful balancing of prognostic information with ethical, moral and legal considerations."

As critical care technology develops further, as more is understood about disease patterns that are responsive to critical care medicine, and as critical care resources become more carefully scrutinized, it is highly probable that these problems will increase.

It is, of course, of paramount importance that nursing activities are included in programmes of research and audit, and this is probably a convenient point at which to turn to a more specific discussion of nursing issues.

The issues as applied to nurses in critical care units

This chapter is largely concerned with the impact of developments in critical care upon nurses – now, and in the future. However, whilst acknowledging this, it has to be remembered that the practice of critical care demands multidisciplinary team work of a high degree, and therefore many of the issues that affect nurses and nursing have implications on a wider scale, or are part of far reaching issues that embrace all the members of the multidisciplinary team. It is therefore the author's belief that, when considering critical care in depth, nursing cannot be entirely considered in isolation.

Indeed, Catalano (1991) suggests that "as medical technology rapidly advances, critical care nurses will increasingly find themselves caught between the life saving benefits of this technology, and the ethical dilemmas created by its use or misuse."

Traditionally, nursing can be divided into four component parts; and it is these that will be used as the basis for discussion, because they embrace many relevant concepts. The four areas are:

1. Clinical practice.
2. Education.
3. Research.
4. Management.

For simplicity, they will be considered individually, but with the over-riding acknowledgement that many areas do overlap, and therefore this could be interpreted as a somewhat simplistic approach.

Clinical practice

"Nursing", states Shuldham (1986), "has undergone great changes in recent times, and it seems likely that in the next few years it will continue to develop and become increasingly complex and demanding . . ."

Kennerly (1990) states that "critical care nursing practice has evolved over the past two decades in response to changes in health care that have served as a driving force in the trend towards nursing specialization."

In particular, reference may be made to the fact that functions which were previously viewed as expanded clinical practice are now commonly accepted as an integral part of daily patient care (Mechanic, 1988).

Critical care nurses must set and demonstrate high standards of clinical practice; keep abreast of current advances in technology and therapeutics, and strive to constantly improve ways of delivering patient care. To do this, they require a vast number of complex skills; and an increasingly diverse base of supporting knowledge. Amongst all this they must maintain the patient's dignity and self-esteem, and foster a humanitarian approach to care; giving due regard to the patients own beliefs and wishes.

Parfitt (1988) suggests that "the conflict of values for the nurse in the intensive care unit is increasingly apparent, for with the emphasis on holistic nursing models of care, there has been increased stress on the need to provide emotional support for the patients".

Yet within critical care areas, technical competence is still the main pre-occupation and nurses (often) support this value system.

There is a requirement for a high degree of efficiency in the technical skills, with the humanistic care taking (a relatively) second place (Parfitt, 1988).

Perhaps, to other disciplines involved in the care of the critically ill patient, this may seem an obvious necessity. But this move of nursing and nurse education towards a holistic view of the patient, with the nurses developing skills to meet individual needs, is creating a situation of conflict; because in many instances, resources have not yet been identified, or skills developed, to make the practice of holistic care functional within the acute clinical situation (Parfitt, 1988).

Virginia Henderson, writing in 1980, in an article aptly entitled 'Preserving the essence of nursing in a technological age', stated "Humane service from health workers is, in the last analysis, dependant on what societies value; nurses are part of those societies and . . . influence those values." Baroness Jean McFarlane wrote in 1982: "there is, I believe, a great need to preserve and use human values in health care, to reduce depersonalisation, isolation and neglect of individuals, but also to develop and use scientific values and competency, especially in nursing."

More recently, Carnevale (1990) takes up the same theme: "High technology", he states, "has established an inevitable and necessary place in critical care". . . . "all of this development has set a stage whereby it is possible for intensive care to focus almost exclusively on the human needs that are measurable, and visible."

Carnevale (1990) states that high technology and humanity can be balanced: "caring is an important ingredient for fostering humanity in critical care. The educational processes necessary to develop the skills of empathy and nurturing must be developed."

The difficulties of time for caring are examined by Masson (1985). She suggests that "whereas medicine is based on the use of tools; nursing is based on the use of self to listen, teach, guide, support, be there – when time is lacking, nurses can perform only technical functions and are unable to nurture." In a profession where the ethic of caring is strong, this can indeed lead to frustration and dissatisfaction.

Previously, perhaps, the clinical role of nursing has tended to be valued less than the administrative role or the educational role; and there has been little incentive for experienced nurses to remain within the clinical field, but instead to pursue a career into management or education.

In the United Kingdom, two publications in the early 1980s – The Royal College of Nursing's *Towards Standards* (1981) and the Department of Health's *Professional Development in Clinical*

Nursing (1982) began to change this, and laid the way for clinical career development – later to be supported by a restructuring of the nurse grading system.

The latter has certainly not been without its problems, but, in itself, it did, perhaps, pave the way for the development of the role of the clinical nurse specialist – a potentially exciting and challenging role especially in the specialist areas such as critical care units. At the time of writing, this development has been slow to occur, perhaps due to the effects of other wider reorganizations in the National Health Service.

The role of the Clinical Nurse Specialist (CNS) has been debated frequently in the literature over the past decade, the original concept being developed in the United States more than 20 years ago (Atkinson, 1991).

Does the role of the Clinical Nurse Specialist have a place in the future of critical care?

Balcombe (1989) has suggested that the CNS should develop patient services for a specific client group; be a clinically-based leader for the nursing team; develop nursing expertise within the unit; provide advice on nursing care and developments; and offer therapeutic counselling for patients and staff.

The Royal College of Nursing (1988) defines the nurse specialist as "someone who demonstrates refined clinical practice as a result of significant experience, advanced expertise, or knowledge of a particular nursing branch or speciality." Furthermore, it is suggested that to claim true status as a specialist, the nurse must be involved in clinical practice, consultation, teaching, management and research.

The CNS must therefore be instrumental in the maintenance of high standards of care and practice in the critical care area. This is achieved by education, involvement in clinical nursing, and involvement in the setting of standards, policies and procedures.

Setting standards for use in the clinical area both helps to evaluate the care provided for patients; and supplies bench marks for use in quality assurance programmes. Such programmes are becoming a fundamental part of health care today. They need to be devised and implemented in conjunction with those involved in the actual hands on delivery of care. Experienced clinical practitioners are in an ideal position to facilitate this.

Boyes (1987) states that "there is a need for the qualified intensive care nurse to be involved in any quality assurance exercise taking place in her unit, and the clinical nurse must have the educational opportunities to prepare her to participate in the formulation of nursing standards that will help to evaluate the care provided."

In addition, Boyes suggests that setting standards for practice will also provide a structure for the orientation of new staff members based on specific competencies necessary for an acceptable standard of practice.

Before moving on to education, two final points are of note. A problem which has traditionally often been quoted as causing difficulties for intensive care nurses is the patient who has been diagnosed as 'brain dead'. But perceptions of this problem vary considerably. Experience in the United Kingdom seems to increasingly suggest that the criteria for diagnosing and caring for the brain dead patient are now so much more well defined that, providing management is appropriate, the majority of nurses have learned to cope with this as part of their work. This has probably been aided to some extent by the development of roles such as that of the transplant coordinator.

However, this is not necessarily so when one considers the continuation of treatment on a seemingly hopeless case. These cases are generally far less clearly defined, and care and treatment of such patients requires a unified approach by the multidisciplinary team (Atkinson, 1988).

Rapin, again from his work in 1987, states that "a decision as to the optimal therapeutic course . . . should be made not by a single physician, but by the team including the nurses."

This philosophy is echoed by Knaus (1988), who suggests that "the complexity of modern intensive care and the amount of information currently available, frequently makes it impossible for one individual to use personal intuitive judgement to decide on the course of treatment. Often the best course of action will only become apparent through a careful balancing of prognostic information with ethical, moral and legal considerations."

The nurse is at the bedside of his or her patient continuously, charged with providing skilled and safe care, in a kind and humanitarian fashion. The nurse may, or may not, have the satisfaction of seeing the patient recover, but in all cases needs to feel involved at all stages in determining the next events in the patient's treatment and care (Atkinson, 1988).

Education

The American Association of Critical Care Nurses (AACN) (1981) describes the critical care nurse as "a registered professional nurse, committed to ensuring that all critically ill patients receive optimal care. . . . To continually refine the practice, the critical care nurse participates in on-going educational activities."

This is said to involve:

☐ Basic preparation.
☐ An advanced knowledge of psychosocial, physiological and therapeutic components, specific to the care of the critically ill.
☐ Clinical competency
☐ The ability to interact effectively with patients, families and other members of the health care team.
☐ The awareness of the responsibility for an environment for safe practice.

Education will be discussed in much greater depth in a subsequent chapter, but it is of necessity to make some introductory remarks here.

Jarvis (1986) suggests that in the same way that nursing is responding to the pressures of society, and undergoing change, so is education. This has become a very complex institution, so much so that Peters (1966) claimed that "education is too complex a phenomenon to be defined."

In the case of critical care nursing, the continuance of sound educational opportunities are seen as essential for several reasons.

Firstly, they increase motivation of staff, and their feeling of involvement in their work – with the ultimate aim of increasing job satisfaction.

Jarvis (1987) stated that "continuing education courses should be provided; so that all nurses . . . have opportunity either to develop their own interests; or to be kept abreast with the latest developments in nursing."

Nurse education does not stop at the end of basic training, and Snow in 1983, wrote that "all critical care nurses have a need for educational offerings."

Critical care nurses must have the underlying knowledge to enable them to adapt to the many changing situations which they are likely to encounter in their everyday practice.

Secondly, as an integral part of the individual development of staff members.

Benner (1982), suggested that "increased acuity levels of patients; decreased length of hospitalisation, and the proliferation of health care technology and specialisations, have increased the need for highly experienced nurses."

Those involved in education are challenged in educating the nurse of the future; to prepare nurses for creativity and flexibility; to teach the nurse not everything there is to learn, but to teach the nurse how to learn – to be "prepared to face change and develop in a flexible way when change occurs." (Boyes, 1987).

It is, perhaps, interesting that this philosophy first arose at the time when Florence Nightingale was writing her notes on nursing, when she stated:

"I do not pretend to teach her – I ask her to teach herself, and for this purpose I venture to give her some hints." (Nightingale, 1859).

Education is necessary to provide the necessary knowledge base to enable the carers to critically appraise clinical practice.

This has already been alluded to in part; but Boyes writes in 1987, how "the clinical nurse must have the educational opportunities to prepare her to participate in the formulation of nursing standards that will help to evaluate care provided." "Education for intensive care practice must therefore be aimed at enabling the trained nurse to relate her education to the realities of clinical practice . . . and to the political climate of the time."

Education is also essential to develop the knowledge and skills necessary to maintain consistently high standards of patient care.

The prime aim of any educational programme has to be to improve the quality of patient care; and these programmes must be evaluated to show the relationship between continuing education, quality of care and cost containment. There is still some work to do in this field, and it is essential that the quality of education programmes is monitored as closely as that of clinical practice.

Finally, education is necessary to enable the practitioner to meet the expectations of his/her patients and their families – which are generally that they should be provided with the highest possible standards of care. In the light of recent government initiatives aimed at increasing available information for patients and their families, this has become even more imperative.

The International Council of Nurses (1973) defines a nurse as: "A person who has completed a programme of basic nursing education and is qualified and authorised in his/her country to practice nursing. Basic nursing education is a formally recognised programme of study, which provides a broad and sound foundation for the practice of nursing and for post-basic education which develops specific competency."

Continuing education has been described by the American Nurses Association as "planned education activities intended to build on the educational and experiential basis of the professional nurse – for the enhancement of practice, education, administration, research or theory development – to the end of improving the health of the public."

As such this encompasses post-basic education, in-service training and staff development programmes. With changing roles has come the recognition that continuing education is essential, and that basic nurse education can only be a foundation.

The current facilities for the education of critical care nurses are universally varied, and consist of a mixture of formal courses of study, planned teaching sessions in-service; staff orientation, *ad hoc* bedside teaching sessions, to name but some, also involving various members of the multidisciplinary team. Other methods include staff interest groups, staff support groups, journal clubs, multidisciplinary seminars and conferences, and the professional organizations (Atkinson, 1990).

International comparisons have, to date – particularly across the continent of Europe – demonstrated wide differences in the length and content of courses to prepare critical care practitioners.

Between 1987 and 1989, a working group of the European Society of Intensive Care Medicine examined the status of critical care nurse training in Europe. Wide diversity was found, and this will need to be addressed in the future with the new

European unity. It may well be that attempting to suggest standards of training which might ultimately be universally accepted across the countries of the EEC and perhaps beyond is desirable (Atkinson and Burchardi, 1990).

Obviously, in the United Kingdom at present, the effects of the outcome of the major changes in nurse education – notably Project 2000 – upon critical care nursing are awaited. Stating the need for a restructuring of the training programme in the United Kingdom, the United Kingdom Central Council states of future nurses:

"Aware of the current policy debates that shape their work, they will need the tools to evaluate their own practice and the skills to argue the case for a particular service and to defend it against criticism." (UKCC 1986).

However, the need for a further level of education is still seen as apparent: "We are not arguing that every practitioner should have all these skills at the end of an initial programme." (UKCC 1986)

These sentiments are concurred with by Durghahee (1990), who suggests that: "Most of the objectives of Project 2000 are likely to be achieved during post-basic training and professional practice, although the foundation must be laid at initial level."

This pattern of training manifests itself as a branch training programme, with progression to various areas. It is unclear at present, exactly where intensive care nursing fits into this pattern – except possibly as part of a critical care module in the adult branch programme – and this is now in place in some colleges of nursing and midwifery. It is vitally important that nurses in training have the opportunity to be exposed to critical care nursing if they wish, as, apart from the fact that it can be a valuable learning experience, recruitment to the specialist areas in the future needs to be considered.

Project 2000 also raises the concept of the health care assistant – to which there has been much attention given in the nursing press. Although there is a defined structure for the training of such personnel, at three levels, nevertheless, the overall level of training is significantly less than that given to our current registered general nurses. Such personnel also exist in several countries in Europe in different forms – the general concept being that of having less definitively trained personnel observing patients or giving care under the supervision of a registered practitioner. In the UK there are currently profound questions and doubts in applying the concept of the health care assistant to critical care nursing.

Is there – in a highly technical and specialist area such as intensive care – a role for the Health Care Assistant (HCA), and if so, what? Ultimately, it is certain that there will be HCAs in intensive care units and other critical care areas, but the role must be carefully defined and monitored. After all, critical care nurses are never merely performing care – they are also using such opportunities to observe, diagnose and report or treat as appropriate.

There are also, at this time, fundamental changes in the financing and administration of our health service which, as well as affecting the way in which patient services are delivered, may well impact upon the availability and organization of education.

Fields (1991), in an article in *Nursing Standard*, stated: "the education and training of health service professionals and non professionals is set to be driven by a market place philosophy, which will exert and endorse competition and control, via rapidly evolving change and reform. New legislation will have profound effects on nurse education, and many concerns relate to the safeguarding of quality and standards and the whole management and delivery of nursing curricula."

Those hospitals in the United Kingdom who have become independent, self-governing hospital trusts are charged with the responsibility for providing training facilities, but how this will work in practice is, as yet, unknown. Will training be viewed as a necessity or a luxury in a system striving for economic viability?

It will, undoubtedly, be up to those who work in such areas to ensure that such training facilities are provided, and this in turn will mean that the profession needs to be very clear about exactly what is required to make the case, and determine appropriate levels of skill mix and education.

Training is a dynamic concept, and the needs of personnel must be regularly reviewed and training programmes modified and updated accordingly. Accreditation criteria for institutions offering training need to be similarly reviewed. This applies not only to nursing education, but to education for other professionals engaged in the practice of critical care.

Gallagher (1991) in an editorial for Critical Care Medicine, writes "our knowledge base and expertise must be similar throughout the country. With today's rapid and proliferative dissemination of information, one has little excuse not to be informed in our chosen speciality."

As regards medical personnel the current situation reflects the fact that, in some countries there is an approved curriculum for an official qualification, in others there are guidelines for training, but no official certification, and in others no guidelines or curricula exist at all.

It is difficult to generalize about the way that intensive care medicine is practised in Europe, because there are marked differences between various countries. These are described by Hillman (1990) in an editorial in the journal *Intensive Care Medicine*. The UK, Ireland and Scandinavia tend to have general Intensive Care Units usually run by specialists, whose primary speciality has been in Anaesthetics. Switzerland and France, on the other hand, tend to have separate Medical and Surgical ICUs. The Surgical ICUs are generally run by specialists whose primary speciality is anaesthetics, and the Medical ICUs are usually run by specialist physicians. There are also other variations, but however these departments are organized, there is an increasing tendency for medical staff in various European countries to become full-time practitioners in intensive care.

The concept of a full-time intensivist, who is not only a clinician, educator and researcher, but also a manager is thus developing – and to support this concept, training schemes are being developed. This may, states Hillman (1990), be a formal training system such as Spain or Switzerland, where supervised time must be spent practising intensive care, followed by a formal examination. Some other training programmes involve recognition acquired in a primary speciality, such as medicine or anaesthetics, followed by an apprenticeship in intensive care medicine.

In addition, the European Society of Intensive Care Medicine hosts a Diploma in Intensive Care examination, with a standardized written paper, and then a viva taken in the country of the candidates choice. This diploma is open to medical graduates, who have completed their training in a basic speciality and, in addition, have had the equivalent of two years full-time training in intensive care. The first candidates have now successfully completed the diploma, and whilst each country will continue to develop the speciality on an individual basis, the aim is to help achieve uniform standards of practice throughout Europe, as well as facilitate movement of medical personnel across national borders.

In the United Kingdom, a standardized examination is currently in the planning stages, and an approved training programme in intensive care medicine is now available in a limited number of centres.

Finally, as regards education – in this case of nurses – what contribution to training can be made by the professional organizations?

Boyes (1987) suggests that "through professional organisations . . . there now exists a unique opportunity to identify the knowledge and skill base from which the intensive care nurse works. These professional organisations can lead the way in identifying standards of practice that will serve to evaluate the specialist care being provided. This effort will not only determine the continuing education needs of the specialist staff providing care, but may also guarantee that the resources for continuing education are forthcoming in the future."

These resources must be guarded.

Research

Having concentrated largely on clinical practice and education, it is appropriate to conclude by offering some brief comments on the place of research and management in critical care, and where we are today. Brevity, however, does not imply that they are considered to be less important, but within the constraints of an introductory chapter such as this, there are only a certain number of issues that can be raised and discussed.

In Western Europe, there are gradually more nurses undertaking first and higher degree courses. This is encouraging, and the fact that many are practising within critical care areas is even more so.

However, if nurses are to be encouraged to critically analyse their practice, then gone are the days of 'we've always done it this way' without any rational supporting theory. Research is a fundamental part of the role if the practice of critical care nursing is to be advanced on a scientific basis.

"The systematic enquiry on which research is based is vital if all other aspects of our work are to be successfully developed." We need to promote awareness of the importance of research for nursing practice (Barrie-Shevlin, 1985).

Nursing research has been defined in numerous ways. Gortner, in 1976, defined it as "a systematic enquiry into the problems encountered in nursing practice and into the modalities of patient care, such as support and comfort, prevention of trauma, promotion of recovery, health education, health appraisal, and co-ordination of health care."

Haughey (1991) suggests that while definitions of nursing research may vary, there is consensus that it is an integral component of the profession. Most importantly, research "provides a scientific base for nursing education, theory and practice." Additionally, research contributes to nursing by providing a data base for decision making, enhancing professional status, improving practice and quality of patient care and fostering professional accountability.

If the benefits of research are to be fully realised, the findings must be utilized in clinical practice. However, before research findings can be accepted, nurses must learn to evaluate them – several authorities well recognize that the fact that a research report has been published does not assure the quality of the research.

A positive attitude towards research engendered early in the critical care nurse's experience, helps to increase motivation to become actively involved in future studies. Nevertheless, again reality is essential, and Moody (1989) suggests that whilst not all nurses may be able, or willing, to be actively involved in research, "it may be sufficient that they seek to acquire, assimilate and apply relevant research findings as a basis for all nursing actions."

The issue of disseminating research findings also needs to be addressed. Previously, studies have tended to be reported in journals which may not be widely accessible to the majority. Such studies need to be published so as to be accessible to many, and, again, the professional associations can have a role to play in this.

Research can be expensive to undertake, and perhaps in the past nurses have shied away from applying to official bodies for funding. This also needs to be addressed; and those with experience need to be prepared to assist others to prepare research prosposals that will stand up to scrutiny, and attract the necessary financial support.

Management

Finally, a brief discussion of management aspects. Today all of us are part of health services that are currently passing through turbulence.

Previously, nurses have perhaps liked to disassociate themselves from management. It is possible that the profession is now paying heavily for this – and this is perhaps just one reason why there are still in the United Kingdom relatively few nurses holding top health service management posts.

Time needs to be taken to take stock and refocus. Tomorrow is another day, and who knows what new challenges it may bring. Managing an intensive care unit today goes well beyond a single physician's or nurse's capabilities – it requires teamwork. There is a growing realization that the critical care director of tomorrow will be spending as much time on personnel and administrative issues as on clinical issues. Several large scale studies are currently underway in the United States and the Netherlands in an attempt to demonstrate a direct association between outcome from the unit and effective administration policies. Many will be familiar with the work of Professor William Knaus and his colleagues in the mid-1980s, where some degree of correlation of these aspects was demonstrated in a study concerning 13 hospitals (Knaus, 1987).

To effectively manage a critical care area today requires a wide range of skills – organization, communication, planning, personnel handling, financial control, to name but a few. It is no use ignoring this, and the nettle, so to speak, has to be grasped.

The current implications of the health service changes in the UK have led to a realization that better data management systems need to be available to support claims and developments.

In 1983, Gregory touched on this in a presidential address to the Society of Critical Care Medicine. In addition, he suggests that there are several things that must be done soon:

☐ We must make known to the public what it is we do, and how it benefits society.

☐ We must examine what we are doing – are we, in fact, benefiting the patient, the family and the nation? Which patients do and which do not do well – and if they do not do well, why?

☐ We must reduce costs – we need to evaluate the cost effectiveness of what we do, and reduce costs where possible.

What is striking about this address is that it was given to an audience in the United States in 1983. In those days, perhaps, it would have been viewed slightly differently in the UK. However, in 1991 that address might just as well have been given in London as in San Francisco. The problems are no longer that different. The issues, so to speak, are no longer the problems, they are the solutions.

One final area relating to management deserves mention at this stage – that of the recruitment and retention of staff. Parrish (1990) reminds us that "staff are the most valuable resource in any organisation and heed needs to be taken of the workforce and the way it is handled in the next decade."

This means that not only the problem of recruiting staff to work in high-tech areas has to be addressed, but also that of retraining them. Undoubtedly, many of the issues already discussed will contribute to this, but a corporate approach needs to be taken of this problem to promote the critical care specialities amongst the profession. More needs to be known about the ways of increasing job satisfaction, preventing disharmony amongst the workforce, and caring and supporting those who, in turn, care.

CONCLUSION

In this introductory chapter, several issues have been raised concerning the current state of critical care and critical care nursing. Some issues will be revisited in subsequent chapters, whilst others may leave questions unanswered. In itself, this is perhaps no bad thing, because the critical care professionals of the future will need to constantly evaluate their practice, develop their skills and knowledge base and direct their efforts to providing care of the highest standard for the seriously ill patients with whose care they are entrusted.

Gallagher (1991) states that "Excellence in patient care must remain in the forefront of all of our activities – the critical care practitioner must call daily on all the knowledge and art of the speciality."

Critical care patients have a mountain to climb. As critical care professionals, our role is to help them to the top. They are, after all, our *raison d'etre*.

KEY TERMS

Critical care

The whole spectrum of high-tech, high-dependency specialist care incorporating, for example, intensive care units, renal units, cardiothoracic surgery ICUs, coronary care units.

Resources

The components which may be utilized in the process of obtaining a specified outcome. Examples in terms of providing healthcare might be beds, theatres, manpower, materials and drugs.

In economic terms, resources tend to relate to the availability of capital and/or revenue finance.

Multidisciplinary team

A team comprising representatives from differing healthcare professions, with the aim of working in harmony to provide optimum care for the patient.

Cost benefit analysis

A measure of the effectiveness and efficiency of a process, in terms of the benefit obtained weighted against the cost of providing the process.

Audit

As defined within the chapter.

Diagnostic related groups

A method of classifying patients into case mix groups. There are currently around 475 DRGs in existence. The system is often used as part of the contract tariff to set charges for patient care for purchasers.

Diagnostic coding

A system utilized to identify individual or groups of diseases. At the time of writing the most commonly used system is the ICD-9 system.

Clinical nurse specialist

The Royal College of Nursing (1988) defines the nurse specialist as "someone who demonstrates refined clinical practice as a result of significant experience, advanced expertise, or knowledge of a particular nursing branch or speciality." Furthermore, it is suggested that to claim true status as a specialist, the nurse must be involved in clinical practice, consultation, teaching, management and research.

FURTHER READING

Intensive Care Society. *Standards for Intensive Care Units*. London: Biomedica, 1983. (There is likely to be an updated version of this work available, by the time the book goes to press.)

Cule, J. An historical view of intensive care. *Intensive Therapy and Clinical Monitoring*. November 1989; 288–293.

Hillman, K. European intensive care. *Intensive Care World*. 1990; 7(2): 75–76.

Intensive Care Society. *The Intensive Care Service in the UK*. London: Intensive Care Society, 1990.

REFERENCES

American Association of Critical Care Nurses. *Core Curriculum for Critical Care Nursing*. Philadelphia: W.B. Saunders Co.; 1981.

Atkinson, B.L. The clinical nurse specialist in intensive care. *Nursing*. 1989; 4(1): 6–8.

Atkinson, B.L. The usefulness of intensive care – the nurses' view. *Care of the Critically Ill*. 1990; 6(3): 93–95.

Atkinson, B.L., Burchardi, H. Education and Training. In Eds. D. Reis Miranda, P. Loirat and A. Williams. *Management of Intensive Care – Guidelines for Better Use of Resources*. Dordrecht: Kluwer Academic, 1990.

Atkinson, B.L. Training nurses for intensive care. *Intensive Care Nursing*. 1990; 6(4): 172–178.

Balcombe, K. Prime time for development. *Nursing Standard*. 1987; 3(17): 36–37.

Barrie-Shevlin, P.D. Creativity, enthusiasm, diplomacy. *Nursing Mirror*. 1985; 160(20): 46–47.

Benner, P. From novice to expert. *American Journal of Nursing*. 1982; 82(3): 402–407.

Boyes, M. Intensive care nursing education. *Nursing*. 1987; 3(16): 593–596.

Carnevale, F. High technology and humanity in intensive care: finding a balance. *Intensive Care Nursing*. 1990; 7(1): 23–27.

Catalano, J.T. Critical care nurses and ethical dilemmas. *Critical Care Nurse*. 1991; 11(1):20–25.

Department of Health. *Professional Development in Clinical Nursing*. London: Department of Health, 1982.

Department of Health. *Patient's Charter*. London: HMSO, 1992.

Durghahee, T. Directions in post-basic education. *Senior Nurse*. 1990; 10(7): 15, 18–20.

Edwards, J.D. *The World in Action: Intensive Care*. Granada TV, 1992.

Fields, H. Nurse education in the market place. *Nursing Standard*. 1991; (29): 33–37.

Gallagher, T.J. Guidelines for care: The time has come. *Critical Care Medicine*. 1991; 19(2): 138.

Gortner, S.R. Research for a practice profession. *Nursing Research*. 1976; (24): 193–197.

Gregory, G.A. Who should receive intensive care? *Critical Care Medicine*. 1983 11(10): 767–768.

Hancock, C. Can it work for patients? *Senior Nurse*. 1990; 10(7): 8–10.

Harris, J. QALYfying the value of life. *Journal of Medical Ethics*. 1987; (13): 117–123.

Haughey, B.P. Something new for Critical Care Nurse. *Critical Care Nurse*. 1991; 11(1): 68–69.

Henderson, V. Preserving the essence of nursing in a technological age. *Journal of Advanced Nursing*. 1980; 5(3): 245–260.

Hillman, K. European Intensive Care. *Intensive Care World*. 1990; 7(2): 75–76.

Intensive Care Society. *Intensive Care Audit*. London: ICS, 1990.

International Council of Nurses; Quadrennial Congress, 1973.

Jacobs, C.J., Van der Vliet, J.A., Roozendaal, M.T., Van der Linden, C.J. Mortality and quality of life after intensive care for critical illness. *Intensive Care Medicine*. 1988; (14): 217–220.

Jarvis, P. *A Sociology of Lifelong Education and Lifelong Learning*. Department of Adult Education, University of Georgia, 1986.

Jarvis, P. Lifelong education and its relevance to nursing. *Nurse Education Today*. 1987; 7(2): 49–55.

Kennerly, S.M. Imperatives for the future of Critical Care Nursing. *Focus on Critical Care*. 1990; 17(2): 123–127.

King's Fund Panel. *Intensive Care in the United Kingdom: Report from the King's Fund Panel*. London: King's Fund, 1989.

Knaus, W.A. An evaluation of outcome from intensive care in major medical centres. *Annals of Internal Medicine*. 1986; (104): 410–418.

Knaus, W. A., Zimmerman, J.E. Prediction of outcome from critical illness. In Ed. I. Ledingham. *Recent Advances in Critical Care*. Edinburgh: Churchill Livingstone, 1988.

Knaus, W.A. The changing challenges of critical care. *Intensive Care Medicine*. 1989; (15): 415–416.

Knaus, W.A. Address to the Intensive Care Society Spring Meeting. April 1991 (Unpublished).

Lenihan, J. The history of intensive care. *Nursing Focus*. 1979; 1(2): 75–76.

Ledingham, I. The N.I.H. Consensus Development Conference on Critical Care Medicine. *Care of the Critically Ill.* 1985; 1(2): 6–8.

Loirat, P. (1990) Evaluation in Intensive Care. In Eds. D. Reis-Miranda, P. Loirat and A. Williams. *Management of Intensive Care Guidelines for Better Use of Resources.* Dordrecht: Kluwer, 1990.

McFarlane, J. Baroness. Nursing values and nursing action. *Nursing Times: Occasional Papers.* 1982; 78(2): 109–112.

Masson, V. Nurses and doctors as healers. *Nursing Outlook.* 1985; 33(2): 70–73.

Mechanic, H. Redefining the expanded role. *Nursing Outlook.* 1988; (36): 280–284.

Moody, M. Developing research based practice. In Ed. P.L. Bradshaw. *Teaching and Assessing in Clinical Nursing Practice.* London: Prentice Hall, 1989.

Nightingale, F. *Notes on Nursing.* London: Harrison & Sons, 1859.

Parfitt, B.A. Cultural assessment in the intensive care unit. *Intensive Care Nursing.* 1988; 4(3): 124–127.

Parrish, A. Managers moving on! *Senior Nurse.* 1990; 10(7): 3.

Peters, R.S. *Ethics and Education.* London: George Allen & Unwin, 1966.

Rapin, M. The ethics of intensive care. *Intensive Care Medicine.* 1987; 13: 300–303.

Royal College of Nursing. *Towards Standards.* London: RCN, 1981.

Royal College of Nursing. *Specialities of Nursing.* London: RCN 1988.

Shuldham, C. The nurse on the intensive care unit. *Intensive Care Nursing.* 1986; 1(4): 181–186.

Smith, T. European health care systems. *British Medical Journal.* 1991; 303: 1457–1459.

Snow, J. Care of the critically ill child. In Ed. K. Stahler-Miller. *Neonatal and Paediatric Critical Care Nursing.* New York: Churchill Livingstone, 1983.

Sprung, C.L. Responsibilities of critical care professionals in setting medical policies for foregoing life-sustaining treatments. *Critical Care Medicine.* 18(7): 787.

Tinker, J. General intensive therapy. In *Intensive Care.* Basingstoke: Macmillan Journals Ltd., 1978.

U.K.C.C. *Project 2000: A new preparation for practice.* London: U.K.C.C., 1986.

2
NURSING MODELS FOR CRITICAL CARE
Helen Ellis

CHAPTER AIMS

This chapter will look at the issue of nursing models in two ways. The first part will review nursing models from the general perspective of all nurses. If a critical care nurse wishes to adopt a nursing model to guide her practice it will be from a range of nursing models that have received attention in the nursing literature. To choose a nursing model, the critical care nurse needs to have knowledge concerning the following:

☐ A definition of nursing models.

☐ The origins of nursing models and the impetus for their development.

☐ The content of nursing models.

☐ The commonly stated advantages and disadvantages of nursing models.

☐ The development of a philosophy for critical care nursing.

☐ The nursing process and care planning in relation to nursing models.

The second section of the chapter will focus upon:

☐ The classification of nursing models to facilitate rational model choices for critical care nurses.

☐ Developing one's own model for critical care nursing.

☐ Adopting and adapting another model for critical care nursing.

☐ Neumans Systems Model and its use with the nursing process for critical care.

INTRODUCTION

Critical care nurses, along with all other groups of nurses, are essentially 'doers'. When asked, 'what is it that nurses do?' most nurses would be hard pressed to come up with anything more than 'we help people'. The majority of nurses throughout their working day act or do things to or for people to help them. If life were uncomplicated this simple statement 'we help people' would be acceptable as it stands. However, nursing involves constant inter-action with people – those that provide other aspects of health care; the managers, politicians and economists who are influential in the delivery of health care, and last but not least, the people who need nursing help. This constant interaction has led to many influences being brought to bear from within and without nursing. It has led to enquiry, introspection and debate about the nature of nursing and the kind of help nurses ought to give to society at large and to the individual people that they meet in the everyday work of nursing. Nursing models are just one of the many influences that we need to consider in the world of critical care nursing.

The nursing process and care planning

Yura and Walsh (1978) identified the nursing process as a problem solving approach and in 1978 as the core and essence of nursing. It is a systematic approach which tells nurses how to go about organizing their work. As an approach to solving problems it rapidly gained acceptance by United Kingdom nurses, albeit with some struggle and much cynicism. By 1977 the General Nursing Council had recognized the nursing process as an important element in educational policy. The four stages of assessment, planning, implementation and evaluation form the essential stages. The foundation is assessment and therein lay our initial problems with the nursing process. The nursing process does not tell you how to nurse or what to assess. Due to a lack of any other framework to guide assessment, nurses rapidly settled on the only one they knew – the medical model. The nursing process became a documentation issue and as long as the nursing report was made out in the format of a care plan and an evaluation of the plan, little thought was paid to the fundamental issue of what exactly are nurses supposed to be assessing to nurse their patients as opposed to purely carrying out medical orders.

Nursing models, which represent a way of thinking about nursing provide a framework for assessment. If the model is concerned with stress (Neuman's System Model) then the nursing assessment of the patient is focused on the identification of stressors in the patient's life. If the model is concerned with the ability of man to adapt and cope with his environment (Roy's Adaptation Model) then the assessment is focused upon the patient's inability to adapt. If the model is concerned with the ability of patients to care for themselves (Orem's Self Caring Model) then the assessment

highlights those areas where the patient is unable to care for himself.

Every nursing model uses the nursing process as an approach to organizing the delivery of nursing care. Some models use an extra 'stage' – the nursing diagnosis. Nursing diagnoses developed as a result of gathering information about patients and analysing the information to reach certain conclusions about their needs and nursing interventions (Field, 1987). For nurses working in critical care, nursing diagnoses such as *ineffective breathing pattern due to . . . ; potential for aspiration . . . ; and decreased cardiac output due to . . .*, would be recommended. The use of nursing diagnoses is an American development and their use has not caught on in the United Kingdom. What has developed is an increasing trend towards standardized or core care plans.

The stress laid upon the individualized approach to patient care and the need for an individualized care plan that recognized each person's uniqueness led to difficulties for many nurses. Martin and Glasper (1986) reported that "there was the difficulty of resolving the paradox between the individual and the universal. In emphasising the uniqueness of human behaviour and experience there was a tendency to understate human commonalities and the legitimacy of agreed nursing protocols." (p. 269). In other words, there were certain nursing actions that were necessary for the majority of patients regardless of their individual needs or family situations. Examples of these are the maintenance of the unconscious person's airway and pressure area care for highly dependent patients in the intensive care unit. The concept of the core care plan was proposed by Martin and Glasper (1986) to be a care plan which nurses could use to highlight individual patient's differences. A core plan would be written and approved by all staff. It would cover all the fundamental nursing activities which have to be done, such as monitoring the ventilator settings, observing the ECG for potentially fatal arrythmias and caring for the patient's physical well-being. The staff could then add to the core plan those aspects of care that uniquely concerned their patient and his family. Time would be saved from excessive written documentation of care and redirected towards nursing actions. The core plan could also act as an audit tool for the unit and enable review of nursing activities and priorities in each critical care setting.

What is a nursing model?

A model is simply a representation of reality. We use models to help us understand the world. An example of a physical model is a plastic heart which comes apart to demonstrate the working mechanisms and their relationships within the heart. A map is a scaled down model of an area of land developed to help us find our way around. Some models, such as mathematical models, are made up of symbols and signs which describe relationships between ideas. Other models have to use words or language to explain ideas such as love, family and government. The use of words and language means that we can communicate with each other about our world. Often we use concepts to communicate with each other. A concept is a shorthand way of painting a complex picture. When we say 'chair' we all understand what this means although there are many different shapes and sizes of chairs. If we speak of 'fear' we generally understand what is meant by this word and react accordingly. Models which use words and language have to do so as they are trying to describe concepts that are not physical, but abstract. They are often known as 'conceptual models'. A nursing model is a conceptual model. It's descriptive function is to attempt to represent what happens when nurses and patients meet in hospital or community settings.

There are many definitions of nursing models. All link practice to theory. Examples are:

☐ "A systematically constructed, scientifically based and logically related set of concepts which identify the essential components of nursing practice together with the theoretical basis of these concepts and values required for their use by the practitioner." (Riehl and Roy, 1980).

☐ "A model is simply a way for nurses to organise their thinking about nursing and then to transfer that thinking into practice with order and effectiveness." (Wright, 1986).

This last definition is probably the most useful one for nurses to think about. There are so many different models, all with competing claims for nursing practice. Nursing models were primarily developed by individual nurses to assist in the teaching of nurses and to guide clinical practice. A physical model which can be handled and taken apart – such as a scale replica of a car – allows us to examine all the different parts to the car, take them out and replace them in different positions to see what would happen. It encourages exploration, experimentation and change. An abstract model – a nursing model – although we cannot touch it, still allows us to do the same. We can ask 'what if' and 'why' and 'when' and think about nursing, the patients, the unit and the outcome of our activities. A nursing model should provide a stimulus and a focus for thought about one's own practice of nursing. It should help nurses to put new ideas into action and to observe and evaluate their effect on the delivery of patient care.

The historical development of nursing models

Why have nursing models developed? Nursing is an activity that has always been based upon action and doing for others. Our activities have been based upon practical skills and we have passed our activities on to other nurses through demonstration, supervision, written rules and procedures. We are traditionally orientated towards the practice or 'doing' of nursing. We remain orientated towards 'doing' but now we are expected to be 'knowledgeable doers'. This chapter does not propose to discuss the nature of nursing knowledge. Carper (1978) has started such a discussion and it is continued by others (Benner, 1984; Meleis, 1985). It is necessary to point out, however, that definitions of knowledge encompass facts, information, understanding and experience (Manley, 1991). The knowledgeable doer needs to continue to 'know how' as well as to 'know why' and to 'know what' (Johnson, 1968). In other words, the knowledgeable doer is able to account for his/her actions rationally and from the perspective of a relevant and well tested frame of knowledge.

The addition of these other forms of 'knowing' to nurses practical skills or 'know how' has been encapsulated by the development of nursing models and nursing theories. It has been argued that nursing in a bid to establish itself as a profession, has focused its energies upon the development of its own theory base for nursing practice. This movement started in the United States of America and was focused through an early article by Dickoff, James and Weidenbach (1968), who argued that nurses must begin to generate their own theory base if they were ever to develop their own goals. They were clear that nursing was a practice discipline and that theory and practice should work hand in hand through the linking factor of research. They argue that "theory is born in practice, is refined in research and must and can return to practice." (p. 415).

Self Reflection:
How do I know what I know?

Nurses began to ask questions about nursing. Traditionally, nurses did not question. We were too involved in the world of our medical colleagues and complied with their model – the so called medical model. The medical model is one particular way to view a problem or a patient. It is a reductionist model which focuses on the individual parts of the body and disease processes affecting a particular part. This is in effect a 'scientific' view of the patient in that the strongest theory or idea holds sway until another comes along to depose it. The opposing way of looking at the world or the patient is that of the 'arts'. This includes the social sciences and the humanities. The arts or the social world view argues that there are many different ways in which to look at the patient or the world, all of equal use. Nurses are beginning to accept this view as one of equal importance to the scientific view and in doing so are beginning to perceive the patient in many different ways. All ways are useful for nursing practice.

Dissatisfaction with the traditional nursing activities which were modelled upon those of their medical colleagues, coupled with a desire to expand nursing roles further, led to the development of more humanistic approaches to nursing care. The thinking nurse began to look away from the medical viewpoint to find a broader nursing horizon. In examining this wider horizon nurses have borrowed from the arts and the sciences – theories on biological and physiological functioning, psychology of a person, social theories regarding family, work, illness and health, to name but a few. It is the application of these borrowed theories by nurses to nursing practice that facilitates the development of a theoretical foundation for nursing. Nursing models assist this process as they help nurses focus on particular issues which directly concern their patients and their practice.

Nursing models were influenced by the existing scientific, philosophical, social, moral and psychological theories existing in the provision of health care at the time of their development. Many models were developed from the late 1950s onwards, although no new models appear to be emerging at the current time. What we have is a refinement of the more popular models and a desire for their adaptation to meet local or specialist nursing needs.

Meleis (1985) presents a useful framework within which to consider the development of nursing models. She classifies nursing models according to the major questions which interested nurses at the time of the model development. The first question was 'what do nurses do'? To answer this question, nurses visualized patients in terms of a hierarchy of needs. When a need is unfilled and when a person is unable to fulfil his or her needs, nursing care is required. Nurses function by helping patients meet their needs. She classifies nursing models developed by Henderson (1966) and Orem (1971) as needs theories. These models are not medically orientated, but tend to reflect Maslow's (1954) hierarchy of needs. Meleis (1985) argues that these models give us a view of the patient that is slightly different but very close to the medical view of the patient as the hierarchy of needs begins with physiological needs and safety needs. It progresses to include other higher level needs such as belonging, love and self-esteem.

Meleis (1985) argues that the needs models are characterized by a focus on problems, nursing functions and an orientation that begins to break away from the medical model. They are still reductionist in approach – a human being is seen as a set of needs, a nurse as a set of functions. There is little emphasis on environment or the patient as a person, and the methods of nurse–patient interaction are not well explained.

A second question which took up nurse theorists

time was 'how do nurses do what it is that they do'? Answering this question focused nursing attention on the interaction which occurs between nurses and their clients. Such models were written by Peplau (1952), Travelbee (1971) and King (1971). Although some of the models did address the needs of people, all interactionists focused their attention on the process of care and on the ongoing interaction between patient and nurse. Their theories were based on interactionism, phenomenology and existentialist philosophy. Meleis (1985) argues that we have learnt much from the interactionist school of thought in that:

☐　Nursing involves help and assistance.

☐　It is an interpersonal process between a person who needs help and one who can give help.

☐　The nurse should clarify her own values in order to give help.

☐　Care is not a mechanistic act, but a humanistic act.

☐　Illness is an inevitable human experience. If a person learns to find meaning in illness, it can become a meaningful experience.

☐　The perception of the patient is important in assessing illness and its meaning.

☐　Nurses intuition and subjectivity are seen to be important.

Many of these ideas are used and discussed today in the clinical setting and aired in pre- and postregistration education and training.

The third question relates to the 'why' of nursing care. The first two questions of 'what' and 'how' are not ignored, but the focus is on the 'why' of nursing care. The why of nursing care is referred to as the outcome approach – goals became important. Theorists such as Levine (1969), Rogers (1970), Roy (1976) and Johnson (1980) saw the goal of nursing care as bringing back balance and stability between the individual and the environment. They based their theories on systems theory, adaptation theories and developmental theories. Their thinking focused on the outcome of nursing care.

WHAT DOES A MODEL TELL US?

Over time the main areas of interest to nurses have generally been agreed to be those of nursing, people, environment and health. These four major concepts are recognized as forming the value base for nursing practice, and as such act as a nursing paradigm. A paradigm can be considered to be the general rules of thumb that guide the practice, management, education and research of any given profession. Many competing paradigms may guide the practice of members of a profession, but there is usually only one paradigm acknowledged by the profession at large, on which the majority of the professionals base their practice (Kuhn, 1969). The nursing paradigm is well described by Donaldson and Crowley (1978, p. 119) who state that "nursing studies the wholeness or health of humans, recognising that humans are in continuous interaction with their environments."

Every nursing model reflects the style, philosophy and experience of the author. It can be hard to pick out the relevant aspects of the model. Without some guidelines to assist the nurse to critically evaluate each model, confusion may easily set in or relevant issues be missed. According to Aggleton and Chalmers (1986), each nursing model will describe or define the following:

☐　The nature of people, definitions of health, environment and nursing.

☐　The causes of problems likely to require nursing intervention.

☐　The nature of the assessment process.

☐　The nature of the planning and goal setting process.

☐　The focus of intervention during the implementation of the care plan.

☐　The nature of the process of evaluating the quality and effects of the care given.

☐　The role of the nurse in patient care in relation to those of other health care workers.

Model analysis is often an exercise that nurses studying for further diplomas and degrees have to undertake. Several frameworks have been developed for model analysis (Thibodeau, 1983; Fawcett, 1984). However, the dry academic study of nursing models needs to be brought to life by their application to practice. The questions are useful for finding out what is in a model and for choosing a model for use in clinical practice.

The pros and cons of nursing models

Nursing models have received a lot of attention in the nursing press and have been reviewed and comprehensively critiqued. Aggleton and Chalmers (1986) suggested that nursing models should provide:

☐ A way of thinking about nursing in general and a way of thinking in a similar way for a group of nurses.

☐ A way of organizing the delivery of nursing care.

☐ Certain skills and knowledge needed by a nurse. In its presentation of the reality of nursing the model should offer information about the beliefs and knowledge underpinning nursing practice, the practice of nursing and its goals.

The advantage in practice of using a model of nursing is that continuity of care is assured and consistent nursing practices are encouraged. Conflict should be reduced within the nursing team if all the team members have accepted the use of the model and all have a common sense of direction.

However, it cannot be said with any certainty that the use of a nursing model will produce these things. One of the major criticisms of nursing models is that they are not valid representations of all aspects of nursing and that they have not been researched in any depth (Silva, 1986; Walker and Avant, 1988). Nursing models are not yet in use to the extent that nurses can show that the use of a model actually leads to a higher standard of care.

Other critics have pointed out that problems inherent in nursing models are those of jargon and different cultural and social values. The use of jargon is frequently used as a criticism by nurses in the United Kingdom. For instance, nurses will not use Rogers (1970) model because they do not understand the use of her complex terminology and jargon. However, it has been pointed out (Chalmers, 1989) that terminology alone should not be used as an excuse for not using a particular nursing model. The cultural and social values of the author may well be different to those of the nurse in critical care, and as such the choice of model needs careful thought. Each published nursing model is essentially a statement of the author's personal beliefs and a synthesis of their thoughts about nursing. Hardy (1986, p. 103) argues that the use of models actually "promotes the view that everyone's world view is the same, that all persons may be assessed in the same way" and pinpoints effectively the major problem with nursing models – they do not reflect all points of view. In fact, the patient's point of view is never considered. She asks "how many of the current nursing models would survive consumer scrutiny?" (p. 106).

Despite these criticisms, nursing models are of use. To kick them out because of the above criticism is also to throw out many useful and stimulating ideas. Nursing models need to be used by both educationalists and practising nurses. By using a variety of nursing models in the curriculum, both tutors and students can explore the many different issues affecting any health care situation. The use of nursing models in practice helps the critical care nurse to use her nursing knowledge in an independent and professional manner. At the level of clinical practice, many models are very similar. They advocate the delivery of a high standard of nursing care that is research based. This involves the nurse in all the day-to-day activities that she always carries out such as pressure area care, nutrition, information giving. At a higher level, the differences between nursing models become more apparent. The models lead a nurse to different assessment formats and introduce her to a range of potentially new and interesting concepts, such as Roy's, 'role function' and concept of 'self', and Neuman's ideas of stressor identification.

Nursing models are not perfect representations of reality, and they will miss out issues which are of relevance in today's rapidly changing health care service. But they can act as a stepping stone towards a clearer definition of nursing and the role of the nurse. To be sure of our professional contribution to patient care the use of nursing models is essential both in practice and education.

Developing a philosophy for critical care

Despite the arguments for and against nursing models, discussion in the nursing literature centred initially on the problem of whether nurses should adopt one nursing model wholesale or take an eclectic approach to the use of nursing models, i.e. take from a range of nursing models the ideas which appeal to them or suit their particular form of clinical expertise or specialism. The issues outlined in the advantages and disadvantages of nursing models apply to the straightforward adoption of a nursing model. There is little evidence to show that nurses in any field of nursing in the United Kingdom have actually done this. What has occurred most frequently is the adaptation of a nursing model for use in specified clinical areas. The nursing literature has examples of specific models being adapted for practice such as Roys Adaptation model (Lewis, 1988) and Neumans Systems Model (Fulbrook, 1991a).

The debate has also moved on to the general acceptance that nursing may well develop further if groups of nurses worked towards developing their own model for nursing. Wright (1986) has effectively debated this point and laid out ideas for nurses who wish to develop their own model for nursing. Many nurses are beginning to do this, and it is standard practice now for the majority of wards or units to have begun the process of model development by developing and owning their own unit or ward philosophy.

A unit or ward philosophy is essentially a statement of beliefs about:

☐ The purpose of nursing within the ward. Virginia Henderson's (1966) well known definition of nursing: "to assist the individual, sick or well, in the performance of those activities contributing to health or its recovery (or to a peaceful death) that he would perform unaided if he had the necessary strength, will or knowledge, and to do this in such a way as to help gain independence as rapidly as possible", is an effective statement which clarifies the purpose of nursing. This definition is often used as a core statement by nurses in all areas of practice. Wright (1986) and the team of nurses working with him in the development of their nursing model considered this to be effective in stating the purpose of their ward philosophy.

☐ People and their health/illness needs – the philosophy usually attempts to demonstrate a holistic approach to people and the nursing care they need.

☐ The ward environment that is developed to assist both nurses and patients.

☐ Significant issues which affect patients and nurses within the ward such as information giving, communication strategies, patient choice, involvement of patients in their treatment and care.
The development of a philosophy for each ward simply has the effect of helping nurses make the conceptual leap into thinking 'nursing' rather than 'medicine'.

To develop a philosophy for critical care units, the staff need to spend time talking and thinking about the work that they do, the goals they hope to achieve with their patients and the environment they work in. Many critical care nurses will recognize that while physical, psychological and social needs are met, priority has to be given to life threatening physical problems and unstable physiological systems. It is this prioritization of needs which lends many critics of critical care units to claim that nurses working within such areas still practice on a purely medical model of care. Nursing models are so broad in their scope that it has to be recognized that not all units can always utilize the complete model in its entirety. For example, Orem (1971) believes that nurses provide help with self-care deficits in three ways – wholly compensatory (doing everything for the patient), partly compensatory (doing only those things that the patient cannot do for him or herself) and supportive-educative (supporting and teaching the patient and his or her family so that he or she can do for him or herself). In critical care units there may frequently be patients who will always require nursing interventions in the wholly compensatory mode, and due to the nature of critical care, patients may well be transferred to other areas before the other modes can fully come into operation.

The development of a critical care philosophy will help clarify the staff's values and may lead to a decision to completely adopt a nursing model or to adapt a relevant model. On the other hand, the staff could decide to develop their own model of nursing which will be ideally suited to the needs of their own unit. In the development of the unit philosophy, ideas about nursing and the values clarified by the group's discussions will be affected by many other factors:

☐ The current organizational issues concerning nursing at the time, e.g. primary nursing, quality assurance, skill mix and staffing levels.

☐ The current professional perspective – accountability, ethical and moral thinking, legal issues.

☐ The changing educational perspectives – Project 2000, PREPP, nursing as a degree based profession.

☐ Ongoing research by nurses and others which affect current nursing practice, e.g. pressure area care, wound healing, pain control, family needs, etc.

All these issues and the myriad of changes occurring with Resource Management and the evolution of clinical directorates will lead to changes in nursing practice in critical care areas, with or without a nursing model.

At the moment, nurses are urged to select the most appropriate model for their work or to develop their own. On the one hand, this encourages creativity and professional decision making, but on the other hand, this could lead to any given hospital using several different models, which could lead to confusion and several different care plans for a patient during one stay in hospital. The other side of the coin which argues for a hospital to use only one nursing model, although leading to simpler documentation and an easily accepted framework for assessment, carries the risk of thinking that there is only one way of looking at people. Essentially, the dilemma is one of professional *versus* organizational requirements.

However, all wards are encouraged to develop their philosophy of care to guide their practice, and to encourage continuing discussion about the relationship between nurses and their patients. A philosophy should not remain static. As new staff come to the ward, discussion should continue and the philosophy should grow and develop over time, accommodating the evolving values of the staff. Needless to say, discussion should take place with all the multidisciplinary team, as shared values should encourage a professional respect between the team members – in reality, it is a team approach which contributes to the successful care of the critically ill patient. A point to note is that many philosophies of care are developed without the input of the patient. Patients and their families come from many different cultures and will hold very different values to the group of nurses working in a critical care unit. Nursing staff must involve patients where possible and their families in their thinking about the unit philosophy. As pointed out earlier, the nursing philosophy should not remain static, and one sure way to the development of a flexible and living philosophy is to involve the patients.

CLASSIFICATION OF NURSING MODELS

Nursing models are usually placed into broad classifications by authors (Fawcett, 1984; Meleis, 1985). Analysis of models usually leads the analyst to pick out the differing orientations and interests of the nurse theorist. The classifications most usually seen are those of developmental models, systems models and interaction models (Fawcett, 1984) although different classifications are used. Meleis (1985), as shown earlier in the chapter, characterizes needs, interaction and outcome theories. It is essential to remember that all nursing models will contain elements from all the broad classifications.

Developmental models

Such models concentrate upon the process of growth, development and maturity of people and societies. The emphasis lies upon change, both of the person and society. Because change is a major concept in developmental models, ideas about the direction of growth, the processes that occur during change, how a person can change and the potential that an individual can reach are all of interest to practicing nurses. Peplau's (1952) model of nursing is often cited as a developmental model.

Systems models

The main features of a systems model are a system and its environment. Systems models grew out of the need for specialists in all disciplines to communicate with each other. The development of systems theory led to a method for looking at general problems that occurred over many specialisms.

A group of assumptions are generally made when using systems models:

☐ That people accept the idea of wholeness – of people and organizations.

☐ A person or an organization is greater than the sum of its parts.

☐ The start of action, movement and growth, can arise from many levels within the system, between the system and the environment and between systems. All parts are independent, yet interact with each other.

☐ One set of circumstances or conditions can lead to different outcomes. On the other hand different initial circumstances can lead to the same outcome.

☐ Communication processes involve the functional use of information and facts.

There are several well known systems based nursing models, e.g. Roger's Life Process Model (1970), Roy's Adaptation Model (1976), Neuman's Systems Model (1980) and Johnson's Behavioural Systems Model (1980). These models would fall under Meleis' classification of outcome theories.

Interaction models

These models concentrate upon individuals in society. The focus lies upon relationships, communication skills and the ability to find a shared sense of meaning in the world. The concept of roles and changes in roles become important along with self-awareness. Emphasis is laid upon individuals being active participants in relationships – partnership becomes an essential ingredient of the nurse–patient relationship. Interactionist nursing models are those of Orlando (1961) and Travelbee (1971).

Table 2.1 outlines the relationship between the nursing process and the different classification of models, showing how the choice of model can influence the approach taken by the critical care nurse throughout the application of the nursing process.

PRACTICAL NURSING IMPLICATIONS OF NURSING MODELS

Developing your own model for critical care

This process involves a significant amount of change, both from the individual's point of view and that of the organization. Outlining a nursing model or framework actually involves the outlining of professional meaning. If the critical care unit staff wish to develop their own model, it can only start if the group have become uncomfortable with the way things are and have become open to change (Rogers, 1990). A variety of strategies are needed to facilitate discussion and airing of anxieties and problems that arise as a result of the proposed changes.

Fulbrook (1991b) has outlined the stages that his intensive care unit went through to adopt and adapt Neuman's systems model. The stages would

Table 2.1 The nursing process in relation to model classification

	DEVELOPMENTAL MODELS	INTERACTIONIST MODELS	SYSTEMS MODELS
ASSESSMENT	Child & young adult physical development. Family status. Coping strategies – family and/or patient. Past hospital experience.	Family relationships. Family and patient roles.	Patients biological/ physiological functioning. Psychological/emotional state of patient and/or family. Social needs of the patient and family – immediate & long-term.
PLANNING	Set goals which allow normal pattern of living and relationships to be restored.	Should be done with patient and/or family. Discuss new role relationships and adaptation of existing ones.	Set short term goals which make clear what is expected of each system.
IMPLEMENTATION OF NURSING ACTIONS	Interventions are educational. A partnership is developed between patient/family.	Both nurse and patient and the family are involved. Interventions may be physically, emotionally based. A trusting relationship develops.	Physiological and physical interventions. Behavioural interventions for psychological systems. Referral for social and/or physical systems/ emotional systems.
EVALUATION	Looking for evidence of growth and change physically, psychologically and socially.	Evaluation mainly by the patient and family. If successful both nurse and patient/family views should coincide.	Assessing whether short term goals have been achieved.

be the same if a unit decided to develop their own nursing model. The initial planning stage involved workshops, discussion groups, literature searching and involvement with other organizational units. This facilitated the development of the intensive care unit's philosophy and the development of care plans. The second phase of implementation required a high level of staff coordination and communication to finalize care plans, assign mentors to the staff, and the actual performance of a trial run. The third stage concerned itself with the development of a formal evaluation tool to evaluate the trial run, the evaluation process itself and the final changes which were needed in the documentation. The adapted model was then

implemented. This kind of preparation requires the commitment of the staff, managers and educational support with a sufficient period of time allocated to such a major change.

Ideas, words and values about nursing from many different nursing models have filtered through to the clinical setting and are increasingly heard in every day use. The use of the term 'self-caring' (Orem, 1971) is now generally accepted, as is the term 'activities of daily living' (Roper, Logan and Tierney, 1983). It is appropriate at this point to ask ourselves whether or not the three broad classifications of developmental, interactionist and systems theories are of use to the critical care nurse. Table 2.1 outlines some ideas for the use of the nursing process bearing in mind the three model classifications. From the experience of the majority of critical care nurses the use of a systems model is usually seen to be the most appropriate for use, although a variety of approaches can be moulded into one critical care model.

Developmental nursing models and critical care

As developmental models are concerned with growth, change and the process of development of people and society the following issues may well need to be discussed by critical care staff:

☐ The impact of increasing technological change on the process of nursing people in critical care units.

☐ The changing ethical and moral boundaries for practice that arise out of technological support.

☐ The development of critical care units and their future roles.

☐ Staff recruitment, development and retention within critical care units.

Interactionist nursing models and critical care

Interactionist models are concerned with the individual. Areas for discussion may include:

☐ The role of the critical care nurse and staff expectations regarding the role of the patient.

☐ Identification of the needs of the family and the role of the patient within that family.

☐ Review of the communication channels and their effectiveness within the unit.

☐ Development of communication skills in all staff members – verbal and written.

☐ The use of alternative therapies within the critical care unit.

☐ The meeting of spiritual and emotional needs within the unit.

Systems models and critical care nurses

Systems models focus on the person and the family both as independent parts and as a whole. The environment is recognized as interacting with patients, their family and friends and staff members. Issues for discussion may include:

☐ A review of physiological aspects of care – monitoring facilities, extended roles, charting observations, reporting changes in the patients condition.

☐ The impact of the critical care environment on patient, family and staff.

☐ The concept of stress and its management in the critical care unit.

☐ Family needs – physical, emotional and social and strategies to meet those needs.

☐ Infection control aspects.

The issues to discuss are endless. What is being promoted through discussion is an awareness of professional issues and an accurately defined framework for nursing practice within each critical care unit. From the discussions a framework for assessment can be developed to suit the priorities and needs of the critical care unit. With reference to Table 2.1, it can be seen that both the science and arts views can be incorporated into a framework for assessment that involves nurses with all the 'high-tech' monitoring and collaborative medical interventions, along with the caring aspects of patient and family interventions. Such a framework leads to the development of an eclectic model, one which takes useful issues from all models and incorporates them into a personal model of care. It is the overwhelming view of many authors (Hardy, 1986; Field, 1987; Kristjansen *et al.*, 1987) that an eclectic approach should be adopted when introducing students to nursing models. One hospital may contain several wards who are all using a different model. The variety in the service side serves to underline an eclectic curriculum.

Make a list of the criteria you would use to help you decide to adopt/adapt a nursing model.

Choosing to adopt and adapt a nursing model

Aggleton and Chalmers (1986) have produced a rational set of questions which ought to be asked when considering which nursing model to use:

- [ ] What assumptions does the model make about people and their health related needs?
- [ ] What values does the model hold?
- [ ] What are the key concepts that the model uses?
- [ ] What relationships are suggested between these concepts.
- [ ] How does the model see the role of the nurse?
- [ ] Does the model present things in a clear cut and understandable way?
- [ ] Does the model have something to say about nursing in the context for which its use is being considered?
- [ ] Is the model likely to lead to better care?
- [ ] Is the model likely to be used in practice?

It is important to ask these kind of questions as adopting a nursing model does mean a commitment to change and all that change entails. Again, the most important question that should be asked first is 'why do we want to change'? Without some thought given to this point we repeat the same problem we had with the nursing process, which was *imposed* on the majority of nurses rather than *proposed* by the majority of nurses.

An example of a nursing model which demonstrates all aspects of developmental, interactionist and sytems models is the Neuman Systems Model. This nursing model has been adapted for use in a critical care setting (Fulbrook, 1991a), and it is not unusual for ENB cc 100 (general intensive care nursing) students to examine their practice in the light of this model.

Neuman's systems model

Neuman's model is well documented elsewhere (Neumann, 1980; Thibodeau, 1983; Fawcett, 1984). A brief overview of the model will be given whilst attempting to answer the questions posed by Aggleton and Chalmers (1986) above.

What assumptions does the model make about people and their health related needs?

Neuman describes 'a person' as a unique individual. Each person grows and develops as a result of the interaction of four sets of factors – physiological, psychological, sociocultural and developmental factors.

Each individual, although unique, has a common core with all other people. All human beings have at their centre a set of factors which are necessary to human functioning. These are genetic makeup, homeostatic mechanisms such as temperature control mechanisms, pH regulation and ego structure. The core has to be protected from stressors. If any stressor penetrated to the core of the individual, death is the likely outcome. Surrounding the core of each person is a series of 'defence lines'. Obviously, these lines cannot be seen, but are used as an analogy to explain how each person keeps well and prevents or copes with stressors. Neuman calls the external line the 'flexible line of defence'. This is a protective buffer that prevents stressors affecting the day to day performance of the individual. The next defence line is the individual's normal line of defence or the day to day level of functioning. When a stressor breaks through the two first lines of defence, internal mechanisms come into play to support the functioning of the person and return them to normal. These factors are called the 'internal lines of resistance'.

Stressors affecting each person can arise from the environment outside the person (extrapersonal stressors), from within the person (intrapersonal stressors) and from between two or more people (interpersonal stressors). Neuman believes that the level of resistance to a stressor is a function of several factors:

- [ ] How long the stress continues.
- [ ] The level of the normal health of the individual.
- [ ] The effort needed to adapt to the stress.

☐ The individual's perception of the stress.

☐ Past coping mechanisms and strategies.

Health is not explicitly defined by Neuman. She states that "Health therefore, is reflected in the level of wellness. If a man's total needs are met, he is in a state of optimal wellness. Conversely, a reduced state of wellness is the result of needs not met" (1980, p. 9). As health is a concept that is still under discussion throughout many different professions, this poor definition serves only to underline this fact. From the perspective of the model, any stressor which penetrates the normal line of defence can cause illness.

What values does the model hold?

The underlying beliefs in the model comes from several disciplines. They are synthesized into the following:

☐ Nurses must be concerned with the whole person.

☐ Each person's response to any stress is unique and therefore acceptable.

☐ It is the role of the nurse to help people reach as stable a condition as possible.

☐ The patients' perceptions of their stress is important, and should be listened to and taken into account during all the stages of the nursing process.

What are the key concepts that the model uses?

The key concepts are those of nursing, man, environment and health. Additionally, the concept of stress is an important one, along with the concept of systems and system interaction. These are all useful concepts for use in the critical care area from the physiological and biological point of view: however, the personal and psychological perspective of staff, patient and family and the social and cultural perspective of all who work or enter the area are additional key concepts for those working in ICU.

What relationships are suggested between these concepts?

The relationship between man and the other three major concepts are well defined. Essentially, each person interacts with the environment continuously. Each person is also a part of the environment. If the person and the environment are in harmony then the person is seen to be healthy. If the individual is not in harmony then he is seen to be ill in that he is not coping with stress from within and without. Nurses are concerned with the environment as a source of stress, the individual as a source of stress and the individual's ability to manage that stress. Nurses can become involved with the individual in wellness or illness states.

How does the model see the role of the nurse?

The role of the nurse is to identify potential stress and either remove it or prevent it from affecting the patient. They will attempt to strengthen the individual's resistance to stress. Neuman identifies three stages of intervention by nurses:

☐ Primary prevention – risk to the person or family structure is apparent, and the nurse acts to prevent the stress affecting the person or family or to strengthen their coping mechanisms if it does affect them.

☐ Secondary prevention – the goals of this intervention are assessment of the effects of stress and the treatment of symptoms. This would be the stage at which many critical care nurses meet their patients.

☐ Tertiary prevention – is aimed at rehabilitation, education and the maintenance of a stable system.

Does the model present things in a clear cut and understandable way?

Yes. However, there is still a conceptual leap to be made. Although critical care nurses have traditionally used the medical model which is essentially systems-based, the move to viewing the person as a whole being who is affected by stressors that nurses can actively alter may require further thought and discussion.

Does the model have something to say about nursing in the context for which its use is being considered?

No. The model was first developed as a basis for curriculum development to demonstrate the breadth of nursing problems that meet nurses in hospital and community settings and to encourage a holistic approach to people. The model can be freely adapted to any nurse setting.

Is the model likely to lead to better care?

This is not known. The problem with all models is the lack of validation through research. The assumption has to be made that by applying any model to practice the changes that occur on a professional, organizational and clinical level ought to lead to an enhanced quality of nursing care and greater patient/family satisfaction. It is argued that the application of a nursing model to clinical practice should stimulate research. The questions posed by the model and arising from the application of the model should foster an environment that encourages research and further developments in the model.

Using Neuman's system model and the Nursing Process

The model can be applied to an individual person or to a family group in the critical care area. The emphasis laid upon systems and their interaction leads first to the inclusion of the family in the critical care experience; and second to a relationship between nurse and patient and family which means that the perceptions of family and patient are important.

The model acts as a framework for the collection of information about each patient and their family. The collection of information can lead to a picture being developed of both patient and/or family and the nurses' perceptions of the situation. Prioritization of problems can then occur and a nursing care plan developed which should reflect this dual perception.

As each individual is influenced by a variety of physiological, sociocultural, psychological and developmental factors, the nurse first considers

these areas, looking for stressors or problems. This means that the physiological aspects of critical care can be considered in as much depth as is needed to stabilize the individual's system. The other three areas can be observed and then clarified further through interaction with the patient and his family. For these areas to be assessed from the point of view of the patient and his family, Neuman recommends that their perception of the problems is identified.

The following form of questions can be asked, either directly to the patient or to the family:

☐ What do you consider to be your major problem at the moment?

☐ How has this problem affected your usual pattern of living?

☐ Have you ever experienced a similar problem before? If so, what was the problem and how did you handle it? Were you successful?

☐ What do you see for yourself in the future as a consequence of the present problem/ situation?

☐ What have you been doing and what can you do to help yourself?

☐ What do you expect the staff in this unit/family to be able to do for you?

The nurse should note his/her assessment of each question. Once these areas have been discussed, the nurse should summarize the situation with the patient through the identification of problems – at the intrapersonal, interpersonal and extrapersonal level. At each level, physical, psychosocial and developmental, problems may be identified. Table 2.2 outlines some possible problems identified with a coronary care patient. Obviously, if the patient can speak for herself, an accurate picture of the patient's view can be obtained and care planning can be negotiated between nurse and patient. Information is gathered from the patient through the above questions and organized by the nurse in such a way that the sources of stress can be identified. Working with the patient, the nurse can identify the main points that concern the patient and incorporate them within the care plan.

Table 2.2 Identification of stressors: Neumans systems model

	INTRAPERSONAL FACTORS	INTERPERSONAL FACTORS	EXTRAPERSONAL FACTORS
A lady admitted to a Coronary Care Unit – nurse and patient perceptions			
PHYSICAL AND/OR PHYSIOLOGICAL PROBLEMS	Chest pain Arrythmias Tiredness Nausea	Cannot look after the family as usual. Have to go sick from work.	Worried about her work which is fairly heavy – on her feet all day.
PSYCHOSOCIAL PROBLEMS	Frightened by the pain Worried about future	Need some help with looking after myself at the moment. Missing the family. Needs to contact her husband.	Need the extra money her work brings in. Children need taking to school and playgroup. A lot of people to contact regarding her stay in hospital – committees and fund raising activities for local charity.
DEVELOPMENTAL PROBLEMS, i.e. FUTURE PROBLEMS	Will I be able to keep my job? Will I be able to look after my children?	Have to arrange for help with children and housework. Husband travels away to work. Family need contacting.	Will have to possibly reorganize her life in the future.

PERCEIVED PROBLEMS
(IN ORDER OF PRIORITY)

PATIENT:	*NURSE:*
Pain	Pain
Nauseated	Arrythmias
Anxious about husband and children	Possible deterioration in cardiovascular system
Feeling tired	Anxiety about present and future – family and job
	Nausea

From this assessment, a care plan can be developed with the patient, highlighting short- and long-term outcomes.

It is interesting to note that on an anecdotal level, students applying such models to their work as part of nursing care studies within intensive care units have found that patients specifically request that the care plan be continued in the general ward environment. The nurse also notes that he/she spends more time actually doing 'nursing' activities rather than delegated medical duties to carry out the agreed care plan.

For the unconscious or sedated patient admitted to an intensive care unit, the nurse may well have to use the family or friends' perceptions. The family's perceived stressors may well include the question of survival, the extent of the pain and suffering being experienced by the patient, their need to be with the patient as well as fears for the future. As the patient is unable to speak for him or herself, the nurse will have to assume that the patient would wish everything to be done that is possible. Obviously, both nurse and family perceptions will coincide where comfort, pain relief and communication needs are concerned. The nurse may well add to this list the need for mechanical ventilation to maintain ventilation and respiration, the patient's total dependence on nursing and other staff for all his physical, psychological, social and developmental needs at the present time, the need for nutrition and hydration, and so forth.

The patient's/family's perception of stressors can be prioritized and compared to the nurses priority list. From this the care plan is written and the levels of intervention identified. The nurse decides to act on the primary, secondary or tertiary level. For most nurses within the critical care area the primary and secondary level may be the main levels of intervention. The primary level for the critical care nurse mainly represents the monitoring and observation that continuously occurs to preempt or minimize future complications – with the mechanical ventilator, sputum retention, arrythmias, and so forth. The secondary level of intervention will involve much nursing activity to do both with the technology as much as the patient and the family. Tertiary intervention will involve continual explanations to the patient and the family regarding nursing and medical procedures; the provision of educational materials and explanations to patient and family at any time during the patient's stay in the critical care unit; follow-up visits to the patient after discharge from the unit, or contact with the family at home following the patient's death.

Evaluation of the care prescribed in the care plan should be evaluated on a shift-to-shift basis due to the rapid nature of change in the critical care unit. Where possible, the perception of the patient and his or her family should be included.

Neumans Systems Model serves as a useful model to demonstrate a framework upon which to base the nursing process. It has its uses for critical care nurses as it is based upon systems theory, and the ongoing use of a systems model in critical care is self-evident. The conceptual leap comes in the application of systems to the patient as a person, their family and the social and cultural environment in which they live and work. Neuman's model helps the nurse to take a wider view of the patient.

SUMMARY

Nursing models have led to a change in the nature and process of nursing. This change has also affected critical care areas. If a critical care unit is using a nursing model, it will have undergone many changes by the time it is up and running. The original model acted as a template for further development, and it is right that models should change as nursing knowledge grows and matures. The impact of nursing models on British nurses has led to many changes in the process of nursing, and their impact has led to similar changes in critical care nursing. Critical care nursing has seen a growing emphasis upon the impact of the intensive care environment on the patient and the family, as well as on the staff who work within them. The focus on the individual and the nature of critical illness has led to a more humanistic approach to care, with the critical care nurse increasingly aware of the patient's perceptions and needs.

Models have encouraged us to take another look at nursing. A model is of use only as long as it encourages nurses to question and move in new directions to deliver a continuing high quality of care for their patients. With this in mind, any model can be utilized by the critical care nurse, but he or she needs to be aware of why a particular model has been chosen for use. If an eclectic approach is required, the classification of nursing models serves a purpose in helping the critical care nurse to choose which model to use for each particular patient at any particular point in their care. The nursing process remains the accepted method of organizing the care critical care nurses give. The relationship between the nursing process and any chosen model is that it enables new ideas and approaches to care to be put into action. Documentation can be in any format as long as it is clear, accurate and relevant to the individual patient. Due to the ever increasing range of nursing activities, the nursing process documentation must remain concise, and the use of a core plan will remain a useful tool for the near future.

Nursing models serve to link the clinical arena to management, education and research. Managers, as part of the multidisciplinary team, have an active role in the development of the critical care unit philosophy and development of the nursing model. As the manager is able to facilitate the development of the critical care unit through a variety of channels, the use of a nursing model leads to clear identification of the nursing roles and activities that occur within the geographical environment of a critical care unit. Within education, many post-registration curricula are developed along the lines of a chosen nursing model. The use of nursing models to teach different aspects of critical care nursing enables the student to focus on such aspects as the patient as a person, the needs of the family, the identification of stress within colleagues, the need for improved bereavement care, and the environment of the critical care area. Research should play an important role in both the validation of nursing models and in the exploration of ideas which will arise from the development of a model in critical care.

The application or adoption of a nursing model in critical care units can help the development of a critical care nurse who is not only a knowledgeable doer, but a nurse who is aware of the moral and professional dimensions of practice within critical care. Nursing models are not the only source of this knowledge, but they act as a resource for all enquiring nurses to reflect upon and enhance their present practice. By using a nursing model, the critical care nurse can start to define what 'critical care nursing' is within the complex arenas of high technology that are called critical care units. The critical care nurse must seriously attempt to use models as a tool for autonomous practice to define the boundaries of professional critical care nursing.

CASE STUDY

A 24 year old man was admitted to the intensive care unit with ascending muscular weakness. He was unable to walk and was having difficulty moving his arms. He was obviously having difficulty in maintaining a conversation and he was obviously very frightened by what was happening to him. A diagnosis of Guillan Barre syndrome was made and as the paralysis rapidly ascended he required ventilation. He was an exceptionally fit person, working in the armed forces in a position of responsibility. He had collapsed whilst on a tour of duty and his wife lived over 100 miles away. They had an active outdoor life and ran a smallholding from which his wife ran a small business supplying produce to local stores. They also rode and he had a dog to which he was very attached.

The course of the syndrome was stormy and he required a tracheostomy, full cardiopulmonary monitoring, renal support and aggressive treatments for several chest infections. He remained ventilated for two months via his tracheostomy and was therefore awake, aware and able to communicate his needs through lip movement, eye movement and clicking of his tongue. He was fully weaned from ventilation after a further three weeks and remained on the intensive care unit a further week to ensure that respiratory difficulties did not occur. He was transferred to the ward with a speaking tracheostomy tube in place, but only able to move his head and shrug his shoulders a little. His wife had visited throughout and also kept her smallholding going to the best of her ability. There was no close family, and only a few friends had been able to visit during his stay on the unit.

You may work on a unit which does not use an explicit nursing model. On the other hand, your unit may have chosen and adapted a specific nursing model. Whichever unit reflects your own, consider the following questions in the light of the above case study.

1. Identify the broad issues which you would need to address to care for this man and prioritize your list.

2. Why are these things important?
   To whom are they important?

3. How do you view your patients? How would you view the man in the case study?

4. Contrast his life before admission to his life following admission. Identify the important concepts (e.g. fear, pain) which may help you in the planning and delivery of his care.

5. Do you consider him to be healthy? Briefly explain your answer.

6. What is your role as a nurse in caring for this man? If the patient was asked about the role of the nurse what do you think he would want?

7. What are your goals for this man and do they coincide with his aims?

8. What role does his wife have to play in his clinical management? How can you facilitate a supportive environment for both of them?

STUDENT LEARNING QUESTIONS

Specifically using Neuman's System Model consider the following points in the light of the above case study.

1. What do you consider to be this man's main problem? How has it affected his usual pattern of living? *Consider your own perceptions and compare them to what the patient may say.*

2. It is clear that he has never experienced a similar problem before, but it may be worth asking him whether he has experienced acute fear and anxiety before? If he has, how did he manage it? *How would you cope?*

3. How long does he think this problem will last for and what does he foresee for himself in the future? *Consider this question for its suitability at this moment and what you would do with the information gained.*

4. What can he do to help himself? *What does this question help you, the nurse, to focus upon?*

5. What does he expect the staff in this unit to do for him? *Compare his perceptions to your own.*

6. Identify the stressors that you would have to consider in care planning from an:
   Intrapersonal focus   the patient as a person
   Interpersonal focus   between the patient and his family and between the patient and health care team
   Extrapersonal focus   between the patient and his present environment.

7. From your list of stressors identify problems that are physical in origin, psychosocial in origin and developmental (change/growth) in origin.

8. Identify priority nursing actions and nursing actions which will need to be considered at a later date. Are you intervening at a primary, secondary or tertiary level?

9. Consider your evaluation strategy from a daily perspective and a long term goal. How do you know whether your intervention strategies have been effective in reducing the patients perceived stress?

KEY TERMS

Nursing theory

A theory is a set of ideas which are linked together in an organized way to help us understand the nature of the world around us. The purpose of a theory is to explain reality and so a nursing theory explains 'nursing'. The purpose of a nursing theory is to *describe nursing, explain nursing activity, help nurses predict outcomes* and *to identify when nursing is needed as opposed to any other health care intervention, i.e. it prescribes NURSING.*

Nursing model

The purpose of a nursing model is to provide a representation of reality. It may not demonstrate all aspects of the real situation. It provides the nurse with a useful framework to think about everyday nursing actions. Because the model is only a representation of reality it can lead to the development of theory – through the generation of questions. A model can allow you to ask *what would happen if . . .* ? A model can stimulate the generation of theory. Theory can confirm that the model is an accurate reflection of reality or it may lead the nurse to change the model if the theory shows that it is an inaccurate representation of reality.

Conceptual model

There are different types of models (physical – small scale replicas of a physical object, e.g. a small boat; maps; mathematical – using symbols to describe relationships and conceptual or abstract – using language as means of describing reality). Nursing models fall into the conceptual type. We use language to communicate the model – on paper and to others.

Practice discipline

It is generally accepted that nursing is a practical profession. It involves 'doing' and 'activity'. The term 'practice discipline' reflects the idea that nurses think about their actions. They use theory and models to help them choose, implement and evaluate useful actions to nurse their patients. Nursing theory and nursing practice are tied together through the discipline of nursing.

Reductionism

This is an intellectual or philosophical way of looking at the world. It involves detailed and in depth study which allows the investigator to break things down into smaller and smaller parts in order to understand them. The way the parts interrelate and function as a whole is not considered important. This is seen in the study of the human body where interest focuses down to genetic structures.

Humanistic

A way of looking at the world from the viewpoint of people; their interests, activities and relationships. The nature of people is of interest to a humanist.

Interactionism

A view of the world which concentrates upon relationships between people and their cultural, social and physical environment. It places emphasis upon such concepts as communication and interpersonal skills.

Existentialism

A way of viewing the world from the individual's perspective. This philosophy is based on the premise that individuals are free, yet responsible beings who grow and develop through the development of their own morality.

Paradigm

The general 'rules of thumb' that guide the practice, education and research in any given profession. Also can be defined as a 'pattern'. Because the paradigm guides the profession it has to be generally acknowledged – either explicitly or implicitly. Many competing paradigms may guide the practice of members of a profession but there is usually only one paradigm acknowledged by the profession at large, on which the majority of the professionals base their practice. It is generally argued that the essential components of a nursing paradigm are *people*, *environment*, *health* and *nursing*.

Philosophy

Philosophy deals with the search for wisdom or knowledge about the world. There are many different ways of understanding and knowing about the world, and different approaches are taken by different people at different stages of any social and cultural development. Any philosophy deals with the most general issues, outlining principles, influences and general activities of a group of people.

Nursing diagnosis

A developing system in the USA by the North American Nursing Diagnosis Association. A nursing diagnosis is a clinical judgement made by the nurse in response to an initial assessment. A Nursing Diagnosis identifies actual or potential problems and allows each nurse to select appropriate nursing interventions to achieve identified outcomes.

FURTHER READING

Perry, A., Jolley, M. *Nursing: A Knowledge Base for Practice*. London: Edward Arnold, 1991.

Robinson, K., Vaughn, B. *Knowledge for Nursing Practice*. London: Butterworth-Heinemann, 1992.

REFERENCES

Aggleton, P., Chalmers, H. *Nursing Models and the Nursing Process*. London: Macmillan, 1986.

Benner, P. *From Novice to Expert: Excellence and Power in Clinical Nursing Practice*. Menlo Park, CA: Addison-Wesley, 1984.

Carper, B.A. Fundamental patterns of knowing in nursing. *Advances in Nursing Science*. 1978; 1(1): 13–23.

Chalmers, H.A. Theories and models for nursing and the nursing process. In Ed. J.A. Akinsanya. *Theories and Models of Nursing*. Edinburgh: Churchill Livingstone. 1989.

Dickoff, J., James, P. Wiedenbach, E. Theory in a practice discipline. Part 1: Practice orientated theory. *Nursing Research*. 1968; 17(5): 415–435.

Donaldson, S.K., Crowley, D. The discipline of nursing. *Nursing Outlook*. 1978; 26(2): 113–120.

Fawcett, J. *Analysis and Evaluation of Conceptual Models of Nursing*. Philadelphia: F.A. Davis, 1984.

Field, P.A. The impact of nursing theory on the clinical decision making process. *Journal of Advanced Nursing*. 1987; (12): 563–571.

Fulbrook, P.R. The application of the Neumans Systems Model to intensive care. *Intensive Care Nursing*. 1991a; (7): 28–39.

Fulbrook, P.R. The application of a nursing model to intensive care: Planning phase. *Care of the Critically Ill*. 1991b; 7(2): 76–79.

General Nursing Council for England and Wales. *A Statement of Educational Policy*. GNC Circular 77/19/A, 1977.

Hardy, L.K. Janforum: Identifying the place of theoretical frameworks in an evolving discipline. *Journal of Advanced Nursing*. 1986; 11: 103–107.

Henderson, V. *The Nature of Nursing*. New York: Macmillan, 1966.

Johnson, D. Professional practice and specialisation in nursing. *Image*. 1968; 2(3): 2–7.

Johnson, D.E. The behavioural system model for nursing In Eds. J.P. Riehl and C. Roy *Conceptual Models for Nursing Practice*. New York: Appleton Century Crofts, 1980.

King, I.M. *Toward a Theory for Nursing: General Concepts of Human Behaviour*. New York: Wiley, 1971.

Kristjansen, L., Tamblyn, R., Kuypers, J. A model to guide development and application of multiple nursing theories. *Journal of Advanced Nursing*. 1987; 15: 142–147.

Kuhn, T.S. *The Structure of Scientific Revolution, 2nd Ed*. Chicago: University of Chicago Press, 1969.

Levine, M. *Introduction to Clinical Nursing*. Philadelphia: F.A. Davis, 1969.

Lewis, T. Leaping the chasm between nursing theory and practice. *Journal of Advanced Nursing*. 1988; (13): 345–351.

Manley, K. Knowledge for nursing practice. In Eds. A. Perry and M. Jolley. *Nursing: A Knowledge Base for Practice*. London: Edward Arnold, 1991.

Martin, L., Glasper, A. Core plans: Nursing models and the nursing process in action. *Nursing Practice*. 1986; 1:268–273.

Maslow, A.H. *Motivation and Personality*. New York: Harper and Row. 1954.

Meleis, A.I. *Theoretical Nursing: Development and Progress*. Philadelphia: J. B. Lippincott Co., 1985.

Neuman, B.M. The Betty Neuman health care systems model: a total person approach to patient problems. In

Eds. J.P. Riehl and C. Roy. *Conceptual Models for Nursing Practice*. New York: Appleton Century Crofts, 1980.

Orem, D.E. *Nursing Concepts of Practice*. New York: McGraw Hill, 1971.

Orlando, J. *The Dynamic Nurse–Patient Relationship*. New York: G.P. Putnam's Sons, 1961.

Peplau, H. *Interpersonal Relations in Nursing*. New York: G.P. Putnam's Sons, 1952.

Riehl, J.P., Roy, C. (Eds) *Conceptual Models for Nursing Practice*. New York: Appleton Century Crofts, 1980.

Rogers, M. *An Introduction to the Theoretical Basis of Nursing*. Philadelphia: F.A. Davis, 1970.

Rogers, M.E.R. Creating a climate for the implementation of a nursing conceptual framework. *The Journal of Continuing Education in Nursing*. 1990; 20(3): 112–116.

Roper, N., Logan, W., Tierney, A.J. *Using a Model for Nursing*. Edinburgh: Churchill Livingstone, 1983.

Roy, C. *Introduction to Nursing: An Adaptational Model*. Englewood Cliffs, N.J.: Prentice Hall, 1976.

Silva, M.C. Research testing nursing theory: State of the art advances in nursing. *Science*. 1986; 9(1): 1–11.

Thibodeau, J.A. *Nursing Models: Analysis & Evaluation*. California: Wadsworth Health Sciences Division, 1983.

Travelbee, J. *Interpersonal Aspects of Nursing*. Philadelphia: F.A. Davis, 1971.

Walker, L.O., Avant, K.C. *Strategies for Theory Construction in Nursing*. Norwalk, New Jersey: Appleton and Lange, 1988.

Wright, S.G. *Building and Using a Model of Nursing*. London: Edward Arnold, 1986.

Yura, H., Walsh, M.B. *The Nursing Process: Assessment, Planning, Implementing, Evaluating, 3rd Ed*. New York: Appleton Century Crofts, 1978.

3
PRIMARY NURSING AND CRITICAL CARE

Kim Manley

CHAPTER AIMS

This chapter will provide the reader with an opportunity to:

☐ Identify the issues involved in practising primary nursing in critical care settings.

☐ Consider the nature of primary nursing in relation to critical care nursing.

☐ Reflect on the values and beliefs central to the practice of primary nursing.

☐ Identify the central components of primary nursing.

☐ Consider the feasibility of practising primary nursing in critical care settings.

☐ Identify the benefits, concerns and actual experiences of practising primary nursing in critical care settings.

☐ Review the problems involved in operationalizing the concept of primary nursing.

☐ Consider the research available regarding patient outcomes and nurses' job satisfaction in relation to primary nursing.

☐ Consider research questions that need to be asked in relation to the practice of primary nursing in critical care settings.

☐ Analyse the attributes of primary nursing as an innovation when considering its implementation.

☐ Review the practical implications for the nurse, team, manager and educator involved in the practice of primary nursing in critical care settings

INTRODUCTION

Primary nursing is one approach to organizing care, a method of matching the needs of patients to the skills of nurses. It is also a philosophy, one which possesses specific values and beliefs about the nature of nursing (Manley, 1990c). The practice of primary nursing in critical care settings in the United Kingdom is in its infancy, assignment of nurses to the total care of patients on a shift-by-shift basis being the method predominantly practised.

It is through the principle of continuity of care that primary nursing can be put into practice. As an organizational approach the off-duty is organized to allow primary and associate nurses to work with the same patient or patients on a continuous basis from admission to discharge. Through this continuity of contact between the nurse and patient a close and therapeutic relationship is nurtured.

In the past, continuity of care in critical care has not been considered a priority (Kaplow, Ackerman and Outlaw, 1989; Worobel, 1981). Staff have been allocated to patients for such purposes as the minimizing of staff stress from the intensity of relationships; providing specific experiences; or in response to requests for specific patients by staff.

It cannot be stated categorically whether primary nursing is better or worse than any other approach to organizing care, although many claims and some evidence exists to support that it is better. It can be argued that it is not a matter of demonstrating whether primary nursing is better or worse than other approaches, but as a philosophy it enables nurses to practise in ways that reflect what nursing may be to them. The benefits to patients if this is so would result indirectly through the greater autonomy, responsibility and subsequently job satisfaction achieved by practising nurses.

Primary nursing may not be an approach that suits every nurse, or one appropriate to every critical care setting, particularly where patients may be transferred out of critical care in less than 24 hours. However, each critical care unit possesses a unique team of nurses who have their own views about what they consider nursing to be.

This chapter suggests that the first step in undertaking a change to primary nursing is to first clarify the values and beliefs held about nursing, and secondly, to select the approach which enables nurses to put these values into practice. Whichever approach is finally selected, nurses who have undergone this process will be clearer of their own views about nursing in critical care, and subsequently through the insights gained will be able to succinctly and confidently articulate those views to others.

The chapter's other aim is to provide insights into primary nursing through considering its characteristics as a philosophy and as an organizational approach, and the benefits and implications of practising primary nursing in critical care. This will enable informed choices to be made, as well as identifying the implications necessary to consider.

MAIN ISSUES

There are four key issues relevant to address when considering whether to practice primary nursing in any nursing setting. These questions are equally relevant to critical care nurses, and are stated below:

1. Is primary nursing congruent with the values and beliefs held about the nature of critical care nursing?
2. Is primary nursing an appropriate and feasible approach to critical care settings?
3. What are the potential benefits of practising primary nursing?
4. What are the implications of practising primary nursing in critical care?

These four issues will now be expanded superficially, but will further be developed in each of the major sections of the chapter.

Is primary nursing congruent with the values and beliefs held about the nature of critical care nursing?

This question is fundamental in that our values and beliefs influence our behaviour (Lancaster and Lancaster, 1982; Fitzpatrick, 1989). But before this question can be answered, several others have to be asked?

☐ What values and beliefs are held about the nature of critical care nursing?
☐ What are the values and beliefs central to primary nursing?
☐ Are the values and beliefs stated in the above two points similar, that is, congruent?

Trying to answer the questions 'what is critical care nursing?', 'what is its purpose?' and, 'how can its purpose be achieved?' is difficult. Each question requires a great deal of reflection on the part of each individual nurse, and then has to be be discussed with others to produce a statement of common and shared beliefs. Only when this process has been undertaken, often over quite a lengthy period of time, can the values and beliefs central to primary nursing be considered to see if they match. To establish this, knowledge of what constitutes primary nursing is needed so an informed decision can be made to consider it further. The central value to primary nursing is that the therapeutic relationship between the nurse, the patient and family is of benefit to the patient. So what is a therapeutic relationship, and what are the implications of developing one? Critical care nurses will need to decide whether they want to develop such relationships, whether they are able to cope positively with them, and what knowledge and skills will subsequently need to be developed?

Is primary nursing an appropriate and feasible approach in critical care settings?

The previous issue may appear abstract; the second is more practical. Having decided that primary nursing is congruent with a unit's philosophy and that it is an approach staff would like to practise, the actual feasibility of practising primary nursing needs to next be considered. The nature of the critical care speciality itself may be an influencing factor, but so too is the organizational environment and the predominant culture and leadership style.

Common concerns include managing the off-duty, and the allocation of the same nurse to the same patient for long periods of time. It is these practical issues that are often raised first when primary nursing is suggested. These genuine concerns can provide barriers and obstacles, but if there is a strong desire to practise primary nursing then such problems can be creatively and innovatively overcome with time.

What are the potential benefits of practising primary nursing?

Many benefits are claimed for primary nursing in other clinical settings. Are these important reasons for practising primary nursing in critical care, and how can these claims be demonstrated? Do the disadvantages outweigh the benefits? What are the disadvantages?

Making explicit the benefits of any service is an essential part of providing cost-effective health care in Britain today. Nurses as the most costly part of the budget need to demonstrate the value of nursing more than ever before. In addition, critically ill patients "need and receive an impressive array of nursing and medical resources. Vast amounts of money, personnel, time, space, and highly sophisticated equipment are expended to provide care and promote recovery." (Dracup, 1987). Intensive care is approximately four times more expensive than routine hospital care (Reigle, 1989). With increasing scarcity of resources, even more questions will be asked about the effectiveness of care being delivered.

Does primary nursing enable the value of nursing to be made explicit by placing nursing on a professional model? Does primary nursing's case strengthen the role of nursing at a time when other options such as healthcare assistants are being considered? What differences are there in patient outcomes when nurses care for patients compared with health care assistants or technicians? Are there longer term implications for the identity and role of nursing? These broader issues are inextricably linked to the issues surrounding the practice of primary nursing.

What are the implications of practising primary nursing in critical care?

What are the implications for the individual nurse, the nursing team, managers, educators and the multidisciplinary team?

The development of a therapeutic relationship with patients and their families probably has the greatest implication for the individual critical care nurse. In the past, nurses rarely cared for the same patients for more than two consecutive shifts. Will individual nurses be able to cope with the greater emotional involvement, and the greater psychological and social support inevitably expected when practising primary nursing? Does practising primary nursing mean being on call? Does it mean that primary nurses are expected to be all knowing? What knowledge and skills need to be developed, and what are the implications for the organizational climate?

THE LITERATURE

Separating the literature from the research on primary nursing in critical care is difficult when there is so little of either about the speciality. However, the division has been made as follows. The content of the literature section is drawn mainly from articles which represent opinions and views concerning the practice of primary nursing in critical care, supplemented by more general literature. Other informal sources are drawn from comments expressed at conferences and on study days, enabling a breadth of views to be expressed.

The research section, in contrast, draws on published research articles or formal research presentations involving research into primary nursing. This includes small or large studies, or studies where the practice of primary nursing may have been a pre-requisite for undertaking research in other areas of critical care practice.

The literature is related to the four issues previously defined by dividing it as follows:

☐　What does the literature indicate primary nursing to be, and how does this relate to the nature of nursing in critical care?

☐　What does the literature state regarding the feasibility of practising primary nursing in critical care settings?

☐　What does the literature identify to be the potential benefits and concerns about practising primary nursing in critical care settings?

☐　What are the implications suggested by the literature of practising primary nursing in critical care settings?

The nature of primary nursing and critical care nursing: the literature

The nature of critical care nursing

Critical care nursing compared with many other nursing specialities has had a relatively short history, the first Intensive Therapy Units (ITU) in the UK opening in the 1960s (Sherwood Jones, 1978). The Royal College of Nursing (RCN) produced its first document concerning Intensive Therapy Units in 1969. This document alludes little to the nature of ITU nursing, concerned more with staffing, nomenclature and staff preparation. However, aspects of the role of ITU nurses could be derived as being concerned with:

"Communicating with mainly unconscious patients
Developing the nurse–relative relationship
Observing patients and documenting these observations
Working within a multidisciplinary team."
(RCN, 1969).

The first extensive survey about what constituted critical care nursing practice was undertaken in the United States in 1979 (Breu and Dracup, 1982) when the responsibilities of ITU staff were identified. These responsibilities were listed mainly in the form of activities, with no stated purpose or underpinning philosophical beliefs about the nature of either nursing or critical care nursing. Although again the concerns of critical care nursing could be indirectly stated as:

☐　"assessment, interpretation and intervention of physiological, and psycho-social data;

☐　teaching patients;

☐　research;

☐　patient care evaluation;

☐　writing and developing of policies." (Breu and Dracup, 1982).

The publications above therefore suggest that intensive and critical care nursing comprises of a series of actions. However, Martha Rogers (1989) suggests that what nurses do is not the same as what nursing is. She suggests that the body of knowledge associated with nursing constitutes what nursing is. An explosion of ideas has occurred generally in nursing during the last two decades in an effort to allude more explicitly to the nature of nursing, its purpose and methods. These efforts have resulted in a multitude of grand theories or conceptual models which make explicit for the first time the values and beliefs held about nursing, and consequently the type of knowledge important to the discipline (Manley 1991b) (see also Chapter 2). Being of an abstract nature, these grand theories can not be tested, their purpose being to provide a philosophical framework for guiding nursing assessment, intervention and evaluation. From these philosophical frameworks, other more specific middle range theories can arise, which may be useful for guiding practice or describing and explaining practice.

Critical care nursing, in common with other areas of nursing, have in the past selected models according to criteria such as simplicity; whether they were known rather than unknown; or because specific models had to be selected for whole departments. Today these trends are being reversed, and philosophical statements of values and beliefs about nursing and critical care nursing are becoming increasingly more common (Warfield and Manley, 1990). Nursing models are now being selected because they are congruent with the values and beliefs held by staff. The organizational approach chosen, too, will also need to be congruent with the values and beliefs held, and made explicit through the specific nursing model or models selected. A feature identified as central to intensive care nursing by Turnock (1989) is the one-to-one relationship that the ITU nurse has with their patient. This is seen to be special and unique to ITU nursing in that the nurse is able to provide all the necessary care to one patient.

The nature of primary nursing

Primary nursing has been described as both an organizational approach and a philosophy (Marram, Barnett and Bevis, 1979; Hegyvary, 1982). Considering the philosophical aspects first, Marram et al. (1979) stated that as a philosophy primary nursing implies that "the patient is central to the focus of the nurse and accountability of nurses for their patients is paramount." Several British authors (McMahon, 1986; Muetzel, 1988; Manley, 1988b) identify that the relationship between the nurse and the patient is an important aspect to primary nursing. This also constitutes one of the key beliefs in relation to intensive care nursing (Manley 1990c). These beliefs can be further expanded:

☐ The nurse–patient relationship is therapeutic, that is, it is of benefit to the patient.
☐ The central focus of nursing is the patient (and their family) not the task.
☐ The development of the personal knowledge of practitioners is essential to the successful practice of primary nursing.

☐ Decentralized decision making can improve the job satisfaction of nurses, if this takes place within a supportive and nurturing environment.
☐ Improved job satisfaction indirectly improves the quality of care for patients.

Many of the organizational concepts of primary nursing centre around the early American writers' definitions of primary nursing (Marram et al., 1979; Manthey, 1980; Hegyvary, 1982). These key concepts have been amalgamated by Ersser and Tutton (1991) into the following four areas:

☐ Particular patterns of responsibility, authority, autonomy and accountability.
☐ Continuity of care.
☐ Care planner as care giver.
☐ Direct communication.

Particular patterns of responsibility, authority, autonomy and accountability

Primary nurses are *responsible* for *the charge* given to them (Goulding and Hunt, 1991). This charge in primary nursing is to forward plan and provide direct nursing care for a (named patient, or) group of patients (Ersser and Tutton, 1991). Nurses in accepting their charge, do so knowingly and willingly.

Accountability focuses on to whom nurses are answerable (i.e. called to account) when undertaking the charge. Hegyvary (1982) considers nurses are professionally answerable to the patient and their family for the nursing care they have provided; to professional colleagues for the standards of care practised; to the employer for carrying out the professional duties expected of nurses; and finally, to the law.

Authority refers to the legitimate power that individuals possess to carry out a responsibility (Bergman, 1981), i.e. the power to act, due to their position, knowledge or situation (Goulding and Hunt, 1991). If primary nurses are to make decisions about care then they need to be given the authority to act. Clinical managers therefore need to be willing to devolve this power to primary nurses (Manley, 1990c), and primary nurses to associate nurses in their absence.

Autonomy refers to independence of action and

the freedom to act. It means that one can perform one's total professional functions on the basis of one's own judgement." (Leddy and Pepper, 1989). It is closely related to the concept of authority.

Continuity of care

Nursing care is continuous, consistent and uninterrupted, around the clock, from shift-to-shift (Hegyvary, 1982). The duration of care is a key point in primary nursing and supports the principle of continuity. Schiro (1980) considers that critical care nurses have always performed primary nursing during their eight-hour shift, but that the objective in primary nursing is to provide "optimum patient care through comprehensive and continuous accountability throughout the patients stay in that unit" (Schiro, 1980). For different critical care specialities the duration of patient stay may vary considerably, from being a matter of hours in the surgical intensive care unit, to weeks in the neurosurgical/medical intensive care unit.

Care planner as care giver

It is the primary nurse who is responsible for planning care for specific patients and for implementing that care when on duty (Elpern, 1977; Marram *et al.*, 1979). This raises two questions: how many shifts does the primary nurse need to work for accountability to be maintained (Anderson and Choi, 1980); and does the primary nurse need to be on call?

According to Fairbanks (1980), 24-hour accountability does not mean that the primary nurse should routinely be on-call. If the primary nurse is off-duty and changes in the patient necessitates changes in the careplan, then the associate nurse is the appropriate person to make them, after seeking advice if necessary from more experienced colleagues. Ciske (1979) considers that being 'on-call' is a total misconception in primary nursing.

According to Manthey (1988), the primary nurse "needs to give enough direct care to assess the patient's status and the effectiveness of the decisions currently in place." Ersser and Tutton (1991) consider that the following factors influence how much direct care individual primary nurses may be able to give:

☐ skill mix of ward/unit
☐ nature of patient's needs
☐ roles adopted by individuals in the team
☐ environmental factors, e.g. geographical position of the patient
☐ the number of hours a nurse works
☐ the acuity of the patient and rapidity of changes in the patient's condition.

The latter influence is also identified by Manley (1990c) as being a major influence in an intensive care unit, where the number of changes in a patient's condition within one shift can be numerous. In such a situation the associate nurse would therefore be expected to implement the necessary changes and inform the primary nurse at the next handover. In selecting the primary nurse for each patient it is important to consider how much direct care the nurse will be in a position to give (Ruzanski, 1981). Within intensive care the night nurse may have just as much opportunity as day staff to develop and maintain a therapeutic relationship with the patient and their family (Manley, 1990c). In Ruzanski's (1981) surgical intensive care unit the off-duty rota was always surveyed prior to appointing a primary nurse, thus ensuring that the amount of direct care that an individual primary nurse could provide would be optimal.

Direct communication

Manthey (1973) and Marram *et al.* (1979) advocate direct communication between the primary nurse and associate nurse as a key concept in primary nursing. This direct communication is later explicitly extended by Manthey (1980) to include all the members of the team, the patient and family.

The concept of direct communication does not include other members of the nursing team who may not be directly involved in care. Such members may need some information about other patients within the ward/unit so that they can respond positively to enquiries. This dissemination of information to non-direct care givers can be achieved in a range of ways; for example, Elpern (1977) held a brief handover for all staff lasting 10–15 minutes when only changes in the patient's condition were reported; in Worobel's (1981) intensive care, a formal handover period was provided in addition to direct caregiver to caregiver handover; and Ruzanski (1981) used brief taped reports, as also suggested by Marram *et al.* (1979). These could be listened to by nurses not directly involved in other patients' care at their convenience.

Self reflection question

List the four key concepts of primary nursing identified by Errser and Tutton 1991:

1)
2)
3)
4)

The nature of the therapeutic relationship: the literature

Developing a therapeutic relationship is central to primary nursing (Manthey, 1988; Manley, 1990c), and so it is important to understand its nature.

According to Hockey (1991), therapeutic nursing is explained "as the practice of those nursing activities which have a healing effect or those which result in a movement towards health or wellness." The outcome of therapeutic practice can therefore be considered to be increased health or wellness. Several conceptual models of nursing, particularly those based on interaction theories such as Peplau (1952), Travelbee (1971) and Orlando (1961) suggest that the activities which produce this effect involve the establishment of a therapeutic relationship between the patient/client and the nurse. Therefore in summary, it appears that it is the relationship which is therapeutic, and the outcome of the relationship strived for is health (Barber, 1991).

Primary nursing as a method of organizing care may give the best opportunity for establishing a close relationship between a primary nurse and the patient, although this closeness is also found between the associate nurses and the patient, and between the primary and associate nurses. The therapeutic relationship itself is seen as the central focus of primary nursing (Manley, 1990c), or the essence (Mead and Adair, 1990) rather than the trappings or its manifestation.

Muetzel (1988), too, considers that the therapeutic process of nursing is achieved through the therapeutic relationship. This is considered to be "suggestive of a purposeful, supportive and healing association between two persons that is interactive and holistic." This relationship she considers has three essential overlapping components:

☐ *Partnership*. This refers to "the working association between two parties in a joint enterprise, and which implies gains for both" (Muetzel, 1988). Partnership therefore suggests a balance of power and equality in the relationship between the nurse and the patient.

☐ *Intimacy*. This "is a closeness at physical, psychological and spiritual levels which suggests a sense of communication between persons that is meaningful and valuing to and of those concerned" (Muetzel, 1988).

☐ *Reciprocity*. This concept suggests that "the nurse too can be the receiver not only of information and cooperation, but also of support and care." (Muetzel, 1988).

Barber (1991) values the theory of symbolic interactionism for explaining the role of perception within a therapeutic relationship. This involves trying to see the world through the patient's eyes and trying to establish their sense and meaning of the world. However, the quality of the therapeutic relationship is also dependent upon how a nurse experiences and positively uses his or her own qualities of self (Barber, 1988). Such awareness requires specialist facilitation (Barber, 1991). This view is also held by Johns (1992a), who supervises primary and associate nurses by helping them to reflect on their practice.

However, Clark (1987) raises the question "Can we hold other nurses accountable for interactions that require them to change their usual way of relating to patients and families? Implementing psycho-social research findings would often necessitate changing our innate and automatic ways of responding."

Drew (1986) identifies how nurses can develop their interactions so that they are perceived as caring, and how to avoid behaviours which may be perceived and experienced by patients as dehumanizing. Drew identified two types of inter-actions: those experienced by patients as exclusion-ary, and those experienced as confirming and enhancing.

Exclusionary interactions in Drew's study de-scribed caregivers from the patient's viewpoint as having the following attributes: lacking emotional warmth, appearing starchy, mechanical, bored, impatient, irritated, flip, superior or preoccupied. Other contributing factors were described as a flat facial expression, lack of eye contact, and too casual an attitude. This behaviour was interpreted by patients to mean that the caregiver had a nega-tive attitude towards them. The patients sub-sequently experienced fear, feelings of shame and anger. They felt hopeless in response and this, they described, sapped their energy. This energy they felt could have been used more productively in the healing process (Drew, 1986).

In confirming or enhancing interactions care-givers were perceived by patients as caring about what happens, liking their work and having perso-nality. Eye contact, lack of haste, and a low and expressive tone of voice were considered extremely important. Patients subsequently experienced feel-ings of hope, comfort, confidence, assurance, and a sense of ease and relaxation. They felt that some sort of energy had passed to them from the care-giver and that this helped them in the healing process (Drew, 1986).

Drew's work therefore supports Clark's view that "through the relationship that the nurse de-velops with the patient, the nurse has the potential to add to the patient's perception that they have the resources to cope with the threatening stimuli pre-sented by a critical illness" (Clark, 1987).

Both Johns (1992) and Barber (1991) focus specifically on interaction skills necessary to facili-tate effective interventions within the therapeutic relationship. Both authors use Heron's (1975) model of 'Six Category Intervention Analysis' as a framework for this purpose. Johns (1992) specifi-cally applies these intervention skills to the practice of an associate nurse. Barber provides insights for carers and suggests how he could have personally benefited from them when undergoing the trauma-tic experience of being a patient in an intensive care unit.

The feasibility of practising primary nursing in critical care: the literature

Little literature exists about the practice of primary nursing in critical care areas, even though there is an abundance concerning other specialities in the UK, particularly those settings which care for elderly people (Pearson, 1988; Wright, 1990), acute surgical patients (Binnie, 1987), and recently a range of other general settings (Ersser and Tutton, 1991).

The earliest mention of primary nursing in criti-cal care settings appears to be in 1978 in the Canadian literature (Medaglia, 1978), where it is described in a coronary care unit. This is followed by American literature concerning critical care set-tings generally (Schiro, 1980), medical intensive care (Worobel, 1981), surgical intensive care (Ruzanski, 1981), and a special care baby unit (Bethea, 1985).

Within the British literature the earliest mention of primary nursing in critical care is in the intensive care unit (Manley, 1988b, 1989), and in the coron-ary care unit (Thompson, 1990), where primary nursing was known to be practised for several years preceeding this publication. More recently, pri-mary nursing has attracted greater interest from British critical care nurses (Manley, 1990a,b,c, 1991b; Constable, 1991; Atkinson, 1991).

However, there is a suggestion that primary nursing is being practised considerably more in American critical care settings than the literature explicitly states. This has been identified from the background of research studies considering aspects of care dependent upon the practice of primary nursing (for example, O'Malley et al., 1991). This observation is further supported by Pasternak (1988), who recognizes that primary nursing is the biggest influence on critical care nursing in the United States in the late 1980s.

Bailey (1981) considers that if intensive care nurses wish to implement primary nursing then the favourably high patient–nurse ratio will allow such a transition to be made more easily than almost any other area. Manley (1990a) reinforces this point when identifying the following factors which make the practice of primary nursing in intensive care easier compared with most other areas:

- [ ] more favourable nurse–patient ratios;
- [ ] consistent nurse–patient ratios on all shifts including at night;
- [ ] all qualified workforce;
- [ ] greater opportunities for autonomous action.

In intensive care, primary nurses have "the most consistent contact with the patient and are best able to assess efficacy of therapies, monitor clinical status and direct the plan of care." (Kaplow, Ackerman and Outlaw, 1989).

Kaplow *et al.* (1989) identify how working 12 hour shifts may make the practice of primary nursing difficult. Twelve hour shifts pose a problem because of the number of days off each nurse has, with, for example, 13 days being worked in each 28 day cycle. This can result in the continuity of care provided by the same primary nurse being disrupted. A solution which maintained maximum off-duty flexibility was the concept of co-primary nursing (Kaplow *et al.*, 1989). Two primary nurses are appointed to each patient working on opposite 12 hour shifts. This means that most of the time the patient is cared for by at least one of the two co-primary nurses. A third nurse, the associate nurse, assumes temporary responsibility for the patient at other times.

The management of the off-duty rota is acknowledged as probably the most difficult obstacle to overcome when considering the feasibility of practising primary nursing in intensive care (Manley, 1990c). A particular problem identified is minimizing the number of associate nurses involved in care (Manley, 1989). Where nurses are practising primary nursing using a conventional three shift system, then the number of nurses potentially involved in care can be higher than in a 12 hour shift system. This problem can be overcome in ITU by allocating all staff to permanent teams (Manley, 1990c), each team being continually responsible for the patient's care from admission to discharge. This approach constitutes team nursing, or 'primary team' nursing as defined by Atkinson (1991), where it is used in a Newcastle ITU. To constitute primary nursing there needs to be in addition a designated primary nurse for each patient within each primary nurse team, the remaining members of the team acting as associate nurses. The off-duty is designed for each team independently, so that one person from each

group is always on duty (Manley, 1990c). However, the skill mix overall for the unit on a shift-by-shift basis needs to be taken into careful consideration. It is this aspect which requires considerable co-ordination.

Within coronary care the staff–patient ratio is different, and a different set of constraints therefore exist. Thompson (1990) considers that in this situation it is pointless to attach a newly admitted patient to a nurse who is due to take the next few days off. To avoid this occurring a flexible system of operating the duty rota has been encouraged. Each nurse prepares their own off-duty rota on the proviso that the agreed minimum number of staff and skill-mix is available on each shift.

The benefits, concerns and actual experiences of practising primary nursing in critical care: the literature

Benefits

The potential benefits claimed for practising primary nursing are considered according to who the benefactors may be:

- [ ] patients
- [ ] families
- [ ] nurses
- [ ] other members of the multi-disciplinary team.

Some of these benefits are supported by research, and these will be addressed in the research section. Here it is the claims in the literature made for primary nursing that will be focused on.

Patients are claimed to benefit from primary nursing because it is believed they receive better quality of care, through the highly personalized (Thomson, 1990) and individual approach it provides; and through the therapeutic relationship that develops with both patients and families (Manley, 1990c). This relationship commences at admission (Schiro, 1980). However, when making judgements about quality it is important to acknowledge the standards against which these judgements are being made. Such standards need to be made explicit as derived from our values and beliefs about the purpose and role of nursing (Warfield and Manley, 1990).

Other benefits to the patient are highlighted by Worobel (1981), who considers that through the day-to-day observation of the same patient the nurse is able to notice subtle changes occurring. This would therefore suggest that earlier intervention may be possible. This type of practical knowledge resulting from many hours of close observation and direct patient care is identified by Benner (1984) in her work on the characteristics of expert practitioners, and which involved the study of intensive care nurses. Finally, Clark (1987) links the benefits of a caring nurse–patient relationship to improved patient morbidity and mortality through the mechanism of assisting patients with effective coping.

Families benefit from primary nursing through developing better communication links with carers, and resultantly are more likely to actively participate in care. This is because primary and associate nurses set out to obtain a greater in depth understanding of the family's behaviour (Schiro, 1980), and more support is subsequently provided to the family (Worobel, 1981).

Clark (1987) suggests that when families are allocated a primary care giver they see this person as a trusted source of information and comfort. This relationship, she suggests, assists both the patient and the family in achieving effective coping. It reduces the feelings of hopelessness which often result from the large number of unknown caregivers in critical care who have access to the patient's body and private reactions sapping the patient's energy.

Nurses can benefit by obtaining greater job satisfaction through devolved decision-making. By being giving control of the work for which they are educated their work becomes more interesting, stimulating and rewarding (Schiro, 1980; Bowman, 1990b). Through having a clearer picture of the unique aspects of their role, areas for research can be spotlighted (Bowman, 1990c).

Other benefits for nurses relate to increased opportunities for; developing personal knowledge (Manley, 1991b), greater decision-making, responsibility and challenge (Manley, 1988b).

Other members of the multi-disciplinary team are said also to value the greater insights gained about patients from the relationship built up by the primary nurse. Schiro (1980) considers primary nursing provides potential for better collaborative practice, and Johns (1992) focuses on the relationship between nurses practising primary nursing and improved colleagueship. Good rapport has been established with all members of the multi-disciplinary team (Worobel, 1981) as a result of practising primary nursing.

A further benefit for both patients and staff identified by Peerbacus and Watson (1991) may be unique to the critical care setting with its 1:1 patient:nurse ratio, that is a reduced risk of cross-infection. If a restricted number of staff give care to only one patient then the risk of cross-infection, for example from Methicillin Resistant Staphylococcus Aureus (MRSA), may be reduced. Secondly, it is easier to account for staff if they themselves require treatment following exposure to a patient with infectious organisms.

Concerns

The concerns of primary nursing frequently voiced include:

☐ The dangers of stress and burnout.
☐ How can the primary nurse be accountable in her absence particularly when he or she goes on leave? (Constable, 1991).
☐ How can other expert's knowledge and expertise be assimilated into the primary nurse's decision-making?

The voiced concerns about stress and burnout often relate to the prospect of caring for the same very sick or challenging patient continuously. Such patients are often in physiological, psychological and social crisis, and their family, too, require considerable support over an extended period, for example, the long-term resident who may be an ITU patient for as long as three months. For staff this may incur the prospect of coming to work and caring for the same single patient day in and day out during a prolonged period.

Constable (1991) considers that stress and burnout are very real in ITU, and can happen before they are recognized. Also, from his personal experience, "nursing a single patient for a prolonged period without a change can be very stressful." Such patients may be for example trauma patients who have a flail chest and require ventilation for a number of weeks. On the other hand, some staff like the intimacy of caring for only one patient as they have more control in ensuring that interventions are consistently applied and evaluated. Additionally, staff feel they really get to know their patients and families very well, which in turn can be less stressful; for example, when communicating with a patient who cannot speak, lip reading becomes much easier if the same nurses are consistently communicating with the same patient. This is because the nurses learn to recognize the unique ways of the patient, which in turn results in less frustration for both the nurse and the patient.

Bowman (1990b) asks "by developing good patient–nurse relationships within primary nursing are we putting nurses in an even more stressful position?" He suggests from his research findings that nurses are less likely to experience stress from the work itself if there is a clear self-directed role which the nurse can control.

Maslach (cited in Pasternak, 1988) considers that although nurses may be proficient in clinical skills, they lack the interpersonal skills needed to deal with intense emotional interactions. If this is true then it may be that stress and burnout relates to deficits in knowledge and skill rather than the practice of primary nursing itself. Practising primary nursing will, however expose such deficits if they are present. Deficits in knowledge and skills, however, is a rectifiable problem which can easily be addressed if the motivation exists to do so.

Experiences

Kaplow, Ackerman and Outlaw (1989) convey their first experiences of introducing co-primary nursing into critical care in the following quotation:

> "At first, resistance to primary nursing from particular individuals was very high, provoked by the effect of change and the increased accountability and commitment demanded. Yet, while some were resistant, other nurses were volunteering, and by the fifth month, all chronic patients were managed by primary nurses and all nurses were reporting positive feelings about the model. Also several patient–family experiences were very rewarding for those involved."

Kaplow et al. (1989) suggest that units should consider mechanisms for considering staff satisfaction and compliance with the method of care delivery. This suggests the need for carefully thought out contingencies in response to problems that may occur.

Many of the concerns and problems experienced from practising primary nursing in ITU were presented by Peerbacus and Watson (1991) at the first national study day presented by Westminster Intensive Care Unit/Nursing Development Unit in 1991. The issues were seen to fall into four areas, as outlined in Table 3.1, and these are further expanded in Tables 3.8, 3.12 and 3.13 of the implications section.

Table 3.1.   Issues related to practising primary nursing in ITU (Peerbacus and Watson, 1991).

Issues for individual nurses

- Accountability
- Care planning
- Stress and burnout
- Opting out
- Relationships
- Handling constructive criticism
- Role change—the nurse coordinating the shift
  —the primary nurse
  —the associate nurse

Issues for management

- Group dynamics of each primary nursing team
- Off-duty
- Isolation and cohesiveness
- Staff awareness
- Senior management support
- Cross infection

Issues for education

- Preparation of staff
- Learning needs of ENB course members

Issues for the multi-disciplinary team

Issues concerning members of the multi-disciplinary team relate to how primary nursing may affect them in their work (Peerbacus and Watson, 1991). However, good preparation and communication with all members of the multi-disciplinary team as a strategy reduced any problems in Manley's (1989) study.

Implications of practising primary nursing: the literature

The section seeks to answer the question what is involved or implied in the implementation and practise of primary nursing? Some of the prerequisites suggested prior to change, and some early experiences of practising primary nursing will be examined, before considering management and educational implications mentioned in the literature.

Prerequisites and implementation issues

Ferrin (1981) identifies a specific list of 'readiness factors' which if met would suggest that the implementation of primary nursing could proceed:

- [ ] adequate registered nurse staffing levels
- [ ] the unit manager's effectiveness
- [ ] an inservice programme
- [ ] an orientation programme
- [ ] a staff evaluation system
- [ ] an effective unit audit system
- [ ] staff competency
- [ ] physicians understanding
- [ ] staff understanding
- [ ] openness of communication.

Worobel (1981) also suggests the following prerequisites are necessary for primary nursing to be practised in intensive care:

- [ ] Staff closely analyse their needs and set specific goals and expectations.
- [ ] Continuous evaluation of primary nursing practice through regular staff meetings, to facilitate discussion and problem solving.
- [ ] Early identification of support systems and resource people.
- [ ] Nursing conferences providing educational support held at least weekly to increase clinical and theoretical skills and knowledge.
- [ ] Availability of appropriate nursing assessment documentation to facilitate collaboration between members of the multidisciplinary team.
- [ ] Time allocated for care planning and documentation. Primary nursing philosophy and process are incorporated into formal unit orientation programmes.

Worobel and Ferrin's suggestions can be further augmented by the issues Kaplow, Ackerman and Outlaw (1989) identified when preparing to practise co-primary nursing in ITU. These included: the assignment of primary nurses; roles and responsibilities; the assignment of nurses to areas within the unit; and the change of shift report. Other issues which arose and discussed over the two years subsequent to the implementation of co-primary nursing are identified in Table 3.2.

It is interesting to note the similarity between these issues and those identified by Peerbacus and Watson's (1991) mentioned earlier (Table 3.1).

In addition to the areas listed in Table 3.2, other projects also resulted suggesting further implications for the practice of primary nursing. These projects (Kaplow, Ackerman and Outlaw (1989)) addressed the:

- [ ] development of a new nursing care plan format, including patient history documentation;
- [ ] initiation of collaborative relationships with nurses in other areas when preparing for transfer of longterm intensive care patients;
- [ ] adaptation of a self-evaluation tool for primary nurses;
- [ ] continuing education conferences on primary nursing;
- [ ] establishment of goals for each year;

Table 3.2. Areas addressed by the ITU Primary Nursing Committee during a two year period of practising co-primary nursing within a 10 bedded Intensive Care Unit (Kaplow *et al.*, 1989).

1 Difficult patient and/or family
2 Orientees
3 Communication between co-primary nurses
4 Burnout from increased investment
5 Scheduling off-duty
6 Problem nurses
7 Resisters
8 Primary nursing scheduling board
9 Patient conferences
10 Updating nursing care plans
11 Change from standardized format to individualized nursing care plans

☐ establishment of unit standards for primary nursing.

Difficulties encountered by Kaplow *et al.* (1989) when introducing co-primary nursing in ITU included:

☐ orientation of new staff, as previously the programme was designed to "provide maximum exposure to a diverse patient population" so these nurses tended to have priority over primary nurses on patient allocation;

☐ disagreement between co-primary nurses concerning which patient they should care for;

☐ lack of a registered nurse interested in presenting patient conferences;

☐ doubling of daily assignment, i.e. being allocated two patients when the primary patient was less demanding;

☐ over-involvement with patient and families around death and dying issues.

Immediate problems experienced on implementing primary nursing by Manley (1989) were considered surmountable with discussion. This highlights the need to have open and flexible communication channels so that problems not anticipated can be quickly addressed as they occur. Problems experienced by Manley included:

☐ obtaining information about patients not being cared for by the primary nurse;

☐ the changing role of senior staff who were unaccustomed to being non-directive and found this initially difficult;

☐ the support primary nurses and associate nurses needed in helping them to be assertive;

☐ supervision and support of more inexperienced staff;

☐ managing the off-duty to enable the same associate nurses to work with the same primary nurse.

The last point concerning the relationship between the primary and associate nurses relates to role theory as identified by Wilson (1990). Wilson considers there to be two models for relationships between the two roles. The first involves the primary nurse having responsibility for the prescription of care and acting also as a team leader with a group of nurses who work collaboratively as associate nurses. The second involves the primary nurse being responsible for the prescription of care, but has no responsibility for team leadership. With this arrangement any one nurse may be selected as a primary nurse to some patients and an associate nurse to others.

Other implications for the introduction of primary nursing relate to using planned change (Manley, 1989). This is not unique to the implementation of primary nursing, and so will not be discussed here.

Management implications

Many authors (Elpern, 1977; Manthey, 1980; Ferrin, 1981; Deiman *et al.*, 1984; Jenkins, 1991) identify the need for complete support, understanding and commitment from nursing management. The environmental culture therefore created by the manager is essential to the success of primary nursing (Jenkins, 1991). It needs to mimic the same attributes of trust, honesty and openness conducive to developing good therapeutic relationships with patients (Jenkins, 1991). Such management relationships are confirming and enhancing rather than exclusionary (Clark, 1987) (see the section on the therapeutic relationship).

Additionally the environment established "must foster behaviour that encourages self-development and independence rather than reliance on the system" (Bowman, 1990c).

Ferrin (1981) states that one of the determinants to successful implementation of primary nursing is the return of "power, responsibility and accountability to the level of practice." This, she states, is incompatible with an authoritarian management style. Bowman (1990b), too, supports this view; "the open style of relationship between the senior nurse and primary nurses must exist if staff are to have confidence to fulfil the role prescribed to them."

Johns (1992) identifies a role for the clinical manager as providing supervision in the sharing and reflecting of experiences from a reflective diary as a collaborative experience which helps people to become increasingly effective in their roles. Also, he identifies the need to create an environment where people are able to give and receive feedback. In summary, the role of clinical managers and their ability, dedication and attitude has been identified as a critical variable in the success of primary nursing (Chavigny and Lewis, 1984).

Educational implications

The autonomy that nurses have when practising primary nursing "has its roots in ongoing education". (Worobel, 1981).

Johns (1992b) identifies four implications of practising primary nursing if primary nurses are to use themselves therapeutically:

☐ nurses need to develop their interaction skills;
☐ nurses need to be sensitive to their own feelings;
☐ nurses need to be able to recognize their need for support;
☐ nurses need a fundamental concern about people.

All of these implications have relevance for both educators and managers and how they can assist staff to fulfil these needs.

Clayton and McCabe (1991) consider that identifying the perceived needs of staff is the most important first step in the educational process, because motivation of staff is a key factor to the success of education. Examples of perceived needs identified by Clayton and McCabe prior to the implementation of primary nursing in ITU include the need for:

☐ "information about primary nursing;
☐ strategies for coping with change;
☐ advancement in the knowledge and skills necessary to enhance patient assessment and care;
☐ enhancement of ability to develop therapeutic relationships with patients and families." (Clayton and McCabe, 1991).

A common need identified by other authors is the development of assertiveness skills (Schiro, 1980; Johns, 1992). Johns (1992) states that many new staff tend to perceive themselves to lack assertiveness and have a need to avoid conflict. Both of these factors, he says, are a deeply engrained social norm. But he identifies both of them as essential to the practice of primary nursing and the carrying out of

responsibility for work. Another need commonly expressed by primary nurses is the feeling that they lacked experience in making good decisions about care and needed help from others (Johns, 1992).

In trying to address such needs, Bowman (1990c) provides an in-service programme which involves 'thinking nursing'; this, he felt, helped in the development of skills which enabled staff to interact confidently with patients, relatives and other members of the health care team. Specifically, Bowman (1990b) considers preparation to practise primary nursing should involve 'good interpersonal skill training' so that staff feel at ease with the closer relationships found in primary nursing. Staff development therefore centres around three key areas:

☐ "developing greater awareness of nursing issues;
☐ developing interpersonal skills;
☐ promoting an ethos of self-development." (Bowman, 1990b).

Clark (1987) identifies the stressors present in critical care nursing generally, and states that nurses need to accept these stressors (as they will always be present in the job), and actively problem-solve to find a solution. She goes on to suggest that there is a need to learn more mature individual and group coping styles, by talking about reactions and observing how others effectively adapt to the day-to-day strain of caring for sick and dying patients, and their families. Such coping strategies are even more essential to develop if additionally practising primary nursing, 'as being open and authentic within relationships with patients exposes nurse to stress' (Johns, 1992). So educational support in developing personal knowledge is essential (Manley, 1990c).

Within practice settings the significance of the therapeutic team in assisting nurses in primary nursing roles to seek and receive support has been identified by Johns (1992). He identifies the need to provide the same sort of reciprocal caring to each other, as to the patient. However, there is also a danger within a harmonious team that a facade of togetherness or teamwork may prevent primary and associate nurses talking to each other about their feelings and resolving their conflicts (Johns, 1992).

Anticipated role change is another topic identified as requiring much discussion. Clayton and McCabe (1991) suggest two areas to consider when preparing for role changes:

1. What preparation can be given to the staff to enable them to function as primary and associate nurses?
2. What effects will result from the change in the clinical managers role?

Within primary nursing, then, staff have different but complementary roles. These roles within the team are collegial rather than hierarchichal (McMahon, 1990; Mead, 1990). Role blurring and role conflict can pose problems when practising primary nursing (Wilson, 1990). One strategy suggested when preparing for these roles includes the development of role descriptions, which act as a source of discussion (Manley, 1989). Other strategies for developing role effectiveness once primary nursing is being practised include the use of reflection under supervision using personal diaries (Johns, 1992), and performing a role analysis which focuses on role expectations (Wilson, 1990).

THE RESEARCH

Research can be defined "as an attempt to increase the body of knowledge by discovery of new facts and relationships through a process of systematic scientific enquiry" (McCleod Clark and Hockey, 1979). Nursing's body of knowledge represents what is currently known about nursing. Therefore, this section tries to address the question, what is currently known about primary nursing specifically in critical care settings?

Kathleen Dracup's (1987) comprehensive review of research studies pertinent to the delivery of nursing care in the intensive care unit between 1975–1985 makes no mention of primary nursing or any other organizational or philosophical approach to nursing.

Pasternak, when considering the research in critical care nursing in 1988, identified primary nursing as a priority in the United States because, "it is the most dramatic and significant factor that currently is influencing the function of the critical care nurse." Primary nursing, therefore, is identified as a relevant area for research in critical care.

Only two published research studies concerning critical care nursing and primary nursing can be identified in the literature (Pasternak, 1988; Manley, 1988b, 1989). One other known to the author has been formally presented and is awaiting publication (Connolly and Gray, 1991). This section will therefore address the research more broadly, and will be augmented by key studies from other settings. It will be divided as follows:

- ☐ Research concerning the operationalization of primary nursing.
- ☐ Research re: patient outcomes of primary nursing.
- ☐ Research re: nurses.
- ☐ Future research questions concerning primary nursing in critical care.

Operationalizing primary nursing: the research

Giovannetti (1986), in her comprehensive review of research involving primary nursing, identified the lack of operational definitions of primary nursing to be the most pervasive problem when attempting to research primary nursing. This means that although researchers state that primary nursing is being practised, there is no way of knowing whether it is actually being practised. Different perceptions and interpretations of what primary nursing is, and modifications made to suit varied clinical setting, result in like not being compared with like. Such a range of interpretation in the use of primary nursing is not a problem in its normal practice, but it does become one if trying to research it as an organizational approach using traditional research methods.

The development of an operational definition would therefore enable specific attributes to be identified which could be observed in practice. If all attributes were present then primary nursing could be said to be practised. But even if this were to be achieved, other organizational approaches with which primary nursing may be compared would also need to be operationally defined. The reason that primary nursing has been so difficult to define is that primary nursing in common with any method of organizing nursing work "represents a whole set of nursing behaviours which can be difficult to isolate and describe as a discrete whole." (Ersser and Tutton, 1991).

MacGuire (1989a) identifies ten principles of primary nursing which she has derived from the literature on primary nursing. If all principles are present then she considers there would be support for the claim that primary nursing was being practised. These principles have been operationalized in an acute medical unit for the elderly, where concrete examples have been developed to illustrate each principle (MacGuire, 1989b).

Mead (1991) identifies 16 dimensions of primary nursing. But instead of drawing on the literature as MacGuire did, she identified her dimensions using a Delphi technique with a panel of 28 experts in primary nursing.

Consider your response to the question

To me primary nursing involves . . .

(Now read on and see if you have identified any of Meads characteristics in your definition)

The dimensions resulting are outlined in Table 3.3.

Both Macguire's and Mead's work are useful for determining whether primary nursing is being practised in any nursing setting including critical care.

How many of the characteristics described by Mead currently can be identified within your unit?

List them:

From the critical care perspective, one study has considered the perceptions of ITU nurses about primary nursing in one ITU practising primary

Table 3.3. The 16 dimensions of primary nursing identified by Mead (1991).

☐ Accountability, authority and responsibility for a caseload of patients
☐ Care delivery centred around individual patient needs
☐ Case load attachment from admission to discharge
☐ Continuity of care
☐ Primary nurse as caregiver
☐ Evidence of a philosophy or value system
☐ Decentralized decision-making
☐ Care plans and care planning which reflect that the primary nurse is the principal organizer of care
☐ Changes in ward organization
☐ Communication pathways which indicate that the primary nurse is the principal organizer of care
☐ Patient/relatives involvement and choice
☐ Skill mix
☐ Evidence of a role change for the nurses involved
☐ Development of collegiate relationships
☐ Patients know their nurse
☐ Visual evidence of a system

nursing (Connolly and Gray, 1991). Nurses were asked what primary nursing meant to them. Half of the staff sample ($n = 26$) clearly stated that "it was about one leader (the primary nurse) and a team (the associate nurses) working together to provide individual holistic nursing care." A quarter of the staff also referred to 'continuity of care' in their answers.

Patient outcomes: the research

A comprehensive review of studies evaluating patient outcomes in relation to primary nursing in all settings up to 1988 is provided by Manley (1989). Ersser and Tutton (1991) also nicely summarize the main research issues concerning the evaluation of patient outcomes in general settings. They identify two hypotheses:

1. Primary nursing increases satisfaction with care.
2. Primary nursing improves the quality of nursing care.

In relation to the first hypothesis, no published research exists considering either patient's or relative's satisfaction with care in critical care settings. Researching patient's satisfaction with care may, however, be inappropriate in some areas of critical care; particularly where patients may be unconscious, unable to communicate or their memory is influenced by a range of factors from the effects of drugs to psychological protection. The effect on families' satisfaction with care is, however, an important area needing to be researched. The underlying premise here would be that families, through developing a continuous relationship with primary and associate nurses, would be supported more effectively. This, in turn, would benefit the patient and enhance the patient's recovery (Clark, 1987). "Philosophically, family members are an integral component of critical care nursing practice" (Tiltler, Cohen and Craft, 1991). However, to demonstrate differences in family satisfaction with care, tools need to be developed which are valid and reliable. Considerable work has already been undertaken during recent years on identifying the needs of families of critical care patients (see Chapter 10). It may be possible to build on or use these tools for the purpose of evaluating families' satisfaction with primary nursing.

In relation to the second hypothesis identified by Ersser and Tutton (1991), only one study in critical care addresses this issue. The research question asked was, "What effect does primary nursing as a method of organizing care in an intensive care unit have on nurse and patient outcomes?" (Manley, 1988a, 1989). This study used the Quality Patient Care Scale (Qualpacs) (Wandelt and Ager, 1974) to measure the quality of care received by patients in experimental and control groups. The study was very small, and although a statistically significant improvement was identified in the experimental group practising primary nursing compared with the control group practising total patient care, it is important to be critical of these results for the following reasons:

☐ The study involved nurses practising primary nursing for a very short period before evaluation of quality took place. Staff are unlikely to have come to terms with new roles in such a short time, and the 'Hawthorne effect' may easily have been responsible for the positive result.

☐ Qualpacs as a tool recommends that a small sample of patients be observed, in an ITU setting this only involved two patients at each observation period from a maximum of 4–5 in each group. If all the patients in the group were long-term (which in fact they were in the primary nursing group), then due to the short duration of the study it would be the quality of care delivered by two individual primary nurses and their associate nurses that was being evaluated rather than the quality resulting from practising primary nursing. This would mean, therefore, that the result was more likely to be influenced by the competency of a small number of primary nurses. Strong support is provided for this argument by research undertaken by Shukla (1981). Shukla raises the level of nurses' competencies in both experimental and control groups until they are the same before introducing primary nursing to the experimental group in a general setting. The quality of care resulting was attributed more to the increased competency than to the practice of primary nursing.

Thus the complexities involved in measuring quality demonstrates the need to have insight into the tools used and how they are used before accepting the results of any research using them. Establishing whether primary nursing actually does improve the quality of care in ITU therefore is a question that still requires answering.

Most studies evaluating primary nursing in the past have involved experimental designs (Manley, 1989). It could be argued that undertaking controlled experimental studies where primary nursing is introduced as an independent variable is inappropriate when considering the quality of care from the consumers's point of view. Alternative research strategies from the social sciences may be more appropriate as these approaches would focus on the 'meanings' and 'feelings' experienced by individual clients and their families. Concepts such as acceptability, access and appropriateness (Manley, 1992) may therefore be more appropriate to consider when measuring quality rather than using tools which measure it externally. After all, understanding the world through the client's eyes' is the basis of the interaction school of thought in nursing

(Meleis, 1985), and this is reflected by interaction-based nursing models and the practice of primary nursing. Research methods too need to reflect underlying values held about nursing and be congruent with them.

Connolly and Gray (1991) considered nurses' perceptions in a small study designed to evaluate primary nursing on two 2 pilot beds of a 5–6 bedded ITU. Staff involved in the pilot ($n = 11$) as well as those not involved but observers to it ($n = 15$) were asked for their perceptions of primary nursing as they experienced it. Aspects relating to quality were considered. Some of the key findings are outlined below:

☐ 91% of pilot nurses, 60% of non-pilot nurses considered the quality of care received by patients had improved as a result of practising primary nursing.

☐ Nobody felt that either communication or quality had deteriorated.

☐ 100% of the pilot nurses, 80% of the non-pilot nurses considered that communication between relatives and nurses within the primary nursing teams had improved compared with before primary nursing was practised.

☐ The predominant reasons given for improvements in quality of care were greater continuity of care, greater knowledge and awareness of patient's condition by nurses, and greater and more effective communication.

☐ 91% of pilot nurses, 47% of the non-pilot nurses felt the relationship between the primary nurse and their patient had improved. 33% considered that it was unchanged. The perception of improvement therefore appears to be mostly from within the nurse–patient relationship.

☐ 82% of pilot nurses, 60% of non-pilot nurses considered that nurses developed a deeper level of understanding of the patient when practising primary nursing.

☐ When asked if primary nursing could provide greater continuity of care to patients in ITU, 82% of pilot nurses definitely felt so, 18% possibly. From the non-pilot group, 60% of staff definitely felt it could, 33% yes probably, and 7% no.

☐ The most predominant advantage of primary nursing identified by both pilot and non-pilot group were improved relationships between nurses/patients/relatives, and between the health care team, colleagues, patients and relatives.

☐ The one major perceived disadvantage was seen to be increased stress levels with long-term patients.

Many of these findings are similar to, and reinforce those found in, studies involving other settings, specifically, improved knowledge of patients (MacGuire and Botting, 1990; Perele and Hentinen, 1989; Sellick *et al.*, 1983), and improved communication (MacGuire and Botting, 1990; Wilson and Dawson, 1989; Sellick *et al.*, 1983).

Nurses' job satisfaction: the research

A comprehensive review of the research in general settings concerning job satisfaction in relation to primary nursing up to the year 1988 is provided by Manley (1988, 1989). Manley's study (1988, 1989) is the first to consider aspects of job satisfaction in relation to primary nursing in critical care. The intention of the study was to establish if a difference in job satisfaction existed pre and post the implementation of primary nursing. However, the length of time between the pre- and post-data collection was far too short, therefore invalidating any difference that may have been observed. Although this methodological problem prevented a difference being demonstrated, some valuable data was collected from both control and experimental groups concerning the job satisfaction of ITU nurses within one large ITU. This data can be interpreted, however, from the perspective of the concepts fundamental to primary nursing.

From a sample of 38 ITU nurses who replied to a questionnaire about their job satisfaction prior to the study taking place, it became very clear what it was that nurses wanted to do more of:

☐ 34 desired increased skills and knowledge
☐ 34 wanted to see more of their work carried through
☐ 31 wanted clearer patient goals
☐ 30 wanted more challenge
☐ 29 wanted to use their initiative more

☐ 22 wanted more decision-making
☐ 19 wanted more responsibility.

Patient improvement was the one aspect unanimously considered to provide the greatest sense of achievement to ITU nurses. The following factors were aspects of the job that they liked least:

☐ hierarchy and petty rules
☐ staff shortages.

When considering these findings, each point is compatible with what primary nursing has to offer in terms of its central concepts and values. The literature supports these findings further; primary nursing was seen to provide greater job satisfaction because there were more opportunities for accountability and fulfilling higher level needs (Carlsen and Malley, 1981); and also more opportunities to accomplish something worthwhile, to participate in decision-making and to set one's own pace (Sellick *et al.*, 1983). Joiner *et al.* (1981) accounted for the higher job satisfaction in their study by stating that "primary nurse's role was more enriched and consistent with job design theory than other nursing modalities." In Britain, Reed's (1988) study also clearly demonstrates higher levels of job satisfaction within a primary nursing ward compared with a team nursing ward.

In Connolly and Gray's (1991) evaluation of a pilot study of primary nursing in ITU, nurses' perceptions about practising primary nursing were considered before and after the pilot. Prior to the pilot, 73% (*n* = 26) of staff were favourable to practising primary nursing, 15% didn't know, and 12% were not favourable. After a six month pilot study using two out of five ITU beds, staff were asked if they wanted an opportunity to give greater continuity of care to their patients: 96% of staff were favourable to the idea, and 4% did not know. This suggested quite a change of attitude, with all staff being even more positive as a result of experiencing the pilot. Additional findings in relation to job satisfaction were:

☐ 100% of the pilot nurses (*n* = 11) considered they experienced a great deal of job satisfaction. Of the non-pilot study nurses, 60% (*n* = 15) experienced a great deal of job satisfaction, 27% experienced a lot, and 6% non at all.

☐ 82% of pilot nurses compared with 13% of non-pilot nurses considered that there were frequent opportunities to give continuity of care to patients. 60% of non-pilot nurses felt there was an occasional opportunity.

Connolly and Gray's (1991) study therefore suggested that for nurses in their unit, primary nursing could provide greater job satisfaction, and this subsequently led the unit staff to implement primary nursing on the three remaining ITU beds. However, this was an evaluation rather than a controlled experimental study, so the results would have been influenced by the staff who volunteered to practise primary nursing in the pilot study. With a controlled experimental design staff would have been selected at random. Therefore, staff motivation in wanting to make primary nursing a success is likely to have been influential in Connolly and Gray's study.

In contrast, Pasternak's (1988a,b) study took place in an intensive and coronary care unit where primary nursing had been established for some time. The research question asked was, 'Is there a relationship between the effective execution of the primary care nursing process and the perceived feelings of isolation–depersonalization that critical care nurses may experience?' Following a descriptive study design, a relationship between the two concepts was demonstrated, but no reference is made to whether this relationship also exists with other methods of organizing care in critical care settings.

Another study in Britain undertaken in an acute setting where primary nursing had been established for a while is that by Bowman, Meddis and Thompson (1990a). The researchers considered nurses' independence and status in primary nursing compared with task-centred practice. Support for the following two hypotheses was demonstrated. Nurses working with primary nursing would (1) feel more independence, and (2) have a higher sense of status than their counterparts in the traditional task-centred environment. Questions relating to independence were concerned with the extent to which a nurse controlled his or her own work. Both groups were asked about the control exerted by clinical managers (sisters and charge nurse) and doctors. In the traditional group 60% (*n* = 20) felt that medical staff had authority over their actions, whereas only 10% ($n = 20$) agreed in the primary nursing group. With regard to status, nurses were asked about the importance of nursing as a health occupation: 55% of the primary nursing group and 35% of the traditional group felt that it was the most important. This study, therefore, by attributing higher status and greater independence to nurses using primary nursing raises again the issues mentioned in the introduction. These issues concern the future development of nursing and highlights how primary nursing itself is inextricably linked to the nature and future development of nursing itself.

RESEARCH QUESTIONS FOR THE FUTURE

There are many areas needing to be researched in relation to primary nursing practice, especially within critical care. This section will therefore identify some research questions that need to be answered; it is by no means comprehensive. Every question answered will lead to a multitude of others which need to be asked.

☐ What relationship exists between primary nursing and the model of nursing selected?

☐ Is primary nursing more cost-effective in critical care? To attempt to answer this question the outcomes of critical care need to be known and agreed. This leads us to another vitally important question:

☐ What indicators of outcome are there in critical care from both a multidisciplinary and nursing perspective?

☐ What impact does the organizational approach have on cross-infection and nosocomial infection rates in critical care?

☐ Do nurses experience greater stress when practising primary nursing in critical care?

☐ What type of stress do nurses experience when practising primary nursing?

☐ Does the degree of stress relate to personal competency and skills?

☐ How can nurses be best prepared for primary nursing?

☐ What educational preparation can be given to reduce any stress?

☐ What are the career outcomes of nurses who practice primary nursing in critical care?

☐ What are the outcomes for families as a result of primary nursing? (Leske, 1991).

☐ How does primary nursing influence the cohesiveness of the multidisciplinary team?

☐ What impact is there on ethical decision making in critical care?

☐ How does practising primary nursing influence the choice of areas research?

☐ How do nurses' coping mechanisms relate to the effectiveness of the nurse? (Pasternak, 1988).

☐ How does primary nursing influence long-term job satisfaction?

☐ How are other nurses used as resources to primary nursing? (O'Malley et al., 1991).

PRACTICAL NURSING IMPLICATIONS

The practical nursing implications will be considered from five perspectives:

☐ The attributes of primary nursing as an innovation in relation to the expected ease of implementation in critical care.

☐ Implications for the individual nurse practising primary nursing.

☐ Implications for each team of primary and associate nurses.

☐ Implications for clinical leaders/managers.

☐ Implications for educators who provide services to clinical practitioners.

The attributes of primary nursing as an innovation

In the United Kingdom, few areas of critical care are practising primary nursing and so consideration of the implications of implementing are briefly considered. The implementation of any innovation can greatly influence its ultimate success. The English National Board (ENB, 1987) suggest a framework for managing change which identifies five broad areas for consideration:

- [ ] the innovation itself
- [ ] the environment for change
- [ ] the users of the change
- [ ] the change agent(s)
- [ ] the change strategies.

These five areas are necessary to consider for planned change prior to introducing any innovation. Planned change is discussed in a range of good texts (Lancaster and Lancaster, 1982; Wright, 1989), and is not unique to the implementation of primary nursing. For this reason only the first area in the ENB framework will be considered; that is, the analysis of the innovation itself. Through analysing primary nursing as an innovation, the ease with which it is likely to be implemented can, to a certain extent, be anticipated, as can prospective areas of difficulty.

Rogers and Shoemaker (1971) consider there to be seven attributes which seem to correlate with successful implementation of any innovation. These are outlined in Table 3.4.

These attributes will now be considered in relation to primary nursing.

Relative advantage The perceived advantages of primary nursing over other approaches to organizing care may be identified from the claims made about it. Such advantages may include for the patient most importantly, better quality of care and better continuity of care; for the staff, greater job satisfaction, which may also provide the organization with positive benefits such as improved staff retention rates and turnover. Subsequently through this mechanism combined with increased quality, more cost effective care can result. In Britain there is some support for this from the Audit Commission's report *The Virtue of Patients* (1992). When focusing on the relative advantages, it is important to also consider possible disadvantages. With an innovation such as primary nursing it may be the disadvantages perceived by staff that inhibit consideration of the advantages. Many of the perceived

Table 3.4. Seven attributes of an innovation to consider before its implementation (Rogers and Shoemaker, 1971).

Relative advantage, this relates to the perceived advantage of the innovation over current practices. One overriding advantage can often provide a sufficient case in its own right.

Compatibility, this relates to whether the proposed change is compatible with the existing values and beliefs held. Changes which are minor and compatible to existing values and beliefs are often easier to implement and are more likely to be successful.

Communicability, this relates to both the ease with which the change can be understood as well as how well the change is communicated.

Simplicity, this relates to how simple the innovation is as a concept and how simple it is to use.

Trialability, relates to whether the innovation lends itself to piloting on either a small or large scale.

Observability, this refers to how noticeable the change may be to observers and participants.

Relevance, this leads one to ask is the change actually relevant?

disadvantages surround misconceptions such as expecting primary nurses to be 'on-call'. Genuine concerns frequently aired include, for example, concern about the long-term care of patients, or the possibility of personality conflict between the patient and nurse, or between primary and associate nurses. These concerns need to be acknowledged and discussed if staff are to openly and seriously consider the advantages of primary nursing and make informed decisions about implementing it. Decisions inevitably will depend on primary nursing's compatibility with the philosophy of the critical care unit, the next factor.

Compatibility For a decision to be made about whether primary nursing is compatible, two areas need to be addressed, the values and beliefs underpinning primary nursing, and the values and beliefs held by the nursing team about the nature of nursing in critical care.

One method used by a team of intensive care nurses together with physiotherapists and the unit's technician to establish common values and beliefs held, combined two processes, a value clarification exercise and the nominal group technique (Warfield and Manley, 1990). The value clarification exercise used centred on the following aspects (Manley, 1992):

☐ the purpose of the service;
☐ the four concepts identified and accepted as central to nursing's domain and included within all nursing models (Fawcett, 1984):
  —The nature of nursing
  —The nature of the individual person
  —The nature of health
  —The nature of the environment of care/society;
☐ how individuals learn as the area was a learning environment for post-registration students, also personal learning and development of staff was highly valued;
☐ the attributes of a good team; nursing and multi-disciplinary.

The value clarification exercise used is outlined in Table 3.5.

The nominal group technique is a technique which allows everyone's values to be collected and built up over time, as it is rarely possible for all staff to meet at once in critical care areas. The value clarification exercise is therefore undertaken in small groups until everyone has participated. All values and beliefs stated are then carried through to the final statement. The total approach used is further outlined by Warfield and Manley (1990) and Manley (1992). The statement of values and beliefs which resulted from this exercise is illustrated in Table 3.6.

Communicability   This relates to both the ease with which the change can be understood, as well as how well the change is communicated. Therefore, how primary nursing is introduced and whether staff are exposed to speakers who are enthusiastic and experienced in the subject will be influential in staff's decisions about implementing it.

Simplicity   This relates to how simple the innovation is as a concept and how simple it is to use. The idea is simple, but the practical implications are complex and therefore require time, also careful and sensitive planning. Staff need to feel they have

Table 3.5. The value clarification exercise used by Warfield and Manley (1990) as the basis of writing a philosophy in an intensive therapy unit (ITU).

I believe the purpose of ITU is . . .

I believe my purpose in ITU is . . .

I believe critically ill patients need . . .

If I was a patient in ITU I would like . . .

I believe families/relatives/significant others of ITU patients value . . .

I believe I can help an ITU patient . . .

As a member of the ITU team I feel valued when . . .

I believe the ITU environment for staff should be . . .

I believe the ITU environment for patients should be . . .

I believe individuals learn best when . . .

What beliefs do you hold about the nurse–patient relationship?

What do you value most highly as an ITU member?

What do you believe makes a good team?

Other values and beliefs I consider important are . . .

time to come to terms with the issues and that they are not going to feel rushed into trying it before they are ready.

Trialability   The smallest pilot possible in ITU where staff–patient ratios are 1:1 is to staff one bed with nurses who will provide care to the patients admitted to it using primary nursing. By identifying maybe six volunteer staff who reflect the skill mix of the whole unit team, a small scale pilot of primary nursing can be undertaken. The off-duty for the staff of this single bed would need to be completed independently. Where staff–patient ratios are higher, (e.g. in the coronary care unit), then the pilot area may need to be slightly larger (e.g. two beds) to make the off-duty easier to manage. In the author's experience, this approach has been very successful because the pilot is well contained, progress can proceed at a rate that the unit staff are comfortable with, and a great deal can be learnt from the first pilot team to assist later teams. The implementation of primary nursing

Table 3.6. Current philosophy (1992) Chelsea and Westminster Hospital Intensive Care Unit/Nursing Development Unit (NDU), London.

We believe our patients to be unique individuals with unique identities and needs, physical, psychological and spiritual. We believe that these needs would be met by nursing care that is individualised and caters for the whole person. This belief also encompasses the family, friends and significant others, held in esteem by the patient.

We aim to assist our patients towards recovery and independence or when this is not possible, to ease their pain and prepare them for peaceful and dignified death. We feel it is important to share the sorrow and pain of a patients death and to help ease others grief.

We believe that the rights of our patients are unassailable. That our care must not be judgemental, based on sound ethical and moral principles. We recognise that the severity of illness experienced by our patients may render them incapable of participating in the decision-making processes which affect their care, and that we, as direct care givers, must serve as our patient's advocate in consultation with family members, acting always in the patient's best interests.

We consider that it is of paramount importance that the patient and his/her family or loved ones, should be kept informed of any changes in his/her condition and care. We feel it is vital to foster good relationships from the outset, facilitated by discussion in an atmosphere of respect, trust and honesty, mindful however, of the patients right to privacy and confidentiality and that the family should be encouraged to participate in the patients care as far as they feel able to.

We believe that the caring environment we provide for our patients should be reflected in our attitudes towards each other and that each member of the team should be valued and nurtured. We also believe that our nursing team is a vital and dynamic force, working for the benefit of our patients and their loved ones. We feel that we are in a privileged position of trust and that this privilege should be repaid by the provision of the highest standards of care, delivered by questioning and motivated staff, who participate in the programme of education within the Unit and accept responsibility for their own development with support and encouragement from senior nursing staff.

from one pilot bed to all 5/6 beds within the Chelsea and Westminster Intensive Care Unit has occurred over a time period of 15 months, and followed the schedule outlined in Table 3.7. This schedule is retrospective, and describes the landmarks achieved as it was important to allow staff to feel that they could progress at a rate at which they were comfortable. The only stage that was predecided in advance was the first evaluation of experiences at one month into the pilot. The educational input necessary for staff to discuss and make an informed decision about whether they wanted to try primary nursing took place over several months preceeding the actual implementation period.

Kaplow, Ackerman and Outlaw (1989) describe their experiences of piloting primary nursing in their ITU where 12 hour shifts was the normal pattern of working. A trial was completed of co-primary nursing with one chronic patient who had "had an oesophago-gastrectomy and was ventilator-dependent." Four co-primary nurses were assigned to this patient for a month, suggesting that it was more team than primary nursing that was being practised. The four nurses had voiced concern about being allocated to this patient, but had pursued an aggressive plan of care, which was adhered to closely and which according to the writers benefited the patient. The trial was then expanded to two patients at the end of the first month.

Observability   This refers to how observable the change may be to observers and participants. What difference does it make? Connolly and Gray's (1991) findings outlined more comprehensively in the research section suggest that staff involved in the pilot as well as those those not directly involved did notice a big difference.

Relevance   Is the change actually relevant? In relation to this point if the claims held about primary nursing and some of the conclusions drawn from research are correct then the relevance to critical care is two-fold. Job satisfaction could be improved therefore increasing the likelihood that staff will be retained as a resource. Secondly, the quality of care, the effectiveness of care and therefore the cost-effectiveness of care may be improved. Both are extremely relevant concerns in today's health care culture (Manley, 1992).

Table 3.7. A retrospective implementation schedule within the Chelsea and Westminster ITU from pilot to full implementation. This followed a period of education and discussion.

Month	Important Landmarks
1	Volunteers identified for first primary nursing team. Team members selected from volunteers to ensure that skill mix was representative of units normal skill mix
	Ground rules discussed and established within team
	Communication channels established within team and with remaining unit staff
	Ground rules discussed and agreed with remaining unit staff
2	First pilot primary nursing team of six staff introduced
	Off-duty organized independently for primary nursing team
	Informal evaluation to take place after one month
3	Staff of first primary nursing team felt that the one month time period was insufficient and wanted to continue for a longer period of time
	Staff felt that team nursing, not primary nursing, was being practised as there was no designated primary nurse within the team for each patient. Team members decided to designate a primary nurse for each patient thereafter
4	Second team of volunteers formed to cover a second pilot bed, following similar preparation as the first team, but also benefiting from the experiences of the first team
5	Formal evaluation study undertaken by Connolly and Gray (1991)
6	Third team of volunteers commenced and underwent the same preparation as identified for the first and second teams
7–15	Three teams continue practising primary nursing, remainder of staff care for remaining patients using total patient care
16	Remaining staff allocated to the two final primary nursing teams

The implications for individual nurses practising primary nursing

Many of the implications and issues involved in practising primary nursing in critical care have been suggested in earlier sections. This section will hopefully provide greater depth and highlight the implications further. Seven issues have been identified by Peerbacus and Watson (1991) for the individual nurse practising primary nursing in an ITU setting. These are expanded in Table 3.8.

Table 3.8. Issues for individual nurse when practising primary nursing in ITU (Peerbacus and Watson, 1991).

Accountability   Nurses initially found accountability for nursing care of patient an added stress, until they became more confident about their own abilities.

Care planning   Care planning documentation did not lend itself so well to the primary nurse's long-term planning as it did to short term planning. This resulted in both the model of care and the documentation of care being reviewed.

Stress and burnout   The potential for this was overcome by encouraging team members to talk about their fears and anxieties and to share responsibilities with team members rather than taking on too much of the workload themselves.

Opting out   It was difficult at times for individual nurses to realize the need to 'opt out' in order for them to have a break from nursing the same patient indefinitely. Also, some nurses expressed the fear that they may be 'losing out' on a variety of experience by looking after one patient all the time (especially if the patient was long term!).

Relationships   To start with, there is/was a tendency to become overprotective of one's own patient. This was overcome by learning to 'share' patients with other nurses and the members of the multi-disciplinary team.

Handling constructive criticism   Constructive criticism was used positively to improve the teams function and standards of care.

Role   Changes in role occurred, staff needed to be supported in this, and provided with opportunities of discussing their experiences.

Clark (1987) acknowledges that if nurses are to maintain the type of relationships that patients view as healing, then nurses must learn how to cope effectively with the stresses that are part of the environment in which they work. Certainly, working as a primary or associate nurse in any setting will involve participating intensely as partners in relationships with patients and families. Learning to cope positively with such relationships will enable both the nurses and the patient to grow from such experiences. This therefore involves individual nurses taking considerable risk in exposing not only deficits in knowledge and skills, but also exposing personal values and beliefs, personal coping mechanisms and sharing personal limitations and strengths. However, these expectations would be the same for all nurses operating within an interaction view of nursing. Meleis (1985) aptly characterizes the interaction school of thought in nursing as an interpersonal process between a person needing help and a person capable of giving help. Nursing considered from this perspective involves forming relationships and the patient's perception is important. Primary nursing relates to this school of thought, and so the implications that Meleis identifies for nurses operating within this approach are therefore equally relevant to practising primary nursing. For nurses to give help they need to:

☐ clarify their own values and become self-reflecting;
☐ use self therapeutically;
☐ be involved in care.

The greatest implication for individuals, therefore, is the development of personal knowledge, that is, knowledge of self (self-awareness).

To nurse patients from an interactive perspective, then, means that nurses would be using the following approaches (Meleis, 1985):

☐ Caring, assisting, helping to find meaning, teaching, counselling, guiding, giving care, gathering information, setting mutual goals.
☐ Deliberate actions not automatic; this needs systematic knowledge to achieve.
☐ Nurturing human potential.
☐ Sensing and perceiving.

☐ Helping to establish meaning.
☐ Validating.

To be able to use such approaches, primary and associate nurses therefore require the appropriate skills and knowledge and feel confident with them. Additionally, they will need to be well supported not just during the period of their initial development, but also in an ongoing way, as such skills can never be perfected. Perfection can only be strived for as one understands the self more. Only through working with the personal self can the professional self develop (Barber, 1991). Two methods may be particularly useful to consider:

☐ Reflective practice.
☐ Peer review.

Both methods can enhance the other; for example, reflection on practice can be undertaken within a peer group using personal journals. Case presentations within primary nursing can also be used to reflect more formally on interventions and goals of practice.

Part of knowing oneself involves recognizing one's limitations. This, in turn, relates to being assertive enough to state when one's personal resources are approaching these limitations; for example, when caring for a patient who is particularly draining over a long period of time. Such issues concerned with 'opting out' of care will need to be thoroughly discussed prior to practising primary nursing. Contingencies will need to be prepared and thought through. One approach which helps nurses in this decision is providing the opportunity of declining to take a primary nursing patient at the beginning of the shift. The role of both the primary nursing team and unit team is to respect peoples' judgement, and to encourage individuals to be honest and open in their judgements. These values can be incorporated within the ground rules of each primary nursing team. In reality, the gesture of support and just knowing that nurses can 'opt out' should they wish contributes to the creation of a caring environment for staff. In practice, the opportunity of 'opting out' of a patient's care is rarely taken advantage of.

The roles of each practitioner need to be explicit, and within the Chelsea and Westminster ITU, role

Table 3.9. The Primary Nurse Role in Chelsea and Westminster Intensive Care Unit (Pritchard and Warner, 1991).

Any member of the primary nursing team may act as primary nurse for a specific patient if they feel confident to carry out this role.

The aims of this role are for the nurse to develop awareness of accountability, responsibility and legal and ethical issues related to patient care. The role will also help the nurse to develop management skills of leadership, decision-making and assessing and planning of long and short term goals related to patient care.

By nature of this role, the primary nurse will also be introduced to the concept of an autonomous practitioner.

The nurse should first consider their availability. If they are about to commence leave, take nights off etc, it may not be appropriate for them to become the primary nurse.

If appropriate the primary nurse should carry out a pre-admission visit and check that a comprehensive assessment is complete and that any pre-operative education is completed.

The primary nurse should complete an initial ITU care plan with clear identification of patients long and short term problems and the required nursing actions to meet these. This should be reviewed or re-written by them when they are on duty, throughout the patients stay. The careplan should be updated and reviewed in the meantime by associate nurses from the team if this is necessary. The primary nurse should make research based decisions over issues such as which dressing to use, etc.

The primary nurse assumes overall responsibility for the patients stay, and is therefore responsible for ensuring that all documentation is complete, that relatives receive adequate support and information and that effective communication is maintained within the team and between other parties, i.e. medical staff, physiotherapists, ward staff, etc. They should also ensure that effective follow-up is maintained, i.e. that the person is visited post-discharge from the unit or that the families are communicated with in the event of death.

Every opportunity should be taken for group discussion over issues and decisions that are to be made, and the team should aim to use external sources of knowledge. If appropriate, the primary nurse should aim to present a summary of the patients stay and management in ITU.

descriptions which have been agreed by all staff, have been particularly useful in helping staff come to terms with role expectations. The role of the primary nurse is outlined in Table 3.9, the associate nurse in Table 3.10, and the primary nursing team co-ordinator in Table 3.11.

In relation to the primary nurse's responsibility for care planning and nursing diagnosis, Kaplow, Ackerman and Outlaw (1989), following the introduction of co-primary nursing, found the need to instigate intermittent nurse care-planning sessions at the patient's bedside. This increased personal assistance to individual nurses who needed to develop their care-planning skills, and also introduced the concept of nursing diagnosis. Patient case conferences were encouraged, particularly where

Table 3.10. The Associate Nurse Role in Chelsea and Westminster Intensive Care Unit (Pritchard and Warner, 1991).

If not acting as the primary nurse, the remaining team members will become associate nurses.

The aims of this role are to develop effective teamwork skills, to develop communication and decision-making skills, and those required to assess, plan, implement and evaluate care in the intensive care setting.

The associate nurse is responsible and accountable for his/her actions and for the care delivered.

He/she should familiarize his/herself with the initial nursing assessment and with the relevant events on the patient's communication sheet. The nurse should assess the patient at the commencement of each shift, and review the care-plan, to ensure that, a) problems and needs are still appropriate to the patient's condition, and that, b) planned care is appropriate to the problem/need identified.

All members of the team are responsible for ensuring effective communication and for having an input into patients care as questioning and innovative practitioners.

The associate nurse should be aware of his/her own boundaries and limitations of practice/knowledge and skills, and be able to seek advice from others when necessary.

Any issues that require team discussion or joint decision-making should be identified by the primary nurse.

Table 3.11. The Role of the Primary Nursing Team Coordinator, Chelsea and Westminster Intensive Care Unit (Pritchard and Warner, 1991).

Each primary nursing team requires an overall coordinator. The purpose of the coordinator is to lead the teams development.

What follows is a brief description of the coordinator's role:

1. Handling recruitment/orientation of staff to primary nursing teams.
2. Facilitating individual performance review of team members.
3. Facilitating development of team members' personal/professional skills and career development (not necessarily to be kept within the team).
4. Coordinating team developments.
5. Fostering communication networks within/between teams (arranging inter/intra team meetings).
6. Evaluating the teams' effectiveness.
7. Facilitating support networks within the team.
8. Delegating areas of responsibility to team members.
9. Liasing with other team coordinators regarding the monthly open days.
10. Facilitating the organization of patient case studies.

the patient had uncommon conditions and/or treatment. Even though Kaplow, Ackerman and Outlaw (1989) had practised co-primary nursing for two years, they still found the need to make long-term provision for assisting primary nurses in:

☐ continuing nursing care-plan workshops;
☐ scheduling the off-duty;
☐ continuing support groups on day shift and initiate another on nights;
☐ providing patient care conferences more consistently.

The team coordinator may, in addition, be a primary or associate nurse. The skills necessary as a coordinator are those required by managers at any level, and involve team building, the introduction of change, and monitoring the team's function as identified in the role description. Opportunities for developing these skills are provided, therefore, at a micro level, and this results in the building of confidence before proceeding to the macro level. It

also has the advantage of providing immediate role modelling to other members of the team. Responsibility of recruitment and interviewing staff to each team when a vacancy results enables the team leader to develop skills in this area with support from senior nursing staff if requested. Personal development and the practice of individual performance review is also devolved to each primary nursing team leader.

The implications for each team of primary and associate nurses

Primary nurses therefore have the support of five other nurses who act as associate nurses to them. Each nurse will have an opportunity to act as a primary nurse at some time. This means that no one nurse carries the responsibility of being a primary nurse all the time. Each team of six nurses develop their own cohesive group and provide considerable support to each other. Each team develop their own unique characteristics and interests, each may try out different practices and may want to use a different model of nursing, for example. Each nurse therefore has the opportunity of being a primary and associate nurse at different times. This means they have the experience of both directing care and implementing someone else's prescription of care. This provides opportunities for both the giving and receiving of feedback which is independent of status. The associate nurse role may therefore be fulfilled for some patients by the team coordinator or the clinical nurse specialist.

For each primary nursing team to develop cohesiveness requires every member's participation in team building, in contributing to the ground rules, and putting them into practice. Communication links need to be excellent because it would be rare for team members to work the same shift. By the very nature of this, each team will look to other teams for mutual support, as it is members of other teams that work the same shift. This in turn contributes to the total cohesion of the unit team as a whole.

The implications for clinical leaders/managers

Communication between each primary nursing team therefore becomes a priority for unit managers in trying to maintain a cohesive unit team, as well as providing a supportive and encouraging environment for each primary nursing team to develop its individuality, be creative and innovative. Kaplow, Ackerman and Outlaw (1989) emphasized the importance of open communication with all members of unit staff. They publicized all minutes so that all staff knew what was going on. Additionally, monthly staff meetings were used as a forum for issues related to perceptions of primary nursing. These monthly meetings became formalized as an ITU Primary Nursing Committee, which continued monthly for seven months before being reduced to 3–4 monthly for the subsequent two years. This implies that in the early stages of practising primary nursing a large investiture in staff meetings and dealing with issues is required, particularly during the first eight months; thereafter, not so many problems and issues arise and so the frequency of meetings can be reduced. This pattern of events has also been found in the author's experience.

Other issues for managers when primary nursing is practised in ITU are highlighted in Table 3.12.

Organization of the off-duty is probably one of the biggest challenges and would be dependent in a general ITU setting upon having an establishment of at least six nurses per bed where the mean patient dependency per month is one nurse per patient. The skill mix of the unit will need to be evenly distributed within each of the teams. An example of the team skill mix within each team at Chelsea and Westminster is as follows:

1 G grade
1 F grade
2 D grades
2 E grades

The implications for educators

The provision of education is an ongoing need within any unit practising primary nursing. It is the author's experience that through practising primary nursing staff become acutely aware of their educational needs and tend to pursue these avidly, continued development becomes a way of life. This view is further supported by the Audit Commission's report (1991), *The Virtue of Patients*, which

Table 3.12. Issues for management when practising primary nursing in ITU (Peerbacus and Watson, 1991).

GROUP DYNAMICS   Each primary nursing team needed time to form and develop as a cohesive group. Members did not initially see themselves as part of a group, they could only see their own personal objectives and were unsure of their role. It was necessary to develop a specific role description.

OFF DUTY   Each primary nursing team needed to ensure 24-hour coverage, so that either the primary nurse or associate nurse were on duty. This required changes in personal off-duty to be made to facilitate this cover.

ISOLATION & COHESION   On occasions team members looking after long-term patients felt they were missing out on other experiences within the unit. Also, by only looking after one patient it was easy to lose touch with what was happening with other patients within the unit. As the team developed, team members learnt to inter-relate and communicate more effectively within the team.

STAFF AWARENESS   There was a need for sensitivity and awareness towards members of staff outside each primary nursing team as each team did not want to be perceived as elite. It was still part of the larger staff group of the ITU. There was also a need to develop each group member's awareness so that individual strengths and weaknesses could be further developed, permitting the realization of aims and objectives.

SENIOR MANAGEMENT SUPPORT   The support and encouragement provided by senior clinical management was considered as invaluable to the developments occurring in each team.

CROSS INFECTION   Due to the limited number of staff caring for one patient, it was felt that there was a reduced risk of cross-infection for patients and also it was easier to account for staff if they themselves needed treatment.

identifies that those areas practising primary nursing have a higher ratio of study days per member of nursing staff than those areas that did not practice primary nursing. Further issues for education are outlined in Table 3.13.

Intensive care course nurses are provided with the opportunity of working either with one team during their time on the ITU, or working with a range of teams. Working within one team provides

Table 3.13. Issues for education when practising primary nursing in ITU (Peerbacus and Watson, 1991).

PREPARATION OF STAFF   Learning about primary nursing in theory is one thing, but in practice it is something that everyone was experiencing for the first time. An information pack was therefore needed to help in the orientation of new staff so that they could learn from each group's earliest experiences.

LEARNING NEEDS OF COURSE NURSES   In the early stages when only three of the six ITU beds were using ENB primary nursing, the ENB course nurses felt they would like to be involved during their allocation to the unit. This choice was left open to the individual course members who could join a primary nurse team for the duration of their allocation or for just a few weeks.

---

a great depth of experience which often also provides breadth of experience over a period of time. Another advantage is that a rich and unique type of support can be provided to individual course nurses when practising within one team. However, course nurses who choose to sample a range of different teams may benefit from experiencing different primary nursing approaches, as well as a breadth of experience; however, this is at the loss of depth obtained from working in the one team. Primary nursing has a great deal to offer to ITU course nurses, and in reality the exact experience is negotiated according to an individual course nurse's identified need and personal choice.

CONCLUSION

In this last major section some of the implications of practising primary nursing have been addressed, many others are found highlighted in the literature and research sections. Therefore, to obtain a comprehensive overview of all the implications, each of the sections need to be read.

This chapter has hopefully addressed all the issues that it sets out to cover. The reader should now be in a position to judge the commitment necessary to practise primary nursing, and the implications for individual nurses, managers and educators if it is practised. It is the author's opinion that to practise primary nursing is to practise the art and science of nursing in it's fullest sense; this is a privilege, and one that places critical care nursing firmly in the nursing camp. Through practising primary nursing the contribution that critical care nurses can offer to the development of nursing generally will become clearly evident. This great richness and potential for the development of nursing within critical care almost seems dormant or unacknowledged until primary nursing is practised. Once unleashed the opportunities of developing nursing become evident, and the benefits that critical care nurses can offer to, and share with colleagues in other nursing settings comes very noticeably to the fore.

CASE STUDIES

Changing to primary nursing

As a senior staff nurse on the 10 bedded surgical intensive care unit for the past two years you are known to be a gregarious and well liked individual. During coffee break one morning you mention in conversation an interest in Primary Nursing. Almost immediately the coffee room is buzzing with excited and enthusiastic support. One staff nurse feels that it could be a good idea but asks, "How would we go about it?"

Take a few minutes and note some of your ideas.

Implications of primary nursing

Karen, a 22 year old serious road traffic accident victim, has been in a coma since admission to your unit three days ago. Her mother and father have maintained a 24 hour bedside vigil. You are assigned to be her primary nurse (before moving on to read the next section): what are the implications for you, Karen and her parents?

STUDENT LEARNING QUESTIONS

1. Identify the implications of practising primary nursing for off-duty rostering in critical care, and further explain why it is beneficial to divide staff into independent teams.

2. Explain the impact on traditional staff roles of practising primary nursing in critical care.

3. Identify the seven attributes of an innovation useful to consider before its implementation and apply these to the innovation of primary nursing.

4. Consider the implications for individual primary nurses and clinical leaders of practising primary nursing in critical care.

5. One of the purposes of primary nursing is the provision of continuity of care. Suggest various ways by which you could evaluate whether continuity of care was being achieved.

KEY TERMS

Autonomy

Independence of action, freedom to act.

Confirming interactions

Interactions where the caregiver is perceived by the client as caring about what happens.

Exclusionary interactions

Interactions where the caregiver is perceived by the client as having a negative attitude towards them.

Grand theory

Theories that define broadly and abstractly nursing from a global and philosophical perspective.

Interaction School of Thought

A school of thought identified by Meleis (1985) which includes those nursing theorists whose models or theories emphasize nursing as an interaction process and the nurse–patient relationship as therapeutic.

Operationalization/Operational definition

A definition in which the attributes of a concept, for example, primary nursing, are sufficiently identified to enable an observer to identify the presence of the concept.

Personal knowledge

Knowledge of self, personal awareness.

Six Category Intervention Analysis

Six different types of interventions identified by Heron (1975) namely, prescriptive, informative, confronting – the authoritative interventions; carthartic, catalytic, and supportive – the facilitative interventions.

Therapeutic relationship

A purposeful, supportive and healing association between two persons that is interactive and holistic (Muetzel, 1988).

FURTHER READING

Barber, P. Caring: the nature of a therapeutic relationship. In Eds. A. Perry, M. Jolley. *Nursing: A knowledge base for practice*. London: Edward Arnold, 1991.

Barber, P. *Who Cares for the Carers?* Distance Learning Centre, South Bank Polytechnic, 1991.

Heron, J. *Six Category Intervention Analysis*. Human Potential Research Project, Centre for Adult Education, University of Surrey, Guildford, 1975.

Manley, K. *Primary Nursing in Intensive Care*. Harrow: Scutari, 1989.

REFERENCES

Anderson, M., Choi, T. Primary nursing in an organisational context. *Journal of Nursing Administration*. 1980; 10: 26–31.

Atkinson, C. Primary team nursing: A new ITU method. *Nursing Standard*. 1991; 6(3): 25–28.

Bailey, K., Gilbert, G., Weber, M., Namur, N., Olson, C. A tool for implementing primary nursing: a colour coded bulletin board. *Supervisor Nurse*. 1981; 12(8): 56–58.

Barber, P. Learning to grow: the necessity for educational processing in therapeutic community practice. *International Journal of Therapeutic Communities*. 1988; 9(2): 101–108.

Barber, P. Caring: the nature of a therapeutic relationship. In Eds. A. Perry, M. Jolley, *Nursing: A knowledge base for practice*. London: Edward Arnold, 1991.

Benner, P. *From Novice to Expert: Excellence and Power in Clinical Nursing Practice*. Menlo Park, CA: Addison-Wesley, 1984.

Bergman, R. Accountability, definitions, dimensions. *International Nursing Review*. 1981; 28(2): 53–59.

Bethea, S. Primary Nursing in the Infant Special Care Unit. *Journal of Obstetrics, Gynaecologic and Neonatal Nursing*. 1985; 14(3): 202–208.

Binnie, A. Primary Nursing – Structural changes. *Nursing Times*. 1987; 83(39): 36–37.

Bowman, G., Meddis, R., Thompson, D. Independence and Status – two different work methods. *Nursing Practice*. 1990a; 3(2): 18–20.

Bowman, G. Developing staff for primary style nursing. *Nursing Practice*. 1990b; 3(4): 17–19.

Bowman, G. Learning From Experience. *Nursing Times*. 1990c; 86 (7): 30–32.

Breu, C., Dracup, K. Survey of critical care nursing practice. Part III. Responsibilities of intensive care unit staff. *Heart and Lung*. 1982; 11(2): 157–161.

Carlsen, R., Malley, J. Job satisfaction of staff registered nurses in primary and team nursing delivery systems. *Research in Nursing and Health*. 1981; 4(2): 251–260.

Ciske, K. Accountability, the essence of primary nursing. *American Journal of Nursing*. 1979; 79(5): 891–894.

Chavigny, K., Lewis, A. Team or primary nursing care? *Nursing Outlook*. 1984; 32(6): 322–327.

Clark, S. Nursing diagnosis: Ineffective coping. II: Planning care. *Heart and Lung*. 1987; 16(6), pt.1: 677–683.

Clayton, J., McCabe, S. Continuing education in an NDU. *Nursing Standard*. 1991; 6(9): 28–31.

Connally, S., Gray, L. Perceptions of Nursing Staff: An Evaluative Study of the Practise of Primary Nursing in Intensive Care. *Westminster Hospital Intensive Care Unit/Nursing Development Unit's first National Study Day*. London, 1991.

Constable, B. Intensive Disagreement. *Nursing Times*. 1991; 87(4): 66–67.

Deiman, P., Noble, E., Russell, M. Achieving a professional practice model. How primary nursing can help. *Journal of Nursing Administration*. 1984; 14(7/8): 16–22.

Dracup, K. Critical Care Nursing. In Eds. J. Fitzpatrick, R. Taunton. *Annual Review of Nursing Research, Volume 5*. New York: Springer, pp. 107–133.

Drew, N. Exclusion and confirmation: a phenomenology of patient's experience with caregivers. *Image*. 1986; 18: 39–43.

Elpern, E. Structural and organisational supports for primary nursing. *Clinics of North America*. 1977; 12(2): 205–219.

English National Board. *Managing Change in Nursing Education*. Section 3. London: ENB, 1987.

Ersser, S., Tutton, E. (Eds) *Primary Nursing in Perspective*. Harrow: Scutari Press, 1991.

Fairbanks, J. Primary nursing. What's so exciting about it? *Nursing*. 1980; 10(11): 55–57.

Fawcett, J. *Analysis and Evaluation of Conceptual Models of Nursing*. Philadelphia: Davis, 1984.

Ferrin, T. One hospital's successful implementation of primary nursing. *Nursing Administration Quarterly*, part II. 1981; 5(3): 44–53.

Fitzpatrick, J.J. The empirical approach to the development of nursing science. In Eds. J. J. Fitzpatrick, A. L. Whall. *Conceptual Models of Nursing (2nd ed.)*. Norwalk: Appleton and Lange, 1989, pp. 427–437.

Giovannetti, P. Evaluation of primary nursing. *Annual Review of Nursing Research*. 1986; 4: 127–151.

Goulding, J., Hunt, J. Accountability and Legal Issues in

Primary Nursing. In Eds. S. Ersser, E. Tutton. *Primary Nursing in Perspective*. Harrow: Scutari Press, 1991.

Hegyvary, S. *The Change to Primary Nursing*. St. Louis: Mosby, 1982.

Hickey, M., Lewandowski, L. Critical Care nurses' role with families: A descriptive study. *Heart and Lung*. 1988; 17(6) pt. 1: 670–676.

Hockey, E. Foreword. In Eds. R. McMahon, R. Pearson. *Nursing as Therapy*. London: Chapman & Hall, 1991.

Jenkins, D. Developing an NDU: The Manager's Role. *Nursing Standard*. 1991; 6(8): 36–39.

Johns, C. Ownership and the harmonious team: barriers to developing the therapeutic nursing team in primary nursing. *Journal of Clinical Nursing*. 1992a; 1: 89–94.

Johns, C. Interacting With Care. *Nursing Times*. 1992b; 88(16): 75–77.

Joiner, C., Johnson, V., Corkrean, M. Is primary nursing the answer? *Nursing Administration Quarterly Part I*, 1981; 5(3): 69–76.

Kaplow, R., Ackerman, N., Outlaw, E. Co-Primary nursing in the intensive care unit. *Nursing Management*. 1989; 20(12): 41–46.

Lancaster, J., Lancaster, W. (Eds) *The Nurse as a Change Agent*. St. Louis: Mosby. 1982.

Leddy, S., Pepper, J. *Conceptual Bases of Professional Nursing (2nd ed.)*. New York: Lippincott.

Leske, J. Family member interventions: Research Challenges. *Heart and Lung*. 1991; 20(4): 391–393.

MacGuire, G. An approach to evaluating the introduction of primary nursing in an acute medical unit for the elderly – I. Principles and practice. *Int. J. Nurs. Stud.* 1989a; 26(3): 253–260.

MacGuire, G. An approach to evaluating the introduction of primary nursing in an acute medical unit for the elderly – II. Operationalizing the principles. *Int. J. Nurs. Stud.* 1989b; 26(3): 243–251.

MacGuire, J., Botting, D. The use of the Ethnograph programme to identify the perceptions of nursing staff following the introduction of primary nursing in an acute medical ward for elderly people. *Journal of Advanced Nursing*. 1980; 15: 1120–1127.

Manley, K. *Evaluation of Primary Nursing in ICU*. Dissertation for Master of Nursing, University of Wales, 1988a.

Manley, K. Evaluation of Primary Nursing in the ICU: Short Report. *Nursing Times*. 1988b; 84(48): 57.

Manley, K. *Primary Nursing in Intensive Care*. Harrow: Scutari, 1989.

Manley, K. Primary Nursing: current research. Applications in ICU. *Nursing Times*. 1990a; 86(7): 32.

Manley, K. The Birth of a Nursing Development Unit. *Nursing Standard*. 1990b; 21(4): 36–38.

Manley, K. Intensive caring. *Nursing Times*. 1990c; 86(19): 67–69.

Manley, K. Intensive disagreement. *Nursing Times*. 1991a; 87(4): 66–67.

Manley, K. Knowledge for nursing practice. In Eds. A. Perry, M. Jolley. *Nursing: A knowledge base for practice*. London: Edward Arnold. 1991b.

Manley, K. Quality Assurance – the path to nursing excellence. In Eds. G. Brykczynska, M. Jolley. *Nursing Care: The challenge to change*. London: Edward Arnold, 1992.

Manthey, M. Primary nursing is alive and well in the hospital. *American Journal of Nursing*. 1973; 73(1): 83–87.

Manthey, M. A theoretical framework for primary nursing. *Journal of Nursing Administration*. 1980; 10(6): 11–15.

Manthey, M. Can primary nursing survive? *American Journal of Medicine*. 1988; 644–647.

Marram, G., Barnett, M., Bevis, E. *Primary Nursing: A Model for Individualised Care (2nd ed.)*. St. Louis: Mosby, 1979.

McCleod Clark, J., Hockey, L. *Research for nursing: A guide for the enquiring mind*. Edinburgh: Churchill Livingstone, 1979.

McMahon, R. Nursing as Therapy. *The Professional Nurse*. 1986; 1(10): 270–272.

McMahon, R. Power and collegial relations among nurses on wards adopting primary nursing and hierachical ward management structures. *Journal of Advanced Nursing*. 1990; 15: 232–239.

Mead, D. Research report: Collegial relationships among primary and associate nurses. *Nursing Times*. 1990; 86(42): 68.

Mead, D. An evaluation tool for primary nursing. *Nursing Standard*. 1991; 6(1): 37–39.

Mead, D., Adair, L. Implementing primary nursing: the essence and the trappings. *Nursing Times' 5th National Conference in Glasgow for Ward Sisters in Association with the King's Fund Primary Nursing Network*, 1990.

Medaglia, M. A coronary care unit implements primary nursing. *The Canadian Nurse*. 1978; 75(5): 32–34.

Meleis, A. *Theoretical Nursing: Development and progress*. Philadelphia: Lippincott, 1985.

Mirr, M. Factors affecting decisions made by family members of patients with severe head injury. *Heart and Lung*. 1991; 20(3): 228–235.

Muetzel, P. Therapeutic nursing. In Ed. A. Pearson. *Primary Nursing: Nursing in the Burford and Oxford Nursing Development Units*. London: Croom Helm, 1988.

Mutchner, L. How well are we practising primary nursing? *Journal of Nursing Administration*. 1986; 16(9): 8–13.

O'Malley, P. *et al.* Critical care nurse perceptions of family needs. *Heart and Lung*. 1991; 20(2): 189–201.

Orlando, I. *The Dynamic Nurse–Patient Relationship*. New York: Putman, 1961.

Pasternak, I. The Effects of Primary Care Nursing and Feelings of Isolation/Depersonalization of the Critical Care Nurse: Part I – Background to the Study. *Nursing Management*. 1988a; 19(3): 112I–112P.

Pasternak, I. The Effects of Primary Care Nursing and Feelings of Isolation/Depersonalization of the Critical Care Nurse: Part II – Results of a Descriptive-Correlational Study *Nursing Management*. 1988b; 19(4): 64Q–64X.

Pearson, A. (ed.) *Primary Nursing: Nursing in the Burford and Oxford Nursing Development Units*. London: Croom Helm, 1988.

Peerbacus, S., Watson, M. 'The implications of practising primary nursing'. *Westminster Hospital Intensive Care Unit/Nursing Development Unit's first National Study Day*. London, 1991.

Perele, M., Hentinen, M. Primary nursing: options of nursing staff before and during implementation. *International Journal of Nursing Studies*. 1989; 26(3): 231–242.

Peplau, H.E. *Interpersonal Relations in Nursing*. New York: Putman, 1952.

Pritchard, T., Warner, J. *Role descriptions for primary, associate nurses and team co-ordinators developed for the Intensive Care Unit*. Westminster Hospital, London, 1991.

Reed, S.E. A comparison of nurse-related behaviour, philosophy of care and job satisfaction in team and primary nursing. *Journal of Advanced Nursing*. 1988; 13(3): 383–395.

Reigle, J. Resource Allocation Decisions in Critical Care Nursing. *Nursing Clinics of North America*. 1989; 24(4): 1009–1015.

Rogers, M. E. Nursing: a science of unitary human beings. In Ed. J.P. Riehl-Sisca. *Conceptual Models for Nursing Practice, 3rd ed*. Norwalk: Appleton & Lange, 1989, pp. 181–188.

Rogers, E., Shoemaker, F. *Communication of Innovations: a Cross Cultural Report (2nd ed.)*. New York: The Free Press, 1971.

Royal College of Nursing. *Intensive Therapy Units*. London: RCN, 1969.

Ruzanski, J. Primary nursing in the SICU. *Nursing Administration Quarterly*. 1981; part 1, 5(30): 21–26.

Schiro, A. Primary nursing in critical care areas. In Ed. K. Zander. *Primary Nursing Development and Management*. Maryland: Aspen, 1980.

Sellick, K., Russell, S., Beckmann, J. Primary nursing: an evaluation of its effects on patient perception of care and staff satisfaction. *International Journal of Nursing Studies*. 1983; 20(4): 265–273.

Sherwood Jones, E. *Essential Intensive Care*. Lancaster: MTP Press, 1978.

Shukla, R. Structure vs people in primary nursing. An enquiry. *Nursing Research*. 1981; 30(4): 236–241.

Tiltler, M., Cohen, M., Craft, M. Impact of adult critical care hospitalization: Perceptions of patients, spouses, children, and nurses. *Heart and Lung*. 1991; 20(2): 174–182.

Thompson, D. At the heart of caring. *Nursing Times*. 1990; 86(19): 70–71.

Travelbee, J. *Interpersonal Aspects of Nursing (2nd ed.)*. Philadelphia: F.A. Davis, 1971.

Turnock, C. A study into the views of intensive care nurses on the psychological needs of their patients. *Intensive Care Nursing*. 1989; 5: 159–166.

Wandelt, M., Ager, J. *Quality Patient Care Scale*. New York: Appleton-Century-Crofts, 1974.

Warfield, C., Manley, K. Developing a new philosophy in the NDU. *Nursing Standard*. 1990; 4(41): 27–30.

Wilson, K. An Associate in Care. *Nursing Times*. 1990; 86(42): 63–64.

Wilson, N., Dawson, P. A comparison of primary nursing and team nursing in a geriatric long-term care setting. *International Journal of Nursing Studies*. 1989; 26(1): 1–13.

Wright, S. *Changing Nursing Practice*. London: Edward Arnold, 1989.

Wright, S. *My Patient – My Nurse: The practice of primary nursing*. London: Scutari Press, 1990.

Worobel, P. Peer Support in implementing primary nursing. *Nursing Administration Quarterly*. 1981; part 2, 5(3): 33–38.

4
TECHNOLOGY IN CRITICAL CARE NURSING

Christopher Turnock

CHAPTER AIMS

In examining the nature of technology it is important to clarify what is meant by the term 'technology'. As McConnell (1990) points out, technology in critical care does not only include the machinery being used to support the patient, but also those human beings who are interacting with this machinery. Therefore, in exploring technology in critical care nursing, it is important to look at it in it's widest sense, that is to look at three main areas: the machinery; the nurse controlling the machinery; and the patient who is attached to the machinery. The general aims of this chapter are to examine issues pertinent to the following areas:

☐ Machinery used in critical care – there are several categories of machines used in supporting critically ill patients. These categories relate to the provision of physiological support, for example ventilators, fluid administration devices or pressure relieving devices; patient monitoring systems, such as cardiac monitors, or arterial pressure monitoring systems; finally computers, which are more and more frequently being integrated with both physiological support systems and patient monitoring systems to attempt to relieve the nurses workload and improve the accuracy of the machinery in supporting the patient.

☐ Effects of technology on the patient – one of the obvious reasons for technological developments in the care of critically ill patients is an attempt to promote the chances of those patients surviving their illnesses. However, there are drawbacks to their use and so we shall explore how technology can influence the patient's well-being. It is important to remember that if we only examine the use of technology in critical care from a physiological perspective, we will ignore the psycho-social implications of the technology for both the patient and their family.

☐ Role of the nurse – critical care nurses are an integral part of the technology found in the critical care unit. They are constantly interacting with both the patients and the machinery surrounding the patient. We shall examine how the critical care nurse needs to achieve a balance between ensuring that the machinery is operating to provide optimal support to the patient, and delivering nursing care that enables patients and their family to cope with the surrounding machinery.

☐ The general purpose of this chapter is to examine the role of the critical care nurse within the area of critical care technology. For developments in the nature of the technology used have had major implications for critical care nurses. This means that critical care nurses continually need to develop skills to be competent in both using the machinery and in meeting the needs of patients and their family.

INTRODUCTION

We are now living in a society where there are constant technological developments, for example the rapid developments that have been made in the use of computer technology in both the home and the workplace. The development of technology in health care starting in the 1950s has led to the growth of critical care facilities which have helped many individuals survive illnesses that would have killed them 50 years ago (Ashworth, 1990). Patients with severe cardiac disorders requiring surgery, or multiple trauma or a host of other critical illnesses are now benefiting from the technological developments of the last 40 years.

THE MAIN ISSUES

The fundamental issue in examining the application of technology to critical care relates to the role of the critical care nurse in utilizing technology to provide maximum benefit for patients in ensuring their survival, whilst trying to minimize the adverse affects the technology has upon the patient.

Underpinning this central issue are a number of other points which need to be analysed, as there are many factors which influence how effective the critical care nurse is in balancing the demands put upon the nurse by both machine and patient. One area relates to the knowledge and skills the critical care nurse has about the machinery being used to support and monitor the patient. Benner (1984) outlines how nurses progress from being novices to experts, and that this process involves the aquisition of knowledge and the development of clinical skills. So, we shall consider how the progression of critical care nurses from being novices to experts relates to their ability to establish the relationship between the functioning of the machinery and the needs of the patient.

Another area that needs to be considered is the way in which technology used in critical care has developed, because these developments have major implications for the critical care nurse. Not only does the use of technology help to promote survival from critical illness, but it may also help the nurse to devote more time to direct care giving. We shall therefore examine ways in which critical care nurses can utilize machinery to take over routine nursing procedures and so focus on the patient and the family.

The implications that the use of technology has for the critically ill patient and family is another issue which we shall examine. The critical care nurse needs to not only be aware of what benefits the technology holds for the patient, but also what adverse effects it has. One important aspect of critical care nursing that needs to be addressed is the role of the nurse in attempting to minimize the unwanted influence that technology has on critically ill individuals.

In a world where the allocation of resources for the provision of health care in both hospital and community settings is under constant scrutiny, and where there is considerable debate about the distribution of funds to support the delivery of care, it is useful to consider how the development of technology influences this debate. As part of this whole debate, we shall examine the way in which technology in critical care has developed, and consider whether the extent to which technology in critical care is given financial support is justified by the benefits that critical care technology can provide to society.

The rest of this chapter will now focus on how the three main categories of technology – patient support systems, patient monitoring systems, and computers, influence the main issue, the way in which critical care nurses use technology for the benefit of the patient, whilst attempting to reduce the adverse effects that the technology may have. This analysis will be related to those issues that have been identified as being important, namely the development and use of technology in critical care, the development of critical care nurses from being novices to experts, and allocation of resources to promote the use of technology in the care of critically ill patients.

THE LITERATURE

Earlier in this chapter, three categories of machinery used in critical care were identified. This section will now focus on these categories, examining the nature of these machines in detail. We shall start by looking at physiological support systems. Within this category of machinery there are two main areas in which machines provide physiological support: firstly for internal and external respiration, and secondly to meet fluid and nutrient requirements.

Respiratory support

The use of mechanical ventilators to support external respiration is widespread in critical care. Table 4.1 indicates a number of critical care disorders which necessitate ventilation to promote the well being of the patient (Turnock, 1990).

The original form of mechanical ventilation involved the use of a negative pressure ventilator, in which the patient's thorax was encased in a shell, and the ventilator then sucks the thoracic cage outwards to create pressure within the lungs that is less than atmospheric pressure. The result of creating a negative pressure within the lungs, is that air is sucked into the lungs, copying the normal mechanisms of respiration. The 'iron lung' that was used for acute cases of poliomyelitis is an example of the negative pressure ventilator.

One major flaw with negative pressure ventilators has been the restrictions they place on patient movement. Consequently, they are rarely used nowadays, though may be used for the overnight ventilation of individuals with chronic respiratory disorders, where the aim of ventilation is to prevent a rise in carbon dioxide levels in the blood. Modern ventilators are based upon the principles of positive

pressure, where the ventilator creates a pressure greater than the pressure within the lungs, so forcing air into the lungs. The positive pressure ventilator bears great similarity to a bellows that is being used to blow air into a patient's lungs.

Positive pressure ventilators can be divided into two categories: pressure controlled and volume controlled.

Pressure controlled ventilators

Hudak, Gallo and Benz (1990) describe the principle of pressure controlled ventilation being that once a preset pressure is reached, inspiration of an air – oxygen gas mixture is terminated. The inspiratory valve is then closed and the patient exhales passively. The use of these ventilators is indicated for children, where there is a high risk of a pneumothorax being caused by high lung inflation pressures during inspiration. This then can be avoided by pre-determining maximum inflation pressure. Pressure controlled ventilators are also useful in weaning adults from mechanical ventilation.

One problem with pressure controlled ventilation is that sometimes critically ill patients may clinically develop less compliant lungs whilst being ventilated. This increase in the 'stiffness' of the lungs can result in a decrease in the volume of air being delivered before the pre-set inspiratory pressure is reached. Therefore, when a patient has lung compliance that is constantly changing, the use of pressure controlled ventilation is not recommended (Hudak et al., 1990).

Volume controlled ventilators

This approach to mechanical ventilation involves the delivery of a pre-determined volume of air–oxygen mixture to the patient. Once this volume is reached, inspiration ceases, the inspiratory valve closes and as with the pressure controlled ventilator, expiration can then occur passively. The volume controlled ventilator has the advantage that the volume of air delivered to the patient is not affected by changes in lung compliance, so the patient will receive a constant volume of air with each breath.

One major problem with the use of positive pressure ventilation is that there is a marked increase in intra-thoracic pressure during inspiration.

Table 4.1 Indications for mechanical ventilation.

Disorders of oxygenation	to ensure that haemoglobin is saturated with oxygen, e.g. acute respiratory failure
Disorders of ventilation	a clinical management decision to promote and maintain appropriate breathing, e.g. following major surgery
Disorders of oxygenation and ventilation	to promote both haemoglobin saturation and breathing, e.g. adult respiratory distress syndrome

This can restrict venous return to the heart, potentially lowering the blood pressure of the ventilated patient. There is, however, an approach to positive ventilation that is claimed to reduce the adverse effects on the circulation which involves the use of High Frequency Jet Ventilation (HFJV).

Large (1987) describes how the HFJV uses a fine catheter to deliver 100–600 breaths every minute. This means that pressure changes within the thorax are minimal. HFJV is used for a variety of critical illnesses, including patients who have suffered chest trauma or during upper airway surgery, though it's more widespread use in critical care has been questioned, requiring further study (Hedenstierna, Rolander and Rasmuson, 1989).

Functions of mechanical ventilation

In addition to being able to breath for a patient, there are a number of functions of the positive pressure ventilator that help to promote respiratory functions and assist in weaning patients off mechanical ventilation. Hudak *et al.* (1990) outline the use of Positive End Expiratory Pressure (PEEP), where at the end of expiration, pressure within the lungs does not return to zero, as one would expect. Instead pressure is kept at a higher, controlled level, so helping to improve gas exchange and prevent alveolar collapse. However, because of the constantly raised intra-thoracic pressure, the danger of seriously compromising venous return, resulting in hypotension is increased. When this pressure is applied throughout the breathing cycle, it is called Continuous Positive Pressure Ventilation (CPPV). It again helps to improve respiratory function (Turnock, 1990), though increases the likelihood of the ventilator having an adverse effect upon venous return.

The use of Continuous Positive Airway Pressure (CPAP) is described by Hedenstierna *et al.* (1989) as helping to improve gas exchange during spontaneous breathing when patients are still attached to a mechanical ventilator. The nature of CPAP is similar to CPPV, the difference being that during CPAP the patient triggers the breath, whereas in CPPV the ventilator initiates and controls breathing. CPAP is of great value, in that it facilitates weaning off mechanical ventilation by helping to

minimize the adverse effects of spontaneous ventilation which can occur during weaning.

CPAP helps to demonstrate an important feature of the modern ventilator, which is its ability to allow patients to breathe through the ventilator as if they were breathing normally. Unfortunately, often because of an underlying chronic respiratory problem or as a result of being ventilated for a long period of time, some ventilated patients who no longer require mechanical ventilation are unable to breathe adequately when removed from ventilatory support. This may result in inadequate oxygenation of the blood.

Additional functions that are used whilst patients breathe spontaneously via a ventilator are Intermittent Mandatory Ventilation (IMV) and Synchronized Intermittent Mandatory Ventilation (SIMV). During IMV, the patient can spontaneously take extra breaths above a volume of breath and rate of breathing that have been pre-set in the ventilator. The ventilator will, however, continue to deliver the pre-set breaths to the patient. During SIMV the patient must create sufficient negative pressure in the lungs during a specified time period to trigger the ventilator to deliver a breath that has been pre-set in the ventilator. As Hinds (1987) points out, SIMV helps to promote weaning as the patient no longer breathes out of synchrony with the ventilator, which can lead to inefficient respiration and patient distress.

Future developments in mechanical ventilation will try to overcome some of the problems with current systems, trying to prevent patients becoming dependent upon the ventilator for respiratory support and to maximize ventilation and perfusion of gases in the lung. Some possible initiatives have been speculated on by Hedenstierna *et al.* (1989), and include the development of techniques to independently ventilate different areas of the lung; use artificial alterations in pleural pressure to create respiratory movement; or the refinement of an artificial lung in which there can be adequate gas exchange. These developments all require detailed development and evaluation before they will become commonplace in the care of critically ill patients.

Whilst the function of mechanical ventilation is to support external respiration, there are also devices whose purpose is to meet the needs of the body's tissues for oxygen. In a situation where there is a breakdown in internal respiration, commonly in critical care situation due to left ventricular failure (Manson, MacKinnon and Moss, 1987), then there are at least two devices whose purpose is to promote tissue oxygenation.

The use of the Intra-Aortic Balloon Pump (IABP) involves the insertion of a catheter into the thoracic aorta, and the balloon contained within the catheter is then systematically inflated and deflated. Hudack et al. (1990) describe how this coincides with the cardiac cycle. Balloon inflation coincides with diastole, increasing aortic pressure and retrograde blood flow back towards the aortic valve. This helps improve blood flow to the myocardium, helping to prevent left ventricular failure due to poor oxygenation of the myocardium.

Once the systolic stage of the cardiac cycle is reached and heart contraction commences, the balloon is deflated decreasing aortic pressure easing blood flow to the body. However, as Manson et al. (1987) point out, for some critically ill patients the IABP is unable to compensate for severe ventricular failure. They go on to outline the use of the Left Ventricular Assist Device (LVAD), which involves the diversion of blood flow from the left atrium to the pump of the LVAD, returning to the circulation via the aorta. In bypassing the left ventricle, the LVAD is claimed to help reduce the pressure in the left side of the heart during both contraction and resting of the heart so relieving pulmonary congestion.

Both the IABP and the LVAD are attached to external devices that control their action. For example, the IABP is attached to a drive system that pumps gas in and out of the balloon, inflating and deflating it. In the case of the LVAD, the blood flows through a pump, blood being driven back into the body by the creation of a centrifugal force. It is important to remember that whilst these two devices are an attempt to promote the survival of critically ill patients with left ventricular failure, the survival of the patient is not assured. The limited experience of Manson et al. (1987), in using the LVAD on patients for whom the IABP has been unable to compensate for the degree of cardiac failure, only two out of five patients survived their time in ICU. The other three patients could not be weaned off the LVAD, highlighting the fact that for many critically ill adults, survival is only because of the supporting machinery, and that once they are removed from the machines they are unable to physiologically support themselves.

Fluid administration devices – the use of devices to control the administration of fluids is commonplace in critical care settings. This is because there is a need to be accurate in the flow rate of a fluid, particularly one being given in small volumes, e.g. 5 ml/hour and which contain drugs that are vital to the physiological stability of the patient. To rely upon regulating this flow with a roller clamp is problematic.

Luken and Middleton (1990) outline potential sources of administration error:

☐ calculating and counting drip rate must be done over a period of time.

☐ changes in plastic tubing – expansion and contraction changes.

☐ changes in back pressure due to blocked cannula, linked tubing or changes in patient venous pressure.

☐ changes in head pressure due to patient movement.

It is clear that all of these factors mean that it is extremely difficult to be accurate when relying upon a roller-clamp to regulate flow rate. Luken and Middleton (1990) identify two categories of gravity fed infusion devices that will provide a more accurately determined flow rate. The first is the drip rate gravity controller, in which a photoelectric drop counter administers fluid based upon drops per minute. The other type is the volumetric gravity controller, in which flow rate is based on administering fluids by millilitres per hour.

The advantages of the volumetric gravity controller is that it can adapt to the fluid type being administered, e.g. aqueous solution, blood product, TPN, whereas the drip rate gravity controller can not do so, except by making complex calculations. Luken and Middleton (1990) argue against the use of the drip rate controller where small volumes of fluid containing vasoactive drugs are to be administered, believing that the administration of drops is irregular, so potentially affecting the critically ill patients cardio-vascular state.

However, the volumetric controller tends to be both more complex to use and more expensive to buy than the drip rate controller (Luken and Middleton, 1990). The only possible way in which fluid administration devices may be developed is in using positive pressure rather than gravity. The potential danger with such a system, is that it may increase tissue damage due to extravasation, as the system continues to infuse fluid despite increased resistance as a result of extravasation.

Patient monitoring systems – The use of patient monitoring systems is commonplace in critical care, ensuring that the nurse is able to constantly and accurately assess patients physiological state, particularly their cardio-vascular and respiratory systems. These monitoring systems can be categorized into invasive, such as arterial pressure monitoring and non-invasive, such as the electrocardiogram.

Invasive monitoring systems are generally concerned with the accurate measurement of pressure, whether it is arterial, intra-cardiac or intra-cranial. Levine (1985) outlines the principles underpinning the measurement of these pressures. This involves the insertion of a catheter into the area in which pressure is to be measured. The mechanical pressure that is being measured is conducted through the fluid filled catheter to a transducer. The transducer is able to convert this mechanical pressure into electrical energy and then sending an electrical signal to a monitor that can convert the mechanical energy originally measured, into a numerical value which can also be represented on the screen of a monitor.

A number of factors can influence reading of pressure made by direct, invasive techniques such as arterial lines. Henneman and Henneman (1989) identify the following factors:

Tapering   – the pressure wave is amplified as it progresses down a tapered tube, or catheter, thus increasing the recorded pressure.

Reflection – when a pressure wave is reflected, such as when an artery branches, then the reflected wave is added to the original wave. Normally 80% of the original wave is reflected and added, though in critical care situations where peripheral resistance is increased, e.g. vaso-constriction, then the amount reflected is increased, so increasing the pressure recorded.

Frequency – monitoring systems vary in their
response   ability to accurately reproduce fast and slow variations in pressure and so represent the wave form detected at the catheter tip.

Damping   – The pressure of blood, clotting, kinking, bubbles, loose or open connections may result in a reduction in the monitoring system's frequency response.

Calibration – Errors in calibrating a monitoring system to a known pressure, such as a column of fluid, will result in the system inaccurately measuring a pressure.

Two common forms of non-invasive monitoring systems are the pulse oximeter and the electrocardiogram. The pulse oximeter, a more recent innovation in critical care, is able to provide the critical care nurse with a constant indication of the state of the patient's cardio-vascular and respiratory systems, by measuring oxygen saturation of blood in peripheral tissue. This monitor is a non-invasive technique giving a continuous measurement of arterial oxygen saturation. The principle of pulse oxymetry is that haemoglobin has distinct light saturation characteristics, based upon the number of oxygen molecules attached to the haemoglobin (Szaflarski and Cohen, 1989).

Arterial blood, due to oxygen saturation has a reddish tint, and will filter out infra-red light, but will allow red light to pass through it. In contrast, venous blood that has a bluish tint due to oxygen reduction, allows infra-red light to pass through, but will filter out red light. The pulse oximeter is able to calculate oxygen saturation of haemoglobin by recording the intensity of light transmitted through a sample of haemoglobin. To do this, the oximeter uses light emitting diodes that transmit light of different wavelengths (corresponding to red and infra-red light) through the peripheral vascular bed of a finger. A light sensitive photodiode receives this light, so measuring the intensity of light transmitted through the haemoglobin.

The other form of non-invasive monitoring involves the use of the electrocardiogram for cardiac monitoring. The placement of three metal plated electrodes, which are surrounded by foam or adhesive paper onto the chest of the patient, allows for the transmission of electrical activity within the heart via a wire cable to an oscilloscope. The oscilloscope is then able to convert this electrical activity into a visual picture of the activity within the patient's heart (Turnock, 1990). The position of the electrodes is important, as these can examine electrical activity from a variety of viewpoints. Schweisguth (1988) outlines the four main positions in which the three electrodes, positive, negative, and earth can be positioned.

ECG lead positions

Lead I: Positive – left shoulder, below clavicular hollow
           Negative – right shoulder, below clavicular hollow
           Earth   – left side of chest, below lowest palpable rib

Lead II: Positive – left side of chest, below lowest palpable rib
           Negative – right shoulder, below clavicular hollow
           Earth   – left shoulder, below clavicular hollow

MCL 1:   Positive – fourth intercostal space on right sternal border
           Negative – left shoulder, below clavicular hollow
           Earth   – right shoulder, below clavicular hollow

MCL 6:   Positive – left side of chest, fifth intercostal space, midaxillary line

Negative – left shoulder, below clavicular hollow
Earth   – right shoulder, below clavicular hollow

These different combinations indicate different aspects of cardiac activity. Lead I shows atrial activity, Lead II represents ventricular activity. Lead MCL 1 may be useful when monitoring patients who have a high risk of cardiac arrest as the position of the electrodes does not interfere with the placement of defibrillation paddles. For the same reason, Lead MCL 6 is appropriate for the patient with a pacemaker (Schweisguth, 1988). It is also important that their position is consistent, facilitating the observation of changes in cardiac function.

Computers – The advent of the computer may help to relieve critical care nurses of some of the more monotonous repetitious tasks they face each day, for example recording observations, measuring fluids and checking equipment (Clifford, 1986). Some recent examples of the use of computers in critical care demonstrate how they can not only monitor and record information about the patients physiological state, but also control physiological support systems.

The direct relationship between monitoring and support is described by Murchie (1987), in which a computer controlled system was developed that could analyse blood pressure waveforms from an arterial pressure monitoring system. The computer is then able to calculate infusion rates of vasodilator drugs in patients with unstable blood pressure.

Smith and Batchelor (1987) describe how a ventilator with an in-built computer can calculate a patient's nutritional requirements. This is done using the principles of indirect calorimetry, in which the ventilator measures oxygen consumption, and by using a pre-programmed value for the patient's respiratory quotient, calculate energy expenditure. As a result, the dangers of providing critically ill patients with too much energy, causing a rise in carbon dioxide which may lead to respiratory distress are avoided.

Whilst computer systems can be used to help the critical care nurse by monitoring and recording the state of physiological systems, particularly cardio-vascular and respiratory systems, it is important to remember that they are not fool proof, and can contribute to errors in pressure monitoring. Pierpont (1987) believes that if there are errors in the monitoring system, due either to system error or human error, the computer is unable to detect or compensate for these errors.

This final point is true of all technology used in critical care, that is to say that it is not infallible, and is only as good as the nurses who use it. In the next section, the research on technology in critical care will be examined. This will help to reinforce the principle that the technology exists to benefit patient care, not to ease the workload of the nurse.

RESEARCH LITERATURE

In recent years there have been a number of studies carried out, in which the purpose was to examine the use of technology in critical care. One area in which some studies have focused has been the effectiveness of technology commonly used in critical care.

For example, Gibbs and Gardener (1988) compared the accuracy of seven different invasive pressure monitoring systems in measuring and recording blood pressure. They found differences in their measurement of a pre-determined pressure, and were able to identify factors that accounted for these differences. The most significant factors related to the adequacy of the dynamic response of the system, and that the simpler the system, the better its performance. The use of extension tubing should be avoided, particularly greater than six inches, as this reduces dynamic response. The existence of air bubbles near to the transducer was found to account for most of the variations in pressure measurement within all seven systems.

The position of the transducer was examined in intensive care patients with either medical problems (e.g. acute respiratory or cardiac dysfunction) or following major surgery. The choice of reference positions at which to place the transducer was either the intersection of the fourth intercostal space and the dependent mid-axillary line or the intersection of the fourth intercostal space and the

sternum. Groom, Frisch and Elliott (1990) found the use of mid-axillary line gave accurate results in the surgical patients who were lying on their backs or their sides. However, the use of the sternum as a reference point for medical patients lying on their side was found to be inaccurate, a finding which is suggested to be due to physiological changes in rolling this category of patient onto their side. This study highlights the need for research into the choice of patient position and transducer position, to ensure optimum accuracy in the direct measurement of arterial pressure.

Another study into the use of pressure monitoring systems, compared the accuracy of the direct (arterial) method with an indirect method (automatic non-invasive oscillometry) (Venus et al., 1985).

Their findings were that in recording a mean blood pressure there was no difference in accuracy between the two machines. However, the direct method was found to overestimate systolic pressure, whereas the indirect method underestimated systolic pressure. Whilst these results were not conclusive, Venus et al. (1985) suggest that either system may be suitable for the routine monitoring of stable patients, but that the direct method is more reliable when patients have a constantly fluctuating blood pressure.

Much of the reported research on the use of patient monitoring systems that focus on their accuracy was conducted when these systems were in their infancy. Many of the problems identified have often been resolved by the systems manufacturers. In contrast, there is little published research on the use of computers in critical care. These differences may well reflect the fact that monitoring systems are now long established, whereas the development of the computer is still in its infancy.

Murchie (1987) describes how a computer system that was used to measure arterial pressure and then determine the rate of infusion to control arterial pressure was compared with manual control of arterial pressure. The study found that for the patients who had their arterial pressure recorded directly by a monitoring system, but relied on the nurse to calculate and determine drug infusion rate, were more likely to have arterial pressure fluctuation outside an optimal range. Whilst this study suggests that the computer is more effective than manual methods in controlling arterial pressure, no data is provided to demonstrate the significance of the findings.

Another area of patient monitoring systems that was identified earlier was that of non-invasive monitoring. Anderson (1982) studied the perceptions of critically ill patients who were attached to cardiac monitors, and found that these patients often had misconceptions about the nature of cardiac monitoring. One subject believed that the monitor acted as a cardiac pacemaker, and was keeping her alive. Often subjects were unaware of the purpose of the monitor, believing that it recorded cardiac function, not a set of electrical events in the heart.

This study also found that it was not unusual for patients to put complete trust in the accuracy of the trace being displayed on the screen of the monitor, unaware of some of the common factors that can result in errors in recording heart rate. Thus, sudden changes in heart-rate due to some innocuous cause such as patient movement, could cause patients to experience great anxiety.

A descriptive study of the experiences of postoperative cardiac surgery patients, conducted by Demeyer (1967), found that the patients also experienced anxiety as a result of feeling tied down by electrocardiograph leads.

A number of studies have examined other ways in which technology can influence the experience of being a critical care patient. One area is in relation to the noise that this technology can create. For example, Hilton (1976) identified a number of sleep disturbing factors when examining the nature of sleep in intensive care unit patients. The study found that equipment noise accounted for only 1.4% of these factors. This conclusion is interesting, especially in light of the work of Redding, Hargest and Minsky (1977), who measured noise levels of equipment commonly used in critical care, and found the following results when measuring the noise levels at the patients heads:

Component Sound	Noise Level (decibels)
Cardiac monitor alarm	71
Ventilator lidal volume	77
Ventilator disconnect alarm	92
Intra-aortic balloon pump	74

These results have particular significance in the light of the finding of Thiessen (1970), that noise levels of 50 decibels or above have a 50% probability of altering the nature of an individual's sleep, either altering the stage of sleep or waking the disturbed individual up.

Hewitt (1970) studied the experiences of 100 patients who had spent time in a surgical intensive therapy unit. Many of these patients remembered little of their stay in the unit, even though not all were ventilated or heavily sedated. However, those who can recollect the experience described features of the unit which they found most worrying, including noise levels from surrounding machinery. This is supported by Badger (1974), who described the personal experience of being a patient in an intensive care unit. Amongst the lasting memories is the high noise level generated by machines and their alarms.

Some of the problems of attempting to ascertain the views of critical care patients on the technology surrounding them are illustrated in a study by Asbury (1985), who used questionnaires to obtain the views of all patients who were admitted to an intensive care unit during a one year period. The data was collected three months after discharge from the unit, obtaining a response rate of 68%. Unfortunately, not only are the views of non-survivors (21% of the unit admissions) not obtained, but a quarter of respondents were unable to recollect their stay in the unit. Furthermore, when asked about their ventilators, a third of the patients who were ventilated remember having their breathing helped by a machine. Exactly the same proportion of those patients not ventilated also remember having a machine assist with their breathing.

This only highlights the problem in ensuring that data collected from critical care patients accurately describes their experiences. Factors such as non-survival, non-recollection or poor recollection of events mean that often an anecdotal account of events can also provide valuable insights into the effects of technology on critically ill patients. Cynthia Smith, an experienced intensive care nurse, is able to describe her experiences of admission to various critical care units (Smith, 1987).

Amongst her observations, she described how background noise can be very distressing, both for the patient and relative. They are unable to interpret the nature of sounds generated by the surrounding machinery. Other problems for her included the effect ventilation had on her ability to communicate, causing frustration at not being able to communicate. She also describes fear when one nurse was undressing her and another was attempting to put electrocardiograph leads on her chest, and was becoming irritated that the cardiac monitor was not working because the nurse undressing her kept knocking the electrodes off her chest.

The effect of ventilation on the communication process is also outlined by Asbury (1985), in which 59% of the patients who recollected their stay in the intensive care unit were worried by not being able to speak because they were ventilated. Ballard (1981) conducted a study which focused on patients in a surgical intensive care unit ranking the degree of stress they felt from 45 identified items relevant to critical care. One of the main stressors related to a feeling of being tied down by tubes, that immobility was caused by the presence of either invasive monitoring systems, or physiological support systems.

Furthermore, the presence of strange machines, or unusual noises were perceived as being only medium stressors. This finding is supported by Asbury (1985), in which the majority of respondents were not concerned by the presence of machinery. A growing awareness of technology and the situation of machinery behind patients may go some way to helping to reduce the degree of stress it causes critical care patients. However, both studies have collected data once the patients can communicate, and are no longer ventilated and heavily sedated, so they are more able to interpret their environment. It is only possible to speculate, but it may be that when critical care patients are sedated and ventilated, the machinery surrounding them may cause anxiety, as they are unable to gain insight into the exact nature of it.

One way in which machinery may well cause these acutely ill critical care patients stress is through a concern of technical failure. Bergbom-Engburg and Haljamae (1988) used both questionnaires and interviews to obtain the views of 304 subjects on their experience as an intensive care unit patient. Approximately 50% were able to recall the experience, and of these 28.5% felt inse-cure for various reasons. Firstly, they were unable to trust the surrounding machinery, fearing that it would break down and they would die. They also felt tied down and restricted in movement by the equipment, including tubes, electrical and monitoring lines and intra-venous lines. Secondly, they also expressed feeling insecure if they felt that they were unable to trust the nurse caring for them. This phenomenon occurred when the nurse paid more attention to the surrounding technology than to the patient. These nurses were thought by the patients to be unskilled, unpleasant and therefore dangerous.

It may be that critical care nurses may also feel uncomfortable when using technology. McConnell (1990) interviewed critical care nurses about using technology and found that a lack of knowledge about technology increased fear in the nurse. The nurses described an expectation that they should be competent in the use of machinery, and that they equated competency with feeling comfortable with the machines. This study also found that there were situations in which technology interfered with the work of the critical care nurse. Machines that were large were described as obnoxious, and that they cluttered the working environment making it more difficult for the nurse to get to the patient.

Another finding of the study was the fact that the surrounding technology competed with the patient for the nurses' time. An unfortunate paradox was identified, in which the iller the patient, the greater the number of machines supporting and monitoring the patient. Therefore the nurses had to find a balance between the needs of the patient and the surrounding technology. Finding this balance was made more difficult by the fact that whilst the machines can make physical care easier, they increased the amount of time the nurses spent explaining the machines to the patients and their family. The additional problem of machine malfunction was also seen as a situation in which technology interfered with the ability of the critical care nurse to give direct care to the patient.

The work of Murchie and Kenny (1988) also identifies from the opinions of critical nurses on the use of automatic computer control of arterial pressure, that technology can have the benefit of helping to save the nurses time. This is because they no longer need to be constantly adjusting the rate of an influsion pump in response to changes in the patient's cardiovascular state, helping to make more time available for other aspects of patient care. Whilst a small majority (51%) preferred the computer system over the old traditional manual methods, concerns were expressed. These related to doubts about the effectiveness of the system to respond to physiological changes in the patient, and also feeling inadequately prepared to use the computer system.

This final point leads us to the end of this section in which there has been an examination of the research literature relating to the use of technology in critical care. There have been a number of studies which have examined the effectiveness of patient monitoring systems, and in particular, identify factors which influence the accuracy of measurements. Other studies have also examined the effects that the technology has upon both the critical care patient and their nurse. One feature of this research is that the technology can produce stress and anxiety in both the nurse and the patient where they are ignorant about the nature of the technology.

Therefore, in the next section we shall analyse the role of the critical care nurse in developing some of the more technical skills required in caring for critically ill patients. One important aspect of this development will be identifying how the critical care nurse finds the right balance between the needs of the surrounding technology and the needs of the patient.

Nursing care

Entry to a critical care environment will introduce a newcomer to a whole plethora or unfamiliar technology. To the inexperienced critical care nurse, the vast array of monitors, ventilators, infusion pumps, computers and other assorted types of machinery can only serve to heighten their fear of being expected to care for a patient who has a high risk of dying. The combination of this sensory overload with the stress of the situation creates a dangerous cocktail. Yates (1983) has identified two ways in which the inexperienced critical care nurse will respond. One response is that the nurse will focus on the surrounding technology, failing to see the patient as their primary concern.

The alternative response is completely the opposite, with the focus of the nurse's attention being upon the patient, so attempting to remove the fear of the unknown by ignoring it. In both responses, we can see that the newcomer to critical care copes with the situation by creating an imbalance in the relationship between meeting the needs of the patient and being competent in ensuring correct functioning of the technology. In creating this imbalance the nurse is behaving as a novice, that the process of becoming an expert in critical care nursing involves a realization that the critically ill patient and the surrounding technology are mutually interdependent.

The increased use of technology in critical care nursing means that to provide effective nursing care, the critical care nurse must be both psychologically fit and technologically competent (Clifford, 1986). To achieve this balance between the 'art' of direct care giving and 'science' created by technology, the critical care nurse must develop both confidence and competence in using the technology to promote the optimum balance between the benefit of the technology of the patient, minimizing the adverse effects of the technology and meeting the non-technological based needs of the patient.

Technology

This section will address ways in which critical care nurses can try to achieve this balance between the needs of the technology and the patient. In examining strategies to balance this relationship, the most appropriate way to use the technology will be considered. For example, Szaflarski and Cohen (1989) describe situations in which there may be inaccuracies in the use of pulse oximetry. These situations include rapidly developing hypoxaemia, lower body temperature, i.e. below 35° centigrade, or other situations where the patient is physiologically unstable, such as shock, severe anaemia or enhanced vasoconstriction. Further problems relate to pulse oximeters reporting high oxygen saturation levels in individuals with high carboxyhaemoglobin levels, therefore their use in monitoring patients with carbon monoxide poisioning or heavy smokers is not appropriate.

Other problems in the use of the pulse oximeter can result from small changes in the position of the sensor, or from other changes in peripheral tissue volume apart from changes in blood volume. These factors can lead to a falsely low reading of oxygen saturation, and in trying to minimize this, manufacturers have slowed down the response of the oximeter (Szaflarski and Cohen, 1989). It is also important that the nurse is aware the patient is at risk of developing pressure sores at the sensor site. The site should therefore be assessed every two hours, and the rotation of digits considered as a preventative measure.

In another form of non-invasive monitoring, cardiac monitoring, there are several actions the critical care nurse should undertake to ensure that there is an accurate visual representation of electrical events in the heart on the oscilloscope. To do this, the three electrodes should be placed in the correct positions, as outlined earlier, and there should be good contact between the skin and the electrode. This helps to eliminate interference to the quality of image on the cardiac monitor.

There may be situations in critical care where a patient is having their blood pressure monitored directly and the nurse is uncertain about the accuracy of the monitoring system. The research discussed earlier (see page 81) does identify sources of error in the direct method of recording blood pressure. The nurse should therefore make sure that the system is free from obstruction or other damping factors such as air, blood or loose/open connections, and when re-calibrating the system ensure that the transducer is at the correct reference point.

Whilst there are potential sources of error in the direct method of measurement, the work of Venus et al. (1985) demonstrates that it is a more reliable method than the indirect method when patients are critically ill. The use of the direct method is particularly appropriate where Korotkov sounds are either diminished or absent, and where the patient is very unstable and requires frequent measurements of blood pressure (Henneman and Henneman, 1989). This has the added advantage of allowing the nurse to monitor the patient without disturbing the patient. Where the patient's vital signs are more stable and blood pressure is being recorded infrequently, then the indirect method becomes appropriate.

Another issue in the use of direct pressure monitor systems relates to the frequency with which the system should be replaced. In reviewing the research literature on infection control practices in the use of intravascular pressure monitoring systems, Keeler et al. (1987) conclude that there is no research evidence to support changing the system unless it has become contaminated, for example where reflux of blood has occurred.

Also, the evidence relating to the frequency with which the solution used to flush the system is changed indicates that it doesn't really matter when this is done. Low contamination has been found when the flush solution has been changed infrequently, i.e. greater than 48 hours, when the bag is empty (Keeler et al., 1987). Whilst these findings indicate that the critical care nurse only needs to make changes to the monitoring system when it has become contaminated, or when the flush solution has run out, it is important to point out that changes to the system should be performed under aseptic conditions.

These findings help to guide the critical care nurse to find the balance between the needs of the patient and the need to correctly monitor the patient's physiological status. The guidelines indicate ways in which the nurse can save time, for example in correctly setting up the monitoring system and the frequency with which the system is changed. There are also recommendations concerning the strategies that should be adopted to ensure that accurate pressure monitoring occurs.

Support systems

In using physiological support systems, there are also guidelines for the critical care nurse which help to maximize the time available to the nurse for direct patient care, whilst ensuring that the system is functioning correctly, and so not putting the patient at risk. Large (1987) outlines three essential aspects to the role of the nurse in caring for the ventilated patient.

First of all, the nurse must be aware of the way in which the ventilator functions. This involves ensuring that the ventilator is delivering the air–oxygen mixture at the correct pre-set parameters, such as volume, rate, pressure and oxygen concentration. Dysfunction alarms, found on all ventilators, should be set at levels that do not endanger the patient if a malfunction occurs. However, the range of these values should not be so narrow, that minor variations in ventilation result in the alarm being frequently activated. This will only result in patient disturbance and distract the nurse from other activities whilst the alarm is silenced and the cause of the alarm activation identified.

There is also the need to observe both the patient and the ventilator for signs of complications. One example is tension pneumothorax, where the patient rapidly develops signs of respiratory distress. There is irregular chest movement and the pressure exerted by the ventilator to inflate the lungs suddenly increases. Other possible causes of respiratory distress include a leak in the ventilator circuit.

The final area of nursing practice relates to patient education and explanation. To ensure that the patient cooperates with the nurse in a way that will promote their recovery, they need to be informed about the nature of the ventilator, especially it's function and the meaning of the alarms. This process should also be extended to the patient's relatives, as they can also play a valuable part in comforting the patient and ensure their assistance during nursing interventions designed to promote respiration, or whilst being weaned from ventilation.

These principles of nursing the ventilated patient can also be applied to caring for patients receiving fluids via an infusion pump. The nurse should choose the appropriate type of pump according to the clinical situation. Drip rate gravity pumps are appropriate for relatively slow influsion where exact precision is not necessary, whereas the volumetric gravity pump is more appropriate where accuracy in administration of fluids is required. The nurse should be able to set the pump to function correctly, and be aware of signs of administration failure.

As these pumps respond slowly to occlusions (Luken and Middleton, 1990), it is important that the nurse is observing for signs of occlusion, or early extravasation. Extravasation can be both painful and traumatic to surrounding tissue, depending upon the type of fluid which is no longer entering the vein, but is instead entering the surrounding tissue. The nurse should carry out constant observations of the infusion site to prevent patient discomfort and to be aware of the potential risk of not receiving life supporting drugs that should have been received through the infusion system.

The patient should be educated about the nature of the infusion and the degree to which it limits movement of the limb through which the infusion is entering the body. This helps to ensure that the patient is no longer frightened to move, and that feelings of being immobilized due to the presence of infusion lines are reduced. These nursing strategies involving the care of the patient who is being subjected to physiological support are aimed at alleviating adverse effects on the patient, whilst trying to maximize the time available to the critical care nurse for providing direct care to the patient and their family.

The patient – There are also a number of ways in which the crtitical care nurse can consider situating technology that may help to minimize the adverse effects that the technology can have on the patient. Hansell (1984) recommends a number of ways in which environmental noise from machines can be reduced. These include the turning down of noise from machines, or that these machines are turned away from the patient's head to reduce the amount of sound they can hear. It is important that these actions do not endanger the patient, that the nurse is still able to hear the alarm and observe monitors for signs of changes in the patient's physiological state.

Other ways in which the effects of noise from machines upon the patient can be removed include an assessment of the position of the machines. The ideal position is one where the patient(s) are subjected to minimum noise levels. The noise from the expiration of gas through a ventilator can be quite disturbing to the patient, and so the nurse must attempt to place the expiratory valve in a position where it is not adjacent to the patient's ear (Hansell, 1984). However, the nurse should be careful that in protecting one patient, they then subject another patient to these undesirable sounds.

The majority of critical care patients are subjected to cardiac monitoring, yet in situations where the patient is aware of the visual trace there is a danger that the patient and relative will focus attention on the trace. This can cause unnecessary anxiety to the patient when false abnormalities occur. The patient and relative need to be informed about the nature of both true and false recording of cardiac electrical activity, and those factors which can interfere with the accuracy of the oscilloscope trace, such as patient movement or lead disconnection. It is also important that the patient is not frightened to cause trace abnormalities by moving and that they feel free to move normally.

It may be appropriate to consider positioning cardiac monitors where they cannot be seen. For example, Kornfeld *et al.* (1968) suggest that they are placed outside a cubicle, and that the monitor is kept silent so that the patient neither hears a constant rhythmic signal sound, nor is aware of any changes to the electrical signal received by the monitor. If patients are not in a cubicle, the monitor should be placed behind the patient's head. Also the nurse should not pay too much attention to the monitor, as this may leave the patient feeling either less important than the machine, or worried that there is a problem with their cardiac function.

Another important aspect relating to the noises emanating from critical care technology is that many patients are not familiar with these sounds and so are unable to interpret them. Smith (1987) describes how on wakening from a period of artificial ventilation, exposure to the plethora of sounds due to critical care technology can be quite bewildering. The nurse needs to help the patient interpret these sounds by informing them about both the source of the sound and its significance. As Bergbom-Engberg and Haljamae (1988) point out, to gain the trust of the patient in both the machinery and the nurse caring for them, the nurse must be able to provide the patient with a full explanation concerning the nature of the equipment surrounding the patient.

As the amount and nature of technology in critical care increases, the nurse must develop ever more complex technical skills (Clifford, 1986). However, they must also be aware of the need to develop their interpersonal skills. This will allow them to provide the patient with an interpretation of the critical care environment to be as real as is possible. The patient should be made aware of some of the benefits of the technology:

Benefits of technology

☐ increases the likelihood of survival from critical illness;

☐ allows the nurse to monitor physiological state accurately;

☐ minimizes nursing interventions, such as recording of blood pressure and so increases the length of undisturbed periods for sleep;

☐ save nursing time which can then be spent on direct patient care.

Awareness of both the need and nature for technology in critical care can help both patient and their relatives to come to terms with the environment. This will then help to promote their co-operation in recovery from critical illness.

The nurse – Working in critical care situations can be very stressful for both novice and expert. There is a need for the nurse to both come to terms with these environmental stressors, and also be able to deliver care which meets the needs of both the patient and the surrounding technology.

Melia (1977) suggests that the creation of regular group meetings can help critical care nurses to examine their work experiences, especially its stressful effects, and so provide the opportunity to air opinions and grievances, as well as discuss the implications of new technology for nursing staff. This support will help the critical care nurse to cope with the stress created by technology.

To provide effective patient care the critical care nurse needs to be both psychologically fit and technologically competent (Clifford, 1986). To achieve this, the critical care nurse needs to be educated in the range of technical skills required for the situation. For the novice in critical care, this involves the provision of support and education from experienced staff, as well as the use of appropriate role models. The purpose of any programme that introduces a nurse to practising in critical care is that they are assisted in making the transition from being a novice to an expert. This allows them to realize how they can achieve a balance between the patient and machine, which not only promotes the patient's survival, but also minimizes the harmful effects the technology may have on the patient.

The process of becoming an expert involves the critical care nurse becoming an excellent technician. They must also pay attention to the physical and psychological effects of the technology on the patient. The nurse needs to recognize that the technology will act as a stressor on the patient. Ballard (1981) points out, to help the patient cope with these stressors the critical care nurse must provide the patient with appropriate information and comprehensive support.

Ashworth (1990) describes the features of the work of a critical care nurse which would suggest that they have mastered the technology used to monitor and support the patient, thus becoming 'expert' critical care nurses. These features include:

☐ reflecting on their observations in relation to their understanding and knowledge developed in critical care to assess the nature of patient–technology interactions;

☐ use the technology as an extension to the nurse's hands, eyes, ears and other senses;

☐ automatically and unconsciously pay attention to this information, reacting quickly to any cues which may have important implications for the patient's welfare.

The process of becoming an 'expert' involves the acquisition of sufficient knowledge and experience to develop an ability to know when something is wrong. This intuition enables the nurse to be aware that something is wrong, despite conflicting information the nurse is receiving from the surrounding technology. One limitation of technology is that it is only as good as the nurse who uses it. The critical care nurse needs to rely upon it to support and monitor the patient, ensuring that it is functioning correctly. However, the expert is also able to collect a wealth of information from both patient and technology, and judge when the patient may be at risk if a false assumption is made in thinking that the technology is functioning incorrectly.

CONCLUSION

The use of technology appears to influence the amount of time a critical care nurse can spend with the patient, the greater the number of machines the less time the nurse has to spend with the patient. The critical care nurse is forced to spend more time assessing data collected from machines, caring for the machines or explaining the machines to the patient (McConnell, 1990). One of the paradoxes in critical care is that the iller the patient is, the greater the number of machines used to support and monitor the patient.

Therefore, the iller the patient, the greater the number of distractions existing to draw the critical care nurse away from directly caring for patients. Marsden (1991) raises another problem in that it is questionable where the patient ends and the technology begins, thus dehumanizing the patients. This is a situation which worsens where the amount of machinery in use increases when the patient is acutely ill. In this situation the patient is likely to be unconscious, sedated or confused, promoting dehumanization. The use of technology can have an adverse effect on patients, particularly when there is a great deal of technology used in the management of the patient.

As Hopkinson (1989) points out, society is entering an era of advances in critical care services, in which the demands for critical care are ever increasing. Yet a recent report by the Kings Fund (1989) has questioned whether the predicted increase in critical care facilities and the obvious costs incurred are warranted. They are currently examining the evidence to support the belief that intensive care units cause a decrease in mortality and morbidity. One problem is that the source of demand for constantly developing critical care facilities will come from both health care professional and a public who are educated by the media to expect such facilities, irrespective of the outcome (Hopkinson, 1989). Both groups require information regarding the benefits of critical care technology and those situations where it's use in patient care is appropriate.

With the development of technology in critical care there is a need to reassess the effectiveness of its use in the management of critical illness. The evidence concerning the benefits resulting from the use of technology in critical illness suggests that there are categories of patients who are likely to benefit from the technology, whilst there are other patients who are not. Certainly, the Kings Fund (1989) believe that critical care is appropriate for patients who have been assessed as being expected to survive or have a good chance of survival. However, where prognosis is uncertain, or if death is very probable or certain, then critical care is considered inappropriate.

Jennett (1990) feels that often technology is even used where it is not necessary in supporting or monitoring the patient. It may be that in a society where resources are not limitless there is a need to assess the most effective use of technology. This involves an assessment of which patients will benefit from the technology and also what form of technology is to be used, where the advantages of using a particular machine outweigh any adverse effects it may have for either the patient or the nurse.

To be effective as a critical care nurse, there is a need to meet both the physical and psychological needs of the patient and to also be a competent technician (Shurdham, 1986). There is often a danger that in coping with the critical care environment, the nurse dehumanizes the patient, regarding them as being inaminate, insensate objects, rather than as immobile, relatively silent people. Taylor (1971) believes that this is particularly so when there is a great risk of the patient dying, where the nurse dehumanizes the patient as a defence against the impending death of the patient. Of course, this behaviour has also been discovered when nurses are caring for dying patients in non-critical care situations, for example, the work of Kubler-Ross.

Often critical care nurses are working in stressful situations, where there are conflicting demands on their time from both patient and the technology. The critical care nurse is told that they must meet all of these demands in difficult and demanding circumstances so that they deliver the optimum level of care.

However, this may not always be possible, especially when the nurse is inexperienced, the patient is acutely ill and where there is a vast array of machines supporting and monitoring the patient. Ashworth (1990) argues that technology alone does not provide good intensive care, that it must be combined with humanity, developing fully the capacities and resources of human beings that the machine cannot replace.

This means that critical care nurses need to maintain the safety, dignity and humanity of the patient, ensure that the technology is functioning correctly and that it accurately monitors the patient, and that both the patient and relative receive adequate explanations concerning the nature of the technology. When critical care nurses become expert in their practice, and are able to combine all these functions, then they will be able to use technology in caring for patients in a way that minimizes the adverse effects of the technology, and which optimizes recovery from critical illness.

CASE STUDIES

Case study one

Terry Banks had been involved in a car accident, resulting in severe chest and abdominal injuries, and needing to be mechanically ventilated. Terry was a mechanical engineer who became very concerned that the ventilator might break down, and that he would not be able to breath.

The presence of the endotracheal tube and the use of sedation made it impossible for Terry to verbalize his concerns, or to ask anybody to explain what the various noises, particularly from machine alarms meant. Terry became extremely worried one morning when a new nurse came to care for him, spending most of the morning looking at the ventilator and rarely speaking to Terry except to inform him of procedures he was about to undergo.

A different nurse came to care for Terry that afternoon, and immediately asked him to squeeze her hand if he was worried about anything. Once Terry gave an affirmative response, the nurse got a pen and paper and helped Terry to write down what he was worried about. She then proceeded to explain to Terry the purpose and function of the ventilator and the nature of the alarm system. Terry finally felt that he could trust the ventilator to provide adequate physiological support.

Case study two

Mary Baldwin was admitted to the coronary care unit of her local hospital after an episode of acute chest pain. At the time of her admission, the unit had been extremely busy and Mary was drowsy because of the analgesia she has been given to relieve her chest pain. Unfortunately, Mary had been given only a brief explanation of the nature of the cardiac monitor to which she has been 'attached' to via three chest electrodes and a cable.

Consequently by the evening of her admission Mary had become afraid to move in bed. This was because every time she moved, the interference to the signal caused the cardiac monitor alarm to be activated. The nurse assigned to care for Mary would subsequently enter the cubicle and without any explanation reset the alarm and tell Mary to lie still. Mary became very anxious, thinking that because the monitor alarm was being activated so regularly her heart condition was deteriorating.

It was only during the night, when another nurse explained to Mary how the alarm was sometimes activated by her movements, that Mary felt happy to move about in bed rather than lie still in one position all the time.

KEY TERMS

Mechanical ventilation

The use of artificial means to transfer air into the lungs.

Internal respiration

The transfer of gases (oxygen and carbon dioxide) between the lungs and the body's cells.

External respiration

The movement of gases (oxygen and carbon dioxide) between the lungs and the atmosphere.

Invasive monitoring

Mechanism for directly measuring pressure inside the body by the use of equipment that will convert mechanical pressure into an electrical signal that can be visually represented on the screen of a monitor.

Non-invasive monitoring

The use of equipment on the outside of the body to measure physiology signs, such as electrical activity in the heart.

Computers

Computers can be programmed to monitor the physiological state of an individual, or to provide appropriate support where physiological imbalance occurs.

STUDENT LEARNING QUESTIONS

1. What is the role of the nurse in ensuring that monitoring systems are accurate in their measurements?

2. In what ways can technology adversely affect the critically ill patient?

3. How can the critical care nurse minimize the effects of technology on the patient and their family, whilst maximizing their safety?

FURTHER READING

Ashworth, P. High technology and humanity for intensive care. *Intensive Care Nursing.* 1990; 6(3): 150–160.

Clifford, C. Patients, relatives and nurses in a technological environment. *Intensive Care Nursing.* 1986; 2(1): 67–72.

Hudak, C.M., Gallo, B.M., Benz, J.J. *Critical Care Nursing.* Philadelphia: Lipincott, 1990.

Smith, C. In need of intensive care – a personal perspective. *Intensive Care Nursing.* 1987; 5(3):116–122.

REFERENCES

Anderson, U.K. In Ed. M.A. Noble. *The I.C.U. Environment: Directions for Nursing.* Boston: Boston Publishing, 1982.

Asbury, A.J. Patient's memories and reactions to intensive care. *Care of the Critically Ill.* 1985; 1(2): 12–13.

Ashworth, P. High technology and humanity for intensive care. *Intensive Care Nursing.* 1990; 6(3): 150–160.

Badger, T.L. The physician-patient in the recovery and intensive care units. *Archives of Surgery.* 1974; 109: 359–360.

Ballard, K.S. Identification of environmental stressors for patients in a surgical intensive care unit. *Issues in Mental Health Nursing.* 1981; 3(1–2): 89–108.

Benner, P. *From Novice to Expert.* Menlo Park CA: Addison Wesley, 1984.

Bergbom-Engberg I., Haljamae, H. A retrospective study of patient's recall of respiratory treatment (2): Nursing care factors and feelings of security/insecurity. *Intensive Care Nursing.* 1988; 4(3): 95–101.

Clifford, C. Patients, relatives and nurses in a technological environment. *Intensive Care Nursing.* 1986; 2(1): 67–72.

Demeyer, J. The environment of the intensive care unit. *Nursing Forum.* 1967; 6(3): 262–272.

Gibbs, N.C., Gardner, R.M. Dynamics of invasive pressure monitoring systems: Clinical and laboratory evaluation. *Heart and Lung.* 1988; 17(1): 43–51.

Groom, L., Frisch, S.R., Elliot, M. Reproducibility and accuracy of pulmonary artery pressure measurement in supine and lateral positions. *Heart and Lung.* 1990; 19(2): 147–151.

Hansell, H. N. The behavioural effects of noise on man: The patient with 'intensive care psychosis'. *Heart and Lung.* 1984; 13(1): 59–65.

Hedenstierna, G., Rolander, C., Rasmuson, S. Mechanical ventilation and monitoring in the year 2000. *Care of the Critically Ill.* 1989; 5(3): 83–87.

Henneman E.A., Henneman, P.L. Intricacies of blood pressure measurement: Re-examining the rituals. *Heart and Lung.* 1989; 18(3): 263–273.

Hewitt, P.B. Subjective follow-up of patients from a surgical intensive therapy ward. *British Medical Journal.* 1970; (4): 669–673.

Hilton, B.A. Quantity and quality of patient's sleep, and sleep disturbing factors in a respiratory intensive care unit. *Journal of Advanced Nursing.* 1976; 1(6): 453–468.

Hinds, C.J. *Intensive Care – A Concise Textbook.* London: Ballière Tindall, 1987.

Hopkinson, R. The future. *Care of the Critically Ill.* 1989; 5(3): 81.

Hudak, C.M., Gallo, B.M., Benz, J.J. *Critical Care Nursing.* 5th Ed. Philadelphia: J.B. Lippincott, 1990.

Jennett, B. Is intensive care worthwhile? *Care of the Critically Ill.* 1990; 6(3): 85–88.

Keeler, C., McLane, C., Covey, M., Smith, N., Holm, K. A review of infection control practices related to intravascular pressure monitoring devices (1975–1985). *Heart and Lung.* 1987; 16(2): 201–206.

Kings Fund. I.C.U. in the United Kingdom: Report from the Kings Fund Panel. *Intensive Care Nursing.* 1989; 5(2): 76–81.

Kornfeld, D.S., Maxwell, T., Momrow, D. Psychological hazards of the intensive care unit. *Nursing Clinics of North America.* 1968; 3(1): 41–51.

Large, W.P. A nursing approach to the use of high frequency jet ventilation. *Intensive Care Nursing.* 1987; 2(3): 112–115.

Levine, S.C. A review of the use of computerised digital instrumentation to determine pulmonary artery pressure measurements in critically ill patients. *Heart and Lung.* 1985; 14(5): 473–476.

Luken, J., Middleton, J. Intravenous infusion controllers. *Nursing Standard.* 1990; 4(29): 30–32.

McConnell, E.A. The impact of machines on the work of critical care nurses. *Critical Care Nursing Quarterly.* 1990; 12(4): 45–52.

Manson, E.K., MacKinnon, C., Moss, S. The left ventricular assist device (LVAD) in refractory heart failure: One year's experience in Edinburgh. *Intensive Care Nursing.* 1987; 3(4): 172–181.

Marsden, C. Technology assessment in critical care. *Heart and Lung.* 1991; 20(1): 93–94.

Melia, K.M. The intensive care unit – A stress situation. *Nursing Times Occasional Papers.* 1977; 73(5): 17–20.

Murchie, C.J. Computer control of arterial blood pressure following cardiac surgery. *Intensive Care Nursing.* 1987; 3(1): 3–7.

Murchie C.J., Kenny, G.N.C. Nurse's attitudes to automatic computer control of arterial pressure. *Intensive Care Nursing.* 1988; 4(3): 112–117.

Pierpont, G.L. Pitfalls of computer use in acute care medicine. *Heart and Lung.* 1987; 16(2): 207–210.

Redding, J.S., Hargest, T.S., Minsky, S.M. How noisy is intensive care? *Critical Care Medicine.* 1977; 5(6): 275.

Rithalia, S.V.S. Never mind the volume, what about the flow rate? *Intensive Care Nursing.* 1988; 4(3): 128.

Schweisguth, D. Setting up a cardiac monitor – without missing a beat. *Nursing.* 1988; 18(11): 43–48.

Shurdham, C. The nurse on the intensive care unit. *Intensive Care Nursing.* 1988; 1(4): 181–186.

Smith, C. In need of intensive care – a personal perspective. *Intensive Care Nursing.* 1987; 2(3): 116–122.

Smith, R.J., Batchelor, A. Metabolic computing. *Intensive Care Nursing.* 1987; 3(4): 160–164.

Szaflarski, N.L., Cohen, N.H. Use of pulse oximetry in critically ill adults. *Heart and Lung.* 1989; 18(5): 444–453.

Taylor, D.E.M. Problems of patients in an intensive care unit: The aetiology and prevention of intensive care syndrome. *International Journal of Nursing Studies.* 1971; 8(1): 47–59.

Thiessen, C. In Ed. B.L. Welsh. *Psychological Effects of Noise During Sleep.* New York: Plenum Press, 1970.

Turnock, C. Demystifying intensive care. *Nursing Standard.* 1990; 4(41): 31–33.

Venus, B., Mathru, M., Smith, R.A., Pham, L.G. Direct versus indirect blood pressure measurements in critically ill patients. *Heart and Lung.* 1985; 14(3): 228–231.

Yates, L. Technology in nursing. *Nursing Focus.* 1983; 5(2): 8.

5

COMPLEMENTARY THERAPY IN THE CRITICAL CARE UNIT

Rachel Ashcroft

CHAPTER AIMS

The plethora of articles concerning the use of complementary therapies in all areas of nursing shows that nurses are realizing the potential of using these therapies in their practice. The main aim of this chapter is to provide information on a limited number of therapies: **acupressure**, **aromatherapy**, **massage**, **reflexology** and **therapeutic touch**. These therapies have been singled out because of their ability to complement the care given to critically ill patients. They are not seen as alternatives to those methods already employed in treating patients but as providing additional support. In this way they can enhance orthodox treatments. Concentration on these five therapies is not to say that other less orthodox methods, of which there are many more, would not be suitable too. But these five appear particularly relevant.

After studying this chapter the reader should be able to:

☐ Describe the concepts of complementary therapy.

☐ Identify the potential uses of complementary therapies in the care of the critically ill patient.

☐ Write an account of the process involved in introducing a complementary therapy into a critical care area.

☐ Describe the potential changes to complementary therapies and their availability after the formation of the Common European Market in 1992.

☐ Show awareness of the legal implications of extending the role of nurses to incorporate complementary therapies.

INTRODUCTION

Complementary therapies are being increasingly explored as potential adjuncts to orthodox medical treatments. Unlike modern medicine, they offer a highly individualistic approach to health, with the emphasis centred on treating the ill person as a whole (holistically), necessitating concentration on more than the physical, making equally important the emotional, psychological and spiritual aspects of ill-health.

Information is presented on the origins of each

therapy, with a brief history of its development. The therapy is then explained in more detail with the inclusion of relevant research which has been done on it. Accounts are given of the use of each therapy in nursing, together with some anecdotal experiences.

The importance of training is highlighted to ensure discriminating and safe use of therapies, and advice is given on developing the incorporation of complementary therapies into current nursing practices, including legal aspects, policy formation and changes resulting from the Common European Market.

THE LITERATURE

Acupressure

Acupressure, also known as Shiatsu acupressure, originates from Japan where it developed from Chinese oriental medicine and acupuncture (Box, 1984). It involves the use of firm and gentle pressure (usually applied by the fingers) on energy points or 'tsubos' which lie on particular energy pathways known as meridians. The meridians run through the body, and each of the fourteen channels is named after a particular organ. Each name refers to a pattern of energy, so the Stomach meridian concerns several processes of digestion, certain mental habits such as worry (which affects digestion) and a number of other functions including some associated with female reproduction (Hare, 1988). The meridians are paired. The seven running up the front are the 'yin' meridians, and those running down the back are the 'yang' meridians. In health, 'yin' and 'yang' energies are balanced and illness results when an excess or deficiency occurs.

Shiatsu aims to restore the balance, by application of gentle pressure at particular points along the meridian lines. These points often manifest as tender areas on the body during illness and usually disappear after treatment.

Box (1984) advocates its use in relieving minor ailments such as frontal headaches, by applying firm pressure to the head at the base of the skull and by pressing for a few minutes on a point between the thumb and first finger. The technique can also be employed to help people suffering from respiratory disease such as asthma, as described by Hare (1988). She believes the intervention is easily incorporated into traditional nursing routines, and provides an alternative to chest physical therapy. Box (1984) suggests the therapy could be included in daily care such as during a bed bath or pressure area care, to facilitate relaxation, improve sleep and relieve pain.

Aromatherapy

As with 'massage', the term 'aromatherapy' is a recent description of a very ancient practice. Since 2000 years BC in China, the earliest documentation available, aromatic essential oils have been noted for their healing properties (Arnould-Taylor, 1990; Davis, 1988; Tisserand, 1990), and evidence exists of their use throughout the Egyptian, Greek and Roman Empires (Arnould-Taylor, 1990).

Through the 18th, 19th and 20th centuries the oils have been used medicinally, aided by increasing scientific investigation into their properties.

The oils are described as life forces, or plant hormones containing the 'personality' of each plant (Tisserand, 1990). They are present in the plant in the form of tiny drops, and methods such as distillation are employed to extract them.

Though having certain similar properties (for example, all essential oils are anti-bacterial), the essences have differing individual effects. They are balancing in nature and are used to maintain mental, physical, emotional and spiritual equilibrium (Davis, 1988).

Treatment methods include compresses, inhalations, baths and most importantly, massage. This latter method combines the effects of massage, touch and essential oils. It represents the most effective treatment technique. Diluted in vegetable oil (usually 2–3% solution; Davis, 1988) the small aromatic molecules pass through the skin to the bloodstream where they are dispersed to all regions of the body.

Apart from the physical effects of the oils, they can also exert a profound psychological effect.

Williams (1989) describes how olfactory nerve fibres are in direct communication with the limbic system of the brain, which is the seat of our feelings and emotions. He believes that odours can affect our moods and our memories.

Interest in aromatherapy as a therapeutic discipline is growing rapidly with many recent articles (for example, Wise, 1989; O'Byrne, 1990; Passant, 1990; Shemesh and Mayo, 1991) reflecting its appeal, especially amongst nurses. The oils are mainly used for treating minor ailments and skin problems (Passant, 1990) and, most especially, stress and emotional difficulties (Passant, 1990; Wise, 1989).

Massage

As one of the oldest forms of treatment known to man, massage has been used for healing in many different cultures – Ancient China, India, Egypt, as well as the Greek and Roman Empires (Maxwell-Hudson, 1989; Arnould-Taylor, 1989).

In the East it has remained an integral adjunct to medicine using an instinctive reaction to 'rub it better', combined with traditional remedies and techniques. In the West, however, such traditional healing has been overshadowed by the scientific revolution and the training and specialization of healers, i.e. doctors (Maxwell-Hudson, 1989). More recently, though, the therapeutic value of massage has once more been recognized and modern massage incorporates new techniques such as 'Swedish Massage', introduced by Per Henrik Ling in the early nineteenth century. This method involves a series of systematic techniques including effleurage (stroking), kneading and pressing areas of soft tissue to bring about relaxation. Usually applied to muscles, it can benefit tendons and ligaments also.

Massage has both a physiological and psychological effect (Davis, 1988; Maxwell-Hudson, 1989; Arnould-Taylor, 1989). During massage the general level of nervous tension is reduced, causing reduced muscle tension, improved circulation, a lowering of both heart rate and blood pressure and it results in a feeling of well-being and relaxation (Jackson, cited by Byass, 1988).

These effects not only heal the body but soothe the mind and strengthen the spirit.

Arnould-Taylor (1989) describes how fast pressure movements speed up the body's physiology, whilst slow, gentle effleurage has a soothing effect, calming the nerves and enabling the patient to relax. Byass (1988) also comments on how massaging a grossly lymphoedematous arm not only encourages lymph drainage, thereby maximizing comfort, but also conveys gentle acceptance through touch. "For patients who create barriers to communication, touch through massage can be a means of bridging gaps without offence or invasion of personal space." It also allows the release of tension and pent up emotions (Byass, 1988; Davis, 1988), so the person is left with a feeling of well-being and energy. As Davis (1988) states, massage can re-educate the individual to be aware of physical stress and tension which normally results from being mentally tense. Once the physical stress becomes uncomfortable, the mind becomes uneasy and so a vicious circle results. Massage can break the chain of events preventing real physical symptoms that are stress induced.

It is important to remember that the giver of the massage can receive positive benefits too. Performing a massage is relaxing and it is rewarding to promote a feeling of well-being in a person who may have little to feel good about (Byass, 1988).

Reflexology or Reflex Zone Therapy

Reflex Zone Therapy derives from an ancient Chinese and Indian diagnostic and therapeutic technique. Hillman (1986) describes how it was rediscovered in the West by Dr. William Fitzgerald, an American E.N.T. specialist in the early part of the 20th century. He described invisible electric currents running through the body to delineate ten major linear zones. On massaging particular points, beneficial effects were seen in other parts of the body.

It was discovered that the hands and feet were especially sensitive areas to the technique. Thus the therapy has traditionally been concentrated in these areas with most reflexologists treating the feet alone.

The technique involves 15 minutes to an hour's massage using the hands in a skilful, specially taught, grip sequence (Evans, 1990). Specific sites corresponding to particular organs are 'massaged' to alleviate symptoms and prevent disease.

As Dobbs (1985) describes, Reflex Zone Therapy is based on several differing hypotheses, none of which is confirmed.

The energy hypothesis

Energy circulates rhythmically via pathways. Through reflexology, blocks in the energy pathways can be removed allowing continuous recirculation.

The lactic acid hypothesis

Lactic acid is believed to crystallize into deposits over the corresponding area of a diseased organ. These deposits can be felt as 'gritty' areas and are tender and painful to massage. Frequent Reflex Zone Therapy breaks down these deposits releasing the energy to recirculate (Hillman, 1986). Wagner (1987) states that this theory has generally been supplanted.

Hypothesis of the proprioceptive nervous receptors

Some researchers believe there to be a nervous connection between certain parts of the feet and hands and organs in the body. Thus treating the hands and feet directly affects the body.

Hypothesis of the endormorphines

Reflexology releases these substances which are known for their ability to activate the immune system and to control pain (Clinical Feature, 1988).

Hypothesis of the relaxing effect

The relaxation caused by reflexology helps remove tension and stress often manifesting itself in physical symptoms.

Psychological hypothesis

Reflexology provides physical contact and allows demonstration of care and concern, thus increasing the persons's feeling of well-being. Certainly, some practitioners believe that a positive attitude towards recovery from the patient can increase the rate of improvement (Hillman, 1986).

Reflexology is suggested to be of value in a wide range of ailments including disorders of the musculo-skeletal system; functional disorders of the respiratory, genito-urinary, lymphatic and endocrine systems and can be used to stimulate circulation (Wagner, 1987).

Reflexology is primarily a treatment that promotes and maintains health by prevention. Wagner (1987) sees reflexology as relaxing and harmonizing allowing the nervous system to calm and the individual to communicate any underlying problems or stresses.

Therapeutic Touch

Therapeutic Touch is derived from the ancient practice of laying-on of hands (Jurgens, Meehan and Wilson, 1987), and is "based on the proposition that the healer can act as a channel transferring energy to the patient" (Turton, 1984). It is not performed within a religious context and the ability to practise it effectively is considered a natural human potential by Krieger (1975). Dr. Dolores Krieger, a professor of nursing at New York University, introduced Therapeutic Touch to nursing. Turton (1984) describes her technique. First the healer centres (assumes a state of meditative awareness) by placing his or her hands two to four inches from the body of the individual. The energy field surrounding the individual is then assessed and mobilized to reduce and redirect areas of tension.

Krieger believes this form of healing to be a natural potential for nurses who are usually strongly motivated to help those that are ill. She also believes that as a tool it is used by nurses in the care of their patients, knowingly or unconsciously (Krieger, 1975).

A small amount of literature discusses the use of therapeutic touch in nursing. Macrae (1979) discussed its role in pain relief. Heidt (1981) monitored its effects on the anxiety levels of hospitalized patients. However, Jurgens *et al.* (1987) describe criticisms of the techniques employed during the research and questions its appropriateness as a nursing intervention.

The appropriateness of a specific complementary therapy is influenced by a number of factors and must be tailored to the specifics of each individual.

The appropriateness of a complementary therapy

As an accountable practitioner the following key questions need to be considered when offering complementary therapies to patients.

1. The patient's informed choice/preference
2. The patient's current condition
3. The plan of Medical Treatment
4. The environment
5. The patient's planned activities
6. The practitioner's skills
7. The practitioner's workload

THE RESEARCH

Much of the research into acupressure has investigated its effects on nausea and vomiting. Stannard (1989) noted reduced levels of nausea in 18 patients receiving cytotoxic drug therapy, after the P6 Nei-Kuon acupuncture point was pressed. The trial resulted in decreased amounts of anti-emetic drugs required, reduced laundry costs, more effective use of nursing time and in some cases patients were discharged earlier. The trial, though not meeting accepted research criteria, indicated to Stannard a need for further research and a randomized controlled trial.

Barsoum *et al.* (1990) performed such a trial on 162 general surgical patients, randomly assigned to receive P6 pressure bilaterally, control treatment with dummy pressure bands, or an anti-emetic injection of prochlorperazine. The severity of nausea was significantly reduced ($p = 0.002$) in patients receiving true acupressure in comparison with both the placebo group and the group receiving routine prochlorperazine. Both these studies seem to confirm the value of pressure at P6

in the control of nausea and vomiting, in clinical conditions in which these symptoms are a problem.

Davis (1988) cites a research study showing that natural pain killing endorphins are produced when specific acu-points are pressed. She states that "both neurochemical experiments and anecdotal accounts support the likelihood of hormonal changes and immune system stimulation from acupressure."

Box (1984) believes acupressure has much to offer nursing and has employed pressure techniques for relaxation and to relieve minor ailments such as frontal headaches. The author's own experience has also found pressure points for headaches and nausea to be effective.

Research concerning aromatherapy remains limited, though this should change as its popularity grows. However, one recent study was undertaken by Chrissie Dunn (1991) in the intensive care unit at the Battle Hospital, Reading: 122 patients admitted to the unit over a 14 month period were randomly allocated to one of three groups. Group one had aromatherapy using grape seed oil, group two had aromatherapy with a 1% solution of lavender oil diluted in grape seed oil, and group three was the control group. The massage took approximately 15–30 minutes, and the control group was given a similar amount of undisturbed time. The massage concentrated upon those areas which are known to be especially relaxing, i.e. outer limbs, back, scalp, although the choice was determined by other factors such as patient's preference, or illness. No significant differences in physiological stress indicators (blood pressure, pulse, and respiratory rate) were seen between the three groups. However, analysis of the behavioural scores (levels of anxiety, general mood and ability to cope in intensive care) showed significant proportions of patients whose anxiety was improved from aromatherapy compared to rest, but no significant differences between the proportions for the aromatherapy and massage groups. Qualitative data was also assessed in some of the patients and yielded such comments as:

"Very relaxing. Helped ease the pain and stiffness in my joints."

"The massage really helped ease the pain I

had, and helped me sleep at night. The smell of the oil helped me feel clean again."

Though small, this study indicates that aromatherapy and massage can help lower anxiety levels and improve an individual's ability to cope whilst in the critical care environment. Perhaps the aromatherapy might have yielded more significant results if the lavender oil had been applied in a greater concentration (3% dilution) or another essential oil had been used. Future studies into the use of aromatherapy in critical care are planned at the Intensive Care Units at the Bristol Royal Infirmary and at the Middlesex Hospital.

Research into the anti-bacterial nature of essential oils has been conducted since 1887. Tisserand (1990) cites a study by Kar and Jaim where lemongrass oil was found to be slightly more effective against *staph.aureus* than *penicillin*, and much more so than *streptomycin*. Tisserand also notes that tea-tree oil is "the single most effective and least harmful anti-microbial oil. Effective against *candida albicans* and *trichomonas vaginalis*." A letter to *The Lancet* (1991) reports the successful treatment of a vaginal discharge by a five-day course of tea-tree oil pessaries, each containing 200 mg of oil. Shemesh and Mayo (1991) also investigated tea-tree's natural antiseptic and anti-fungal properties, by treating various skin disorders and moniliasis of the throat and mouth with 1% tea-tree lozenges, 5% cream and pure oil. Of the 50 patients, 49 were cured of their monilial condition after one to four weeks. Shemesh and Mayo (1991) recommend that "tea-tree oil offers a natural, less expensive, effective alternative to currently used drugs" for such conditions, and that "its side-effect profile is superior to most products currently prescribed."

Wise (1989) has found lavender oil to be effective in the relief of migraine after surgery, and uses it in conjunction with rose-geranium as a pre-operative bath to sooth anxiety. She also comments that leaving essential oils in boiling water near a bed promotes deep breathing in her experience. This has obvious benefits for those recovering from anaesthetic. Helen Passant (1990) has also found lavender useful for migraine and for aiding sleep. On her ward, caring for elderly dementia patients, there has been a dramatic reduction in the use of conventional sedatives since essential oils have been incorporated into nursing care. She also notes how the use of oils has changed the ward atmosphere, "making it less clinical and more homely."

Though massage has been used for centuries and its benefits are widely known, there are relatively few research studies examining its use within nursing. Longworth's study (1982) on normotensive college students found slow-stroke back massage resting and relaxing, and causing lower generalized muscle tension. A similar study by Simms (1986) assessed the effect of slow-stroke back massage on six female patients with breast cancer, who were receiving radiotherapy treatment. Such patients are known to have high anxiety levels associated with fears of disfigurement, burning and of being surrounded by large complex machinery. When compared with a control intervention of lying down for a similar period of time, those receiving the back massage reported fewer symptoms of distress, higher degrees of tranquillity and vitality, and less tension and tiredness.

Results from the measurement of physiological changes after massage appear less conclusive. Dunn's (1991) study produced no significant difference in physiological parameters after massage. In contrast, Ashton (1984) describes "a profound state of relaxation induced by massage with which the breathing deepens, the heart rate slows, blood pressure lowers and the parasympathetic nervous system moves towards a correct balance." White (1988) also quotes sources suggesting that the relaxation induced by massage deepens breathing, reduces oedema, enhances blood and lymph circulation and aids a decrease in pain.

Some of the data available concerns the massage of neonates, especially those that are pre-term. Many critical care units nurse sick babies, and massage has been shown to have profound effects on their health. It has been estimated that they are handled 130 times in every 24-hour period (Wolke, 1987), causing sleep disruption, bradycardia, apnoea, behaviourial distress and other problems (Pohlman and Beardslee, 1987). A study at Missouri University on 16 babies found that only 15.4% of contacts were involving comforting touch, and those babies that were ventilated received the fewest number of comforting touch contacts (Paterson, 1990).

One study by Field *et al.* (1987) involved 40 pre-term infants, 20 of whom received massage/passive movements for 15 minutes, three times a day for ten week days. A control group of 20 received no stimulation. Clinical and behavioural variables were measured. The results showed a greater weight gain and superior performance on development assessments across the first six months for the group of infants who received the massage. This was thought to be due to an increase in somatotrophic or growth hormone. This study concluded that "regardless of the underlying mechanism, providing massage for pre-term neonates appeared to be a cost-effective form of facilitating their growth and development." An earlier study by Taylor (1983) describes the massages carried out on babies in the Unit where she worked. She believes the infants responded positively to deliberate gentle handling and that if taught properly massage can help relax the parents and increase their confidence in handling the baby. Other studies not statistically conclusive have highlighted the mother's (parent's) increased pleasure in giving massage.

Though objective evidence of the therapeutic value of massage is scanty, individual reports from individuals describe a feeling of improved well-being and of feeling relaxed and rested.

As with most other complementary therapies there is no specific research pertaining to critical care, but reflexology has been used successfully as an adjunct to treatment in oncology nursing, with cystic fibrosis sufferers and for post-natal problems.

In her article, Barbara Zeller Dobbs (1985) describes how she and two colleagues decided to practise reflexology with terminal oncology patients. Specifically, they assessed its potential in "diminishing fear of loneliness and isolation; contributing to decreased pain; providing an opportunity for patients to receive physical contact in an acceptable, non-aggressive way; facilitating the presence of loved ones and/or care givers; and promoting a state of relaxation." Seven terminally ill patients formed the basis for the study, and were cared for several months before their death. Reflexology was used purposefully to decrease pain that broke through the relief provided by their analgesic medication. Other beneficial effects also appeared: "Patients expressed feelings of being less aban-

doned and the families expressed satisfaction at seeing that something painless existed that could help their relative. In three situations we taught a relative how to use reflexology and the benefit seemed to have been as important for the relative as the patient."

When Sarah Wynn in a clinical feature (1988) used reflexology she found it suitable in relieving some of the symptoms associated with cystic fibrosis especially shortness of breath and chest pain. She says "most of the time, patients don't know the intricacies of the treatment, but are relaxed and have some of their symptoms relieved." To quote one young sufferer: "At first I didn't know which part represented which organ, but it was still working. There is no way it can be psychological. It helps me get my breath back straight away and the chest pains subside within half an hour. If my chest feels very tight, it helps me cough up a lot of sputum." Another area of nursing where Reflex Zone Therapy can provide relief from problems is midwifery. Though usually far removed from critical care nursing Evans' (1990) use of reflexology has its own relevance. She describes treating the zones relating to kidney, bladder and solar plexus for 20 minutes in those women having difficulty passing urine post-delivery. Evans describes treating several mothers successfully, thus avoiding catheterization. She has also successfully relieved the discomfort caused by wind. The babies are not forgotten. When restless, they are settled with a gentle stroking of the feet in the zones of the intestines and solar plexus, to help soothe them.

Research into therapeutic touch has been mainly concentrated within the framework bound by valid scientific methodologies and this has led to criticisms. Krieger's (1975) study indicated the possibility that therapeutic touch may have the potential to raise haemoglobin levels, but the study's research methods were criticized for not yielding scientifically valid results. Heidt (1981) reported a significant decrease in situationally induced anxiety in hospitalized cardiovascular patients who received therapeutic touch compared with patients who received casual touch or verbal interaction. Again, criticisms were levelled at the study, in which Heidt herself provided all the treatments. One study by Fedoruk, as cited by Jurgens *et al.*

(1987), reported a significant decrease in a physiological indicator of stress in premature infants in an intensive care unit, when they received therapeutic touch compared with a mimic treatment or simply the presence of a nurse. In another study, therapeutic touch or a mimic were assessed for reducing abdominal pain. Findings showed the standard narcotic analgesic to be much more effective, and no significant difference emerged between therapeutic touch or a mimic. In general, research into therapeutic touch seems to provide little evidence either for or against its benefits beyond a placebo.

Research methodologies and complementary therapies

It seems appropriate to discuss the importance of scientific validation in complementary therapy research because the verification of benefits such therapies have to offer continues to be a contentious issue. Though there appears to be little doubt that people do benefit from complementary therapies, these results are not easily accounted for by conventional Western scientific measurements. Until the criteria for conventional measurements are improved in scope, it seems doubtful whether complementary therapies will attain any recognition. The British Medical Association reviewed six major 'alternative' techniques in 1986 concluding that alternative remedies had no scientific basis, were based upon untheoretical assumptions and could not be recommended (BMA, 1986). Arguments against this dismissal focused on the invalidity of the tests which employed methods based on the medical model. Therapists rejected these as inappropriate.

It can be argued that traditional quantitative research methodologies consider only parts of the whole, in direct opposition to the principles of holism, that the whole is greater than the sum of its parts. Perhaps consideration of both quantitative and qualitative methodologies would yield a research basis that was reflective of the whole (Bockman and Reiman, 1988).

Traditional medicine has generated the need for results that can be replicated and generalized to groups other than the sample and this has led to reducing the phenomenon to be studied into smaller parts easily controlled and manipulated in laboratories. Nursing also seems to have emulated such models, rejecting qualitative studies in favour of quantitative ones. But qualitative research is needed to explore those human phenomena about which little is known and which cannot be broken down into small pieces without losing sight of the whole, or for those that are too esoteric for examination in the laboratory. Quantitative research, in contrast, generates new knowledge in basic sciences, explores etiologies and predicts outcomes of intervention and care.

One solution to the problem, advocated by Professor Christine Webb of Manchester University, is the use of the 'action research process' which incorporates a variety of research methodologies, and specifically provides findings that are easily incorporated in patient care. Such a process could help meet the need for appropriate research methods which are sensitive to the practice of complementary medicine. Another necessity is for cooperative projects between orthodox medical researchers and complementary practitioners.

PRACTICAL NURSING IMPLICATIONS

The research base concerning the benefits of complementary therapies is growing, but at present little data directly relates to their use within nursing, especially in the critical care environment. Despite this, I believe critical care units could benefit enormously from the incorporation of unorthodox therapies into nursing care, provided they are implemented cautiously and their use is well evaluated. Though the results of research into some therapies is inconclusive, most appear to profit the patient and, more importantly, positively affect the 'quality of life' of many individuals as revealed by the anecdotal data. Perhaps it is this intangible benefit that accounts for the recent increase in popularity of 'alternative' treatments.

For a brief moment remember (if you can) the first time you entered a critical care unit. For most of you this will have taken place as part of your work as nurses. Perhaps you were still a student nurse, or it was your first day as a staff nurse on a unit. Can you remember how you felt, the sounds, what caught your eye (apart from the bright lights), the impressions the medical and nursing staff made on you? For each of you memories of, and responses to, this event will be unique and will vary according to the reason for being there, previous experience and the environment itself. My memories include: feeling daunted by the number and sophistication of the machinery around the beds; adjusting to the loud alarms and the continual cycling noises from the ventilators; and noticing the staff looking knowledgeable and busy, charting recordings, administering drugs and performing chest physiotherapy, amongst other things.

In recalling your feelings when entering a critical care unit you will probably find them similar to those experienced by relatives and patients. As nurses, however, we have the advantage that some aspects at least of the environment are familiar to us. Relatives, on the other hand, may never have seen or been in a critical care unit, enhancing the stress from the environment and adding to anxieties about their loved one.

Equally stressed may be the patients who, on admission to the unit, suddenly find themselves in isolated, alien and noisy surroundings, cared for by busy nursing and medical staff concerned with recording endless observations and administering a plethora of drugs and fluids. The patient may be unable to talk, see or hear clearly, and may be completely immobilized because of the illness, drug therapy or simply terrorized by the thought of dislodging any of the multitude of drips or monitoring equipment attached to them. Often they may be experiencing pain, and all this whilst separated from relatives and friends for long periods of time.

Research exploring patients' recollections of their critical care experience has highlighted stresses including difficulty resting and sleeping, pain and discomfort, physiotherapy, management of tubes, immobility and thirst, among others (Ballard, 1981; Wilson, 1987). It has been suggested (Anderson, cited by Simpson *et al.*, 1989) that coronary care unit patients experienced isolation, shock, disbelief and memory loss for the first 24 hours, compared with intensive care patients who remembered mainly noise, nightmares and helplessness. Pain and immobility were common stresses to both types of patients whilst cardiac patients highlighted increased anxiety due to the monitoring system. The researchers' suggestions were to focus nursing care on alleviable stresses whilst helping patients cope with those that are not reducible.

Physical contact communicating reassurance and caring is a potential way of reducing the stresses of being in critical care. But the need for physical contact (McCorkle, 1974) is often not met (Barnett, 1972), perhaps due to lack of time or because depersonalizing the individual reduces the personal stress we feel as nurses and carers. Even when touch is used it is rarely expressive (Weiss, 1986), and this can add to the patient's feelings of isolation and alienation.

One explanation for lack of expressive touch involves Maslow's hierarchy of needs. Hudack *et al.* (1986) state that "the need for a sense of security to allay anxiety is always present but that it is superseded by more basic needs", for example, at a time of low cardiac output or difficulty in breathing. Thus in critical care, meeting physical needs is a priority and once that has been achieved then the nurse, as patient's advocate, can help the individual attain security, a sense of belonging, and self-esteem. The nurse is then able to facilitate the patient's adaptation to the situation allowing the energy bound up in stress to be utilized effectively. Examples might include aiding the patient to synchronize with the ventilator, helping the patient relax enough to sleep or promoting effective coughing to remove sputum.

Supporting the individual physically, using outside interventions of medication, technology and interaction to conserve energy, reduce physical requirements and allow recovery but necessitate some loss of control for the patient, which in turn can lead to feelings of insecurity. Individuals may feel unsafe about the equipment surrounding them and its reliability, the unfamiliarity of being in hospital, or even the competence of the nurses caring for them.

All the complementary therapies previously considered can help reduce stress and anxiety and increase the individual's sense of well-being and self-esteem. They can be used effectively to promote security and help meet the critically-ill individual's human needs, whatever the stage of illness, overnight post-operative management, short-term recovery from illness, long-term recovery after multi-system failure, or in the terminal stages.

Massage, with its soothing and calming influences, can reduce anxiety, promote sleep, perhaps with a reduction in the amount of sedatives used, and bring comfort. Abdominal massage can relieve wind and constipation, toning the gut and improving its functional ability. Combined with aromatherapy, muscular aches, pains and cramps can be eased and can temporarily alleviate the discomfort associated with oedematous limbs.

Aromatherapy can both stimulate and sedate. Particular combinations of oils can promote sleep, help relieve aching joints and encourage deep breathing and expectoration after an anaesthetic. Certain oils may also be important natural treatments for *candida albicans*, often a problem for patients with a suppressed immune system, or on large amounts of antibiotics. Psychologically, too, use of aromatherapy can lift the mood of patients and improve their feelings of well-being.

Reflexology has been used to relieve urinary and sputum retention as well as discomforting constipation. Acupressure has been demonstrated to be effective in reducing the pain from headaches and in stopping nausea, especially if acupressure bands are applied. Therapeutic touch, though found to be inconclusive when researched, forms an important component of all the other therapies and can aid relaxation and perhaps bring about healing.

Training

Many of the complementary therapies require considerable training if they are to be used safely and effectively. The training usually consists of completing a minimum number of theory and practice hours and successfully passing written, practical and sometimes oral examinations. Once entry requirements are passed, many therapies have registers identifying competent practitioners. Courses range from weekends spread over from six months to three years to intensive week-long training sessions leading to qualifications varying from diplomas to degrees and PhDs.

A good training is essential to give a sound knowledge base in the subject. Fears are that the individualistic basis for certain therapies could be lost in the overgeneralization of treatments given by enthusiastic nurses, who have not enough knowledge to use the treatments discriminatingly (Rankin-Box, 1991). Box sees training through appropriate bodies as essential especially with the proposed legislative changes in 1993 and free trade throughout the European Community.

Until recently, training standards have fluctuated from establishment to establishment with it being possible to become a public practitioner with minimal training. Other countries such as Italy, Germany and Holland have legal guidelines, and advice is given on all aspects of practising complementary therapies. In Britain we, too, need to have national standards of training agreed by all parties if complementary therapies here are to survive the formation of the European Market. Wright (1991) believes nurses can enhance the standing of 'alternative' therapies in society because they provide such a force for change. He adds, though, that nurses must be seen to be adhering to standards of training and be instrumental in deciding standards within the NHS by way of policy formation, for example.

How to develop the use of complementary therapies in nursing

☐ Explore the information available on the different complementary therapies through the literature, searching current journals, or perhaps by organizing a study day or seminar and inviting guest therapists or practitioners.

☐ Having raised awareness about certain therapies, then select one for your nursing area remembering that some represent systems of medicine, such as acupuncture and herbalism; some are more diagnostic, such as iridology and others, such as aromatherapy and massage, are primarily therapeutic in nature. In selecting a therapy concentrate on its specific application to critical care. Review current research and assess how it might enhance patient care.

☐ Begin to search out possible training establishments and courses remembering that to be used effectively a high standard of training is necessary. If a course interests you check that it is properly validated.

☐ Explore the legal implications of using complementary therapies at work by contacting your union or the United Kingdom Central Council for advice. Further professional indemnity insurance may be needed.

☐ Prepare relevant information concerning the therapy chosen including a brief resumé, pertinent research and the reasons for its proposed integration in patient care. Allow discussion amongst colleagues by presenting the data at a multidisciplinary meeting. Any discussions must include relevant research so that the benefits to be gained by a therapy's use are highlighted. Take into account the research methodology used as this can significantly affect the research findings.

☐ Investigate the existence of a regional health policy for the integration of complementary therapies into practice and, if one does not exist, consider helping to develop one. At present, Bath is the only authority to have developed a policy (Armstrong and Waldron 1991).

☐ If you discover a suitable course then become a qualified practitioner. Note that until recently nurses often funded themselves; this can be costly, both in time and money. It may be hoped, however, that having convinced your manager of the benefits of being able to offer complementary therapies to patients, unit funds or at least study leave might be available.

☐ Once you qualify, be prepared to undertake research in your area to enhance the credibility of your practice. Further research is necessary if complementary therapies are to become an integral aspect of professional nursing practice in the future.

CONCLUSIONS

The ever increasing technology of critical care can make it possible to lose sight of the patient. Refocusing on the person as an individual can be achieved by using complementary therapies as a natural extension to good nursing practice. Some therapies, though inappropriate in caring for the acutely ill, can be of great benefit to individuals recovering and preparing to leave the unit, also to relatives, dying patients and the staff, too.

The public are becoming increasingly aware of complementary methods of healthcare, and many people are expressing an interest in receiving such care in conjunction with orthodox systems of treatment. For this reason, it is important that nurses have a basic knowledge of the different benefits offered by these therapies and how they might be incorporated into nursing practice. For this to be achieved there is a need for more research. To be able to say that it has helped a patient, but not to be able to give the extent or predict outcomes, invites uncertainty – a feature of many of the interventions we use daily at work. If used carefully there are few indications that such therapies are harmful and many individuals are convinced that they can help. Compared to many of today's accepted procedures, unorthodox practices are not life threatening or invasive. Incorporated into care they can help balance the scientific knowledge acquired through modern technology with the intuitive knowledge of the art of healing which has been enjoyed throughout mankind's history.

CASE STUDIES

Case study one

Clare Davis is a student in her early 20s who has been admitted to a critical care unit with status asthmaticus. This is her first admission to hospital and she is acutely anxious, has markedly, laboured breathing, tachycardia and diaphoresis.

Infusions of Aminophylline and Salbutamol are already being administered in conjunction with continuous Salbutamol nebulizers, though in Clare's distress she keeps removing the mask because it irritates her. She sits hunched on the bed, shoulders and back tensed with stress, further constricting her chest by her body's position.

By massaging Clare's shoulders and back with Camomile (anti-spasmodic) and Frankincense (decongestant, antibacterial, slows and deepens breathing) aromatherapy oil (3% dilution), it was slowly possible to encourage her to relax her shoulders and control her breathing. She was also continuously supported through touch and vocal encouragement to calm her.

After some minutes Clare began to relax and her breathing gradually became less laboured. Later, having avoided intubation, she was transferred to a general ward to complete her recovery.

Afterwards, she commented on how useful the aromatherapy massage and breathing instructions had been in relaxing her. She feels herself becoming tense and starting to panic as soon as the asthma begins, and realizes this exacerbates the problem. She agreed that perhaps relaxation and breathing control exercises might improve her ability to cope during future asthma attacks, and hoped to find a yoga class to attend.

Case study two

One afternoon I was asked to help the mother of a young baby who was very sick on the critical care unit. The mother, Ann, had been unable to sleep since her young son had been admitted two days previously. She was very anxious, tearful and in desperate need of sleep. It was suggested that an aromatherapy massage might help her relax and Ann agreed to 'give it a try'.

She was made comfortable on the overnight-stay bed on the unit, not far from her son, and after explaining what the massage would involve I mixed some Lavender Oil (3% dilution) to relax her and promote sleep. As the massage of her feet proceeded she commented on how she felt as though she was being relaxed from the head downwards, which corresponded to the reflexology areas I was pressing as I massaged her. Before the end of the massage she was deeply asleep and awoke six hours later feeling calmer, more rested and able to cope.

KEY TERMS

Holistic medicine

Concentrates on treating the ill person as a whole, making the physical, emotional, psychological and spiritual aspects equally important.

Complementary therapy

Provides additional support to the orthodox method of treating the critically ill.

Acupressure

Involves firm and gentle pressure applied to the energy points (tsubos) lying on the meridians.

Meridians

Are 14 channels running through the body each named after a particular organ, e.g. stomach meridian.

Aromatherapy

Is massage, inhalation and baths using essential oils.

Essential oils

Are aromatic oils extracted from plants and trees.

Massage

Is a series of systematic techniques including effleurage (stroking), kneading and pressing of soft tissue to bring relaxation.

Reflexology

Massage of particular points of the body which benefits other parts of the body – especially feet and hands.

Therapeutic touch

The laying on of hands or healing considered a natural human potential not performed within a religious context.

Action research process

Incorporates a variety of research methodologies and specifically provides findings that are easily introduced into patient care.

FURTHER READING

Arnould-Taylor, W.E. *The Principles and Practice of Physical Therapy. 2nd Ed*. Cheltenham: Stanley Thornes, 1989.

Arnould-Taylor, W.E. *Aromatherapy for the Whole Person*. Cheltenham: Stanley Thornes, 1990.

Davis, P. *Aromatherapy an A–Z*. Saffron Walden: C.W. Daniel and Co., 1988.

Hudak, C., Gallo, B.M., Lohr, T. *Critical Care Nursing: A Holistic Approach. 4th Ed*. Plymouth: J.B. Lipincott Co., 1986.

Maxwell-Hudson, C. *The Book of Massage*. Colchester: Ebury Press, 1989.

Tisserand, R. *Aromatherapy for Everyone*. London: Arkana, 1990.

Wagner, F. *Reflex Zone Massage. The Handbook of Therapy and Self-help*. Glasgow: Thorsons, 1987.

Williams, D. *Lecture Notes on Essential Oils*. London: Eve Taylor, 1989.

REFERENCES

Armstrong, F., Waldron, R. A complementary strategy. *Nursing Times*. 1991; 87(11): 34–35.

Ashton, J. In your hands. Holistic health 6. *Nursing Times*. 1984; 80: 54.

Ballard, K. Identification of environmental stresses for patients in a surgical intensive care ward. *Heart and Lung*. 1981; 3: 89–108.

Barnett, K. A theoretical construct of the concepts of touch as they relate to nursing. *Nursing Research*. 1972; 21(2): 103–110.

Barsoum, G., Perry, F.P., Fraser, I.A. Post-operative nausea is relieved by acupressure. *Journal of Royal Society of Medicine*. 1990; 83: 86–89.

B.M.A. *Alternative Therapy: A report of the Board of Science and Education*. London: BMA., 1986.

Bockman, D., Reiman, D. Qualitative versus quantitative nursing research. *Holistic Nursing Practice*. 1988; 2.

Box, D. Made in Japan. Holistic health 3. *Nursing Times*. 1984; 80: 139–140.

Byass, R. Soothing body and soul. *Nursing Times*. 1988; 84(24): 39–41.

Dennerley, M. The nature of I.C.U. nursing. *Nursing*. 1991; 4(26): 30–32.

Dobbs, B.Z. Alternative health approaches. Oncology Nursing 6. *Nursing Mirror*. 1985; 160: 41–42.

Dunn, C. Staying in touch. *The International Society for Quality Assurance in Health Care*, Washington, DC. 1991; May 29–31.

Evans, M. Reflex zone therapy for mothers. *Nursing Times*. 1990; 86(4): 29–31.

Field, T., Scafidi, F., Schanberg, S. Massage of preterm newborns to improve growth and development. *Paediatric Nursing*. 1987; 13(6): 385–387.

Hare, M.L. Shiatsu acupressure in nursing practice. *Holistic Nursing Practice*. 1988; 2(2), May: 68–70.

Heidt, P. Effect of therapeutic touch on anxiety level of hospitalized patients. *Nursing Research*. 1981; 30: 32–37.

Hillman, A. Zone Therapy. *Nursing*. 1986: 6: 225–227.

Hillman, A. Alternative medicine – an introduction. *Nursing*. 1986; 1: 26–28.

Jurgens, A., Meehan, T.C., Wilson, H.L. Therapeutic touch as a nursing intervention. *Holistic Nursing Practice*. 1987; 2(1): 1–13.

Krieger, D. Therapeutic touch: the imprimatur of nursing. *American Journal of Nursing*. 1975; 5 May: 784–787.

Lancet. Letter. *The Lancet*. 1991; 337 (8736): 300.

Longworth, J.D.C. Psychophysiological effects of slow stroke back massage on normotensive females. *Advances in Nursing Science*. 1982; July: 44–60.

Macrae, J. Therapeutic touch in practice. *American Journal of Nursing*. 1979; April.

McCorkle, R. Effects of touch on seriously ill patients. *Nursing Research*. 1974; 23(2): 125–132.

O'Byrne, J. The smell of success. *Nursing Standard*. 1990; 4(47): 23.

Passant, H. A holistic approach to the ward. *Nursing Times*. 1990; 86(4): 26–28.

Paterson, L. Baby massage in the neonatal unit. *Nursing*. 1990; 4(23): 19–21.

Pohlman, S., Beardslee, C. Contacts experienced by neonates in intensive care environments. *Maternal-Child Nursing Journal*. 1987; 16(3): 207–226.

Rankin-Box, D. Proceed with caution. *Nursing Times*. 1991; 85(45): 34–36.

Ryman, D. The sweet smell of success? *Nursing Times*. 1984; 80: 48–49.

Shemesh, A., Mayo, W.L. Tea-tree oil – natural antiseptic and fungicide. *International Journal of Alternative and Complementary Medicine*. 1991 (Dec); 11–12.

Simms, S. Slow stroke back massage for cancer patients. *Nursing Times and Nursing Mirror*. 1986; 82: 47–50.

Simpson, T.F., Armstrong, S., Mitchell, P. Patient's recollections of critical care. *Heart and Lung*. 1989; 18(4): 325–332.

Smith, M. Healing through touch. *Nursing Times*. 1990; 86(4): 31–32.

Stannard, D. Pressure prevents nausea. *Nursing Times*. 1989; 85(489): 33–34.

Taylor, P.S. Massage in a special care nursery. *The Australian Nurses Journal*. 1983; 12(7): 42–45.

Turton, P. The laying on of hands. Holistic health 4. *Nursing Times*. 1984; 80: 47–48.

Webb, C. *Day Conference on Complementary Therapies*, Manchester, 1991. Northern Institute of Complementary Therapies.

Weiss, S. The language of touch. *Nursing Research*. 1986; 28(2): 76–80.

White, J.A. Touching with intent: Therapeutic massage. *Holistic Nursing Practice*. 1988; 2(3): 63–69.

Wilson, V. Identification of stressors related to patients' psychological responses to the surgical intensive care unit. *Heart and Lung*. 1987; 16: 267–273.

Wise, R. Flower power. *Nursing Times*. 1989; 85(22): 45–47.

Wright, S. *Day Conference on Complementary Therapies*. Manchester, 1991. Northern Institute of Complementary Therapies.

Wolke, D. Environmental neonatology. *Archives of Disease in Childhood*. 1987; 62(10): 987–988.

Wynn, S. Reflex zone therapy. *Nursing Standard*. 1988; 2(17): 28.

Section 2
EDUCATION AND MANAGEMENT IN CRITICAL CARE NURSING

This section examines fundamental issues in the institution which influence the care of the critically ill adult. Emphasizing practical skills throughout, the chapters in this section look at the contribution of education and management to the delivery of quality care.

6
EDUCATION FOR CRITICAL CARE NURSES

Helen Ellis

CHAPTER AIMS

The aims of this chapter will be to highlight the balance needed between training and education. Many educational changes are facing critical care nurses, in the immediate present and over the next decade. As professional nurses, critical care staff are faced with the problem of how to respond to the needs of the patient and families who come into their care. They need to decide upon the balance of education and training required to perform their role competently, effectively and in a cost-effective way, yet retain the insights that experience, problem solving and accountability bring to their practice. To achieve this clarification the chapter will deal with:

☐ The problem of what critical care nurses need to know, i.e. the problem of training 'needs' and 'continual professional education'.

☐ The impact of the educational changes arising from P2000 and PREPP.

☐ Flexible pathways for professional education.

INTRODUCTION

The debate surrounding the issue of professionalization of nursing has been linked to the two key words 'education' and 'training'. Training on the one hand argues that nurses have always been in an apprenticeship system, learning practical skills in the clinical setting from those already practising, or as Fish and Purr (1991) put it, "sitting by Nellie." Education, on the other hand, calls for each nurse to practise from a broader base. To be a professional, the nurse requires knowledge from a range of theoretical framworks – physiology, sociology, psychology, to name but a few. A nurse's standing as a professional requires the additional knowledge to practise with due regard to the moral, legal and professional aspects of the work in any clinical setting. This knowledge is seen to be ongoing, and is not necessarily learnt from her peers in the clinical setting. Defining the terms 'education' and 'training' enables critical care nurses to clarify their professional standing within the multidisciplinary health care team.

IMPLICATIONS IN PRACTICE

Although many changes affect the critical care unit from the outside, there are training and educational implications that need to be addressed from within the unit:

☐ the current status of specialist training courses;

☐ the development of a clinical learning environment;

☐ the role of the mentor and preceptor as an expansion of the role of the critical care nurse.

All staff involved in critical care nursing will need to maintain an interest in the education of critical care nurses, both as providers and recipients of training and education. An educated and trained group of nurses can:

☐ achieve a high level of job satisfaction through their increased understanding and involvement in critical care work;

☐ provide a motivated group which attracts and retains new staff;

☐ deliver a consistently high standard of care to the patients and families who come into their units.

This vested interest in education for critical care nurses occurs against the backdrop of rapid medical and technological changes in the field of critical care, and a wider backdrop of changes in the funding and resourcing of all health care workers.

Education versus training

Education – the act or process of acquiring knowledge; the knowledge or training acquired by this process; the act or process of imparting knowledge; the theory of teaching and learning; a particular kind of instruction or training (*Collins Dictionary*, 1988).

Training – the process of bringing a person to an agreed standard of proficiency by practice and instruction (*Collins Dictionary*, 1988).

These two definitions accurately reflect the core dilemma facing those nurses who are striving for the education of critical care nurses. Training is a basic foundation to enable the work of a critical care unit to continue, and many clinical nurses are adept at a range of clinical skills. However, the definition of education would describe a critical care nurse as someone who gains knowledge, and in so doing 'learns' what to do with that knowledge. For many nurses the critical care unit is the arena in which they practise nursing or teach others how to practise nursing. Yet there exists a real

division between those nurses who 'can do' and those nurses who 'can do' but also know 'why they do as they do'. This division highlights the impact of both training and education – and is clearly distinguished by Fish (1989), who discriminates between training as 'learning from practice' and education as 'learning through practice'.

The nurse who is trained in critical care nursing will have many complex and technical skills to hand, acquired from observation and continuous practice under supervision until he or she is able to perform the skills alone. The more the skills are repeated, the more proficient the nurse becomes. This can lead to efficient nursing as long as the skills are appropriate to every new situation. On the other hand, the nurse who is educated in critical care nursing performs nursing activities in such a way that he or she learns from the situation – something which is "of more significance than the ability to repeat the original activity" (Fish, 1989). By learning through practice, the critical care nurse can adapt to new situations using a range of skills and move on to becoming an expert nurse, one who has a wide perceptual grasp of the situation to hand (Benner, 1984). Fish and Purr (1991) astutely observe that the professional dilemma facing nurses is that the training and educational needs of nurses have never been clearly thought out and articulated.

What does the critical care nurse need to know?

Any new nurse entering the critical care unit begins a new career phase where new skills will have to be learned. Both old and new skills will need to be applied within a new environment, and in very different situations than before, and the nurse will have to begin to incorporate them into a comprehensive framework for practice through experience and reflection. It is generally accepted that the clinical skills aspect of critical care nursing will come first. Clinical staff are generally more concerned with workload, and take the pragmatic view that the work needs to be done, and to do the work certain practical skills are necessary.

Johnson (1968) points out that "knowledge differs in kind not amount. It is the difference between *knowing that* and *knowing how*, and *knowing why*, and *knowing what*." The 'knowing that' relates to the theory underlying practical skills, and the 'knowing how' relates to the skill itself, i.e. practical knowledge. Any new nurse facing the critical care unit with its complex machinery, alarm systems and highly dependent patients, and faced with a group of nurses who can deal with the surrounding technology with varying degrees of competency, will be fired with the desire to know how it all works. Many nurses report that on beginning work in the critical care unit they are unable to focus on the patient until the technology is assimilated and it begins to sink into the background (Fitter, 1987). Learning how to move and handle the critically ill patient who is attached to and invaded by the machinery becomes paramount. Until this is mastered, the nurse cannot begin to concentrate upon the patient as a person and begin to try to meet their complex emotional needs. Once 'knowing how' is mastered, 'knowing that' can be concentrated upon, and the nurse begins to seek for explanations and reasons for the practice. As soon as the nurse understands the theory underlying the practice, he or she can begin to 'know why' certain practices are maintained, and as a consequence can begin to make choices in the application of clinical practices to different and changing patient situations. The difference between *knowing that* and *knowing how*, and *knowing why*, and *knowing what* leads to the development of autonomous clinical practitioners.

It can and does take time for the four aspects of knowledge to become inextricably linked in any area of nursing practice. Benner (1984), in a study of critical care nurses, highlights the stages that nurses pass through to become 'expert' in their field. Five stages are identified from novice, advanced beginner, competent, proficient through to expert.

☐ The novice has rule governed behaviour. As they lack experience of the situations they face, they can only fall back on rules. Benner argues that the following rules can actually prevent successful nursing as the rules cannot tell a nurse how to prioritize tasks or how to do them.

☐ The advanced beginner is coping better than the novice. This a nurse who has had enough experience to be able to grasp certain aspects of situations. The advanced beginner is still needing support from more experienced nurses.

☐ The competent nurse is one who has been in similar situations for at least two years. Such nurses can cope with and manage the situations that arise within their speciality.

☐ The proficient nurse can understand the situation as a whole. Decision making is more effective and requires less painstaking thought than before.

☐ The expert nurse does not depend on rules or guidelines. With a large amount of clinical experience under the belt, such a nurse demonstrates an intuitive grasp of a situation and can concentrate immediately and directly on the problem at hand. According to Benner (1984), the expert operates from a deep understanding of the total situation.

In the development of her ideas regarding expert clinical nurses, Benner and Wrubel (1982, p. 13), in an earlier paper, summed up the development of skilled knowledge, pointing out that the "beginner must rely on a deliberative analytical method to build the clinical picture from isolated bits and pieces of information. The expert has the skill and the option to grasp the situation rapidly, to see the whole." To progress from the novice stage, with its narrow focus on training in procedures and skills, the critical care nurse needs an education.

Benner's study (1984) was based on the Dreyfus model of skill acquisition, and is underpinned by the idea that theoretical knowledge (*knowing that*) and practical knowledge (*knowing how*) are different. The value placed upon the different forms of knowledge by nurses has been very different, with the highest value placed on the theoretical knowledge and the practical knowledge given low esteem. Benner's work begins to stress the importance of practical knowledge. This knowledge is skills-based, and comes from a large amount of experience. Nurses who are expert will have attained a high enough theory level and synthesized this with their practical experience. In fact, both forms of knowledge are important. What nurses need to know is how to synthesize their theoretical knowledge with their practical knowledge, and in the context of the wider issues in health care apply it to professional autonomous decision making.

It is hard to distinguish between education and training for the registered nurse. There will be times when both are needed, and a balance needs to be achieved between the two. From the perspective of the organization, there is a clear relationship between training and needs. As a critical care unit caters for critically ill patients who are highly dependent upon nursing staff, there are specific training needs. Such needs are those involved with the management of patient care in a highly technological environment, e.g. setting up a ventilator, being able to perform endotracheal suction, being able to lift an unconscious patient, being able to pass a nasogastric tube. The unit needs staff who can perform these skills with dexterity, effectiveness and efficiency. Critical care staff wish to be able to perform the required skills. By doing so, they can demonstrate their value to the unit and rapidly become part of the team and gain a sense of belonging.

The relationship between the organization and education is not so clear. Education implies that learning has occurred. Education will take place within the critical care unit in formal or informal ways. Staff may attend in-service programmes, discussion groups, study days and conferences, or simply learn from their previous experience through reflection. Learning cannot be controlled. It is hard for the manager who is attempting to provide both training and education to find a balance. Because training is objectively assessed and monitored, and it does help to get the work of the unit carried out, the trap is to fall into the provision of funding of study time which is seen to provide for training needs only. Benner's work has highlighted the importance of practical clinical know how, yet the nurse cannot progress to the expert stage until he or she understands as an individual the crucial difference between training and education. Education requires reflection and thought to learn and grow as a professional. Many critical care nurses who appear to be highly skilled in their work struggle to explain the theory underpinning their practice – they do not know what the ventilator

readings mean, they find it hard to interpret the changes they observe in their patients. What is wanted is the ability to think constructively about their practice, reflect upon it and learn from it. This ability can be stimulated from within the critical care unit through the development of a stimulating learning environment, or by specialist support through courses and attached educational staff. These issues are developed further in the chapter.

P2000 – A new preparation for the future critical care nurse?

Project 2000 is a significant change affecting pre-registration training for first level nurses. It emphasizes the need for education as well as training, in that education is seen as the "preparation of reflective autonomous practitioners" (Fish and Purr, 1991). It began as a project in 1984 under the auspices of the United Kingdom Central Council (UKCC) to clarify the education and training needed for the professional nurse of the future. The project looked towards the 1990s and beyond, and so took its name. After lengthy and detailed consultation with the professions of Nursing, Health Visiting and Midwifery, the final proposals were laid out in 1986 in its major report, *Project 2000: A New Preparation for Practice*. The factors which led to this review of the preparation for practice were those of demographic change, a need for a cost-effective delivery of health care and a shift towards the prevention of ill health and a community-based health care provision. These are factors which will affect the critical care nurse in the future.

The changing demographic patterns predicted for the 1990s and beyond centred upon the problems that the profession would face in recruitment. It was predicted that the number of school leavers would fall, and that nursing would be in direct competition with other forms of employment for these people. To maintain a flow of people into the profession and to maintain a steady number of nurses, the UKCC identified three areas which would need attention:

- [ ] registered staff wastage;
- [ ] wastage during training and on completion of training;
- [ ] nurse returners.

These areas are of importance to critical care units as they cannot afford to lose registered staff who have the experience and skills suited to the needs of the critically ill patient and their family. In times of staff shortage or periods of intense activity in the critical care unit, the units have to look towards the use of bank nurses who may have returned to nursing after a break of service. Along with staff retention, all critical care units need to attract new staff, and are increasingly coming into competition with other areas in the hospital for the newly registered nurse.

The UKCC took the view that the future for the nursing profession would be composed of a single level of registered nurse who would provide care with the help and support of advanced or specialist practitioners and support workers. This view is slowly being recognised through the growth of national vocational qualifications (NVQs) as a competency based training for health care assistants. The role of health care assistant in the critical care area is being scrutinised and many critical care units may find that these 'new' staff members will be replacing or supplementing registered nurses. It is beyond the scope of this chapter to pursue this issue, but further data will be needed to analyse the impact of NVQs on critical care nursing. It is probable that all competencies in nursing practice will be related to the NVQ scheme in the future,

Predicting the future is a hazardous occupation. Many of the predicted issues expressed during the development of P2000 have not developed as expected. The nature of registered staff wastage, considered to have its origins in dissatisfaction with terms and conditions of employment, and alternative attractive careers, has altered to one of reduced nursing budgets, ward and hospital closures and staff redundancy. The economic recession has encouraged many professionals to remain in their present jobs and the newly qualified nurse is having trouble finding employment on a long term basis. P2000 is also undergoing evaluation with many concerns being expressed regarding its administration, student support and effectiveness for clinical practice. However the basic premise of P2000 will remain, as nursing education continues to look to the future and responds to rapidly changing clinical needs. Whatever the outcome of P2000

evaluation, the future critical care nurse will have experienced a different preparation for practice than the core of registered nurses, who are presently working in them, and the mix of staff will take many years to work through. Their preparation will be one focused on the concept of health; on the prevention of ill health and the promotion of good health. This preparation may appear to contrast oddly with the work of the critical care unit with its focus on the physiological stabilization of the critically ill or injured person. However, within the institutionalized setting of the general hospital, the movement of the person towards health is supported by a broad multidisciplinary approach, and the work of the critical care nurse will form only a small part of this overall system.

Registered staff who have not experienced Project 2000 preparation have expressed their concern over their ability to work with or manage this 'new breed' of nurse. The Project 2000 nurse ought not to pose a problem but rather a challenge. To meet this challenge, many nurses have long been aware of the need for a continuing education in nursing. Davies (1990), in a report for the English National Board, outlined issues relating to broad employment trends within nursing, and proposed educational strategies for consideration. Basing her thoughts upon Handy's work (1984), she outlined five key principles which are easily related to the education of registered nurses:

1. All nurses will want and need more education at many different times in their career.
2. Nurses can learn in many different ways and nursing therefore needs many different ways of assessment.
3. Learning can happen in any setting.
4. Nurses should have more scope to arrange their own pattern of learning.
5. The health service must recognize its role in the provision and facilitation of learning.

These issues are in the process of being addressed by the profession, and the following sections on PREPP, Credit Accumulation Transfer Schemes and the Accreditation of Prior Experiential Learning will reflect these issues.

PREPP – Implications for critical care nurses

The Post Registration Education and Practice Project (commonly known as PREPP) was a long overdue review of the needs of registered nurses, and a recognition that education is the necessary ingredient in the many processes that are at work forming the professional nurse. PREPP has been before the profession and the UKCC since the late 1980s. In May 1989, the Educational Policy Advisory Committee had certain recommendations approved by Council – namely that a major project on post-registration education and practice should be initiated. The recommendations emerged from a recognition of four elements influencing the overall practice of nursing today:

☐ educational provision and policy;
☐ requirements for continuing competence to practise;
☐ the meeting of health needs;
☐ changing health and social policies.

It was recognized that there was a pressing need for explicit Council standards relating to the whole area of post-registration education and practice. Post-registration practice and education is affected by the prevailing health and socio-economic policy. Underlying all of the above issues is the role of the UKCC in protecting the public through its responsibility towards standards of education and practice.

The PREPP report (1990) was grounded in an ethos of change. The overwhelming conclusion of the PREPP report was that the "professions are profoundly affected by an environment of rapid change. What is needed above all else, therefore was a strategy for coping with uncertainty." The change will be experienced through the changing demographic trends, altered epidemiology, changing life styles and health inequalities and the impact of the NHS and Community Care Act 1990. Briefly, the demographic trends show that the proportion of elderly people in the UK is expected to increase further, and the report cites a 1990 Joseph Rowntree Foundation Report which stated that the birth rate since 1973 has fallen below that needed to maintain the population size. If the birth rate remains low, the labour force will rapidly decline after 2006. The number of school leavers is forecast

to decline at record speed, with a reduced pool of entrants into nursing. As patterns of disease alter, the nursing profession must change to keep abreast of altered health needs, and as social change continues the profession must change to accommodate altered health promotion strategies and become increasingly involved in political debate and policy.

The working parties developed a model to show the three main planks of the PREPP project, which are surrounded by the UKCC's standard framework. A working group was set up to examine each of the three themes of:

☐ the nature of professional practice;
☐ the process of professional education and development;
☐ the requirements for continuing competence for practice.

The working groups provided a paper for discussion and debate within the professions to test reaction. Road shows were held, the proposals regarding the model were discussed and debated throughout the profession. From this came *The Report of the Post Registration Education and Practice Programme*, with its recommendations for the maintenance of a quality service provided by educated registered nurses (see Table 6.1).

The overall response to the nine recommendations was one of overwhelming support. But what are the implications for critical care nurse? The following points are made to show that change in such a wholesale way will not be easy and that critical care nurses need to be flexible in their responses and start thinking about and discussing the proposals in the PREP document and the latest consultative document on the Proposed Standards for Post registration Education (1993).

☐ Proposals 1 and 2 outline the need for support when entering a new workplace, both for the new practitioner in his/her first employment and for the nurse who changes career pathways. At present, the support of new staff in critical care units may be formally recognised within individual hospitals or may not be recognised at all. The quality of the support will vary, now and in the future, according to the present clinical conditions at the time, such as workload, staffing levels and the expertise

Table 6.1. The PREPP proposals.

1. There should be a period of support for all newly registered practitioners to consolidate the competencies of learning outcomes achieved at registration.
2. A preceptor should provide the support for each newly registered practitioner.
3. All nurses, midwives and health visitors must demonstrate that they have maintained and developed their professional knowledge and competence.
4. All practitioners must record their professional development in a personal professional profile.
5. During the three years leading to periodic registration, all practitioners must complete a period of study or provide evidence of appropriate professional learning. A minimum of five days of study leave every three years must be undertaken by every registered practitioner.
6. When registered practitioners wish to return to practise after a break of five years or more, they will have to complete a return to practise programme.
7. The standard, kind and content of preparation for advanced practice will be specified by the Council. Advanced practitioners must have an appropriate Council-approved qualification recorded on the register.
8. To be eligible to practise, individuals must every three years:

   □ submit a notification of practice;
   □ EITHER provide verification that they have completed their personal professional profile satisfactorily; OR show evidence that they have completed a return to practise programme; and
   □ pay their periodic fee.

9. Practitioners after a break of less than five years returning to practise using a specific registered qualification shall submit a notification of practice and, within the following calendar year, provide verification that they have completed their personal professional profile satisfactorily.

Recommendations 1 and 2 were statements of good practice, and recommendations 3–7 were intended to be statutory requirements.

of the current staff. This recommendation will formalise the period of support that a new nurse receives when she enters a critical care unit. However, it is not a guarantee of 'quality' support.

□ Preceptorship is developing with the advent of courses specifically developed for such a role (In a following section this role will be discussed in more detail). The educational and service implications involved in the development of this preceptor role are numerous, with staff needing to be released for study time to prepare for the role, and educational staff needing to prepare for the study time, both in the college and clinical setting. The preceptor role will require monitoring and many staff may well experience role strain with the formal addition of this role to their ongoing clincial and personal development.

□ The council has accepted the recommendation of the project that a minimum of five days of study leave every three years should be allowed for each practitioner. It is sad that education and training for post registered nurses has in the past had low profile. Unlike our medical colleagues, study leave has not been regarded as a requirement for practice by managers or by nurses themselves. Obviously such a requirement would need extra staff and finance. The UKCC has ruled that the employer will have to foot the bill for mandatory continuing education (Tattam 1991) and further discussions are pending with the government over funding and legislation. it is not known what form the managerial issues will take e.g. will extra staff be supplied to cover mandatory periodic refreshment or will critical care units run short staffed? These points continue to be debated.

The PREP Project (1990) and is allied report on the Proposals for the Future of Community Education and Practice (1991) provided the basis of the third report on the Proposed Standards for Post Registration Education (1993). The PREP proposals, although not fully in place or underpinned by full financial support, seem to be generally accepted by the profession. Proposal 7 opened the way for the debate over the nature of advanced practice and the remaining proposals have been subsumed into the concepts put forward by the 1993 report. This report proposed a model for post registration education which rests upon three areas of practice – primary, specialist and advanced.

(Midwifery is explicitly recognised as a separate profession with three identified areas of midwifery practice – primary, enhanced and advanced). The model has received a critical response from the profession and confusion reigns over the proposed classifications and their appropriate academic preparation.

The impact of these reports on critical care nurses will take time to be seen in practice. However, they should provide a bench mark for a minimum standard of educational development. The individual nurse and the unit manager will need to decide upon the nature of that development – will it be through training for a new skill or will it be broader based education? The development of a reflective practitioner will be through reflection, and the use of a personal journal. These activities are reflected in the development of the English National Boards' Higher National Award which, along with PREPP, makes use of a flexible approach to continuing education.

Flexibility in education

At the same time that work was being carried out on PREPP (under the auspices of the UKCC), the English National Board was funding a three year training and education project which has culminated in the ENB Higher National Award – a system of education study and attainment based on a number of themes and validated through centres of higher education to degree level and beyond. A framework for Continuing Professional Education was developed, based upon a training needs analysis which attempted to uncover the professional educational needs of nurses, midwives and health visitors (Larcombe and Maggs, 1991). At the heart of any continuing education programme lies the divide between 'needs' and 'wants'. The skills and the education that nurses need to carry out their role may not coincide with the nurse's individual wants or desires. It was recognized that there are various factors influencing the continuing education of nurses:

☐ the organization's goals and its monitoring of the goals;

☐ the manager's needs for a trained workforce;

☐ the professional's training needs and professional desires;

☐ the availability of courses in general and the availability of specific required courses to meet identified needs;

☐ the availability of staff to attend courses.

Despite these factors, Larcombe and Maggs (1991) recommend that there should be a close relationship between the employer and the employee, with both being sensitive to the other's requirements. Although individual nurses need specific skills, they also need a professional perspective from which the skills can be used. Professional nurses have to make decisions about the use of their skills in relation to patient care every working day. Continuing professional education for nurses has to take this into account, and provide a variety of avenues for nurses to learn new skills, update old ones and enlarge their professional perspective.

The framework is considered to be a "flexible system for the organisation and delivery of continuing professional education." This framework consists of ten key characteristics or aspects of nursing that each professional nurse must master so that a high standard of care can be delivered to their patients. Table 6.2 outlines the ten key characteristics which are combined to culminate in the Higher Award. The key characteristics have been applied to the critical care nurse, but are the same for any practitioner in any field of practice. The 'framework', or ten key characteristics, is generally being used as a template upon which to develop courses leading to the Higher Award – a degree for nurse practitioners. This award is viewed as an academic (the level of study required will be to first degree level) and a professional award.

Using the framework, critical care nurses can identify, together with their managers and associated educational staff, the particular educational or training needs both for the unit and the individuals concerned. Each nurse can take a different route and method of study within a flexible time limit. Whether or not the critical care nurse decides to study for the Higher Award, the vision for the future is that all professional continuing education will develop in a system of modules for which nurses can gain academic credits.

Table 6.2. The ten key characteristics of the framework for continuing education (adapted for critical care nurses).

1. Professional accountability and responsibility within the critical care unit.
2. The development of specialist skills and knowledge relevant to critical care.
3. The development of a research base for practice in critical care.
4. The ability to work in a multidisciplinary team.
5. The ability to be innovative and flexible in critical care nursing practice.
6. The understanding of the process of health promotion and preventative policies within the critical care unit.
7. The ability to act as a mentor/preceptor for learners and junior staff.
8. The ability to take informed decisions regarding the availability of resources for individual patient care.
9. Evaluation of patient care and participation in unit audit.
10. The management of changing practices within critical care.

Modules or individual programmes can be developed to suit a range of clinical needs, both for training and education. The underlying aim is that they will prevent repetition in courses. Each module will demonstrate clearly stated course content and objectives, and will be allocated a certain number of academic credits. Each student can then accumulate credit towards the Higher Award from a whole variety of learning experiences and in a variety of subject areas. This system is often referred to as the CAT (Credit Accumulation and Transfer) system. It allows for learning, wherever it occurs, and provided it can be assessed, to be considered for credit towards university degrees. Whilst nurses and their managers are planning to meet service needs, professional needs can also be met, and nurses can take a personally planned route towards the achievement of a degree. Within this system critical care nurses could transfer their accumulated credits towards another course of study without having to repeat course work.

Learning can also be assessed on a professional basis. Many critical care nurses acquire skills, knowledge and expertise through many different experiences, through paid and unpaid work, and through attendance at study days and conferences. This learning through practice can be incorporated into the routes for professional and academic qualifications. Systems are being developed to provide for Assessment of Prior Learning (APL) and the Assessment of Prior Experiential Learning (APEL). The difficulty lies in matching prior learning and previous experience to some form of quantifiable standard. A document will be needed within which the critical care nurse can keep a record of his or her own learning and clinical experiences, in such a way that it acts both as a record of recognized learning, but also as a reflective record of clinical practice. Both the UKCC and the ENB have developed portfolios for the clinical nurse. The ENB portfolio is linked to the Higher Award and the UKCC portfolio is awaited, but may well be a simple record of achievements to provide a record for mandatory periodic refreshment.

The place of specialist critical care courses

Despite the changes occurring in pre-registration nurse training, the latest UKCC proposals and the work of the National Boards to provide a coherent strategy for continuing professional education, the specialist critical care courses continue, although in different forms according to the relevant National Board. All subscribe to the need for a planned progression of knowledge, and a reduction in repetitive learning. It is recognized that the courses dealing with critical care nursing in one form or another are well established, and generally, provision of these courses is adequate compared to other specialities such as general surgery and medicine, where no courses, as such, exist. Despite this, there is a continuing shortage of critical care nurses with their specialist certification working in critical care units. To change this balance the government in 1990, made available additional funding to enable extra training places. There is as yet no evaluation of the effect of this intervention. However, demand for the critical care course remains high, yet many staff cannot get secondment from their employer due to the impact of resource management and the need for cost cutting exercises in line with government directives.

For each ENB critical care course there is an outline curriculum produced by the board, although many are out of date. In recognition of the changing educational needs an ENB circular (1989/27/AS) gave guidelines for fundamental changes in the structure and nature of critical care courses. The length of the critical care courses was to be reduced to 24 weeks, with the theoretical content making up at least a third of this period. This was in recognition of two factors. First, critical care managers were finding it difficult to release staff for six months to attend a specialist course on full secondment, and were unable to afford a replacement. Secondly, it was recognized that many staff come to the courses with wide clinical experiences and they did not need the longer clinical input. Due to the increasing difficulty experienced by staff in gaining secondment to critical care courses, the Board felt that part of the practical placement should be held in the course members own unit. Each course is approved by the ENB through an educational officer who visits the centre prior to course validation by the Board. A variety of criteria arc assessed, such as the ratio of course members to registered staff; the size and workload of the critical care unit; the number of staff able to act as mentors; and the educational facilities for course members and staff education and training.

Critical care course curricula are being redesigned across England and Wales to meet the changing educational needs of the professional nurse. In the circular it was pointed out that there should be no repetitive learning across the critical care courses on offer in one centre. The pattern tends to be one of a common core curriculum which all critical care course nurses will study, with branches off to the relevant specialism, e.g. accident and emergency nursing, intensive care nursing. This core and cluster approach has been interpreted in different ways, and individual colleges have developed a variety of methods and routes to achieving a diploma or degree in critical care nursing.

It would appear that with the development of the Framework for Continuing Professional Education and the development of CAT systems that the existing critical care courses will continue, but in such a way that they fit into the new systems being devised. The existing courses could simply be cre-

dited with a number of credit points which the successful course member can then accrue against further studies. The courses may become more modular, with the course members taking modules as required over a designated time period. Each module may be credited and built into an individual package for continual professional learning. This would recognize the individual critical care nurse's level of clinical experience and previous learning. A more flexible approach will need to be taken as schools of nursing have now amalgamated into Colleges of Nursing. Each college may include two to four previous schools. Colleges of Nursing are now in the process of further amalgamations, and in a variety of ways are linking up with centres of Higher Education, either as associated colleges or as departments of nursing within the higher centre. The amalgamations may mean that the number of centres running set 24 week courses has been reduced; yet demand for the courses remains high. A flexible, modular approach is the route for the future to manage the level of demand that currently exists in the clinical setting for such courses.

The critical care unit – a learning environment?

Within the five principles described by Davies (1990) are two points of relevance to the critical care unit; that nurses can learn in many different ways; and learning can happen in any setting. The influence of the clinical learning environment for nurses has always been recognized, but through the impact of the student nurse as a apprentice learner and therefore as an essential part of the workforce. The debate over student or worker status for student nurses has resolved itself through the Project 2000 proposal for student status. Many critical care units may not take student nurses, others may see them for a relatively short time during their three year programme. Despite this, the development of a clinical environment in the critical care unit which encourages learning is of equal importance for students and registered staff.

In 1977, Bendall pointed to a fundamental flaw in the structure of nurse education as it was then and to a certain extent is so today, when she said that "those who were to be the official teachers were removed from the practising role, but a training programme was drawn up with an emphasis on learning by experience in a service context." Kitson (1985) points out that this split between service and education left nursing education in a "position of weakness", for while it teaches theory and identifies necessary skills, "the unspoken assumption is that you cannot learn about nursing without 'doing nursing'." This experiential aspect of learning to be a nurse, either at the student level or at registered nurse level, is strongly influenced by the clinical staff and the clinical learning environment that develops from the values held by the clinical staff and their willingness to teach, supervise, assess and mentor new staff.

The teaching role of the clinical staff has received much attention after the Report of the Committee on Nursing (1972) pointed out that "there is a fairly large body of opinion which is not satisfied with the amount of quality of instruction on the wards from staff nurses and sisters" (para. 21). Although the Committee felt that "every qualified nurse or midwife should in some sense be an educator", it appears that the main responsibility for ward teaching stems from the ward sister. The organization of work within a critical care unit is different to that of a general ward with respect to the high level of patient dependency and the staff:-patient ratios. The main responsibility for teaching may well lie with a number of sisters/charge nurses and senior staff nurses. Various research projects have outlined the teaching role of the sister, and these will be applied to the teaching role of the experienced nursing staff in the critical care unit.

To provide an effective teaching role the critical care nurse must:

☐ Be a role model. Orton (1981) set out to examine the role of the ward sister in relation to student nurse learning on the wards. Her review of the literature confirmed her view that "the ward sister is the most influential person dominating the scene." Gott (1984) demonstrated that the behaviour of clinical role models was more influential on the development of student nurses than that of teaching staff.

☐ Teach the new nurse in a variety of ways, using the clinical experience to help the new nurse learn. Fretwell (1982) recognized that the

teaching responsibilities may be demonstrated through role modelling, active teaching (such as designated 'teaching sessions') and covert teaching (through experience and feedback).

☐ Attend courses to enable nurses to effectively recognize and develop their own teaching skills and to utilize the clinical environment as an effective learning tool.

The clinical learning environment was mentioned by Revans in 1964, who indicated the need for an environment in which nurses could ask questions about the patients and their own studies. Orton's (1981) study emphasized the importance of a good learning climate, and was illustrated by earlier studies undertaken by several other authors (McGhee, 1961; MacGuire, 1969; Davies, 1971; Bendall, 1975). Orton's work established that for wards which fell at either end of a continuum running from 'high student orientation' to 'low student orientation', the concept of a ward climate existed as "an identifiable, psychological reality for students on whom it had a very powerful effect." Those wards which had a high student orientation demonstrated an approach consisting of teamwork, consultation and an awareness of the needs of learners by senior staff. This was further verified by Fretwell (1982) who found that in an ideal learning climate the sister was democratic, patient-orientated and saw the students as learners rather then workers. Fretwell's learning environment was one of teamwork, negotiation and communication.

The points highlighted by the various studies can be taken for the critical care unit. Many critical care units have more than one sister/charge nurse running the unit. Experienced staff nurses are also forming part of the core team of staff who need to be working towards the establishment of a learning environment. It is more than the provision of educational facilities, such as blackboard, slide projector or overhead projector. The learning environment within the critical care unit is created through supportive and interested staff who recognize the value of educating other staff as well as themselves. A positive learning environment can lead to staff retention and development. In the past, nursing officers considered that two years was the expected amount of time that a staff nurse ought to stay on one ward. Once the two years was up it was thought that any nurse 'worth her salt' ought to move on for promotion. This led to the stable core of staff having to continually start over with new staff development. With changes within the nursing profession such as primary nursing and resource management, it is unavoidable, but it is desirable that staff stay and pursue clinical and professional development for the benefit of the ward and the patients on that ward. Their contribution to the learning environment can enhance the training and education of all staff.

Teaching roles in critical care – the mentor and preceptor

It is generally accepted that clinical practice and education for clinical practice should be closely linked. Yet there is discussion in the nursing literature regarding the theory–practice gap (Orton, 1981; Ogier, 1982; Alexander, 1982). The closure of the theory–practice gap is directed towards ensuring that what is learned in both the classroom and the clinical setting corresponds, and that knowledge gained is validated through research. Up until the 1980s the role of the clinical teacher was developed to act as a stepping stone between theory and practice. Not an easy role, it suffered from the conflicting demands of the service and educational sides of the health service. At the same time in the clinical setting there was a degree of support present in the wards from the senior staff. This support tended to be unstructured, and varied tremendously in its process and goals. As the role of the clinical teacher shrank the teaching and educational role became focused on the ward sister.

The emphasis laid upon the ward sister's role in teaching is increasingly being spread over a wider area. With the ENB (1987) recommending that each learner nurse should have a mentor on each ward to support and to facilitate learning, the concept of mentor slipped into everyday use for student nurses and for nurses on post-registration courses. The recommendations of the PREPP report now concentrate on the development of a 'preceptor' role for the newly registered nurse or the nurse in a new clinical environment. However, there is still debate as to the role of a mentor and a description of both the mentor and preceptor role will require clarification (Burnard, 1990; Morle,

1990). For the purposes of this chapter, the term 'mentor' will relate to nurses either at pre-registration level or undertaking post-registration courses, and the term 'preceptor' will relate to the support of a new nurse within the critical care unit.

Examining the mentor role, it appears that there is little consensus as to what it is and how it usefully can be defined (Morle, 1990). In the United States the term 'mentor' was seized upon as a means of reducing reality shock (Kramer, 1978) which occurs when the values instilled in the newly registered nurse by the school come into conflict with the bureaucratic values of the workplace. It was pointed out that the typical, informal, *ad hoc* orientation to the workplace led to rapid staff turnover, early burnout and a lack of professional satisfaction at all levels of nursing (Shamian and Inhaber, 1985). The word 'mentor' was taken from the economic business schools where many successful business people attributed their success in the world of business to the presence of a mentor throughout their apprenticeship and consequent life.

In applying it to the world of nursing the concept of mentorship requires a different definition, as it is rare for a nurse to have one mentor throughout his or her career. Consequently, the role of a mentor was described in many different ways, and it was interchangeably used with that of 'preceptor'. As Burnard (1990) points out, the term mentor has been in general usage in the United Kingdom since the 1980s with little clarification of the role. In the United States, the term 'nurse-preceptor' is used to describe a unit-based nurse who carries out one-to-one teaching of new employees or nursing students in addition to her regular unit duties (Shamian and Inhaber, 1985). It is related to the teaching role within every nurses' work where a skilled practitioner helps a less skilled/experienced practitioner to achieve professional abilities appropriate to their role. In the United Kingdom the ENB has variously described mentor for student nurses as a 'wise reliable counsellor', an 'experienced, trusted advisor' (1987) and as 'supervisors, assessors and if possible, mentors' (1988).

Shamian and Inhaber (1985) reviewed the literature in the United States relating to the role of mentor/preceptor. They identified the following functions:

☐ to orientate the new nurse to the unit;
☐ to function as a teacher and a role model;
☐ to plan a programme for the new nurse;
☐ to carry out an evaluation of the new nurse's progress;
☐ to socialize the new nurse to the philosophy of the unit, to integrate him or her into the team and to inform relevant personnel of progress.

The mentor/preceptor role was seen to decrease as the new staff member became more confident and skilled in the role. The mentor/preceptor steps back and acts more as a resource person. The above functions are generally those of relevance to the critical care staff member acting as a mentor to the nurse on a post-registration course such as the ENB 100 (general intensive care nursing) course. On such a course the mentor role is of a short duration of two to six weeks. Due to the intense nature of such courses, the mentor will not become solely a resource person. All the above functions will be compressed into the short time scale. Such is the additional pressure of taking on a mentorship role that many units utilize a team approach to mentorship. One course member may have two or three unit staff allocated. One will be recognized as having the final responsibility for the support of the course nurse, one will act as mentor when the first mentor is off duty or has to work night duty, and the third may well be a fairly junior unit member who is observing the role.

The preceptor role outlined by the PREPP proposals will relate to a longer period of time – up to six months. In many critical care units there already exist in-house training programmes which all new staff undertake. These programmes may be formalized with the appointment of a sister with responsibility for new staff development, or be informal with a senior staff member overseeing and demonstrating particular skills that the new nurse needs to know. The aim of the preceptor is to ensure that the new staff member functions effectively and efficiently as a team member. The emphasis may well be on training, rather than education, as a pragmatic approach is needed to quickly develop a staff member who can work alone without constant supervision.

Who can be a mentor?

Shamian and Inhaber (1985) summarize the attributes of a mentor/preceptor as:

☐ a nurse who has years of experience
☐ a nurse who demonstrates leadership skills
☐ a nurse with the ability to communicate clearly and effectively
☐ a nurse with decision making abilities
☐ a nurse with an interest in professional growth.

If one went from the above points, it may be difficult to find enough nurses with all the skills required! There are few guidelines as to who can be a mentor. For post-registration courses, those staff who hold the same awards may act as mentors. Many staff have not been able to attend a specialist post-registration course in critical care nursing, and it is now being recognized that staff with many years experience can still act as mentors. All mentors are encouraged to gain extra teaching qualifications such as the ENB 998 (Teaching and Assessing) course, but the development of the mentor/preceptor roles still requires planned programmes. Shamian and Inhaber (1985) recommend that mentors/preceptors:

☐ should attend workshops in order to prepare for the role;
☐ have a role description;
☐ have ward-based manuals to explain the role and functions of the preceptor;
☐ should receive some kind of reward for the role as it requires preparation, practice and expertise.

The development of the mentor and preceptor role within critical care could have benefits for both the identified mentors/preceptors and the unit as a whole. For the individual nurse it could:

☐ provide a way of teaching nursing care strategies and facilitate the development of personal and social skills;
☐ enable the clinical role of the staff nurse to be

expanded through the addition of educational and training skills;

☐ enable personal reflection and a recognition of further educational needs.

For the unit as a whole the roles could:

☐ clarify the philosophies and values of the unit staff;

☐ assist in personal development plans and staff appraisal;

☐ encourage the development of an educational learning climate which encourages all staff to progress and develop;

☐ lead to a higher standard of care which is both demonstrated and articulated by all staff.

Shamian and Inhaber (1985) argue that such roles can only improve the situation all round:

☐ the college of education wins as its students are better prepared;

☐ the hospitals may gain due to improved staff retention and development;

☐ the mentor/preceptor wins as he or she grows professionally;

☐ the new nurse wins as adjustment to the new unit is smooth and uncomplicated.

At the present there has been very little research into these roles in the United Kingdom. It appears to be self-evident that the role is beneficial, and as such it will continue in all clinical settings.

Anecdotally, the development of the mentor role has led to an extra burden being placed upon the clinical staff. Staff shortages, rapid throughput of patients and a numerous array of changes having to be managed throughout the health service are all combining to form extra pressures upon the clinical work of the staff, which is essentially the care of patients. Although the student and post-registered nurse on a course receives the bulk of theory in the classroom, it has to be applied and refined through practice. The mentor is needed to facilitate this. For the new nurse working in a critical care unit with its bewildering array of technology and highly de-pendent patients, the preceptor role is essential to enable rapid transition from novice to at least that of the competent nurse. The preceptor role for the support of new staff members may well prove to be an effective tool for staff retention and develop-

ment. The emphasis laid upon the clinical unit as a learning and developmental environment is a fixed one, and staff will have to continue to juggle their roles. The development of the mentor role for learners and the preceptor role for new staff may well be the foundation upon which future stan-dards of clinical practice will rest.

CONCLUSION

For the development of a critical care nurse who is skilled in his or her field, learns through and from practice and is able to function as an autonomous professional nurse, both training and education are needed. The novice critical care nurse requires a training to help him or her function as part of a team. To move on to a higher level of expertise the critical care nurse needs experience. Experience does not mean that the nurse has to work for a certain number of years in one unit, or be placed in a senior position. "Experience means living through actual situations in such a way that it informs the practitioner's perception and under-standing of all subsequent situations" (Benner and Wrubel, 1982). The gaining of such experience needs an education. Many people need time and support to be able to reflect on practice, it is a skill which will not come easily to all nurses. Through attending study days, conferences and studying for higher degrees, nurses can develop this skill. The art of reflection will need to be incorporated into more courses and discussions as all staff will be required to reflect on their practice to assess their continuing educational needs.

A problem to be faced by all course organizers and staff in clinical placements, is the need for supernumerary status for the learner – whether the learner is at a pre- or post-registration stage of their career. Fish and Purr (1991) recognize this need, and reinforce the point that learning can occur if the learner has time to observe, question and reflect upon the clinical environment around him/her. For many critical care nurses, on specialist courses or at the beginning of their work in the unit, there is simply not the time to do this, and frequently the learner is having to act as part of the team due to staff shortages. Constraints on the learning experi-ence in any critical care unit arise from periods of work overload and staff shortages. Both these constraints frequently reduce the nurse's role to one of observing machines, giving medications and coping with patient crises. Having a high level of inexperienced or new nurses can also lead to staff fatigue, and the core of experienced nurses can only teach skills at a basic level through demonstration and role modelling.

The development of new frameworks for continuing professional education will need a lot of time and energy invested in them from clinical staff, managers and educationalists. Whilst new frameworks are being developed, ongoing training and educational needs have to be met. Underlying the recognition of such needs is the concept of quality assurance. It is recognized that by training and educating the clinical staff, the goals of the organization can be met – namely the provision of a quality service and a high standard of clinical care. The organization has to balance the achievement of these goals with the professional needs of the staff. Training and education have to occur in an environment which provides support, goodwill and recognition of the professional needs of the staff. If staff are developed into autonomous professional practitioners, they have to be allowed to practise as such.

The clinical environment has to cater for the training and educational needs of a number of nurses who will be at different stages of their development. Whilst recognizing their professional wants, the manager has to balance these against the critical care unit's needs for trained staff. In a cost effective health service, staff will probably have to be selected for specified skills training. Education and training have to balance against cost – the aim of the service being to achieve the highest standard of care for the lowest cost. For the first time in nursing history we have a proposal from the UKCC that the employer will pay the cost of the minimum five days periodic refreshment over three years. Whilst this may not seem a lot, it is a beginning. However, the responsibility for continuing education remains within the remit of the individual nurse.

The opportunities for critical care nurses to achieve their individual training and educational needs are now far wider than ever before. Critical care nurses will be able to choose their own routes through to higher education and the holding of one or more degrees. As flexible routes open up, learning will expand. The more the critical care nurse learns and the more he or she reflects on practice, the higher the quality of care delivered to the patient and his family will be.

CASE STUDY

You are a staff nurse, working in a busy adult intensive care unit. Attached is a four bed high dependency unit. Over the five years that you have worked in the unit you have undertaken the ENB 100 (general intensive care nursing) course on a six month secondment in a college which used two different intensive care units and a cardiac unit. You are now half way through a nursing degree which you are fitting into your busy home life with some financial support from your manager. You have not been successful in your application for study leave to continue your studies.

Your unit also runs the ENB 100 and you frequently act as mentor to the course members. Student nurses also visit the unit for three to four weeks at the end of their P2000 course. Having just returned from a two week holiday you return to work to find that you are nominated mentor for an ENB 100 course nurse, who started her unit allocation two days ago; two student nurses have been in the unit for a week and you note that a new staff nurse is starting on the unit in two weeks time in his first job – on a six month contract. Looking at the off duty you note that you are 'in charge' twice this week due to staff shortages.

STUDENT LEARNING QUESTIONS

Bearing in mind the above case study and your experience of your own clinical setting:

1. Consider why the ENB 100 nurse, the student nurse and the new staff member are on the unit and list for all three, the role of clinical practice in the learning experience.

2. Why does the ENB 100 nurse require clinical practice?

3. What can your unit provide from an educational, professional and clinical point of view for the student nurses?

4. For all three people, identify:
   The practical experience your unit can offer the student.
   The theoretical perspectives your unit can offer.
   The kind of practical experience you know your unit can offer.

5. Identify ways in which your unit:
   Can offer these experiences
   Can encourage learning through practice

6. What can be better learnt in practice rather than in a classroom?
   What can be better learnt in a classroom rather than in practice?

7. Should different staff members be allocated to mentor/precept these students?
   What are you looking for in an ENB 100 mentor/a P2000 mentor?

8. What are the needs of the new staff member over the first six months?

9. Using your thoughts from the above questions, devise a programme that would benefit any new staff member coming onto your unit.

KEY TERMS

Mentor

Historically, Mentor was the advisor of the young Telemachus in Homer's Odyssey and his role encompassed elements of guardianship, tutoring and support. Classic mentoring provides an informal link between two people who are willing to work with each other and provide wise advice, with no financial gain on either side. Various subroles have been identified in a mentoring relationship. They are those of 'advisor', 'teacher', 'counsellor', 'guide and networker', 'role model' and 'sponsor'. The benefits gained from such relationships are obviously attractive, and a more formal mentoring provision has grown up within the nursing profession. Formal mentoring within nursing has not taken into account the willingness of the more able or 'wise' nurse to act as a mentor, and in fact many students are assigned mentors with little thought for the true nature of mentoring. Inevitably, these relationships are time constrained and related to specific clinical scenarios and outcomes.

Preceptor

The functional element of mentorship deals with the practical issues of teaching, instruction, support and advice giving. This is preceptorship. It is related to the teaching role within every nurse's work wherein a skilled practitioner helps a less skilled/experienced practitioner to achieve professional abilities appropriate to their role.

Autonomy

The freedom to make discretionary and binding decisions consistent with one's scope of practice and freedom to act on those decisions. The major consequence of autonomy is accountability or the ability to be answerable for what one has done, to stand behind ones decisions and actions.

Supernumerary

The word supernumerary is exactly what it states – extra to numbers. It is frequently used when discussing sheltered practice and real practice. Students need the freedom to learn to solve problems in a sheltered environment. A sheltered environment is one in which support is given to the student to such an extent that he or she has time to think about practice without worrying about 'getting the work done'. The clinical setting can be a sheltered environment if the student has contact with a supervisor and is supernumerary.

Primary practice

A term which encompasses nursing practice from initial registration to the point at which further specialist and advanced education and practice is recognized through professional and academic qualification.

Specialist practice

Practice within a specialist arena, e.g. intensive care nursing. The practitioner must hold a relevant qualification.

Advanced practice

Advanced practice is externally reflected in the attainment of higher qualifications and promotion. The advanced practitioner has to demonstrate a range of skills which incorporate direct care, education, research, management, involvement with health care policy making, and development of strategies.

Consultant practice

A term which was considered under the initial PREPP report. It was considered to be a natural progression for some but not all of the advanced practitioners. The consultant nurse is seen to be pioneering new roles, charting new territory, and acting as an authoritative resource.

Reflection

This word encompasses the concept of consideration or thought. Reflection is a mental exercise that deals with perceptions and sensations, ideas and thoughts. Reflection is vital for learning through practice. Reflection-in-action and reflection-upon-action are core needs for professional practice. Reflection is the prime role for supervisors – of themselves and in promoting it in their students.

APL

Accreditation for Prior Learning: an academic exercise which allows students to be given academic credits towards a present or future course of study. Students have to demonstrate that they can meet all or some of the learning outcomes of the course they wish to undertake. This has to be done prior to the course or prior to the relevant module. This is done through the development of a portfolio and through the auspices of an APL assessor.

APEL

Accreditation for Prior Experiential Learning: an academic exercise which allows students to be given academic credits towards a present or future course of study on the basis of past professional/clinical experience. The student has to demonstrate that they can meet all or some of the learning outcomes of the course they wish to undertake and that this prior learning has occurred through previous clinical practice. This has to be done prior to the course or prior to the relevant module. This is done through the development of a portfolio and through the auspices of an APEL assessor.

FURTHER READING

Benner, P. *From Novice to Expert: Excellence and Power in Clinical Nursing Practice.* Menlow Park, CA: Addison-Wesley, 1984.

Davies, C. *The Collapse of the Conventional Career.* Project Paper 1, English National Board, 1990.

Fish, D., Purr, B. *An Evaluation of Practice Based Learning in Continuing Professional Education in Nursing, Midwifery and Health Visiting.* Project Paper 4, English National Board, 1991.

Handy, C. *The Future of Work.* Oxford: Robertson, 1984.

Morton-Cooper, A., Palmer, A. *Mentoring and Preceptorship: A Guide to Support Roles in Clinical Practice.* Oxford: Blackwell Scientific Publications, 1993.

REFERENCES

Alexander, M. F. Integrating theory and practice in nursing: Parts 1 and 2. *Nursing Times.* 1982; 78(17/18): 65–68, 69–71.

Bendall, E. *So You Passed Nurse.* London: Royal College of Nursing, 1975.

Bendall, E. The future of British nurse education. *Journal of Advanced Nursing.* 1977; 2: 171–181.

Benner, P., Wrubel, J. Skilled clinical knowledge: The value of perceptual awareness, Part 1. *The Journal of Nursing Administration.* May 1982 p. 14.

Benner, P. *From Novice to Expert: Excellence and Power in Clinical Nursing Practice.* Menlo Park, CA: Addison-Wesley, 1984.

Burnard, P. The student experience: Adult learning and mentorship revisited. *Nurse Education Today.* 1990; 10: 349–354.

Collins Concise Dictionary of the English Language, 2nd Ed. London: Collins, 1988.

Davies, J. *An Evaluation of First Line Management Training Courses for Ward Sisters in the Manchester Region.* Centre for Business Research, University of Manchester, 1971.

Davies, C. The collapse of the conventional career. Project Paper 1, English National Board, 1990.

English National Board. Circular 1987/28/MAT *Institutional and Course Approval/Reapproval Process, Information required – Criteria and Guidelines.* 1987, London: English National Board.

English National Board. Circular 1988/39/APS *Institutional and Course Approval/Reapproval Process, Information required – Criteria and Guidelines.* 1988, London: English National Board.

English National Board. Circular 1989/27/AS, *Guidelines for the Development of English National Board Certificate Courses in General Nursing,* 1989.

English National Board. *Framework for Continuing Professional Education for Nurses, Midwives and Health Visitors: Guide to Implementation.* English National Board, 1991.

Fish, D. *Learning through Practice in Initial Teacher Training.* London: Kogan Page, 1989.

Fish, D., Purr, B. An Evaluation of Practice Based Learning in Continuing Professional Education in Nursing, Midwifery and Health Visiting. Project Paper 4, English National Board, 1991.

Fitter, M. The impact of new technology on nurses and patients. In Eds. R. Payne, J. Firth-Cozens. *Stress in Health Professionals.* London: Wiley, 1987.

Fretwell, J. E. *Ward Teaching and Learning,* London: Royal College of Nursing, 1982.

Gott, M. *Learning Nursing.* London: Royal College of Nursing, 1984.

Handy, C. *The Future of Work.* Oxford: Robertson, 1984.

Johnson, D. Professional practice and specialisation in nursing. *Image.* 1968; 2(3): 2–7.

Kitson, A. Educating for quality. *Senior Nurse.* 1985; 3(4): 11–16.

Kramer, M. *Reality Shock: Why Nurses Leave Nursing.* London: Mosby, 1978.

Larcombe, K., Maggs, C. Processes for Identifying the Continuing Education Needs of Nurses, Midwives and Health Visitors: An Evaluation. Project Paper 5, English National Board, 1991.

MacGuire, J. M. *Occasional Papers on Social Administration, No. 3: Theshold to Nursing.* London: Bell, 1969.

McGhee, A. *The Patients' Attitude to Nursing Care.* Edinburgh: Churchill Livingstone, 1961.

Morle, K. M. F. Mentorship – Is it a case of the emperors new clothes or a rose by any other name? *Nurse Education Today.* 1990; 10: 66–69.

Ogier, M. E. *An Ideal Sister?* London: Royal College of Nursing, 1982.

Orton, H. D. *Ward Learning Climate.* London: Royal College of Nursing, 1981.

Report of the Committee on Nursing. Chairman Professor A. Briggs. London: HMSO, 1972.

Revans, R. W. *Standards for Morale: Cause and Effect in Hospitals.* London: Nuffield Provincial Hospitals Trust/Oxford University Press, 1964.

Shamian, J., Inhaber, R. The concept and practice of preceptorship in contemporary nursing: A review of pertinent literature. *International Journal of Nursing Studies.* 1985; 22(2): 79–88.

Tattam, A. Nursing Times news. *Nursing Times.* 1991; 87(47): 5.

United Kingdom Central Council. *Project 2000: A New Preparation for Practice.* Report From UKCC. London: UKCC, 1986.

United Kingdom Central Council. *The Report of the Post Registration Education and Practice Project.* London: UKCC, 1990.

United Kingdom Central Council. *Report on the Proposals for the Future of Community Education and Practice.* 1991; London: UKCC.

United Kingdom Central Council. *The Councils Proposed Standard for Post Registration Education.* 1993; London: UKCC.

7
MANAGING THE CRITICAL CARE UNIT
Belinda L. Atkinson

CHAPTER AIMS

This chapter is concerned with the management aspects of the critical care unit. For simplicity, the intensive care unit is used as the basis for discussion, but the principles referred to are relevant to all types of high-care, high-tech critical care areas.

The chapter will consider the following key issues:

☐ definitions of what management is – and what an intensive care unit is, and what it is not;

☐ whether management matters, and who should manage;

☐ the importance of audit;

☐ the recruitment and retention of staff;

☐ the place of the intensive care unit in the internal market mechanism.

INTRODUCTION

The health service, as we know it, is in the middle of radical change. Self-governing trusts, contracts and the internal market, quality monitoring, clinical audit and resource management are but some of the issues with which we are having to concern ourselves increasingly.

Lack of experience in dealing with some of these issues, major reorganizations of hospital management structures, demographic aspects and the apparently ever increasing need to curtail financial resources are some problems currently being experienced by health care professionals. Additionally, many of these problems are not solely the concern of the United Kingdom – they occur in one form or another in many countries of the world.

The Briggs Committee (1972) stated that "Good management is a precondition of good care" – which emphasizes that good management is essential if patients are to receive an appropriate and acceptable level of care. It could be argued that this need has never been more paramount than in the current health service climate of today.

The chapter will probably raise more questions than provide answers; but if this is so, and managers and practitioners are encouraged to critically appraise their current systems and develop a vision for the future, then this can only be a good thing. For it is only by developing such a vision that we can be prepared in any way for what lies ahead. In essence, the unexpected is as common as the predictable in the intensive care unit; and indeed, "crisis is the norm, not the exception" (Bailey, 1985).

What is management?

Vaughan and Pillmoor (1989) describes management as "the art of getting work done through people." Like work, or many other things, management can also be considered as a process, with a series of interrelated steps. These include such elements as planning, organizing, leading and controlling. There also has to be something about forecasting, coordinating, delegating, teaching, counselling and development, to name but a few more components. It is a dynamic process, changing over time to meet the local needs of the organization, and often society generally. In short, to quote from Fielding and Berman (1990), "management is not a neat or tidy business."

Dixon (1990) in a workshop for managers, described the intensive care unit (ICU) as a "complex place to manage", and there is also a growing realization that a critical care director of tomorrow will be spending as much time on personnel and administrative issues as on clinical issues.

To manage a critical care area today requires a wide range of skills – organization, communication, planning, personnel management and financial control – to name but some. The resourcing and development of these skills are essential to ensure that critical care managers are adequately prepared to face today's challenges.

What is an intensive care unit?

Intensive care may be broadly defined as "a service for patients with potentially recoverable conditions, who can benefit from more detailed observation and treatment than is generally available in the standard wards and departments" (Intensive Care Society, 1990).

It is usually reserved for patients with potential or established organ failure. The Intensive Care Society (ICS) definition suggests that an ICU should offer the facilities for diagnosis, prevention and treatment of multiple organ failure. The most commonly supported organ is the lung, but an ICU should offer a wide range of facilities for organ support. This will require a multidisciplinary team approach, and the highest possible standard of nursing and medical care. A nurse to patient ratio

of one-to-one should be the minimum, and the services of a full time medical resident are essential (ICS, 1990).

A similar definition is suggested by the Association of Anaesthetists (1989): "Intensive care is defined as a service for patients with potentially recoverable disease who can benefit from more detailed observation and treatment than is generally available in standard wards and departments."

Furthermore, an intensive care unit is "an area to which patients are admitted for treatment of actual or impending organ failure who may require technological support (including mechanical ventilation) and/or invasive monitoring." (Association of Anaesthetists, 1989).

Leigh (1985) describes the main purpose of an intensive care unit as "the delivery of the highest possible quality of care to gravely ill or injured patients to restore them to active life as soon as possible."

In contrast, a high dependency unit (HDU) is an area offering a standard of care intermediate between the general ward and full intensive care unit (ICS, 1990). The HDU should not manage patients with multi-organ failure, but should provide monitoring and support to patients at risk of developing organ system failure. An HDU should be able to undertake short-term resuscitative measures, and might provide ventilator support for a short time, prior to the transfer of a patient to the ICU (ICS, 1990).

The HDU does not need, and should not provide, a full range of support services. It would normally function with a nurse to patient ratio of one-to-two, and does not require the exclusive services of a full time resident doctor (ICS, 1990).

In recent years, the emergence of more HDUs has led to some controversy and difficulties. Generally, these issues arise around the manpower levels of such units, the general dependency of the patients and the case mix. Particular difficulties can arise where the HDU is combined with the ICU; making manpower resources difficult if HDU beds become utilized as ICU beds.

Intensive care has also traditionally been divided into various levels of care. The actual method of categorization appears to vary from country to country, but the type of system used is as follows (Miranda *et al.*, 1990):

Level one – intensive care – such as is found in a university hospital, and is comprehensive. There is constantly a physician/director available, and the nurse to patient ratio is one-to-one or greater. A wide range of clinical measurement equipment is available.

Level Two – intensive care units are characteristic of district general hospitals, and may provide limited invasive monitoring and therapeutic interventions, such as assisted ventilation. There must be ready access to a physician/director, and in-hospital cover is provided by a physician who is skilled in life support and airway management. In such units, the nursing ratio is generally lower, and ranges from one-to-two, to one-to-four.

Level Three – represents speciality units in small community or rural hospitals, providing noninvasive arrythmia monitoring and basic cardio-pulmonary resuscitation, but does not meet the definition of an intensive care unit.

The application of these definitions varies from country to country, and indeed in some countries (particularly in Europe) the scales are reversed – that is, level one represents the most basic level of care, and level three the most comprehensive level of care. There is currently much discussion taking place as to the distribution of intensive care units and resources – whether all hospitals should have an intensive care unit, or whether manpower and expertise should be concentrated into regional and sub-regional centres.

What size should an intensive care unit be, in terms of bed numbers? Generally speaking, the number of beds allocated for intensive care, should be related to the size and workload (both in terms of numbers and case mix) of the hospital concerned. In 1978, Tinker suggested that a common ratio is one ICU bed for every 100 acute beds (with an additional one or two if the hospital has a cardiothoracic or neurosurgical department). Units having fewer than six beds are uneconomic, while those with more than twelve are difficult to manage – eight being the optimum number (Tinker, 1978).

More recent guidelines have been published by the Association of Anaesthetists (1989) and the Intensive Care Society (1990), leading to some changes in the basic recommendations. Some aspects have changed in terms of patient case mix – for example, more sophisticated cardiothoracic and neurosurgical techniques have tended to lead these areas to make their own provision for specialist intensive care services. Similarly, the advantages of grouping seriously ill children together in their own specialized environment are now well recognized (British Paediatric Association, 1987, 1992).

This has tended to lead to fragmentation of intensive care services into specialist areas, leaving the traditional ICU serving a very much more generalist function. However, this does not appear to have reduced demand.

With the advent of more sophisticated technology and therapeutics, the demand on intensive care resources has increased – "intensive care has been a victim of its own success – patients are now surviving, who would not have done so ten years ago, and, in many cases, we are still treating them with the same resources" (Edwards, 1992).

This has, in turn, led the recommendations regarding the number of ICU beds to rise from 1% to 2% of acute hospital beds (ICS, 1990). In addition, patient throughput has been assessed in terms of a unit's economic viability, and it has been recommended that a minimum of 200 patients per year is needed to sustain this (Association of Anaesthetists, 1989). This has obviously led to some difficulties in that, while it may be ideal to concentrate patients together in specialist regional centres, the reality is that such centres generally do not have the capacity and/or resources to handle all patients for whom intensive care may have been deemed appropriate.

The question is often raised as to whether intensive care is a speciality in its own right or not. Again, this varies throughout the world; and has been a question of much debate. In some countries, intensive care is recognized as a defined speciality, with practitioners dedicated within it. In others, it is seen as an off-shoot of other specialities, most commonly of anaesthetics (Dudley, 1987).

It is only relatively recently within the United Kingdom that a training facility has been set up for medical practitioners with a specific interest in intensive care. This is a two-year programme, which is currently available only in a limited number of centres, and which, while containing certain essential requirements in terms of experience, is also tailored to the individual doctor's previous clinical experience. There is also the ability for these practitioners to retain their parent speciality, should they wish (or need) to return to it in the future.

Jennett (1990) describes intensive care as "a strange hybrid". For some, he states, it is a discipline, for others a way of organizing certain activities, for yet others a technological package. It is suggested (Jennett, 1990) that an intensive care unit is a place, but that many activities commonly associated with such a unit can also be done in recovery rooms, high dependency areas and even ward side rooms. The question is asked as to when does care become intensive? Some insist on making a distinction between intensive care and intensive therapy. What *is* common to both is intensive attention – on the part of both doctors and nurses.

Does management matter?

Having considered what intensive care is, it is now appropriate to consider some of the more specific areas of management.

Firstly, does management actually matter? This is, indeed, difficult to substantiate scientifically, but attempts have been made or are being made to do so. One of the classic attempts was incorporated in a study by Professor William Knaus and colleagues in the USA in the mid-1980s (Knaus, 1986). Knaus studied 13 intensive care units, and compared the predicted outcome, measured by APACHE (Acute Physiology and Chronic Health Evaluation) scoring with the actual outcome. Those hospitals performing better than expected, appeared to have certain common features, which seemed to correlate with a degree of effective management practice. Some of those features were:

Correlates of effective ICUs

1. Agreed and acceptable guidelines and policies for the admission, care of and treatment of critically ill patients.
2. An ongoing education process for nurses and others working in intensive care units.

3. Recognized directors of medical and nursing care and good liaison between them (Knaus, 1986).

The study findings suggested a positive correlation between the patient outcomes from the unit, and good management practices. However, generalizations cannot be made based on a single study, and this study now needs to be replicated in other centres, and in other countries.

The study also underlies the importance of direction and communication as essential attributes of the modern ICU manager. In addition, there is also something about the empowerment of others to assist in achieving shared goals.

Who should manage the intensive care unit?

The next question that arises is the debate as to who should manage the ICU? There is little doubt that, due to the complexity of the service, managing an intensive care unit today goes well beyond a single physician's or nurse's capability – it requires exceptionally well coordinated teamwork; and a fundamental need to ensure that there is adequate means of representation for all disciplines involved in intensive care practice. Alone, this will require well developed interpersonal and coordinating skills on the part of the ICU manager.

There is a dichotomy. On the one hand, the treatment and care of critically ill patients requires a well-versed medical practitioner to lead and coordinate the team and the contributions to care by other disciplines. On the other hand, the largest part of the workforce will be nurses, and one of the key activities nursing, therefore sound leadership of the nursing team is required. Leigh (1985) suggests that "intensive care is, above all, nursing care, and so an expert nursing staff, strongly led is essential."

The ideal is identified medical and nursing leaders, but undoubtedly, the relationship between them must be harmonious, with mutual respect for each others position and an open-minded attitude to discussion and problem-solving. Important also is a shared vision of the way forward and development of the ICU.

There are undoubtedly some areas of management where it is relatively clear which discipline is involved. There are other areas where the division of responsibility between the consultant and manager needs to be clearly defined, with particularly good interdisciplinary collaboration. These areas have been listed by the Intensive Care Society (1990) as being:

- [ ] operational policies
- [ ] equipment management
- [ ] staffing
- [ ] health and safety at work
- [ ] hospital and medical administration
- [ ] liaison with other hospital departments
- [ ] research
- [ ] teaching
- [ ] audit.

In the United Kingdom today, an increasing number of hospitals have now adopted the clinical directorate management model. In effect, this means that the hospital services are divided into directorates, each headed by a service director – who is usually a consultant.

The consultant will be assisted by a service manager (who may be from a variety of backgrounds) providing the day-to-day management function. In some directorate systems a separate role of business manager is identified. There will undoubtedly be a need to provide sound nursing leadership and advice, and as mentioned above, a fundamental need to ensure that all disciplines represented in the unit are part of the communication strategy. However the system is organized, one cardinal rule must be remembered; if value of any kind is to continue to be placed on the multidisciplinary teamwork of critical care, then the unique contribution of each discipline and individual must be recognized.

The ICU interface

Hopkinson (1990) suggests that intensive care units can be regarded as operating with three distinct levels of responsibilities and control – technical, managerial and institutional.

The technical aspect serves the primary function of delivering medical and nursing care to the critically ill. The managerial level provides resources and overall operational direction to the technical. At the institutional level, the ICU interfaces with the demands of health authorities, patients, managers and other specialities.

The Intensive Care Society (1983) have described two different patterns of clinical referral. The consultant-in-charge of the intensive care unit may have complete clinical responsibility for all patients admitted to the unit. This begins when the patient is admitted to the unit and ends when the patient is referred to another consultant on discharge from the unit. The consultant who originally admitted the patient to hospital may continue in a consulting capacity, with other specialists being asked for advice where appropriate.

Alternatively (and this seems to be the more common model in practice), the patients may be admitted to the intensive care unit under the care of their admitting consultant, and remain so throughout their stay on the unit. In this case, the ICU consultants will be acting in consultation, with other specialists being called in when necessary.

This pattern may well vary, depending upon the size of the ICU and the specialities being catered for. However, it is evident that whichever model is utilized, the importance of good communication between the specialities involved cannot be emphasized enough.

Admission and discharge policies

The use of admission policies relative to patients in intensive care units remains a difficult topic.

McLachlan (1984) stated that an admission policy is necessary to make sensible use of an expensive resource, and that it is also conducive to good management practice.

The criteria for admission to ICUs suggested by the King's Fund Panel (1989) have already been outlined in Chapter 1. The need for additional supporting research and data collection was clearly stated; and, in addition, the panel recommended that "each ICU should prepare a set of guidelines setting out criteria for admission to the unit to help doctors and other staff determine priorities for treatment" (Kings's Fund, 1989).

Despite the fact that it is difficult to lay down specific rules concerning the admission of a patient to the ICU, the Intensive Care Society (1990) also advocated the use of a formal policy for the admission and discharge of patients. In addition, it was suggested that all admissions should be agreed with the consultant in charge of the unit at the time, particularly if all resourced beds are currently occupied. Due to the fact that any admission to the ICU requires nursing services, discussion must also take place between the admitting consultant and the senior nurse in charge of the unit.

Although perhaps now dated, the admission guidelines of Tinker (1978) are still very much applicable, largely due to the underlying concepts which they represent. These are:

Admission guidelines

1. The physiological disturbance should be judged to be reversible.
2. Patients should not be admitted solely for 'heavy' nursing.
3. There may be a problem where acute on-chronic illness is concerned, and the possible outcome of treatment must be considered in depth.
4. Age, though a necessary consideration, should never be the sole reason for refusing admission to the ICU.

The King's Fund Panel (1989) discussed the concept of benefit, stating that "benefit should be assessed not only in terms of survival, but also in terms of the quality of life." The same group also contended that the ability to provide a more accurate prognosis than is possible at present would help to avoid some of the conflicts which arise, and suggested that severity scoring systems may have a good deal to recommend them, provided they are not applied rigidly in individual cases. The panel concluded that: "selection for intensive care should be based on broad concepts of prognosis, derived from statistical analysis of comparable cohorts of patients backed up by sound clinical trials."

Discharge of the patient from the ICU has to be considered from several perspectives, with the aim of providing 'seamless' care. Again, the criteria for discharge from ICU are those suggested by the King's Fund Panel (1989). The panel envisaged four broad situations:

1. The patient has recovered and is stable.
2. The immediate threat has been alleviated, but the patient remains at risk unless under close observation.
3. The immediate threat has been alleviated, but the patient is expected to die shortly.
4. Death is agreed to be imminent, even if intensive care is continued.

The panel suggested that patients in the first category should be discharged as soon as possible, whilst those in the second may be discharged or retained in the ICU, depending upon the needs of other patients and the available facilities elsewhere in the hospital. The last two categories are perhaps somewhat contentious, but it is generally considered inappropriate to transfer patients to ward areas who are expected to die imminently.

Nursing staff often feel particularly strongly regarding this matter, because they have developed a relationship with the patient's family and often feel that they are letting the family down if they are not present to support them at the time of bereavement. However, it goes without saying that competing pressures in the ICU for beds, or indeed in the general ward areas, will inevitably affect this decision.

At the time of discharge, good liaison between the staff of the intensive care unit and the receiving ward is always an important factor. This not only enhances the standard of care given to patients, but is also a vital communication link between the two areas involved. It may well be that in the future we shall see the advent of discharge scoring systems similar to those currently used for the admission of patients to ICU.

Critical care audit

This has already been referred to in Chapter 1. However, the subject is of such importance that some aspects will be revisited here.

The King's Fund Panel (1989) highlighted the deficit of information regarding critical care practice, and specifically intensive care. Similarly, the Association of Anaesthetists (1989) state that "there is not much information about the number of units and their utilisation" and also that "it is recognised that intensive care is expensive both in manpower and resources. These should be used efficiently, but hitherto little information has been available upon which to base the future provision of these services."

There are many forms of audit – both at local and national level. What is important, however, is the fact that careful unit audit is a prerequisite of national audit, and therefore the need for agreed procedures exists (ICS, 1990).

Data is required at several levels. Firstly, there is what might be termed the macro level – used as an indication of the overall activity of a unit. Details might include:

- ☐ Number of admissions per day/month/year – overall, by speciality, by district of residence, age, sex, and so on.
- ☐ Time of day of admission.
- ☐ Midnight bed state and/or occupancy rates.
- ☐ Patient dependency scores.
- ☐ Disease classifications.
- ☐ Survival rates.
- ☐ Discharge data.

Additionally, into this category could be placed information regarding financial performance. Increasingly, more sophisticated data is available in this respect, and with close scrutiny of all aspects of the service becoming increasingly prevalent, it is vital that this information is used prudently. Financial information is generally divided into staff and non-staff expenditure, and can give fairly detailed information regarding expenditure against particular items, e.g. drugs and disposables usage.

Secondly, data is required at the micro level, and here the reference is to data concerned with individual patients and their treatment. Obviously some of this data may well contribute to the macro level previously described. Here, it is essentially clinical audit that is the subject of the discussion.

Clinical audit is central to the whole audit process, and this can be very detailed. The need to develop this aspect of practice was detailed in the Health Service Act 1990. While many medical practitioners voiced concern at this, it has to be suggested that this type of clinical audit was perhaps being developed in critical care already – partly as a result of the King's Fund recommen-

dations. The minimum data set will include demographic information, disease classification, severity of illness and outcome (ICS, 1990). Also relevant are details of individual therapies, their cost-effectiveness and morbidity due to them.

As part of the audit process, many units have regular audit meetings, which are multidisciplinary in nature. These are an important forum, not only for discussion regarding clinical problems, but also for wider debates concerning ethical issues, management and resourcing issues, and so on.

Clinical audit is vitally important if we are to justify the existence and development of the critical care specialities in the future. The King's Fund panel (1989) state that "the absence of data on workload, outcome and costs, and the heterogeneity of ICU's, make it evident that any recommendation about a future provision must be highly speculative." We have been warned!

NURSING MANPOWER ISSUES

Recruitment and retention of nursing staff

The discussion will now turn to the issues related to the recruitment and retention of nursing staff for critical care units – particularly how staff are best retained, the potential effects of demographic changes, and the potential effects of other changes, for example educational changes, upon manpower in the critical care areas. It is recognized that there are other groups of staff in the intensive care unit, with whom the manager may be involved, for example, technical staff and administrative/clerical staff. However, as nurses form the largest part of the ICU workforce, the discussion here will centre upon them.

In essence, all managers and senior staff would do well to heed the words of Parrish (1990) who reminds us that "staff are the most valuable resource in any organisation, and heed needs to be taken of the workforce and the way it is handled in the next decade."

The stage prior to recruitment is human resource planning – which is generally concerned with planning what staff are needed. Nelson (1989) describes human resource planning as having five stages or units of consideration. These are:

Nelson's five stages

1. The starting point – that is, a clear understanding of the current situation to determine whether, and if so what, change is necessary.
2. Higher productivity or more staff – that is, can existing staff be better deployed to cope with the workload, or are more staff actually necessary?
3. Planning for change – the prediction of future needs, which involves being clear as to the plans for the development of the service managed, and translating these into requirements for different staff. Obviously, in critical care there is a complicating factor here, in that it is necessary that managers are also aware of the implications for their service of developments in other user services.
4. Putting the plans into context – that is, within the continual process of labour turnover, changing clinical practices, technology and changing workload.
5. Supplies of labour – the state of the labour market and, for example, the effects of demographic changes (Nelson, 1989).

If it is assumed that the planning of manpower requirements is as this process, then it can also be understood that the recruitment, selection and induction processes are concerned with finding the necessary staff, and settling them into their jobs. Nelson (1989) states that "often, though not invariably, these processes are to do with recruiting a single employee, which though not difficult takes time to do well."

Most readers will be familiar with the recruitment process from one side of the fence or the other, and therefore it is not intended to elaborate here. Briefly, the stages are as follows:

1. Drawing up the job description and person specification.
2. Identifying the grade of the post, and conditions of work and service.
3. Planning the necessary advertisements.
4. Screening and short listing the applicants – also dealing with enquiries and informal visits.
5. Interviewing and selecting.
6. The appointment process.
7. The induction of the new employee.

Technically, the recruitment process is not complete until the induction of the new employee has been undertaken to the satisfaction of both manager and employee.

The critical care unit manager and senior nursing staff should be involved in the recruitment of all nursing staff for the unit. Good recruitment is essential to promote harmonious working relationships within the unit, and to maintain the balance of appropriately qualified staff. The manager should be aided in staff selection by the senior nursing staff, i.e. senior clinical nurses, sisters, charge nurses. This not only gives them an introduction to the techniques of interviewing, but also enables them to participate in the selection of the staff they will be working with and supervising on a day-to-day basis (Atkinson, 1987).

Is there an 'ideal' critical care nurse? This is a difficult question to answer because the ideas of individual managers vary, and, indeed, different nurses will be 'right' for different units. However, the author has changed her thoughts little over the years, and still fosters a belief that there are some generally desirable criteria which contribute towards the success of individual critical care nurses. These are:

Desirable attributes of an ITU nurse

☐ A sound base of nursing knowledge and clinical skills.

☐ The willingness to learn.

☐ The ability to remain objective in difficult situations.

☐ The character and ability to work well as a team member.

☐ The ability to maintain high standards of care with meticulous attention to detail.

☐ Initiative, ingenuity, stamina and, appropriately, a sense of humour.

☐ Motivation towards this type of work and a reasonable insight into it (Atkinson, 1987).

Intensive care units should have an orientation and in-service training programme for new staff, and, where appropriate, this should also include a general orientation to the hospital concerned. The programme needs to be reviewed at regular intervals to ensure that it is in line with current practices and policies in the unit. Similarly, staff who are expected to act as mentors or facilitators for new staff should be aware of the responsibilities of their role, and appropriately trained to undertake them. Nelson (1989) states that "left to their own devices, more new staff leave an organisation or get into bad habits in the first six months, than in any other period of their employment. Both factors cause organisation problems and cost a great deal; and both are avoidable."

Demographic changes also have effects upon staff recruitment, and the 'demographic' time bomb is frequently talked about. In essence, this appears to have been a very slow bomb to defuse. However, it is known that in the United Kingdom there is currently a shortage of 18 year olds, and that the prediction of a reduced rate of entrance to basic nurse training is becoming true – and it follows that, one day, this will catch up with the speciality areas. It is necessary, therefore, to consider innovative ways of recruitment, and the discussion will now focus briefly upon these aspects.

Because of the decline in the number of school leavers suitably qualified to go into training, Conroy and Stidson (1988) concluded that the National Health Service would need more than 60% of the appropriately qualified female school leavers, mainly for the health care professions, in the mid-1990s. Fittall and Thompson (1992) state that, clearly, workforce strategy will need to include a move away from this reliance on recruiting 18 year old school leavers. In addition, the same authors suggest that the recent re-structuring of the National Health Service is likely to cause shifts in service demand, and therefore demand for staff, away from the major centres; and that, also, boundaries between the roles of staff are already breaking down – this is likely to be further encouraged as a result of the drive to reduce junior doctors' hours.

How can this be dealt with? Innovative ways of recruitment should include flexible shift patterns, alterations in shift patterns where practical to suit local needs, and formal job sharing arrangements. For the manager, this may well be difficult as the balance is often a fine line between the needs of the unit and the needs of individuals. However, if the reward is long serving, satisfied, good employees, then this is a small price to pay. Many critical care areas have, perhaps, previously been rather restrictive in terms of flexibility of hours offered to employees. However, this practice is changing, not only as a result of the need to provide equal opportunities, but also because of the need to recruit and retain suitably qualified staff.

Much can be gained from a formal job share arrangement. However, to be most successful, this arrangement should not merely consist of two part-time staff sharing the equivalent number of hours. Formal liaison between the two staff involved needs to be worked out so that both have optimum opportunity to contribute to the unit, and to support each other. To encourage communication between such individuals, the rota pattern adopted needs to ensure that they work together on several occasions during a month so as to promote continuity. There is little doubt in the author's mind that job sharing, where properly instituted, can be of great benefit to any critical care area not only in terms of manpower, but also in terms of the expertise that two individuals can bring to the post.

Flexible shift patterns are also essential to encourage and enable those nurses who perhaps have been previously trained in the critical care specialities and then left to have families to return to work. Such shift patterns may need to include restricted hours, fixed shifts on a regular basis, or avoidance of certain unsocial hours, e.g. night duty. This can be difficult for the manager to deal with, not only in terms of the restrictions that such hours may place on rota patterns, but also in terms of ensuring equity between all staff in the critical care unit. However, there is no doubt that if we look to the future, and consider the problems caused by a reduction in supply of trained nurses, we may well need to rely far more heavily on such employees, despite the problems that their restricted hours may bring.

Additionally, there is little doubt that if employees are satisfied that they have adequate child minding arrangements for their families, they will then be able to devote themselves more fully to the hours they are at work, even if these are on a limited basis, and therefore gain increased job satisfaction and commitment.

No discussion of recruitment today would be complete without mention of the need to promote equal opportunities. This applies to a wide range of potential employees, but most notably includes such features as racial discrimination, discrimination because of family commitments, sex, disability, etc. Most personnel departments now undertake scrupulous equal opportunities monitoring, and the results of this should be fed back to managers on a regular basis. In line with personnel policy, most application forms have now been modified to remove such features that might now be termed to be discriminatory. These may include provision of a photograph with the application form, details of the applicant's dependents, and so on.

Return to work courses have now been popular in the health service for the last few years. These are of particular relevance to the critical care areas because these are areas which have traditionally experienced rapid change.

In practice, it is often found that employees even only having the minimum break for family commitments may experience difficulties on returning to work. Therefore flexibility and innovation in terms of such programmes is essential to encourage such nurses to return and continue to practice in the critical care specialities.

Some hospitals are now practising retainer schemes, which, in outline, are a formal scheme to keep the employee in touch with the hospital whilst he or she is not practising due to family commitments or other circumstances. There is usually a maximum time limit on such schemes, but providing the employee agrees to this there is also a commitment in terms of the hospital in providing updating and educational programmes.

How do we keep staff? A lot of emphasis has been placed on the recruitment of staff, but still more needs to be placed upon the retention of such staff in the critical care areas. Excessive turnover is not cost-effective, and is extremely time consuming for managers.

It is generally accepted that most aspects of retention have something to do with making the unit a 'nice' place to work in, and, in turn, ensuring that staff feel that their contribution to the overall work of the unit is valued. This may sound rather simplistic, but it is undoubtedly the underlying issue.

It may, in turn, mean making sacrifices – for example, several units have given up a senior nursing post to provide a staff development sister/ charge nurse. This has undoubtedly helped to reduce staff turnover in some areas by providing support and advice on a variety of issues, to various grades of staff – particularly at times where they may be at their most vulnerable; for example, new staff, or those who have perhaps just finished their post-basic training course.

The value of adequate orientation to a new workplace cannot be over-estimated. All critical care areas should have an orientation and in-service training programme for new and more experienced staff, and this needs to be reviewed at regular intervals to ensure that it is in line with current practices and policies in the unit. The 'buddy' system of orientation has been tried with some success in many units. This involves attaching a new member of staff to a more experienced one for orientation and training programmes. Many critical care areas now have formal education programmes aimed at nurses of various experience, and the development of these is to be encouraged because they can normally accommodate the flexibility needed to ensure that as many staff as possible from a particular unit are able to participate.

Performance review is also an important aspect of staff retention and development, and one which has perhaps, historically, not been good in the health service.

Previous forms of documentation have perhaps been rather inappropriate and subjective, and sometimes completed for the wrong reasons and have, in this respect, been counter-productive. However, individual performance review has been concentrated on by personnel departments considerably more recently, and it is necessary to ensure that those carrying out the process are competent, so that the exercise is received as constructive. The individual performance review programme essentially consists of:

Individual performance review programme

1. The employee's view of his/her job and its strengths and weaknesses.

2. The employer's view of the employee in that job, with the identification of necessary areas of development as well as strengths and weaknesses.
3. The agreeing of objectives for the employee.
4. The identification of action necessary for the achievement of such objectives, together with the identification of those involved in assisting the employee to achieve them.

The performance review is a confidential exercise between the reviewer and the employee, except where agreement is reached from the employee for other individuals who might be of assistance to him or her, to be informed where necessary.

The employee is given a copy of the agreed development plan, and review dates are set up on a regular basis. In addition, in most systems the employee has the right to discuss the review with a 'grandparent'. This is normally the manager once removed from the person who actually carried out the review.

The mechanism of linking performance to pay for certain grades within the health service structure is still somewhat contentious, but may well be set to increase. Similarly, the full implications of the rights of self-governing trust hospitals to set their own pay levels and conditions of service, in order to attract staff, have yet to be realized.

Levels of nursing staff

The appropriate number of nursing staff for a critical care area is still a topic which is hotly debated, and has been examined in some detail by a working group set up by the Intensive Care Society (1990), and more recently by a similar group (ICS/BACCN, in publication). Telfer (1984) summarizes the findings of the previous group, and states that "the group decided that it was necessary to have some kind of scoring system to calculate the nursing workload of a particular patient", and the following broad categories were suggested:

☐ Category 1 – patients who require close supervision, but not necessarily the continuous presence of a nurse at the bedside.
☐ Category 2 – patients who require a nurse at the bedside continuously for the 24 hour

period. It is generally accepted that, in practice, this group will form the majority of patients in the intensive care unit.
☐ Category 3 – the most seriously ill patients; for example, those with multiple organ failure and/or those on multiple support systems. It is generally assumed that for a large part of the nursing shift two nurses will be required, and that the presence of one nurse only is generally insufficient for patients in this category. (Intensive Care Society, 1990.)

In the calculations, a number of assumptions were then made. Assuming a $37\frac{1}{2}$ hour working week, it was calculated that to provide a nurse at the bedside for 24 hours a day would require 4.5 wte (whole time equivalents) nurses per bed. It was then calculated that a further 22% of nursing time would be required to cover factors such as holidays, sick leave and study leave. In fact, Reis-Miranda *et al.* (1990) suggest that to cope with all eventualities the figure required is nearer 25%. A figure of 22% raises the requirements to 5.5 nurses per bed. It was also suggested that it may be necessary to provide extra staff to help with turning, meal breaks, supervision and teaching, and that the nurse in charge of the shift should be supernumerary in terms of workload requirements.

This latter provision has often been difficult to attain, and it is undoubtedly true that in many smaller units the nurse in charge is expected to take a patient case load as well as supervise the running of the unit. Studies by the working party at the time of their investigation showed that out of 52 units who returned questionnaires, the vast majority fell below the recommended 5.5 nurses per bed. This problem has since been compounded in many instances by recruitment difficulties, with the results that many units have experienced considerable difficulty in maintaining an optimum number of critical care beds open, with adequate and safe levels of nursing care. Telfer (1984) stated that "nurses in ICU should not be expected to carry the responsibility of caring for critically ill patients, without adequate numbers, and in particular no circumstances should ever arise when pressure of work means that patients receiving mechanical ventilation are left unattended."

There are many factors that will affect the ideal number of nursing staff for a particular critical care unit, and it is therefore difficult to be prescriptive and lay down absolute guidelines – indeed, to do so would be naive in approach. Factors such as the layout of the unit, the available medical cover, the experience of the nurses involved, the provision of a post-basic nurse training course and so on, all contribute in different ways to determining the optimium level of nursing resource.

Sensitive critical care managers will need to be able to identify the optimal levels of staff for their units, and be able to present a well informed and statistically supported case for increases where the present numbers fall short of those necessary for good care. Like many other things, this ability is becoming more important at a time when finance for health care is becoming proportionally less in a climate which is increasingly competitive.

The management of staff morale

Because of the nature of work in critical care areas it is important that efforts are made to maintain good staff morale. In the experience of the author there are three basic areas which seem to cause the most problems for critical care unit staff:

Areas of concern for ITU staff

1. Poor staffing levels.
2. Ethical/moral problems surrounding the care and treatment of individual patients.
3. Being moved out of the unit to other areas in the hospital when the unit is quiet. (Atkinson, 1987).

In respect of the first, staffing levels, these are very much the concern of the manager. If there are problems with the recruitment and retention of staff for a particular unit, then it may be necessary to carry out a proper investigation to attempt to determine the causes.

There is no doubt that difficulties in the recruitment of critical care staff are a problem of today, and many units are being forced to close beds and/or work with poor staffing resources. At a local

level within a particular unit, there needs to be good communication between all disciplines, so that the real extent of the problem can be examined and appropriate efforts made to resolve it. The decision to close critical care beds should obviously be taken as a last resort because undoubtedly the number of times where problems have been caused by shortages of critical care beds has increased within recent years, and this has not escaped the notice of the media. Closing beds is obviously not an ideal state of affairs, but the other side is that it may tide the unit over a difficult period, improve staff morale, and therefore possibly prevent further staff losses.

There is no doubt that communication is a major adjunct in maintaining good staff morale. Staff have a great need to be kept informed of developments and problems, and given opportunities to air their views. Undoubtedly, difficult periods of recruitment and heavy workload can be alleviated greatly by adequate exchanges of information, and a concerted effort by all disciplines to maintain the team spirit. Experience has shown that, provided staff are kept informed and feel valued, their tolerance of heavy workload can be fairly high over a sustained period of time. Recently, more attention has been paid to the causes of stress and psychosocial problems amongst unit staff.

In the author's own unit, an employee assistance programme has been instituted to give staff the opportunity for one-to-one discussions, or discussion on a group basis. It is difficult to make provision for this sort of service as what may be suitable for one employee, may be found to be vastly unsuitable for another. However, the experience has been that, in general, this type of programme can work well within the critical care areas.

Inherent in intensive care work are the moral and ethical problems surrounding individual patient care. As technology becomes more advanced, so the complexity of these problems increases. There is no doubt that multidisciplinary ward rounds and case conferences may help to some extent, but above all there needs to be a sensitivity between team members, to identify when colleagues may have particular problems dealing with a situation (Atkinson, 1987). Previously, this has always been considered to be a prime need of the more junior members of the team, but it has to be remembered that the more senior members of the team also need this support, and it is generally up to the manager to ensure that a forum is available to facilitate this. Experience has shown that there is much to be gained from enabling senior members of the team to meet with those from other units, to exchange ideas, problems and solutions. In turn, managers themselves are not a bottomless pit of emotional and psychosocial support, and all managers need to recognize the need to develop their own support mechanisms.

The movement of staff out of critical care areas when the unit is quiet always poses difficult problems. In the current financial climate it is likely that this may well happen more, as health authorities look to their own, rather than the use of agency staff. However, managers must always bear in mind that staff who are working in this type of environment need to have periods to 'wind down' from time to time, and also to apply themselves to teaching, projects and other clinically related pursuits which may not always be possible when the unit is busy, and the demands on the staff are greater.

The critical care unit in the internal market system

We now turn to a discussion of some of the financial aspects of critical care management.

With so many changes in health service finance in recent years, it is necessary to consider the place of critical care in the internal market system of providing health care. Although this has existed for some time in the United States, it is still reasonably new here in the United Kingdom. It is also necessary to consider how critical care is 'marketed' and what the place of business planning is.

Firstly, where does critical care fit in? The cost implications for critical care are undoubtedly significant, and perhaps give rise to many controversies regarding the use and abuse of the service.

It is perhaps unclear exactly what critical care costs, and there are several studies in the United Kingdom seeking to address this problem at present. Traditionally, it has always been considered that the cost of keeping a patient in the critical care unit, is roughly three to four times that of keeping a patient in a general ward per day.

Limited local studies in the United Kingdom seem to show that a patient costs more during the first 24 hours after admission, and that this as a general rule tends to decrease subsequently. In reality, this is to be expected as most invasive procedures are carried out within the first 24 hours. However, there are obviously exceptions to the rule where specialist treatments (e.g. haemofiltration or extracorporeal membrane oxygenation) are instituted subsequently. It is also known that certain drugs and therapeutic treatments are very expensive, and their use needs therefore to be carefully monitored.

Critical care, and intensive care particularly, tends generally to be marketed as a support service to other more directly marketable services, and very rarely directly in its own right, although this varies from hospital to hospital. This means that in the future, most intensive care budgets will be derived from the services using them, and therefore it has to be certain that the cost charged to purchasers adequately reflects the intensive care unit cost.

This, in turn, means that it will be essential to have good information available regarding cost and expenditure, and at the time of writing considerable work still needs to be done in this area.

Critical care areas are no longer defined as core services meaning that a hospital is not under an obligation to provide them. The effects of cost saving measures by provider units to enable competitive pricing have yet to be fully realized, but the implications could be profound.

How do we market critical care? It is likely with difficulty. If provider units want to be cost competitive, there is a real risk that they might reduce their usage of costly, high-tech areas. Whether this is of benefit to the patient is, of course, another argument. Essentially this is where audit is important – and critical care managers must work at data collection aimed at supporting the benefits of critical care practice. It is probable that general intensive care areas may be at most risk here – there is perhaps likely to be less of a problem in respect of intensive care units which are designed to support specialist, highly marketable services, for example cardiac surgery.

What of the relevance of the business planning process? Although this is relatively new to the health service, it has now been for a few years an established concept.

It is by no means a simple task, and to ensure commitment to it, business planning needs to involve as many relevant people as necessary. Business planning may well be new to the health service, but it is well established in industry, and it has been encouraging to see the assistance given to the health care service by industry in terms of training and the sharing of experience in this respect.

Business planning generally involves the following concepts:

1. The strengths, weaknesses, opportunities and threats (SWOT) analysis, i.e. the identification of strengths, weaknesses, opportunities and threats to the service. It is helpful to undertake this to focus the mind at the start of the business planning process, and also to encourage the consideration of positive attributes for the service as well as the purely negative ones.

It becomes clear here that it is essential that the manager is aware of potential developments in other services which may have implications for the intensive care service. For instance, if the surgical services decide to commence liver transplantation, then there is obviously a big implication for the provision of an intensive care service. In practice, it can sometimes be quite difficult for the critical care manager to ascertain what everybody else is up to!

2. The setting of objectives – short term for the year in question; and then longer term, for the next three to five years. The important thing about the setting of objectives, as those experienced in this process will already know, is that they must be easily quantifiable, measurable and achievable. There will be some objectives that have to be set in line with the core objectives of the organization concerned, and there will be others that are specifically relative to the provision of the critical care service.

3. Development bids – these are normally submitted a year in advance of the requirement for a release of funds. The development bid process is complex with large amounts of information currently being required. One of the difficulties of critical care is that because of the unpredictable nature of this speciality itself, it can sometimes be very difficult to provide adequate infor-

mation in the depth necessary. Often one is using the 'best guess' or a projection based on current use. Again, it is helpful to know of the plans of other services and how these may cause changes to the critical care service in the future.

4. Cost improvements – it is a mandatory government requirement that all services make 1% cost improvements annually, which has to be submitted as a formal proposal in their business plan. In addition, locally, individual organizations may demand a greater percentage of cost improvement.

Again, in respect of critical care, there is often very little surplus to easily determine which part of the budget the cost improvement may be made in.

5. Quality assurance initiatives – these for many services are often related to the contracting of their service to the purchaser. Obviously, these are therefore not so easily quantifiable in terms of many critical care areas, but nevertheless the need to monitor quality aspects of the service is important.

It is likely that, in the near future, we will see the development of service user contracts for intensive care, and indeed, those hospitals who already have well developed management and financial arrangements are working towards these at present. Essentially, this means that the ICU services will be sub contracted, and the user clinical services will be charged – either by patient numbers or bed days used – or a combination of both. Undoubtedly, business planning is indeed a complex process, but it is one that managers will need to become competent at to state their claim on resources in the future.

The critical care manager

To conclude this discussion of critical care management, we should take time to consider what makes a good critical care manager. Of necessity the manager has many roles – administrator, clinical expert, facilitator, representative of the unit, counsellor, liaison officer – to name but a few. For all of these the manager must be adequately prepared.

It is generally recognized that management development in the health service has been slow to develop, particularly for nursing staff. However, in recent years there has been an increase in opportunities available and most managers will be expected to have completed not only a first line, but also a middle management course, and in some cases a senior management course. Of benefit during this training they will have come into contact with other disciplines, and this is undoubtedly helpful in broadening the outlook of the specialist nurse manager, and in casting new light upon differing problems.

Critical care managers must keep themselves up to date by participating in further education opportunities, so that they may advise and guide others. They must always be aware of education opportunities available for their staff to enhance their performance and further their careers generally.

The manager may have a teaching commitment, both in the formal sense, and, particularly where they are from a nursing background, as a clinical expert. It is necessary to develop a wide knowledge base, so that they may be used as a resource. Liaison with the College of Nursing should be close to ensure that the optimal learning environment exists in the unit, and managers must encourage their trained staff to be an active part of this environment. In cases where the manager is not from a nursing background, this responsibility is usually designated to a senior clinical nurse. Whether clinically based or not, managers must remember that they also teach by example, and will be seen as a role model, for example in terms of how they organize their work, deal with other disciplines and departments, and communicate with staff, patients and relatives.

The administrative functions of the manager are many, but essentially they will need to maintain the record keeping and clerical function for the unit. To do this, all managers must have adequate secretarial/clerical support. They, or another designated person, are responsible for records, such as annual leave, sickness and study leave, the personnel aspects such as appointments and terminations, and generally a whole myriad of other paperwork. In the past, nurses have traditionally tended to shy away from paperwork, but experience has proved that proper organization of this at management level will not only contribute to the efficient running of the service, but may well be essential in terms of justifying resources for the future.

Managers are also the spokesperson for their unit. To do this effectively they must be sure that they are representing the true views of their staff, achieved by good consultation with them, and secondly, they need to have a good working knowledge of the speciality, so that they can cast an objective and an informed view on the problems encountered.

Critical care managers are also responsible for ensuring that standards are set and maintained, and that policies are defined and adhered to. In both respects, they need the help and advice of their senior nursing staff.

CONCLUSION

It is tempting for nurses to always think of management as being the province of 'others'. Perhaps this is where mistakes have been made in the past, and it is now time to re-think this. Management today is a dynamic and complex process because nurses are part of health services that are currently passing through turbulence and experiencing rapid change. This to the experienced airline pilot, and likewise to the experienced critical care nurse, is clear air turbulence – the sort that is very difficult to see in advance, and once in it has to be dealt with – for pilots for the comfort and safety of their passengers, and for nursing managers for the well-being and security of their staff.

It is now necessary to take stock and refocus. Tomorrow, as the saying goes, is another day, and who knows what new challenges and opportunities it may bring. Recognizing opportunities is exciting, and the manager's own opportunities in helping to shape the future are extensive.

Bennett (1991) reminds us that the future will arrive, whether we are well prepared or ill prepared for it. How do we measure our success? By being prepared, by anticipating possibilities, by using current potential to the full, and by actively participating in today, so that we are ready to face the challenges of the future (Bennett, 1991). Undoubtedly, whatever the future of critical care nursing (and management) may be, it will be within the context of rapid change, diversity, new knowledge and new horizons (adapted from Rogers, 1988).

KEY TERMS

Trust hospital

A hospital which, as a result of the Health Service Act (1990) has additional powers for the management of its own affairs and the control of its finances. In addition, Trust hospitals have the powers to establish their own contracts. Such hospitals are still accountable to the Department of Health.

Contract

The basis for a service agreement between a purchaser and a provider. The contract may be one of several types and there may be particular stipulations attached regarding, for example, quality aspects of the service provision. The contract is likely to specify the quantity of services to be provided, the quality of care to be delivered, and the cost (or price) of this care.

Quality

Quality tends to be considered in terms of degrees of excellence. However, it is difficult to define because it tends to be subjective in nature, i.e. what is quality to one person may not be to another. There are generally considered to be four differing perspectives of quality in health care – the users, providers and purchasers of services, and the public. Quality definitions may depend upon individuals' prior expectations and may, in addition, change over time as quality is not an absolute concept.

Audit

This is generally considered to refer to the process of systematic and critical examination, e.g. of the planning, delivery and evaluation of nursing care. Medical audit refers to critical analysis of the quality of medical care, including the use of protocols, procedures and resources and their effects on patient outcomes. Clinical audit tends to be used to refer to audit in which a multidisciplinary approach is taken.

Internal market

A new method of financing the delivery of health care since April 1991, in which a purchaser–provider split is the basis – with the aim of making the service more businesslike in its approach. Purchasers are in essence the health purchasing commissions, general practitioner fundholders and the private sector. Providers are many, but are basically divided into the public and the private sectors, and encompass hospital, community and other services related to health care.

Resource management

This term includes the planning, implementation, control and monitoring of the use of resources. The ideal is that clinicians and others will become more involved in the management and decision making aspects of their service delivery and accountable for its use and cost. This is achieved by providing better and more relevant patient-based information systems, which are more readily available to those for whom their use is relevant. In most hospitals this is being achieved by the use of computerized facilities based on integrated local area networks.

Management

As defined in the text.

Intensive care unit

As defined in the text.

High dependency unit

As defined in the text.

Case mix

Grouping together of patients who can be identified by similar clinical features and/or demands on resources.

FURTHER READING

Reis-Miranda, D., Loirat, P., Williams, A. (Eds.). *Management of Intensive Care: Guidelines for Better Use of Resources*. Dordrecht: Kluwer, 1990.

Birdsall, C. *Management Issues in Critical Care*. St. Louis, MI: Mosby Year Book, 1991.

Nelson, M. J. *Managing Health Professionals*. London: Chapman and Hall, 1989.

Fielding, P., Berman, P. C. (Eds.). *Surviving in General Management: A Resource for Health Professionals*. Basingstoke: MacMillan, 1990.

Spurgeon, P., Barwell, F. *Implementing Change in the NHS*. London: Chapman and Hall, 1991.

Vaughan, B., Pillmoor, M. (Eds.). *Managing Nursing Work*. London: Scutari Press, 1989.

REFERENCES

Association of Anaesthetists. *Intensive Care Services – provision for the future*. London: Association of Anaesthetists, 1989.

Atkinson, B. L. Management of the intensive care unit. *Nursing* (3rd Series). 1987; 16: 584–589.

Atkinson, B. L. The current state of critical care. *Intensive Care Nursing*. 1991; 7(2): 73–79.

Bailey, R. D. *Coping with Stress in Caring*. Oxford: Blackwell Scientific, 1985.

Bennett, J. A. On to the future. In: Ed. C. Birdsall. *Management Issues in Critical Care*. St. Louis, MI: Mosby Year Book, 1991, p. 366.

Briggs, A. *Report of the Committee on Nursing*. London: HMSO, 1972.

British Paediatric Association. *Report of a Working Party on Paediatric Intensive Care*. London: B.P.A., 1987.

Conroy, M., Stidson, M. *2001 – The Black Hole NHS*. London: Department of Health, 1988.

Dixon, M. *Management Workshop for Service Managers*. Southampton General Hospital, 1990. (Unpublished.)

Dudley, H. A. F. Intensive Care: a speciality or a branch of anaesthetics? (Editorial). *British Medical Journal*. 1987; (294): 459–460.

Edwards, J. D. *Documentary – The world in Action*. Granada Television, 1992. (Unpublished.)

Fielding, P., Berman, P. C. (Eds.). *Surviving in General Management: A Resource for Health Professionals*. Basingstoke: MacMillan Education, 1990.

Fittall, B., Thompson, V. Thinking beyond the next vacancy. *Senior Nurse*. 1992; 12(6): 19–20.

Hopkinson, R. B. Director of ITU? *Care of the Critically Ill*. 1990; 6(3): 89–91.

Intensive Care Society. *Intensive Care Audit*. London: ICS, 1990.

Intensive Care Society. *Intensive Care in the UK*. London: ICS, 1990.

Jennett, B. Is Intensive Care Worthwhile? *Care of the Critically Ill*. 1990; 6(3): 85–88.

King's Fund Panel. *Intensive Care in the United Kingdom*. (Chair: J. G. G. Ledingham.) *Anaesthesia*. 1989; (44): 428–431.

Knaus, W. An evaluation of outcome from intensive care in major medical centres. *Annals of Internal medicine*. 1986; (104): 410–418.

Leigh, J. M. Who should manage the intensive care unit? *Intensive and Critical Care Digest*. 1985; 4(1): 8–9.

McLachlan, G. The intensiveness of care. *Nursing Mirror*. 1984; 159(10): 42–44.

Nelson, M. J. *Managing Health Professionals*. London: Chapman and Hall, 1989.

Paediatric Intensive Care Society. *Standards for Paediatric Intensive Care*. Bishops Stortford: CCI Publications, 1992.

Parrish, A. Managers moving on! *Senior Nurse*. 1990; 10(7): 3.

Reis-Miranda, D., Loirat, P., Williams, A. (Eds.). *Management of Intensive Care: Guidelines for Better Use of Resources*. Dordrecht: Kluwer Academic, 1990.

Rogers, M. E. Nursing science and art: a prospective. *Nursing Science Quarterly*. 1988; (1): 99–102.

Telfer, A. B. M. Choosing the right number. *Nursing Mirror*. 1984; (3): 11–12.

Tinker, J. General intensive therapy. In *Intensive Care*. Basingstoke: Macmillan, 1978.

Vaughan, B., Pillmoor, M. (Eds.). *Managing Nursing Work*. London: Scutari Press, 1989.

8
STRESS AND BURNOUT IN CRITICAL CARE

Netta Lloyd-Jones

CHAPTER AIMS

This chapter will identify major categories of coping strategies to provide an overview from which readers may develop a broad-based repertoire, thus aiding cognition (and hopefully application) of coping styles which are appropriate to individual situations which arise. The aims of this chapter are to:

☐ provide an understanding of the concept of stress and the associated theory;

☐ dispel some of the myths which have become popular in recent years;

☐ present an overview of coping strategies which may be drawn upon by carers;

☐ place in context the role the individual may play in controlling their own level of stress, within organizational and educational issues.

INTRODUCTION

It is without doubt essential to include a chapter regarding stress and coping in a book such as this. Not only has the term stress developed popularity within health care terminology, but also within that of the general public. The term is used almost glibly, and there is a great danger of it becoming meaningless, with consequently little or no action taken to deal with the problem.

Nursing literature and research in relation to stress has often failed to clarify the theory behind any discussion presented. This may have contributed to many of the 'myths' associated with stress which have arisen over the last few years. It is hoped that this chapter will help to dispel some of these. For example, the general notion that stress is something that happens *to* you, and happens *to you more often* when working in critical care is still expressed by carers within this speciality.

There is increasing literature which suggests that stress is linked to both disease and illness. For example, physical and cognitive stimuli have been linked to cardiovascular and neuro-endocrine responses (Burchfield, 1985; cited by Broome, 1989). Whilst the relationship between stress and the development of disease is not yet fully understood, stress appears to play a major role in health/ill-health, and is costly to both the individual, industry and society (Sutherland and Cooper, 1990). Broome (1989) argues that not to include some dimension of stress as part of any understanding of a disease process and its treatment is a serious and potentially damaging omission.

The effects of stress, therefore, are too great and widespread to ignore, and it is appropriate to address the subject in relation to carers of critically dependent patients.

An individual's coping ability is regarded as an important variable between stress and its effects. It is all too often expressed that suffering from stress indicates an inability to cope. This implication of weakness in an individual prevents the positive outcomes of stress from surfacing, and restricts the investigation and application of appropriate strategies.

Historically, earlier research of the 1970s and 1980s addressed the debate regarding whether critical care nursing was more, less or equally stressful than other nursing environments. However, most of these studies presented conflicting findings, and many of them suffered from poor theoretical guidance and other design weaknesses.

Clarification of the theoretical approach to stress is therefore outlined in the early part of the chapter. Coping is often viewed as a 'strength' and as something which appears to be closely linked with personality, but before exploring variables such as this, a clear understanding of the various strategies which may be employed is necessary. The need for a comprehensive repertoire is discussed.

There appear to be many variables which influence the coping strategy selected, for example, personality characteristics, or the social support available and actively sought. The 'unique body of knowledge' that we seek for our profession is beginning to emerge in relation to transactional stress and coping theory. Correlationships appear to exist between certain variables, but as yet no causal, predictive picture has been shown. For example, outcomes related to selection of specific coping strategies remain uncertain.

Nursing must always remain a practice-based profession, and it would be inappropriate not to discuss practical nursing implications. This section has been subdivided as follows:

☐ individual approaches to coping;
☐ the role of education and training.
☐ organizational and managerial issues.

It is hoped that this provides a wide view of the complexity of the subjects concerned, yet still provides an adequate resource for individual nurses to begin broadening their own coping repertoires, and to be able to implement appropriate changes in their own place of work.

DEFINING STRESS AND COPING

Whilst many definitions of stress have been discussed and debated in a plethora of literature since the early 1930s, it is necessary to clarify what is meant by terms used within this chapter. There are three models of stress which predominate:

1. Stimulus model.
2. Response model.
3. Interactional model.

Stimulus-based model

This model implies stress as being something external to which an individual is exposed. Examples may be extreme environmental temperatures or the intensive care environment. The result of such exposure is often described as strain (see Fig. 8.1).

Typical disruptive responses may be headaches or anxiety. Early research into stress aimed to identify sources of stress in work environments, aiming to improve industrial productivity, and a stimulus-based model allowed for this theme of source identification. However, criticisms of this simplistic view are apparent. The lack of allowance for individual varied responses to stimuli and a single term 'stress' describing a multitude of various noxious stimuli makes the term stress almost meaningless. A second criticism is that no guidance is offered to predict which stimuli will cause stress, or to suggest how individuals cope with stress.

Response-based model

The main conceptual domain of this model is the manifestation of stress. The response of an indi-

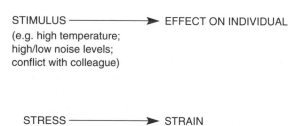

Figure 8.1.

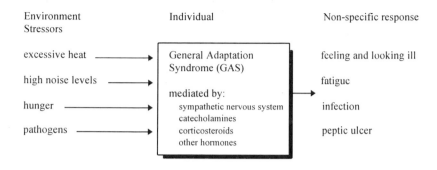

Environment Stressors	Individual	Non-specific response

Figure 8.2. General Adaptation Syndrome (GAS) (Selye, 1976).

vidual to a stimulus (stressor) can be described as a set of physiological responses aiming for restoration of homeostasis. Selye (1976) described a general adaptation syndrome (GAS) which is well accepted as reflecting these responses (see Fig. 8.2). A generalized activation of the sympathetic nervous system occurs, resulting in increased catecholamine secretion, together with hypothalamic and pituitary activation increasing glucocorticosteroid production (see Fig. 8.3). Selye (1976) believed that three stages of the stress response could be determined. The sudden exposure to a stressor produces an alarm stage which prepares the body for 'fight or flight'. However, in contemporary society, this is often inappropriate and disadvantageous when neither aggression release or physical activity are required.

If the stressor persists, and fight or flight have not been the choice of action, then a second stage of resistance results. The symptoms of the alarm stage improve and successful adaptation may result. During this phase, resistance to other stressors is reduced. The final stage is one of exhaustion. This follows an unrelenting demand for adaptation which eventually depletes all energy reserves. Collapse or even death may result. Bodily responses may be specific such as a measles rash, or nonspecific such as general aches or pains. Selye (1976) described stress as "the non-specific response of the body to the demands made upon it." He also recognized that not all stress is harmful, and that the same stress which makes one person sick can be an invigorating experience to another. This model

also is open to criticism in that the individual is regarded as a passive recipient to stressors and is limited to physical (not psychological) stressors. Selye's work, however, has done much to clarify understanding of the physiological response to stress, which is often invaluable to the critical care nurse.

Transactional model

The work of the psychologist Lazarus (1966) supplemented the work of Selye. Lazarus believed that fundamentally the concept of stress referred to *relations* between an organism and the environment rather than either the organism or the environment alone. Such transactional views are more contemporary, and have developed the theme

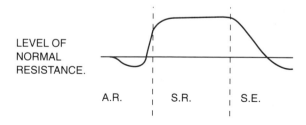

A.R. – ALARM REACTION
S.R. – STAGE OF RESISTANCE
S.E. – STAGE OF EXHAUSTION

Figure 8.3. The triphasic course of the stress response (Selye, 1976).

of an individuals' ability to act on his environment, and also are more useful in providing guidelines for the study and management of stress. A transactional model considers three conceptual domains:

☐ the source of stress;
☐ mediators of the stress response;
☐ manifestations of stress.

Stress is therefore most usefully viewed as

"a dynamic, interactional process rather than a single event or a set of responses. In essence, stressors make some sort of demand ... (physical or psychological) which requires the individual to assess and understand the situation, and then to respond to it."

(Broome, 1989, p. 25.)

A *demand* is an internal/external stimulus which is perceived by the individual as requiring an adaptive response. The perception of the demand by an individual will influence the degree of stress experienced (Fig. 8.4). This will also effect how an individual will cope with the perceived demand. *Coping* may be defined as "a response carried out by the individual and appraised by him as either satisfactorily or unsatisfactorily affecting the demand in the desired direction." (Clarke, 1984a.)

Stress will be experienced if there is a mismatch between perceived demand and perceived ability to cope with meeting the demand. This demand/coping imbalance (stress) is often functional in that it leads to an improved ability to cope.

Lazarus (1966) believed that appraisal of the demand (primary appraisal), appraisal of coping ability (secondary appraisal) and appraisal of effectiveness of coping (reappraisal) were vital stages in defining and managing stress. These stages of a transactional model of stress are similar to those of the nursing process, and may therefore be useful as a guide for coping with patient's stress and that of

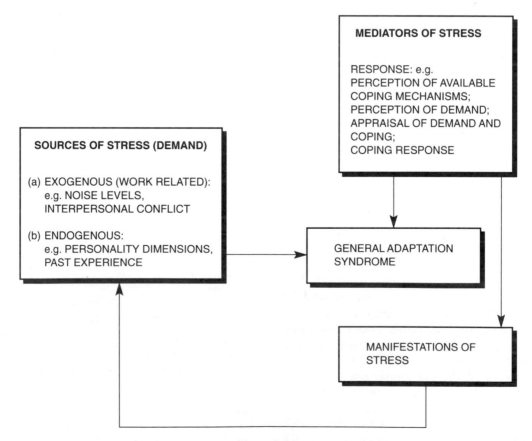

Figure 8.4.

the individual nurse (Bailey and Clarke, 1989, p. 23).

IDENTIFICATION OF STRESS

Albrecht (1979) advocates the use of 'self-monitoring'. This is giving close attention to physical sensations of your own body, which enables individuals to distinguish between positive stress (producing moderate anxiety symptoms) and when mismatch between demand and coping is present. For example, the tachycardia and tachypnoea experienced when dealing with a cardiac arrest situation may not be a mismatch, but the normal response of the body in preparation for 'fight' – fighting for the patient's life.

BURNOUT

> "the word evokes images of a final flickering flame, of a charred and empty shell, of dying embers and charred ashes." (Maslach, 1986, p. 3.)

Whilst manifestations of stress may be short-lived, as effective coping develops or demands reduce, the final stage of the GAS, exhaustion, may result. Burnout may be equated with this stage as it has been described as a syndrome of emotional exhaustion, depersonalization and reduced personal accomplishment (Maslach, 1986). Freudenberger first coined the term in 1975, describing negative self-concepts and job attitudes with a loss of concern and feelings for clients. There is apparent general agreement as to the symptoms of burnout: emotional exhaustion, detachment, boredom and cynicism, impatience, depression and loss of purpose have each been described (Maslach, 1986; Wessels et al., 1989; Bailey and Clarke, 1989). Anyone in a caring profession may be a candidate for burnout as they may be often so busy caring for others that their own needs are neglected. Bailey (1985) suggests that burnout is a progressive stress process by which a previously committed professional helper disengages from work as a result of the appraised stressful transactions experienced within the job.

Avoidance of emotional investment in patient care may be self-protective when perceived coping ability does not meet the perceived demand of patient needs. Distancing or detachment may be early signs of burnout in the critical care nurse. Technical care may be given, but the more in depth professional care is avoided. Self-protection from strain in this way may be effective initially but may develop into a stage of complete emotional detachment, and a cold indifference to patient needs results. Distancing may also produce a loss of a sense of identification or commitment which creates a vicious circle (Lazarus and Folkman, 1984).

A reduced sense of personal accomplishment with feelings of inadequacy and low self-esteem may be indicative of prolonged fluctuating exposure to demand-coping mismatch. If such symptoms become continuous, then recovery may take a long time, even with professional intervention (Biley, 1989). Burnout can therefore be interpreted as a lack of usual social standards, an estrangement towards fellow man, with accompanying physical and behavioural reactions to occupational stressors. The prevalence of this phenomenon in nursing, least of all in critical care, is not easily determined. This may be due to staff suffering from this syndrome leaving before colleagues observe that there is a problem, or that individuals regard their symptoms as a weakness. Such a syndrome may also be difficult to observe as the term suggests a static state rather than a process.

Coping strategies

Coping has already been defined as an individual response aimed at satisfactorily affecting the demand in the desired direction and attempts to manage, master, tolerate or alter the events so that they are not so threatening (Lazarus and Launier, 1978, in Bailey and Clarke, 1989, p. 44). Such a response or attempt may take different forms. Lazarus (1966) distinguished between direct (problem-focused) action and palliative (emotion-focused) actions. These have been categorized further as direct coping, indirect coping and palliative coping (Bailey and Clarke, 1989).

Direct coping

The individual attempts to deal with the demand by direct action aiming to alter the situation into one which is less threatening. Coping actions may change over time as the appraisal of the demand alters. Appraisal of the changes achieved by direct actions will enable the individual to perceive the change and reappraise the need for action.

Indirect coping

Circumstances may arise when direct coping may not be appropriate. People are often confronted with situations which have to be endured, for example, experiencing bereavement. Emotion-focused strategies may be useful in this type of situation. Lazarus and Folkman (1984) suggest that cognitive emotion-focused coping leads to a change in the way a demand is perceived without changing the objective situation. This may give rise to self-deception. Hope and optimism may be maintained, but denial of fact and implication may result by, for example, refusing to acknowedge the death itself.

Palliative coping

Behavioural emotion-focused strategies may be palliative, such as engaging in physical exercise for distraction, or by altering the physiological response to the demand by methods such as relaxation techniques, for example, guided visual imagery (Capel and Gurnsey 1987; Murgatroyd and Woolfe, 1982). Palliative coping, also like indirect coping, does not lead to mastery of the event, but to reduction in the individually perceived or experienced threat. It is usually only temporary, and allows time for the formulation of more therapeutic coping strategies. Such coping strategies include crying, self-controlling (inhibition of one's feelings), confrontational approaches and denial.

Palliative coping has been described as being both harmful and initially effective. Temporary reduction in stress may be produced when this coping is used, but may lead to greater stress experienced at a later date, as the demand has not changed and may still need to be faced. Several forms of palliative coping may lead to increased risk of psychological or physical illness. Psychological defence mechanisms such as denial, repression (prevention of painful thoughts from entering conciousness) or projection (placing blame for dif-

ficulties onto others) may produce emotional ease in some individuals/situations (Lazarus and Folkman, 1984, p. 134). However, such distortion of reality is considered inherently maladaptive. Malignancies may be associated with general emotional inhibition, denial and repression (Sutherland and Cooper, 1990, p. 131). Psychological disorders such as phobic anxiety states, and obsessive compulsive neuroses have also been described as a result of maladaptive coping (Dally and Harrington, 1975). Biley (1989) cites Brown and Birley (1968) as interpreting schizophrenia as a result of demand-coping mismatch.

Judicious use of humour may be effective in stress reduction. One often hears 'you've got to laugh or else you'd cry'. However, outsiders may be surprised or disgusted at some of the things critical care nurses find amusing. Hay and Oken (1972, in Crickmore, 1987) explain that it is natural to develop this type of behaviour in a group of young people working together, as a tolerable working atmosphere is maintained. It has been claimed that humour has a deeper spiritual function which allows the assertion or reassertion of perspective by providing different viewpoints without negating the validity of any alternative opinions (Price and Murphy, 1985). They cite Storlie (1979) as believing humour to be a necessity when matters are most serious.

One must be aware that humour may also be a result of disengagement from emotional involvement and may be evidence of indirect or palliative coping, and may suggest maladaptive methods of coping are being employed. Coping therefore includes "strategies for engagement and involvement as well as strategies for increased control and distance" (Benner and Wrubel, 1989, p. xii), and as Harris (1989) states, coping involves the perception of stress, the conditioning factors and situational supports affecting cognitive appraisal of the stress, and the assessment and eventual selection of the coping mechanism from the person's repertoire.

Stabilities in coping may exist in that preferred modes in relation to similar circumstances may be apparent (Lazarus and Folkman, 1984, p. 130). These may be viewed as particular personality characteristics. However, there is much debate over the nature of personality which requires further discussion.

Personality

The term 'personality' has many conflicting theories and definitions. Personality has been defined as "that which causes behaviour to be consistent in different situations" (Hyland and Donaldson, 1989, p. 45).

It may be possible to predict social behaviour (such as that of coping behaviour) if some knowledge of personality is present.

There is much controversy over whether personality characteristics/traits are stable enduring styles of behaviour or whether they are transitory dynamic states/moods being measured. Opposing views are that personality traits may exist and develop, or that behaviour may be socially learned (Mischel, 1986).

The term is popularly used to refer to either social skills (for example, 'personality problems' implying a lacking of social skills) or outstanding impressions (such as 'an aggressive' or 'submissive' personality). Maslach (1986, p. 62) defines personality as "the essential character of an individual, the mental, emotional and social qualities that combine into a unique whole." These traits are often displayed as opposing extremes on a continuum (see Fig. 8.5).

The intraversion-extraversion continuum was described by Eysenck (1963). He suggested that groups of co-related traits could be defined in this way. Extraverts are seen as sociable, cheerful and talkative, whilst intraverts are quieter, shy and more withdrawn. He believed this to be due to intraverts having a higher level of cortical arousal. Most people are somewhere in the middle of the continuum and may be described as ambiverts.

Personality judgements may be influenced by implicit personality theories. However, the perceiver's ideas of related traits lead to an over-generalization of overall personality. For example, the trait of concientiousness may incorrectly be associated with punctuality. Labelling of colleagues (or patients) with types of personality may adversely influence the support (or care) they receive. Personality has been thought to influence the amount of stress experienced, and it is necessary to include particular aspects in this review. Maslach (1982) believes that particular aspects are especially significant in relation to burnout. Interpersonal style, method of handling problems, expression and control of emotions and self-concept may influence whether burnout will result. Bailey and Clarke (1989, p. 40) outline intraversion/extraversion, problem confrontation/avoidance, repression/sensitization and self-reliance/dependance continuums as being relevant coping styles. However, they argue that personality influences on coping styles employed are strongest when ambiguity exists. Personality traits, therefore, may not be reliable for determining coping responses, as situational and time effects are not considered. Situations influence specific behaviours despite underlying traits (Mischel, 1986). In spite of this, the 'person factor' is considered to influence the amount of stress experienced. Sutherland and Cooper (1990) describe how personality characteristics/behaviour patterns, past experience, needs, values and ability, life stage characteristics, demographic effects, physical condition, and social support are some of the many factors which influence individual vulnerability to stress.

Locus of control

Rotter (1966) is attributed as having described this personality characteristic, and refers to the perceived degree of personal control over a given situation. An *internal* locus of control indicated high perception of individual control, whilst an individual with an *external* locus of control believes that they have little influence upon the situation presented.

Internals are said to be more able to deal with frustration, are less anxious, and more concerned with achievement than those with an external locus of control. Psychological adjustment and coping ability are more successful in *internal* people. This

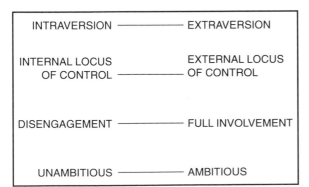

Figure 8.5. Examples of personality traits.

may account for interpersonal relationships being a particularly highly rated stressor in critical care, as relationships with 'superiors' such as medical staff or nursing management may be seen as being externally controlled and are therefore more stressful.

Externals are more likely to be compliant and prone to persuasion. Such a negative belief about one's capacity to have any control in a situation . . . can discourage essential problem-focused efforts (Lazarus and Folkman, 1984, p. 160).

Hardiness

Kobasa, Maddi and Kahn (1982) describe the 'hardy' personality construct as incorporating traits of commitment, control and challenge.

- ☐ Commitment may be defined as being fully involved in an undertaking, rather than disengaging oneself.
- ☐ Control is the belief of being able to influence the course of events (see locus of control).
- ☐ Challenge involves the expectation that life will change and personal growth will be stimulated.

It may be suggested that people who generally possess these traits experience less stress, as they are more able to perceive themselves able to cope. As the term stress is being used as meaning the mismatch between perceived threat and perceived ability to cope, then this is appropriate. Kobasa (1988, in Boyle *et al.*, 1991) stated "A hardy person's sense of control encourages development of an extensive coping repertoire."

If coping is viewed as a function of personality (Argyle, 1983), then it may be assumed that individuals differ not only in the way that they perceive threat but also in the way in which they cope.

Personality traits are described as being stable, and not related to situational effects; however, this is generally unhelpful when predicting behaviour. It is probably more useful to view personality as that which is 'released' to outsiders, in a staggered kind of way (Burnett, McGhee and Clarke, 1984, p. 218).

If personality labels are applied to nurses or patients, inappropriate support or care may result. Therefore the concept of personality may only be useful at a particular time and for a specific situation. This negates the concept of personality in itself (Bailey and Clarke, 1989, p. 41).

Social support

Social support is generally thought of as comprising of three components – emotional support, instrumental support and informational support (House, 1981). *Emotional* support enables emotion-focused coping by directing action or thoughts to control undesirable feelings resulting from stressful interactions. *Instrumental* support enables direct coping by focusing on the problem and removing or altering circumstances perceived to be threats. *Informational* support enables perception-focused coping by altering the meaning of a situation by reducing its perceived threat. Lazarus and Folkman (1984) outline the possible positive and negative effects of social support. Whilst on the one hand positive prevention, coping and recovery may result, the opposite may arise. For example, if social support is promoted as being effective and necessary, those with little social support may feel further isolated or lonely, and therefore experience more stress. This may be demonstrated by a new member of critical care nursing staff finding difficulty in gaining a sense of belonging within a large highly skilled, knowledgeable team. Social support is more usefully viewed as a resource which may be tapped to meet social demands.

The knowledge that social support is available for use affects the way in which a stressor is perceived and the coping strategy is adopted. Such a socially learned response may be developed within a supportive working climate which has been suggested to reduce perceived job stress and improve psychological and physical health.

Work colleagues may be the most valuable resource in relation to reducing or preventing burnout. In particular, a colleague in a similar situation may have insight into an individual's problem, and may provide a useful measure against which individual response may be gauged (Maslach, 1986). When comparing social support to self-help coping strategies, Murgatroyd and Woolfe (1979) suggest that group support may be effective when self-help strategies have failed. This may be particularly relevant where complex sets of relationships are present, such as in critical care nursing where there is potential for conflict and ambiguity. Such situations highlight the need to seek social support from peers. The general feeling of staff being 'in this together' (collective coping) may account for the many informal networks of support which arise during meal breaks, providing opportunity for airing moans and groans (and many humorous conversations) and allowing the off-loading of stress to the whole team, in return for group support. Whilst this structure may provide an adaptive resource, it also contains potential dangers in that denial and distancing may be encouraged, and cliques may develop which prove to be counter-productive.

REVIEW OF THE RESEARCH

Early reports had been largely anecdotal and were based on much subjective information. Most of the research into stress in critical care nursing during the 1970s and 1980s addressed the debate regarding whether critical care was more, less or equally stressful than other nursing environments. Such comparative studies had produced conflicting results. The hypothesis that working in critical care is more stressful (stimulus-response) than working in other areas has been both supported and rejected. This demonstrates why models of stress have developed towards the transactional view. The measurement of the presence of stress in a particular environment does not reflect contemporary opinion of stress being demand-coping mismatch. It is not difficult to accept that particular environments are not stressful in themselves and are not solely responsible for the degree of stress experienced by an individual. Summers (1989), following a random survey of nurses in critical care ($n = 181$), dispelled the notion that working in critical care contributes to job stress. However, clarification of theory development is required, and an overview of comparative study assists in determining current theories of stress.

Comparative studies

Cronin-Stubbs and Rooks (1985) investigated 296 critical care and ward nurses from three hospitals. Using the Staff Burnout Scale for Health Professionals (SBS-HP) (Jones, 1980), and the Nursing Stress Scale (NSS) (Gray-Toft and Anderson 1981), they determined that greater job stressors were experienced in critical care over ward areas. However, critical care nurses were experiencing less stress than their ward colleagues. The conclusions drawn from this study are somewhat contradictory and confusing, which reflects difficulties with the stimulus-response model. In approaching 96 nurses from six units (2 ICU, 2 HDU and 2 non-ICU), Keane, Ducette and Adler (1985) used the SBS-HP and the Hardiness Scale developed by Kobasa et al. (1982). This includes measuring locus of control (Rotter's Locus of Control Scale, RLCS, 1966). Whilst job stressors were not measured, burnout, hardiness, control and challenge were found to be *equal* in ICU and non-ICU nurses. Those who demonstrated higher levels of burnout were more external in their locus of control.

Much of the other comparative research presents conflicting findings. This appears to be due to not only poor theoretical guidance, but also other design weaknesses such as poor sampling and use of invalidated tools. Harris (1989) highlights the vagueness and overusage of the term stress which severely restricts generalization and clarity of findings. Nevertheless, studies such as these and those shown in Table 8.1 reinforced the need for theory development, and changed the emphasis from determining *which speciality* is more stressful, but *how* may the mismatch between perceived demand and perceived coping ability be reduced.

Table 8.1.   Examples of studies comparing ICU and non-ICU nurse stress (adapted from Harris, 1989).

Stress more in ICU	Stress equal	Stress more in non-ICU
Lewandowski and Kramer (1980)	Cronin-Stubbs and Rooks (1985)	Maloney (1982)
Beyers et al. (1983)	Keane et al. (1985)	Kelly and Cross (1985)
	Maloney and Bartz (1983)	
	McCranie et al. (1987)	
	Cross and Fallon (1985, in Bibbings, 1987)	
	Stehle (1980) review	

Occupational stressors

Various studies have been undertaken to determine what occupational stressors arise within critical care. Classifying stressors into intrapersonal, extrapersonal and interpersonal categories assists in clarifying stressors cited in research (see Table 8.2), including specialities of ICU, CCU, Renal and Trauma nursing.

Intrapersonal stressors (which arise from within an individual) include meeting needs of patients and their families, lack of knowledge/skill, and rapid decision-making.

Extrapersonal stressors (which arise from out-side an individual) include staff/patient ratios, excessive workload, shift-work, noise levels and increasing legal implications of the role.

Intrapersonal stressors include conflict with other health care staff, poor communication with senior nursing and medical staff, and uncertainty concerning patient treatment.

Unit management is suggested to be related to burnout. Vincent and Billings (1988) concluded that if unit management is perceived as poor, then burnout levels increase, particularly in relation to emotional exhaustion. (The results from this American study ($n = 150$, from four hospitals) may not be generalized to work in the UK, but personal

Table 8.2. Occupational stressors for nurses working in critical care areas.

Intrapersonal stressors

Lack of support in dealing with death/dying	1, 3, 10, 11
Life stresses	5, 8
Meeting needs of patients and significant others	1, 3, 6, 10, 12
Lack of knowledge/skill and rapid decision-making	1, 2, 3, 4, 7, 9, 10
Responsibility for patients' lives	2, 7
Role conflicts	7, 13
No sense of support	13

Extrapersonal stressors

Shift work	6, 7
Workload, staff-patient ratios, amount of physical work	1, 2, 3, 6, 7, 9, 10, 12
Equipment failure, new technology	1, 10
Noise levels	1, 3, 5, 9
Increasing legal implications of role	2, 7
Physical layout, work environment	3, 4, 9, 12
Unit management	4, 13
Lack of time to give emotional support	6
Dealing with interruptions and new admissions	6

Interpersonal stressors

Communication between staff members	1, 2, 4, 9, 12
Communication between staff and other departments	1, 3, 4
Uncertainty concerning patient treatment	1, 4
Communication with senior nursing/medical staff	1, 2, 3, 4, 9, 10, 12, 13
Dealing with 'difficult' or 'demanding' patients	6
Dealing with inexperienced physician	10

Key

1. Huckabay and Jagla (1979), 2. Coghlan (1984), 3. Norbeck (1985a), 4. Vincent and Billings (1988), 5. Topf and Dillon (1988), 6. Dewe (1989), 7. White and Tonkin (1991), 8. Cronin-Stubbs and Rooks (1985), 9. Kelly and Cross (1985), 10. Ehrenfeld and Cheifetz (1990), 11. Davidson and Jackson (1985, in Biley, 1989), 12. Cassem and Hackett (1972, in Biley, 1989), 13. Nichols, Springford and Searle (1981, in Biley, 1989)

experience suggests that similar findings may be discovered in a replicated study.) Burnout has been linked to noise levels in critical care. Irrespective of noise sensitivity, noise induced stress increases the level of burnout (Topf and Dillon, 1988).

Many variables affect the stress response, and consideration of other independant variables such as social support, demographic influences, coping strategies and personality traits require further investigation to propose predictive guidelines for practice.

Job satisfaction and social support

Job satisfaction (see Table 8.3) was investigated in two studies by Norbeck (1985a,b). The growing concern for nurses' well-being initiated sampling of 180 and 164 nurses in the two studies. Norbeck found that if job stress was perceived as high, then job dissatisfaction increased together with psychological symptoms. Low social support (emotional and instrumental support) also increased job dissatisfaction and high perceptions of job stress. It is

Table 8.3.   Job satisfaction and social support.

Study	Year	Sample	No. of hospitals	Research tool(s)	Outcome
Norbeck	1985a	180	8	Stressful factors in ICU (SF in ICU) (Huckabay and Jagla, 1979) Nursing Job Satisfaction Scale (Atwood and Hinshaw, 1985) Brief Symptom Inventory (BSI) (Derogatis and Spencer, 1982, Cited in Norbeck, 1985a)	Increased perceived job stress decreases job satisfaction and increases psychological symptoms
Norbeck	1985b	164	8	Norbeck Social Support Questionnaire (NSSQ) SF in ICU BSI	Poor social support increases risk of job stress and job dissatisfaction
Boyle et al.	1991	103	1 (6 units)	SBS-HP (Jones, 1980) Hardiness Scale (Kobasa et al., 1982) House & Wells Social Support Scale (HWSSS) (House, 1981)	Level of social support predicts level of burnout
Cronin-Stubbs and Rooks	1985	296	3	Nurses Stress Scale (NSS) (Gray-Toft and Anderson, 1981) SBS-HP NSSQ Life Experiences Survey (LES) (Saronsen et al., 1978)	Low social support increases stress experienced
Dear, Weisman, Alexander and Chase	1982	234 (ICU) 868 (non-ICU)	2	Job Descriptive Index (JDI) Autonomy Scale (University of Michigan) Rotter's Locus of Control Scale (RLCS)	Autonomy is the strongest determinant of job satisfaction. Strongest determinants of turnover are younger age, lower educational level and low perceived autonomy. Job satisfaction and turnover – ICU = non-ICU

well recognized that an inverse relationship exists between job satisfaction and staff turnover which is of great concern not only in nursing but in the general labour force. In nursing, staff turnover appears to be increasing, and Harris (1989) suggests that this is "mostly related to interference with the autonomy and practice of professional nursing."

Dear, Weisman, Alexander and Chase (1982) compared ICU nurses to non-ICU staff in relation to job satisfaction and turnover (voluntary resignations and not dismissal or retirement). They determined that perceived level of automony was the strongest predictor of turnover, and that this is linked with level of education and a younger age. ICU nurses equalled non-ICU nurses in levels of job satisfaction and turnover.

Using multiple regression analysis, Boyle, Grap, Younger and Thornby (1991) supported Cronin-Stubbs and Rooks' suggestion that social support may be an effective predictor of burnout. Work-related social support was more beneficial than outside sources, and they concluded that social support may therefore be situation-specific. Lees and Ellis (1990) also indicate that work-related social support has great importance in relation to occupational stress.

Coping

"Coping methods are the key mediators in the nurse's stress reaction." (Harris, 1989. p. 12).

An Australian study by Kelly and Cross (1985) described coping behaviour and levels of stress in 102 intensive care and ward nurses. Despite ICU nurses experiencing greater stressors (e.g. work space, unit management, noise levels) ward nurses experienced greater stress. However, coping behaviour was not measured but described, and this design weakness prevents generalization of the conclusion that ward nurses favour palliative coping strategies such as crying. Contrary to this are two Australian studies by Coghlan (1984) and White and Tonkin (1991). Whilst the validity of the questionnaire used within both studies is not determined they describe that indirect and palliative coping strategies are preferred by critical care staff. Occupational stressors highlighted are predominantly extrapersonal in nature.

Using data collected during workshops on 'Cop-ing with Stress', Ehrenfeld and Cheifetz (1990) categorized four distinct coping modes which were employed by critical care nurses ($n = 264$ from cardiac units throughout Israel).

☐ Active problem-solving (direct coping)
☐ Diverting responsibility (palliative coping)
☐ Passivity or avoidance (palliative coping)
☐ Indirect activity (indirect coping)

Whilst this was acknowledged as not being a definitive statistical study, results indicate a relationship between coping mode and emotional in that the only mode employed associated with positive feelings was that of active problem-solving. This is also supported by Ceslowitz (1989): using Maslach's Burnout Inventory (MBI) (Maslach and Jackson, 1981), and the Ways of Coping scale suggested by Lazarus and Folkman (1984), high levels of burnout were associated with palliative coping and lower levels of burnout associated with seeking social support and active problem-solving. Ceslowitz concluded that if the threat is conceived as being amenable to change, or coping resources perceived as being adequate, then less burnout is experienced (see Table 8.4).

Many negative feelings and behaviours may be associated with restrictive coping strategies. Feelings of guilt or inadequacy, low morale, absenteeism, lowered productivity, arguing, scapegoating staff, busy behaviour, intolerance of others and defensiveness may all be indicative of palliative or indirect coping being in operation. The typical 'busy gait' of a critical care nurse allows an internal locus of control over a situation, which will reduce feelings of inadequacy. This avoidance or self-controlling coping increases the risk of burnout. In critical care especially, physical avoidance or reduction in patient contact is difficult to achieve as patients cannot be left unattended. However, emotional detachment, such as that described in burnout, may be an unfortunate alternative.

Dewe (1989) explored the transactional view of stress across nursing groups, measuring the stimulus-response relationship in terms of excess demand (tiredness and/or tension). The study ($n = 1801$ from 29 New Zealand hospitals) found that:

☐ different work stressors do not produce different levels of tiredness or tension;

Table 8.4.   Coping.

Study	Year	Sample	No. of hospitals	Research tool(s)	Outcome
Kelly and Cross	1985	102	2	Questionnaire (Bailey, Steffen and Grout, 1980)	Ward stress more than ICU stress. Ward staff favoured palliative coping strategies
Boyle et al.	1991	103	1 (6 units)	SBS-HP Hardiness Scale (Kobasa et al., 1982) Ways of Coping (Lazarus and Folkman, 1984) HWSSS (House, 1981)	Problem-focused coping not related to burnout. Emotion-focused coping increased level of burnout
Coghlan White and Tonkin	1984 1991	73 53	3 2	Questionnaire (Coghlan, 1984) Questionnaire (Coghlan, 1984)	Critical care staff did not employ active or direct coping strategies
Ehrenfeld and Cheifetz	1990	264	Most cardiac units in Israel	Workshop discussion	Active problem-solving – the only coping strategy to produce positive feelings. Coping mode employed influences the emotional response
Ceslowitz	1989	150	4	Maslach's Burnout Inventory Ways of Coping (adapted)	Direct coping reduces level of burnout. Self-controlling, confronting or avoidance strategies increase burnout. Higher burnout = less control
Dewe	1989	1801	29	Questionnaire (to measure 'demand')	Charge Nurses used more direct coping than EN's or Staff Nurses. EN's used more palliative and indirect coping than Staff and Charge Nurses. Level of demand cannot be predicted by stressors themselves

☐ frequent stressors may produce tiredness and/or tension;

☐ charge nurses used more direct coping strategies than staff and enrolled nurses;

☐ enrolled and staff nurses use palliative and indirect coping more frequently than charge nurses.

This is also supported by Lees and Ellis (1990); however, more information regarding variables such as stressor duration and coping strategies appears to be required before predictive guidelines may be defined.

Demographic variables

Bartz and Maloney (1986) compared 89 nurses (ICU and non-ICU) in one American army medical centre using MBI and a job diagnostic survey. They determined that demographic variables such as age, gender status and length of experience were predictive of level of burnout. Older women of civilian status with less than degree level education experienced less burnout. The specialist sample chosen prevents generalizing these results as other studies seem to dispute links between age and level of burnout (Boyle *et al.*, 1991; McCranie *et al.*, 1987; Topf, 1989).

These variables do not appear to have predictive qualities in relation to stress or burnout, and further research may not be appropriate at this time.

Hardiness

The investigation of this personality trait has gained recent popularity, and appears to be partly due to the conflicting results of comparative studies reviewed earlier, notably that of Keane *et al.* (1985). The studies reviewed here (see Table 8.5) do not enter the debate on whether hardiness is a personality trait or whether it may be learned. They address whether hardy characteristics may be predictive of level of burnout experienced. Keane *et al.* (1985) used the SBS-HP and a Hardiness Scale (Kobasa *et al.*, 1982), and concluded that higher levels of burnout were associated with a non-hardy personality. To determine whether hardiness moderated the impact of perceived job stress on the level of burnout, McCranie, Lambert and Lambert's (1987) study used an adapted Hardiness Scale, the Tedium Scale (Pines and Aronsen, 1981),

and the Nursing Stress Scale. Keane *et al.*'s conclusions were supported – less hardy individuals experienced high levels of burnout.

In relation to coping modes, Boyle *et al.*'s (1991) study indicates that hardy individuals are more likely to seek social support, use direct coping strategies and are less likely to use purely emotion-focused (indirect) coping.

However, as symptoms of burnout have been already outlined as including detachment, depression and low self-esteem, then it seems hardly surprising that low hardiness increases burnout. When hardiness is measured together with other variables, such as social support and coping strategies, a more predictive picture may emerge (Topf, 1989).

PRACTICAL NURSING IMPLICATIONS

"Obviously the quality of patient care depends greatly on those providing it. The psychological stage of the staff will, in part, determine how effective they are." (Bishop, 1981, in Crickmore, 1987, p. 20).

This section of the chapter is intended to provide useful guidance in dealing with stress and coping. Three approaches have been identified as pertinent:

Table 8.5. Hardiness.

Study	Year	Sample	No. of hospitals	Research tool(s)	Outcome
Boyle *et al.*	1991	103	1 (6 units)	SBS-HP Hardiness Scale (Kobasa *et al.*, 1982) Ways of Coping (Lazarus and Folkman, 1984) HWSSS (House, 1981)	Increased hardiness reduces the use of palliative/indirect coping. Personality hardiness negatively related to burnout
Keane *et al.*	1985	96	2	SBS-HP Hardiness Scale (Kobasa *et al.*, 1982)	ICU stress = non-ICU stress. Low hardiness increases risk of burnout
McCranie *et al.*	1987	107	1	Hardiness Scale Tedium Scale (Pines and Aronsen, 1981, Cited in McCranie *et al.*, 1987) NSS	Low hardiness increases level of burnout

☐ how individual nurses may help themselves;
☐ the role of education and training;
☐ organizational and managerial issues.

It is often all too easy to blame the organization or individual members of staff for the stress that is experienced. However, individuals are able to do much to reduce their own levels of stress, which may in turn influence both the team and managerial approaches.

Individual approaches to coping

The most important factor in relation to coping style is the ability to identify stress in oneself (and others), and to be able to determine an effective, appropriate coping strategy. Identification of stress has been outlined in the literature and research review, and this may have helped readers to recognize situations, feelings and reactions associated with stress.

It is now necessary to discuss in more depth how these may be coped with more effectively.

Direct coping strategies

Coping directed at the demand itself such as planned problem-solving or maintaining up-to-date skills and knowledge (e.g. in Advanced Life Support) has been shown to produce positive feelings and be negatively related to burnout (Ehrenfeld and Cheifetz 1990; Ceslowitz, 1989).

A problem-solving approach consists of seven main stages (see Fig. 8.6).

These stages are similar to those of the nursing process and are therefore familiar to us. However, in relation to stress and coping they appear to be most effective, yet least used.

Problem-solving
Problems are concerned with choosing the *best* method towards a solution (Adair, 1979). When adopting this kind of approach, a redirection towards internal locus of control results, and focusing on the problems produces activity, both of which account for the positive feelings and stress reduction.

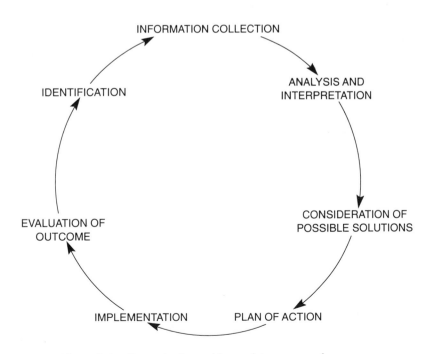

Figure 8.6.   Stages in the problem-solving approach.

Identification and definition of problems may not be as simple as it sounds. Problem-solving skills are drawn from resources such as range of experience, application of knowledge and the ability of self-control and self-awareness. These and other factors such as situational characteristics may influence problem recognition as they affect information gathering and interpretation. Also what may seem to be the problem may only be a symptom of the problem. For example, a nurse who is always late for work, and therefore is always allocated the 'easiest' patient, may not be 'lazy' or 'thoughtless' or 'uncaring', but may have problems outside of work such as childminding difficulties. Specific definitions of problems will only be accurate if appropriate *information* is collated and interpreted. (Defining problems in terms of solutions may lead to varying interpretations, and it is more useful to be specific.) Relevant knowledge and experience must be utilized to consider all possible causes and perspectives. For an effective plan of action to be developed, appropriate *interpretation* of information must be achieved. Discussion with other staff at this point may help to prevent narrow individual perceptions.

Solutions may be analytical and/or creative. The generation of as many possible solutions will permit elimination of those which would not be 'in character', and also allow judgments in relation to their feasibility, practicability and reliability (Garofalo-Ford *et al.*, 1979). Management techniques such as force field analysis may help in determining choice of solution together with consideration of personal risks, benefits and priorities. It may also be useful to consider the positive and negative consequences of *each* of the options that have been suggested (Bond, 1986).

The *planning* and *implementation* stages, in relation to patient care, can be expressed in physiological or behavioural goals, yet in relation to general problem-solving a wider interpretation is necessary. Planning action aimed to alter/reduce the demand may not have the goal of eliminating the demand altogether. Direct nursing care often requires elimination of the problem as the goal, for example, a painfree state. In problem-solving for stress management, the goal may be only to reduce the 'pain' or to only feel it on Fridays! Plans must include *how* the problem will be dealt with.

Following implementation of the plan of action, *evaluation* of the outcome must be undertaken to determine whether the desired changes have resulted.

Example of using a problem-solving approach

Situation: a junior nurse is caring for a patient with acute renal failure and peritoneal dialysis (PD) is in progress. The nurse feels that the nurse in charge (NIC) is not giving her the support she needs, as she has little experience with PD.

Problem identification
Information collection:
  What information is required?
  Consider the following questions (and others) which may be appropriate to gain pertinent information.

☐ Is the problem solely with the nurse in charge?
☐ Which other people affect the junior nurse's feeling of lack of support?
☐ What other roles/priorities does the NIC have?
☐ What reasons may there be for the lack of support? (e.g. time, capability, awareness.)
☐ Do other staff feel the same way?
☐ How is the specific situation influencing feelings and behaviour?

Depending on information gained, the problem may be identified as one or more of the following:

☐ Lack of knowledge and skills (in junior nurse and/or NIC).
☐ Communication problem between junior nurse and NIC (the nurse in charge is not aware of the junior nurse's lack of experience with PD.)
☐ Other priorities of the nurse in charge.
☐ Other influences outside work.
☐ Others.

Thus the initially perceived problem may be defined as four or more specific problems.

Consideration of possible solutions
For each of the problems identified a list of possible solutions may be made, for example, for the problem of communication solutions may be:

a. Leave the patient and tell the NIC that more support is needed.
b. Confide in another staff member.
c. List the skills the junior nurse possesses in relation to caring for the patient.
d. Identify others who may be able to help.
e. Moan about NIC at coffee time.
f. Resign on the spot!
g. Gain help from a colleague regarding PD.
h. When NIC comes to the bed area hit her on the nose!
i. Discuss with NIC at a later stage how to improve knowledge and skills.

Planning and implementation
Prioritize – which solutions would not be feasible, practical or reliable? Time and situational factors will influence choice. It may be most practical to initially seek support from an alternative source. However, evaluating this chosen solution may highlight the need to discuss development of knowledge and skills with NIC at an appropriate time to reduce stress in a future similar situation. It may also be necessary to discuss support in general terms if the situation is not an isolated incident.

Creative problem-solving has been emphasized as an adaptive stress management technique, but it is important to point out some weaknesses of the approach.

It is tempting to try too hard to find the 'right' solution, and if tired or upset, inappropriate decisions may be made. The strategy also requires time and effort which may result in delaying action. This may result in escalation of the problem and an ensuing risk of increasing levels of stress or burnout.

If implementing the plan of action becomes difficult, then it may be easy to feel disheartened, and full implementation may not be achieved. Bureaucracy may also restrict the opportunities for using problem-solving strategies (Dewe, 1989).

Maslach's (1986) suggestion of "working smarter not harder", reflects direct coping. Organizational skills such as setting achievable goals may prevent large problems from becoming overwhelming. Doing the same thing differently, and possibly more efficiently, avoids rigid routines. Both of these may provide challenge and may help to develop the concept of control.

Other direct coping strategies appear more familiar such as the application of pressure to prevent haemorrhage or clearing a patient's airway. This indicated that nurse education had traditionally emphasized biomedical skills over and above psycho-social skills of patient (and self) care. However, the unique knowledge base for the nursing profession is developing to incorporate skills and knowledge and skills related to holistic care.

Palliative coping strategies

Palliative coping strategies may be emotion-focused, and behavioural responses vary between increased physical activity (e.g. exercise or hyper-activity), crying, denial or relaxation techniques.

Examples of palliative coping strategies

crying	detachment
smoking	withdrawal
increased alcohol intake	projection
snacking	physical exercise
humour	relaxation
denial	meditation
self-controlling	yoga

These have been described as mal-adaptive, providing only temporary relief with the likelihood of greater stress being experienced later on, and possible links with psychological disorders such as schizophrenia or phobic anxiety states. Consequently, palliative coping strategies have more recently been given less attention. However, it is apparent that many 'palliatives' are essential in allowing some 'time-out' from a situation and are used frequently by more junior members of staff (Dewe, 1989). Particularly in critical care many problems may not be changeable (e.g. death of a patient) and palliative strategies which are immediately effective seem legitimate. However, if other strategies are not subsequently employed then individuals may be at risk.

As stated, individual nurses may help to reduce stress in themselves. Relaxation techniques have achieved wide popularity, and those such as progressive relaxation, deep relaxation or meditation are reputedly beneficial to health. Responses are highly specific to the individual and if relaxation is successful enhances feelings of well-being, peacefulness and a sense of control. Physiological signs of success include a decrease in blood pressure, heart rate and respiration. As with all skills, these techniques require practice, and each individual may prefer different techniques. It must be remembered that it isn't *what* is done that matters but that each individual develops *their own way* of achieving physical and mental relaxation.

Before you read the two particular favourites outlined on these two pages, a reminder . . . sleep is not always relaxation. Too much sleep may be indicative of detrimental stress; for example, successful relaxation for half an hour may be more effective than an extra four hours sleep.

Once an individual becomes skilled in practices such as these, it may be possible to achieve instant or momentary relaxation. This is most useful in dealing with on the spot situations which are likely to produce the stress response. For example, role conflicts such as that of patient advocate and criti-

---

Physical relaxation exercise

N.B. Please read through carefully before attempting the following exercise.

SITTING (on an armless chair or stool)

HANDS: Let your arms dangle by your sides or between your knees; shake your hands hard, as though shaking off water.

SHOULDERS: i. Pretend you are a string puppet and your shoulders are being pulled up, just a little. Quickly imagine the strings have been cut, and your shoulders fall.
                          Pretend you are carrying two heavy suitcases and feel your shoulders being pulled down; drop the cases.
                      ii. Using your shoulders, fold them forward six times (don't cheat and use your upper arms only!). Then back six times.

NECK: i. Pretend your neck is broken and let your head drop forward; imagine it becoming heavier and heavier; raise it slowly.
                          Lower your head gently to your right; feel it sinking further and further, by its own weight; raise it slowly. Do the same to the left.
                      ii. Pretend your neck is made of flexible rubber; turn it from side to side trying to look behind you, three or four times each way.

ANKLES: Remove your shoes, cross your knees and slowly rotate each ankle in turn, several times in each direction.

THIGHS: Sit with your knees together. Press your thighs against each other; quickly release them and allow your legs to flap apart.

STANDING (Stand with your feet slightly apart, arms by your side.)

ARMS: With feet apart, rapidly shake or twist both arms in their sockets. Let your arms hang straight down while you do this and you will feel the upper muscles wobble. (This is the Olympic swimmers exercise.)

ARMS AND   i. Imagine they are not your arms, but a long heavy, floppy scarf, quite lifeless and
SHOULDERS: unable to move itself. Start turning your body from side to side, gently at first, and the scarf will gradually lift and flap around your body.
                          Repeat this rhythmically several times. (WARNING! To avoid becoming giddy, shut your eyes, or else keep your head and eyes still.)
                      ii. Raise your arms loosely in front of you to shoulder height. Let them drop so that they swish past your body. Swing them up again in front.
                          Repeat several times.

Mental relaxation exercise (Adapted from Maslach, 1986)

A quiet room and comfortable position is essential for this exercise.

1. Prevent active thoughts (mind-racing) by 'thought-stopping' techniques such as verbalizing the word 'no' when thoughts are persistant. Self-commands such as this can be repeated many times whilst remaining physically relaxed. Silent 'no's' may be used when active thoughts become less persistent.

2. Visualize a place in which you have felt warm relaxed and happy, such as a sunny day during a favourite holiday or day out. Concentrate on the details of the scene you have visualized. For example, the colour of the sky, the shape of the clouds and the texture of the grass.

3. Think of what you felt happy about. Where did you go/what did you do next? (e.g. a gentle walk along the cliff, or beach, or sitting on a bench in a park in the sun. Visualize the route you took.

4. Feel the warmth your body experienced – notice which parts of your body are warm, is it your face, . . . or hands, . . . or back?

5. Turn to face the source of the warmth and remain physically relaxed. Gradually racing thoughts will disappear, when this has occurred enjoy the scene for a few moments.

6. Slowly let a grey/black 'nothingness' take over the scene. Dispel all the detail you have focused on so far.

7. Finally, let blue colours intrude upon the nothingness. As these colours enter your mind, concentrate on the *feeling* you are experiencing.

cal care nurse. Instant relaxation can be achieved in 30–60 seconds and may be employed during a quick coffee break. Using your in-built muscle memory in this way does not prevent the stress response, but it helps prevent this response from interfering with successful functioniong (Albrecht, 1979).

Other palliative strategies

Crying, smoking, increasing alcohol intake, denial, detachment or projection are also palliative coping strategies. These may be recognized as effective temporary measures, and experience suggests that they are frequently employed by critical care nurses, but as far as the individual is concerned, monitoring the extent to which these types of behavioural response are being employed will help to identify which other strategies would be useful.

This appraisal of the situation (likened to Lazarus and Folkman's secondary appraisal, 1984) involves evaluating which coping options are available and which may be most effective in producing the desired result. The answer will not usually solely be a palliative strategy.

Indirect coping strategies

Indirect coping strategies have particular use when dealing with situations which are not amenable to change. Care of a dying patient or unsuccessful resuscitative attempts may be extreme sources of stress in critical care.

Instances such as these led to the initial belief that critical care areas were more stressful than other areas. However, coping strategies such as emotion-focused indirect coping appears to be effective in such situations. For example, when the death of a patient appears inevitable, a strategy that is often adopted is that the impending death is accepted and the death is then viewed as a welcome release from pain and discomfort. In this way the role of the nurse changes from being a 'life-saver' to one of promoting a peaceful death (Henderson, 1966).

Death has been reappraised as no longer being the problem/threat (as it is not amenable to change), but that providing a dignified pain-free death is something within the scope of the skilled critical care nurse.

Reappraisal also assists when stress has been perceived in an exaggerated way, often due to strong emotional reactions resultant from past experience and ingrained habits. Taking criticisms too personally reduces perceived ability to cope with the demand. Reappraisal and 'standing back' from the situation may allow objectivity into a strongly subjective viewpoint and therefore reduce the strength of the emotional response. Employing logic and reason in an appropriate way may produce increased perception of coping ability.

Albrect (1979) described a *rethinking* technique as substituting a new, more useful thought for the stressful one. For example, an inexperienced nurse whom one may find particularly frustrating may produce thoughts such as 'She's terrible, she can't do anything!'. Substitute the thoughts that 'No, she is merely doing what she is able to with her level of knowledge and experience, at this time'. This substituted thought may give the direction to offer appropriate support in place of demonstrating exasperation. This not only assists in managing stress more effectively, but may provide a more long-term solution to a problem for both the individual nurse and her new colleague.

This technique is comparable to the 'language of choice'. Substitution of the words 'choose not to' for 'can't' may reduce stress as perception is altered. For example: 'I can't go to break . . . we're *too* busy'. 'I choose not to go to break . . . we're *too* busy'. Other substitutions may be 'and' for 'but'; for example: 'But I'll be too tired to go out'. 'And I'll be too tired to go out'.

Finally, the individual can do much to develop particular interpersonal skills to cope with stress more effectively. Skills which assist in dealing with interpersonal conflict (a frequently cited stressor) include assertiveness, the giving and receiving of support, and saying no.

> "Complex communication skills may be learned, but may not be used or maintained without ongoing training and supervision." (MacGuire, 1990).

So it is necessary to remind ourselves of the need to practise and develop communication skills.

Finally, other methods that the individual may employ include actively seeking instrumental or emotional social support either at work or outside; this is negatively related to burnout in female nurses (Norbeck, 1985b; Boyle *et al.*, 1991; Ceslowitz, 1989).

Physical exercise is associated with reduction in anxiety scores (Morgan, 1987), and in some units, team exercises have been implemented as warm-up procedures at the beginning of the shift (Fletcher, 1987).

It is therefore important to take responsibility for initiating the process of sorting out individual stresses (Bond, 1986), seeking out appropriate coping strategies and resisting the temptation to blame other people or things. Monitoring the level of stress in self (and in peers) must also be undertaken as those who are in the best position to know the staff are those who are in the most contact with them.

The role of education and training

The frequently cited extensive knowledge base required by critical care nurses is of vital importance in both influencing perception of demand and perception of coping ability. Clinical knowledge and skill assists in direct coping strategies related purely to the *clinical* nature of nursing. As clinical knowledge and skill increase, perceived internal locus of control may increase, which in turn may increase ability to deal with situations which may cause stress (Keane *et al.*, 1985). Nevertheless, in relation to the management of stress, the application of theory to practice is not so easy (the complexity and continuing development of stress theory partly restricts such application).

Dewe (1989) asked individual qualified nurses how their training had helped them cope with the pressures of their work. Many nurses replied that they had learned that stress was unavoidable, and that training had helped them "come to terms with how they felt", and in Ehrenfeld and Cheifetz's study (1990), only 33% of nurses applied knowledge of active (direct) coping strategies to practice. The continued diligence in preparing nurses for dealing with the stressor death and dying may be evident in that nurses who have been educationally prepared for dealing with this stressor tend to view it as challenging, rather than threatening (Norbeck, 1985a). This also supports the argument that hardiness or at least one aspect of the concept (challenge) may be learned.

Expedient evaluation of the effectiveness of the many techniques which may be employed is difficult owing to individual preferences.

Organizational and managerial issues

"Work-related social support from peers reduces emotional strain, either by doing something about the source of stress or by getting you to cope with it more effectively." (Maslach, 1986.)

A difficulty in promoting a supportive group or team often evident in critical care nursing is that of numbers of staff. For example, in large ICUs there may be many staff (even if not meeting appropriate staff/patient ratios), and often too many for effective team building to materialize. Lack of peer support and poor communication may result. It is essential that consistency of professional support, if not from peers but from more senior staff, is given. This is inherently linked to the management style of charge nurses. Two-way communication and the fostering of mutual trust and support are themes which continually arise when people management is discussed.

The most important word in relation to stress and organizational issues is *communication*. An open, two-way communication style will encourage active involvement of all levels of staff in the decision-making process, and an awareness of the role of nursing administration and or clinical directorates. Regular group meetings led by individuals with good chairing skills facilitate open communication and may include liaison with psychiatrists (Holsclaw, 1965, in Crickmore, 1987). However, the recommendation for a counsellor to be attached to the ward/unit was not rated highly in the study by Kelly and Cross (1985). Nevertheless, the lack of availability of a comprehensive network of counselling services may have much to do with the levels of stress currently being experienced in critical care.

Guidelines for staffing levels produced by the Intensive Care Society (ICS) in 1979 are long out of date. It is hoped that new guidelines currently being investigated by the ICS and the British Association of Critical Care Nurses will help to solve this problem.

Selection of staff for critical care is often difficult when nurse shortages in general are problematic. Keane *et al.* (1985) suggested that although hardiness scales were too weak to use in the selection procedure, the concepts of commitment, control and challenge would be useful to explore at inter-

view. Identification of staff who are more at risk of burnout enables more support to be given (Biley, 1989).

There have been many managerial solutions proposed to help deal with staff stress. Rotation of staff between critical care areas and other less stressful areas has been suggested (Fletcher, 1987; Wimbush, 1983; Crickmore, 1987). However, determining which areas are less stressful is less easy than first imagined (e.g. ICU stress = non ICU stress). In 'Life Stresses', it also seems that changing jobs may be an additional stressor and this idea has not been received with enthusiasm (Kelly and Cross, 1985), despite the insistence that no 'blaming the victim' or stigma should be attached to individuals who may feel the need for temporary transfer or rotation of duty.

Alternating the frequency and intensity of patient care may also go some way to reduce work stress, but this must be sensitively achieved by consulting individual nurses. For example, the rapport and strength of a relationship which may develop between the nurse, patient and relatives may provide job satisfaction in an individual, despite the intensity and frequency of stressors related to the patient and care required.

The concept of primary nursing is often resisted due to it being viewed as providing no escape from specific long-term patients, but the philosophy of primary nursing may provide many answers for reducing the stress experienced.

Work patterns such as 4 × 10 hour shifts have also been suggested, and there are still some advocates for 12 hour shift patterns. These may be attractive in some ways in that more days off-duty may be gained, but generally other factors such as social commitments and resistance to change influence non-acceptance of such schemes.

A frequent expression of job dissatisfaction is that specialized units often only come into contact with patients who are highly dependent, and that staff have little or no contact with patients (or relatives) after transfer from the unit. Patient follow-up programmes and good interdepartmental liaison may help providing a less pessimistic view of effectiveness of service provided than may be apparent.

Workspace and noise levels are particular environmental factors which are positively related to work stress or burnout, both of which may be addressed by appropriate planning and organization.

Although not proven through research, much evidence exists to suggest that workplace health promotion programmes can have a positive impact on employees (Pencak, 1991). Murphy (1984) suggests that worksite-based health promotion programmes for staff may be easily incorporated into existing orientation programmes and in-service training, do not have to disrupt the work routine, and may be effective in dealing with work and non-work stressors. Work-related social support has advantages as outlined previously, and may be appropriate to formalize this support within an organization.

Finally, a word of caution: many of the proposed methods of stress reduction have not been systematically implemented and tested to evaluate their use and effectiveness. Stehle (1980) noted a lack of evaluative research, and this is still true today.

CONCLUSIONS

The contemporary view of stress has developed the theme of an individual's ability to act on his environment and proposes that it is not solely the source of stress that is important, but that mediators of the response also play an important role in the level of stress experienced. Occupational sources of stress have been well publicized in relation to critical care, and may be categorized as interpersonal, intrapersonal and extrapersonal in nature. However, comparative studies of critical care nursing and other areas reveal that there are many mediators of the stress response other than that of the area itself. Factors associated with this include social support, the coping strategy employed, and personality characteristics such as those of hardiness.

Burnout, defined as a syndrome of negative self-concepts, with a loss of concern and feelings for patients (equivalent to the exhaustion phase of the GAS), has been linked to variables such as low social support and indirect and palliative coping strategies. It is interesting to note that in Dewe's (1989) study, senior staff more frequently used direct coping strategies than junior staff. This raises the question as to which came first, the coping strategy or the senior post? Developing skills in

using direct coping strategies such as problem-solving may assist in the level of stress experienced, and produce more positive feelings towards the demands placed upon critical care staff (Ceslowitz, 1989). However, whilst direct coping strategies seem to be more effective long-term, the use of indirect and palliative strategies are most useful to 'buy time' for appraisal of the situation and to select a more adaptive strategy. Therefore, developing a wide ranging repertoire of appropriate effective coping strategies is suggested to deal with the many and varied demands of critical care nursing.

The role of education and training is particularly important in relation to stress and coping. Traditionally, emphasis has been placed on biomedical skills and knowledge. Nursing education must increasingly incorporate the knowledge and skills of an holistic philosophy which should include factors which influence coping ability.

Organizational and managerial issues are many and varied owing to the complexity of the concepts of stress and coping, and that of the health care organization itself. Many of the studies reviewed here state the importance of effective communication, and diligence in both managerial and educational personnel to develop trusting and supportive relationships cannot be overemphasized. Optimum staffing levels and skill mix, a reduction in noise levels, counselling networks, and alternating frequency and intensity of patients cared for may each go some way towards reducing staff stress. However, providing only one of these (or other), solutions may have little impact.

In the present climate of financial constraint and scarce resources, it may appear that investment in the health and development of critical care staff has low priority, but if staff health is ignored, then the problems discussed here will surely escalate.

Finally, in relation to developing a 'unique body of knowledge' much of the research to date remains descriptive or explanatory. Prediction or prescriptive levels of theory remain only possibilities which require further study, and if nursing is to continue as both an art and science, then the theoretical framework for research into stress and coping must be open to change. As Pearson and Vaughan (1986) state, a theory "once proved beyond reasonable doubt, . . . is considered to be a law. Until that time individuals must make knowledgeable judgements about the theories they accept."

CASE STUDIES

Case study one

Megan Rees is a 22 year old nurse who worked as staff nurse for six months prior to moving to an eight-bedded ICU where she has been for nine weeks. On a late shift she is asked to care for Joanna Johnson, a 30 year old patient who has been diagnosed as having brain-stem death following a road traffic accident. Both sets of brain-stem death criteria have been completed, and her husband, aware of Joanna's wishes, has consented for her heart, lungs and kidneys to be procured for donation. Joanna has been booked for theatre for five hours time and is physiologically stable. Her husband has gone home. It is the first time that Megan has nursed a patient of this type and although she understands the procedures involved and is competent in delivering the technical care required, she feels uncertain as to how to 'cope' with caring for Joanna for the next few hours. The unit is quite busy and other staff are not readily available. Megan decides to view the situation as being a positive one, in that the immediate task is to prepare Joanna for theatre so that her wishes may be met and others benefit from her death.

Joanna is transferred to theatre successfully, and afterwards, Anne, the sister in charge, speaks to Megan, praising her for the care she gave Joanna in such circumstances. Anne asks her how she is feeling, and Megan becomes very tearful. They speak for some time talking through how they both feel and they discuss different ways they each use to cope with situations like this. Together they draw up a plan of action to help Megan develop further skills and knowledge to assist her in the future.

Case study two

Martin, a charge nurse in a surgical high dependency unit, has been concerned over the apparent shortage of staff which will be present when three of his staff leave in two weeks time. He has completed the duty rotas and there are 12 out of 21 shifts where there is insufficient cover according to predictions based on likely patient dependency scores, skill mix, and theatre time booked. He arranges to discuss this with his senior nurse. He has investigated the following options:

- ☐ planned assistance from staff from other wards;
- ☐ temporary requested transfers of two staff from a ward which is closing;
- ☐ reduction in booked theatre time until staff recruitment is achieved;
- ☐ discussion with the manager of the intensive care unit regarding admission of patients to ICU instead of HDU;
- ☐ closing HDU beds.

STUDENT LEARNING QUESTIONS

The following questions are presented to help you reflect on the content of this chapter:

1. Describe the transactional model of stress and identify the three domains this model encompasses.

2. What three types of coping strategies may be employed in stressful situations? Write down four examples of each of these coping strategies. Which coping strategies did Megan employ during the shift and later on discussion with Anne, the sister in charge?

3. Consider the environment you work in, and identify factors which may influence risk of burnout.

4. Which coping strategies result in positive feelings both from the literature presented and from your own experience?

5. Think of a situation when you felt stressed at work. Plan each stage of the problem-solving approach applied to your example.

KEY TERMS

Stress

A mismatch between perception of a demand and perception of ability to cope with the demand.

Demand

An internal or external stimulus which is perceived as requiring an adaptive response.

Coping

An individual response which either satisfactorily (or not) influences the demand (to a perceived less threatening demand).

Direct coping

Action is directed at the demand itself with the aim of altering the situation into a less threatening one. For example, using a problem-solving approach.

Indirect coping

Changing the way a demand is viewed so that it seems less threatening. A cognitive reappraisal resulting in a changed perception. For example, seeing death as a welcome release from pain.

Palliative coping

A reduction in the perceived demand through the use of strategies such as crying or denial. The demand is not altered. This coping response allows the 'buying of time', to select a more effective coping strategy.

Burnout

A syndrome of emotional exhaustion, depersonalization and reduced personal accomplishment. Symptoms include loss of purpose, boredom and cynicism; impatience or depression may also be present.

Locus of control

The perceived degree of personal control over a given situation.
    An internal locus of control indicates a high perception of individual control.
    An external locus of control indicates a low perception of individual control.

Personality hardiness

A construct incorporating personality traits of commitment, control and challenge.

FURTHER READING

Maslach, C. *Burnout – the cost of caring.* New York: Prentice Hall, 1986.

Bailey, R., Clarke, M. *Stress and Coping in Nursing.* London: Chapman and Hall, 1989.

Benner, P., Wrubel, J. *The Primacy of Caring.* California: Addison-Wesley, 1989.

Lazarus, R. S., Folkman, S. *Stress, Appraisal and Coping.* New York: Springer, 1984.

Murgatroyd, S., Woolfe, R. *Coping with Crisis,* London: Harper and Row, 1982.

REFERENCES

Adair, J. *Training for Decisions.* Aldershot: Gower, 1979.

Albrecht, K. *Stress and the Manager.* London: Prentice Hall, 1979.

Argyle, M. *Psychology of Interpersonal Behaviour,* 4th Edn. London: Penguin, 1983.

Atwood, J. R., Hinshaw, A. S. Nursing Job Satisfaction Scale (NJS): A program of testing and development. *Research in Nursing and Health.* 1985; 8: 321–328.

Bailey, J., Steffen, S., Grout, J. The stress audit: Identifying the stressors of ICU nursing. *Journal of Nurse Education*. 1980; 19(6): 15–25.

Bailey, R. *Coping with Stress in Caring*. Oxford: Blackwell, 1985.

Bailey, R., Clarke, M. *Stress and Coping in Nursing*. London: Chapman & Hall, 1989.

Bartz, C., Maloney, J. P. Burnout amongst ICU Nurses. *Research in Nursing and Health*. 1986; 9(2): 147–153.

Benner, P., Wrubel, J. *The Primacy of Caring*. California: Addison-Wesley, 1989.

Beyers, M., Mullner, R., Byre, C. S. *et al*. Results of the nursing personnel survey. Part 2: RN vacancies and turnover. *Journal of Nursing Administration*. 1983; 13(6): 16–20.

Bibbings, J. The stress of working in intensive care: a look at the research. *Nursing*. 1987; 15: 567–570.

Biley, F. C. Stress in High Dependency Units. *Intensive Care Nursing*. 1989; 5(3): 134–141.

Bishop, V. Stress in the ICU. *Occupational Health*. 1983; 537–543.

Bond, M. *Stress and self-awareness: a guide for nurses*. London: Heinemann, 1986.

Boyle, A., Grap, M. J., Younger, J., Thornby, D. Personality, hardiness, ways of coping, social support and burnout in critical care nurses. *Journal of Advanced Nursing*. 1991; 16(7): 850–857.

Broome, A. K. (Ed.). *Health Psychology Processes and Application*. London: Chapman & Hall, 1989.

Burnard, P. How to reduce stress. *Nursing Mirror*. 1985; 361.

Burnett, R., McGhee, P., Clarke, D. D. (Eds.). *Accounting for Relationships*. London: Methuen, 1984.

Capel, I., Gurnsey, J. *Managing Stress*. London: Constable, 1987.

Carnevale, F. A. A description of stressors and coping strategies among parents of critically ill children. *Intensive Care Nursing*. 1989; 6(1): 4–11.

Ceslowitz, S. B. Burnout and coping strategies among hospital staff nurses. *Journal of Advanced Nursing*. 1989; 14: 553–557.

Chen, Y. Psychological and social support systems in Intensive and Critical Care. *Intensive Care Nursing*. 1990; 6(2): 59–66.

Chyun, D. Patients' perceptions of stressors in ICU and CCU. *Focus on Critical Care*. 1989; 16(3): 206–211.

Clarke, M. Stress and coping constructs for nursing. *Journal of Advanced Nursing*. 1984a; 9(1): 3–13.

Clarke, M. The constructs 'stress' and 'coping' as a rationale for nursing activities. *Journal of Advanced Nursing*. 1984b; 9(3): 267–275.

Coghlan, J. An analysis of stress in ICU's in Melbourne. *Australian Journal of Advanced Nursing*. 1984; 1(3): 27–32.

Crickmore, R. A Review of stress in the ICU. *Intensive Care Nursing*. 1987; 3: 19–27.

Cronin-Stubbs, D., Rooks, C. A. The stress, social support, and burnout of critical care units: the results of research. *Heart & Lung*. 1985; 14(1): 31–39.

Dally, P., Harrington, H. *Psychology and Psychiatry for Nurses*. Sevenoaks: Hodder & Stoughton, 1975.

Dear, M., Weisman, C., Alexander, C., Chase, J. The effect of the intensive care unit nursing role on job satisfaction. *Heart and Lung*. 1982; 11(6): 560–565.

Dewe, P. J. Stressor frequency, tension, tiredness and coping: some measurement issues and a comparison across nursing groups. *Journal of Advanced Nursing*. 1989; 14: 308–320.

Dunbar, F. *Psychosomatic medicine*. New York: Hoeber, 1943.

Ehrenfeld, M., Cheifetz, F. R. Cardiac nurses coping and stress. *Journal of Advanced Nursing*. 1990; 15: 1002–1008.

Eysenck, H. Biological basis of personality. *Nature*. 1963; 199: 1031–1034.

Fletcher, J. Stress management. *Intensive Care Nursing*. 1987; 3: 56–60.

Freudenberger, H. J. *Burnout: the High Cost of Achievement*. New York: Doubleday, 1980.

Garofalo-Ford, J. A., Trygstad-Durland, L. N., Nelms, B. C. *Applied Decision-making for Nurses*. St. Louis, MI: C. V. Mosby, 1979.

Gray-Toft, P., Anderson, J. G. The Nursing Stress Scale: Development of an instrument. *Journal of Behavioural Assessment*. 1981: 3(11).

Harris, R. B. Reviewing nursing stress according to a proposed coping-adaptation framework. *Advances in Nursing Science*. 1989; 11(2): 12–28.

Henderson, V. *The Nature of Nursing: A definition and its implications for practice, research and education*. New York: MacMillan, 1966.

House, J. S. *Work Stress and Social Support*. Reading: Addison-Wesley, 1981.

Huckabay, L. M. D., Jagla, B. Nurses stress factors in the ICU. *Journal of Nursing Administration*. 1979; February: 21–25.

Hyland, M. E., Donaldson, M. L. *Psychological Care in Nursing Practice*. Harrow: Royal College of Nursing, 1989.

Jones, J. W. *Preliminary test manual: The Staff Burnout Scale for Health Professionals* (SBS = HP). Illinois: London House Press, 1980.

Keane, A., Ducette, J., Adler, D. C. Stress in ICU and non-ICU nurses. *Nursing Research*. 1985; 34(4): 231–236.

Kelly, J. G., Cross, D. G. Stress, coping, behaviours, and recommendations for Intensive Care & Medical/Surgical ward registered nurses. *Research in Nursing and Health*. 1985; 8: 321–328.

Kline Leidy, N. A structural model of stress, psychosocial resources and symptomatic experience in chronic physical illness. *Nursing Research*. 1990; 39(4): 230–236.

Kobasa, S. C., Maddi, S. R., Kahn, S. Hardiness and Health: A prospective study. *Journal of Personality and Social Psychology*. 1982; 42(1): 168–177.

Lazarus, R. S. *Psychological Stress and the Coping Process*. New York: McGraw-Hill, 1966.

Lazarus, R. S., Launier, R. Stress related transactions between persons and environment. In Eds. M. Pervin, M. Lewis. *Perspectives in interactional Psychology*. New York: Plenum Press, 1978.

Lazarus, R. S., Folkman, S. *Stress, Appraisal and Coping*. New York: Springer, 1984.

Lees, S., Ellis, N. The design of a stress management programme for nursing personnel. *Journal of Advanced Nursing*. 1990; 15(8): 946–961.

Lewandowski, L. A., Kramer, M. Role transformation of special care unit nurses: a comparative study. *Nursing Research*. 1980; 29(3): 170–179.

Lloyd-Jones, N., Winter, F., Lightfoot, J. *Confidence in the Classroom: An open learning package*. 1988. (Unpublished.)

McCranie, E. W., Lambert, V. A., Lambert, Jr. C. E. Work stress, Hardiness and Burnout Among Hospital Staff Nurses. *Nursing Research*. 1987; 36(6): 374–378.

Macguire, P. Can communication skills be taught? *British Journal of Hospital Medicine*. 1990; 43: 215–216.

Maloney, J. P. Job stress and its consequences on a group of intensive care and nonintensive care nurses. *Advances in Nursing Science*. 1982; 4(2): 31–42.

Maloney, J. P., Bartz, C. Stress tolerant people: intensive care nurses compared to nonintensive care nurses. *Heart and Lung*. 1983; 12(4): 389–394.

Maslach, C. *Burnout – The Cost of Caring*. New York: Prentice Hall, 1986.

Maslach, C., Jackson, S. E. The measurement of experienced burnout. *Journal of Occupational Behaviour*. 1981; 2: 99–113.

Mischel, W. *Introduction to Personality*. New York: CBS College, 1986.

Morgan, W. P. Reduction of state anxiety following acute physical activity. In Eds. W. P. Morgan, S. E. Goldston. *Exercise and Mental Health*. Washington: Hemisphere, 1987.

Murgatroyd, S., Woolfe, R. *Coping with Crisis*. London: Harper & Row, 1982.

Murphy, L. R. Occupational stress management: a review and appraisal. *Journal of Occupational Psychology*. 1984; 57: 1–15.

Norbeck, J. S. Perceived job stress, job satisfaction and psychological symptoms in critical care nursing. *Research in Nursing and Health*. 1985a; 8: 253–259.

Norbeck, J. S. Types and sources of social support for managing job stress in critical care nursing. *Nursing Research*. 1985b; 34(4): 225–230.

Pearson, A., Vaughan, B. *Nursing Models for Practice*. London: Heinemann Nursing, 1986.

Pencak, M. Workplace health promotion programmes: An overview. *Nursing Clinics of North America*. 1991; 26(1): 233–240.

Price, D. M., Murphy, P. A. Emotional depletion in critical care staff. *Journal of Neurosurgical Nursing*. 1985; 17(2): 114–118.

Robson, M. *The Journey to Excellence*. Wantage: M.R.A. International, 1988.

Rotter, J. General expectancies for internal versus external control of reinforcement. *Psychological Monographs*, (1 Whole No. 69), 1966.

Saronsen, I. G., Johnson, J. H., Seigel, J. M. Assessing the impact of life changes: development of the Life Experiences Survey. *Journal of Clinical Psychology*. 1978; 46: 932–934.

Selye, H. Rev. *The Stress of Life*. New York: McGraw-Hill, 1976.

Sponholtz, P. An ICU responds: Accept your limitations. *Journal of Christian Nursing*. 1986; 3(3): 23–24.

Stehle, J. L. Critical care nursing stress: The findings revisited. *Nursing Research*. 1980; 30(3): 182–186.

Summers, S. Job stress in critical care nurses. *Nurse Educator*. 1989; 13(3): 26–33.

Sutherland, V. J., Cooper, C. L. *Understanding Stress*. London: Chapman & Hall, 1990.

Thornton, S. Stress in the neonatal ICU. *Nursing Times*. 1984; February 1.

Tomlin, P. J. Psychological problems in intensive care. *British Medical Journal*. 1977; 2: 441–443.

Topf, M., Dillon, E. Noise induced stress as a predictor of burnout in critical care nurses. *Heart & Lung*. 1988; 17(5): 567–573.

Topf, M. Personality hardiness, occupational stress and burnout in critical care nurses. *Research in Nursing and Health*. 1989; 12(3): 179–186.

Vincent, P., Billings, C. Unit management as a factor in stress among intensive care nursing personnel. *Focus on Critical Care*. 1988; 15(3): 45–49.

Wessels, D. T. Jr., Kutscher, A. H., Seeland, I. B., Selder, F. E., Cherico, D. J., Clark, E. J. (Eds.). *Professional Burnout in Medicine and the Helping Professions*. New York: Haworth, 1989.

White, D., Tonkin, J. Registered nurse stress in ICUs: an Australian perspective. *Intensive Care Nursing*. 1991; 7(1): 45–52.

Wimbush, F. B. Nurse burnout: its effect on patient care. *Nursing Management*. 1983; 56–57.

9
EVALUATING CRITICAL CARE

Penny Irwin

CHAPTER AIMS

The aims of this chapter are:

- [ ] to introduce the critical care nurse to the full range of evaluation in nursing including reflection in practice, evaluation of care plans, quality assurance and research;

- [ ] to identify the main issues in evaluating care in critical care nursing;

- [ ] to explore the different strategies and techniques used in quality assurance and their relevance to critical care nursing;

- [ ] to explore the implications for practice;

- [ ] to give some guidance as to how some of the quality assurance methods may be used in critical care;

- [ ] to whet the appetite of all critical care nurses to further explore the many dimensions of evaluating care.

INTRODUCTION

The evaluation of nursing care is the process by which the value of care given is judged against the results it achieves. It asks the questions: 'Is it appropriate?' 'Is it effective?' 'Is it good?' and 'What is good care?'.

In intensive care, as in other acute specialities, evaluation starts subliminally as part of the reflective clinical decision making process where interventions may be tried in rapid succession to achieve the desired result in terms of the comfort and stability of the patient. More formal evaluation occurs as the nurse evaluates the care plan and the effects of the interventions prescribed in relation to the goals set. If the progress achieved towards the

goals is consistent with what the nurse judges to be good, the interventions will probably remain the same. If, however, they are not, action will be taken to prescribe other interventions which it is believed will speed progress towards achievement of the goal.

Two other major methods of evaluation in nursing are Quality Assurance and Research. Both are very necessary in intensive care. Quality assurance evaluates the care to a group of patients as part of the routine review of the unit activity. It involves monitoring whether care is given according to preset standards, and evaluates whether it achieves the desired results. In many ways this is similar to the nursing process, because if the desired standards are not met or the desired effects not achieved then action is taken to rectify it. In both the nursing process and quality assurance the desired effects of care are identified in advance, and are therefore known, so that the process of evaluation determines to what extent they were achieved.

Research asks a question about what the results might be. The results of the phenomenon under scrutiny are usually unknown or in dispute. The purpose of the research will be to identify unknown aspects of patient responses to illness, new treatments, interventions, hospitalization, grief or other experiences.

At any stage in the routine evaluation of nursing, whether it be during reflection, the nursing process or quality assurance, a question could be identified, which merits systematic examination through research. Research extends the body of knowledge on which practice is based, thus enabling the nurse to know the best interventions to achieve certain results. This should influence standards of practice and the type of interventions used.

The evaluation of care can therefore be viewed as involving aspects of reflection in decision making, the review of individualized care in the nursing process, the review of care to a client group and research.

The aim of this chapter is to familiarize the intensive care nurse with the principles of evaluating care from all these perspectives, with particular emphasis on quality assurance and the varied methods of approaching it.

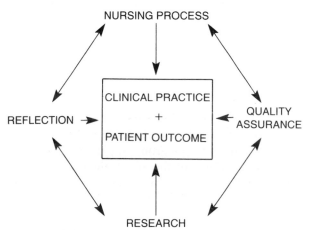

Figure 9.1.   The dimensions of evaluation.

THE MAIN ISSUES

The main issues surrounding evaluation of care at whatever level are:

☐ Why should care be evaluated?

☐ What should be evaluated?

☐ How should it be evaluated?

☐ Who should do it?

Why?

In 1984 the World Health Organisation (WHO) declared in *Health for All* by the year 2000 that "By 1990 all member states should have built effective mechanisms for ensuring quality of patient care within their health care systems" (Target 31 – WHO, 1984). In recent years, a number of changes have occurred in the health care systems of most countries aimed at meeting this target. The focus is to improve the outcomes of care for all patients through regular review and evaluation.

In intensive care one of the most striking features of evaluation for health care managers has been its high cost. Controversies abound over the costs and benefits of treatments. Ill effects, such as loss of the patient's dignity, autonomy, and privacy can be cited in arguments about the possibilities for survival. Review of survival rates in terms of years is no longer regarded sufficient vindication for treatments, without some indication of the quality of life achieved as well.

It is therefore crucial that treatments and interventions are evaluated against the results they achieve, and that improvements are constantly sought. Unless there is evaluation of care to identify the benefits there is no other measure but its financial costs (Maxwell, 1990).

What?

In intensive care, perhaps more than in any other branch of nursing, the success of treatment is dependent upon the multidisciplinary approach. The regular review of medical treatments through effective medical audit and research is a necessary pre-requisite for effective medical clinical decision-making. Nursing care in this highly sophisticated technical environment requires a similar process. Poor nursing can destroy the effectiveness of advanced treatment, just as poor medicine or ward organization can destroy the benefits of high quality nursing care.

It is therefore essential that nursing interventions and their effects are regularly reviewed. Any aspect of work in the unit can be the subject for review from the most complex elements of patient care to the most simple arrangements for keeping the unit running smoothly and effectively. Hence the organization, the equipment, the staff, the care given and the results for patients can all be the object of monitoring and evaluation.

How?

How the evaluation of nursing in intensive care is done will depend to a very large extent on the philosophy of the unit. The model of nursing used inevitably influences the way in which care is evaluated as part of the nursing process. Similarly, the values of the unit will influence the choice of methods in quality assurance, and perhaps the research methods chosen. Quality assurance may be carried out in a variety of ways, as will become evident in the literature review. There will be aspects of it which are continuous, such as the monitoring of indicators like pressure sores and infection, while others may be intermittent and use packages; or there may be methods which are locally devised as part of standards setting (RCN, 1991). The approach and instruments chosen must be appropriate to the phenomenon being measured, whether it be patient care, nursing competencies, equipment safety or relatives' satisfaction with the information they were given.

Issues relating to the choice of each tool when evaluating the care to a group are similar in quality assurance and research. They are:

- ☐ *Validity*: The validity of instruments for the construct, subject, situation.
- ☐ *Frequency*: Associated with the validity of the instrument itself is the frequency of its use. In the nursing process the review date for one

situation is totally inappropriate for another, because some aspects of care require more frequent evaluation, while others need time for the effects of an intervention to become apparent. Similarly, in quality assurance and research choices have to be made as to whether something is monitored constantly or reviewed at intervals, and what those intervals should be.

- ☐ *Sample size and type*: Some aspects of care will need to be monitored across total populations of patients, whilst others can use samples. The sample size should be sufficient to give results that would be representative of the entire population.
- ☐ *Reliability*: The reliability of the instruments used and whether or not they measure the same over time, and with different observers is of crucial importance for the results to mean anything.
- ☐ *The inter-rater reliability* when two or more observers are used.
- ☐ *Overall approach*: Whether quantitative techniques are appropriate, or qualitative. This will be discussed further in the section on research.
- ☐ *Criterion or norm-referenced*: Whether the evaluation of care should be criterion referenced vs. norm referenced.
  - —*Norm-referenced* evaluation rates performance relative to the performance of other subjects in some well-defined comparison or norm group. The key feature is the variance between the scores and the different ranges of scores.
  - —*Criterion-referenced* – to determine whether a subject has reached a pre-determined set of targets/behaviours/set of criteria.
- ☐ *Prevalence vs. incidence*: Whether in collecting statistics of particular indicators the prevalence or the incidence should be used.
  - —*Incidence* of a condition expresses the proportion in a population developing a condition. Put another way, the incidence indicates the number of times the problem (e.g. number of patients with pressure sores in a year) occurred compared to the total number of people or times it could have done

(e.g. number of admissions to the unit over a year).

—*Prevalence* of a condition expresses the proportion of population suffering from a condition. Prevalence can measure the number of people with a particular problem at any one time, e.g. once a week or a point prevalence once a year. If these figures are used over time it becomes evident that the prevalence score is much less accurate because some cases could be counted twice, while others may be left out of the system. Prevalance is what is commonly measured because of the difficulties associated with getting accurate incidence figures, particularly in hospitals with restricted access to information technology.

The important thing to be aware of is that rates of a particular condition (e.g. pressure sores in ITU) can vary depending upon how the original data was collected (Crow, 1981). This has particular relevance when judging the performance of different units or hospitals, and is one of the difficulties associated with norm-referencing when currently data is collected in a variety of ways.

Who?

Whatever methods are used one of the arguments surrounding evaluation of care is who should do it. In terms of every-day care there is general acceptance that the patient's bed-side registered nurse should be the one to evaluate the care at the level of the individual. However, when care is evaluated on a wider level there are still prevailing arguments as to who should do it. Traditionally, it has been seen as a higher management duty, i.e. the top-down approach. In recent years it has been identified as something that all professional nurses should participate in as part of a system of peer review, i.e. the egalitarian or 'bottom-up' approach. The issues surrounding both approaches will be reviewed in the literature and research sections, and are part of an ongoing debate in nursing as it progresses towards professionalism.

THE LITERATURE

The literature review will be divided into the four sections concerning the different types of evaluation, i.e. reflection in decision-making, evaluation as part of the nursing process, quality assurance and research. The reader should bear in mind: why do it; what to look at; how best to evaluate; and who should be doing it, in each section.

Decision-making and reflective practice

Clinical decision-making is the process of making choices about actions which will have certain results. To make such choices intelligently, the practitioner has to evaluate the current situation. One of two approaches may be adopted – the rational or the phenomenological (Harbison, 1991).

The rational method involves an analysis of the situation with the choice of action being made in a logical way with explicit rationale. In rationalist theories the decisions are made using a logical step-sequence (such as a decision tree) which identifies the different elements in the situation with their costs, benefits and harms. In such a way, practice can incorporate research and accountability be assured.

However, there are limits to the use of such a method, for instance in crisis situations, when there is no time to reduce the situation to its elemental parts before making a decision. Those who expound the phenomenological approach say that experts in practice see patterns in situations, based on their knowledge and experience, and that they make decisions quickly in accordance with cues they identify in the situation. This does not mean that he or she resorts to ritual at the first opportunity, but rather that the practitioner can adapt to rapidly changing patient situations and take the right action at the time to achieve the desired result for the patient. This is perceived as intuitive decision-making, and is something that comes from years of practice and knowledge accumulated from similar situations or paradigm cases (Benner, 1984). The work of Schon (1983, 1991) indicates that this level of performance is best developed by nurturing the ability to critically reflect on the effects of decisions made so that uncertainties and limitations to expertise can be acknowledged and rectified.

Nursing process

The functions of evaluation in the nursing process are to:

☐ Identify the progress towards the goals, and when they are met.

☐ Provide further information for the reassessment of patient's needs.

☐ Discover which nursing actions are the most effective in solving particular nursing problems. (Hunt and Marks-Maran, 1986).

Evaluation can only be effective if the nursing process is properly carried out. The patient's assessment should therefore facilitate the accurate diagnosis of nursing problems for which achievable and measurable goals can be identified and appropriate care prescribed.

If the nursing diagnosis is those problems which can be described as uniquely nursing and for which nursing care must be prescribed, there is sometimes a problem in intensive care with this, because many of the patient problems have implications for all members of the multidisciplinary team. The nursing diagnosis emphasizes the independent role of the nurse, whereas the dependent or interdependent role is often the one in evidence. Although it has been argued that nurses need to identify what nursing does in this environment to cost out what nurses do (Guzzetta and Dossey, 1983), the argument will no doubt grow for multidisciplinary care planning and patient centred notes in specialities where this is a particular problem.

Whatever the nature of care planning, regular evaluation should take place on pre-set dates and/or times to identify the progress towards the goals set. To do this all aspects of problem under review or the care plan should be evaluated:

☐ Is the initial assessment still valid?
☐ Do the problems/needs identified still reflect what is going on with the patient?

☐ Are the goals still valid and are they realistic?
☐ Are the nursing interventions working? And are they still appropriate?
☐ Is the time allowed before evaluating the results of care realistic? (Hunt and Marks-Maran, 1986.)

Audit of nursing documentation and medical notes is one method of evaluating the care patients receive and the knowledge and expertise of the staff (Hunt and Marks-Maran, 1986). Has the patient been individually assessed? Have problems been identified and are they appropriate to the patient? Has care been planned in the light of the problems identified? Are the goals realistic? Is there evidence of them being regularly reviewed, and is there evidence of evaluation taking place? There is a general problem with auditing the quality of care using the documentation – the care may have been good at the time but have been poorly documented, and not all care that is documented has necessarily been given. There is evidence however that in the hospitals where documentation is regularly audited for the quality of the care planning and evaluation that these elements improve dramatically as action plans incorporate education to improve deficiencies. This has the important result that audit of the care itself is made easier. Those units wishing to use their notes to audit care should therefore address their attention first to the quality of the way in which care is documented.

Quality assurance

How quality assurance is implemented and used will depend upon the model on which the strategy is based. The tools available to work within a strategy are increasing all the time. This section contains an introduction to some of the major theories underpinning quality assurance (QA), and which form the basis of QA strategies, and reviews methods which could be used in intensive care.

Definition of quality assurance

"Quality Assurance is a process in which achievable and desirable levels of quality are described, the extent to which these levels are achieved is measured, and action to enable them to be reached is taken" (HMSO, 1988, p. 12).

Different aspects of quality assurance

Quality assurance incorporates two other important dimensions with which it is sometimes used synonymously. These are quality control and quality improvement.

Quality control is the process of checking a sample of the product or service to ensure high standards. It began in the First World War munitions factories and checked products at the end of the line, and then threw out those which did not reach the standard. This incurred waste. Quality assurance works differently in that its methods are to ensure quality at each stage of the process of production or service, and therefore demands the commitment to high quality of all those involved in the process. In health care the quality control function is performed by risk management and some aspects of audit in checking standards of safety. Whilst quality assurance can include quality control it also incorporates quality improvement.

Quality improvement relates to objectives and projects which are oriented towards future improvement in the service, and focuses on the client and the service he or she wants.

What is good care?

The dimensions of quality health care have been described by Maxwell (1984) as:

- [ ] Access
- [ ] Relevance to need
- [ ] Effectiveness (for individual patients)
- [ ] Equity (fairness)
- [ ] Social acceptability
- [ ] Efficiency and economy.

These dimensions can be the foundation for assessing the quality of a service, and therefore for standards and contracting (Rainbow pack).

The principles of quality assurance

1. *Define* the standards of care.
2. *Measure* what happens in practice against the standards

3. *Take action to improve* where deficiencies are identified.

This can be demonstrated as a cycle (see Fig. 9.2).

Donabedian model

Donabedian (1966) identified three perspectives from which health care could be measured:

1. *Structure* – factors affecting the material, social or intellectual environment of care (buildings, equipment, staff competence, etc.).
2. *Process* – activities to provide care.
3. *Outcome* – results of care for the patient.

Whilst the model differentiated these three perspectives, Donabedian acknowledged the importance of linking them together in the final analysis to identify the causes of certain outcomes. This reflects the same principles, therefore, as evaluation of an individual's care in the nursing process, that whilst interest will no doubt focus upon the progress towards the goal, the totality of the plan and how it works needs to be considered in context.

Wilson model

This model (Wilson, 1987) provides a practical working framework for quality assurance throughout a hospital.

1. *Principal functions* – Each department is recommended to identify its principal functions (usually numbering about five or six). Possible principal functions in all branches of nursing include:

- [ ] assessment and planning
- [ ] direct nursing care
- [ ] patient education/psychological support of patients and relatives
- [ ] staff/student education
- [ ] maintaining a therapeutic environment
- [ ] co-ordination of care.

2. *Indicators* – The unit should then identify its quality indicators. These are measurable variables which relate to the department's performance. They can be positive or negative, and sometimes their significance will not be clear until they have been investigated. They can relate to structure, process or outcome. The model identifies three types of indicator:

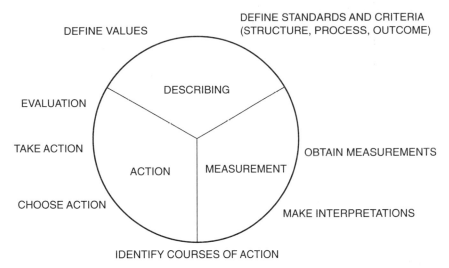

Figure 9.2.   The quality assurance cycle (after Lang, 1976).

(i) Risk indicators – will normally be patient-centred, and indicate areas of high risk requiring regular monitoring, e.g. infections, pressure sores, returns to theatre, accidents, complaints.

(ii) Leading/key indicators – areas which are not so high risk but which nevertheless are a guide to the unit's performance (e.g. sickness and absence, staff turnover) and which would be recorded monthly.

(iii) Descriptive indicators – which may come to light through audit on a periodic basis, e.g. period of fasting before surgery; relative's opinions of information they are given: patients' opinions of their stay in ITU.

3. *Evaluation* – the QA programme will include obtaining information from four different sources:

P – patients
A – audits
I – indicators
X – outside experts

4. *Report* – All QA activities should be reported on. Wilson recommends that a report should be brief and answer five questions:

Question	Report headings
(i) What did you look at?	FOCUS
(ii) How did you look?	METHOD/ MEANS
(iii) What did you find?	FINDINGS
(iv) How is that significant?	SIGNIFICANCE
(v) What are you going to do about it?	ACTION/ FOLLOW-UP

Methods of measurement

The techniques used in quality assurance to measure the quality of care and its effectiveness are similar to those used in research, and in the same way need to be valid and reliable for the purpose they serve. They include:

- [ ] Direct observation of care
- [ ] Review of documentation
- [ ] Patient/relative questionnaires or interviews
- [ ] Review of complaints
- [ ] Staff questionnaires/interviews
- [ ] Post care staff conferences
- [ ] Measurement of the nursing competencies
- [ ] Statistical information regarding indicators
- [ ] Checklists
- [ ] Equipment, e.g. sound level meters.

The quality assurance tools to be outlined below illustrate how these different methods are used. As is evident from the Chris Wilson model, no one way of measuring care is sufficient on its own. For most tools to work they use a mixture of methods for data collection and a variety of sources. Which methods should be used will depend upon the situation, who is involved and the sensitivities of the subject matter. When information is sought, and by whom are discussed below.

Retrospective audit
This is performed after the episode of care under review. It could be after discharge from the Intensive Care Unit, or when the patient has gone home, or even several years after the stay in intensive care, if effectiveness in terms of survival and quality of life were being examined. The methods used could be audit of notes, relative/patient questionnaires/ interviews and review of other sources such as computerized data.

Concurrent audit
This is carried out during the episode of care under review. Techniques used could include observation, patient/relative interviews/questionnaires in the middle of the patients' stay, and review of notes regarding current care such as care plans.

As is evident in the section below on quality assurance tools, a mixture of retrospective and concurrent audit is helpful.

Peer review

Internal audit may be done as something by higher management using a 'top-down' approach; or as part of a system of peer review, where nurses review the practice of each other. The issues surrounding both approaches will become evident during this chapter, and are part of an on-going debate in nursing as it moves from being a hierarchically dominated to a collegiale profession.

Peer review can be defined as the judgement and review of practice by equals from the same profession or setting according to predetermined criteria of what constitutes good practice. In nursing this means nurses reviewing the practice of those in the same area of clinical practice and themselves being reviewed. However, on a wider level it could mean a whole hospital being reviewed by professionals from other hospitals. This happens in the accreditation audits discussed below. The advantages of peer review are that the reviewer or auditor has professional or clinical credibility, understands the environment he/she is auditing, and can make meaningful judgements on the information available.

The use of 'developmental evaluation' has become particularly popular in the way quality assurance techniques are used (Pearson, 1987). It involves an evaluator, whether from within the unit or from outside, feeding back the results of the audit in such a way that the staff in the unit can receive the information positively and develop an action plan from it.

Structure tools

The King's Fund Organisational audit
The King's Fund Organisational audit (1991) identifies the organizational standards by which a hospital should operate. The standards are British versions of those used in Canada and Australia for hospital accreditation. They were first piloted by the King's Fund in 1989. There are standards for all departments in an acute hospital, including the Intensive Care Unit. The standards cover seven main areas of hospital management in each section:

Organizational standards
Philosophy and objectives
Organization, policies and procedures
Staffing
Staff development and education
Facilities
Patients' rights
Evaluation and quality assurance

The audit is repeated every three years, and is carried out by outside observers made up of practising senior acute hospital staff.

The main benefit of it for staff is that it provides a validated framework of good management practice that ensures the unit is run in the best interests of patients. The way a unit is organized can have profound effects on the outcomes of the care it provides. This will become evident in the section on research.

BS 5750/ISO 9000 is the organizational standard for institutions more commonly used in commerce. However, it is increasingly being used by some departments associated with health care, whether it be GP surgeries, laundry departments, pharmacies and some hospitals. The standards are very detailed and cover all aspects of management and service in the organization, including the standards for suppliers of goods and services to the organization. Once an institution has BS 5750 the clients/consumers are guaranteed a particular standard of service.

Process tools

In nursing, quality assurance tools have been developed which mainly examine the *process* of care. The tools reviewed below are Phaneuf's audit, QUALPaCS, ITU Monitor, and the Dynamic Standards Setting System (DySSSy).

1. *Phaneuf's audit* is a retrospective audit of patients' notes following discharge, and although it originated in America (Phaneuf, 1976) it is used in some centres in Britain (Bradshaw, 1987; Sale, 1990). The notes of 10% of the patients who have been discharged from a ward are reviewed each month against pre-set criteria to identify the quality of care they received. The areas of care reviewed include:

- [ ] Application and execution of legal medical prescriptions
- [ ] Observation of symptoms and reactions
- [ ] Supervision of the patient
- [ ] Supervision of those participating in care
- [ ] Reporting and recording
- [ ] Application and execution of nursing procedures and techniques
- [ ] Promotion of physical and emotional health by direction and teaching.

The ratings given following audit are given according to the score achieved and range from 'excellent' through 'good', to 'incomplete', to 'poor' and finally to 'unsafe'.

2. *QUALPaCS* The Quality Patient Care Scale (QUALPaCS) was developed from the Slater competency scale at Wayne State University, USA (Wandelt and Ager, 1974). The Slater competency scale assessed the competency of the nurse, while QUALPaCS concentrates on the care received by a group of patients.

It is a scale with 68 items or criteria, which are divided into six sections covering the following aspects of care:

1. Psychosocial individual.

2. Psychosocial group.
3. Physical.
4. General.
5. Communication (between professionals regarding patients).
6. Professional implications.

Non-participant observation of nurse-patient interactions is carried out by two nurse observers over a period of two hours. It is recommended that there are two assessors to reduce the risk of observer bias, and that periods of observation are repeated at different times of the day, and on different days (Wiles, 1987; Sale, 1990). The sample size recommended is 15% or five of the patients, and those selected should be representative of the ward as a whole. The charts and records of the patients observed are also examined as part of the exercise, which brings the amount of time the assessors are on the ward to three hours.

The scale allows each item to be rated and scored as follows:

Rating	Score
Best care	5
Between	4
Average care	3
Between	2
Poorest care	1

In most centres in Britain the QUALPaCS assessments are carried out by peer review (Wiles, 1987; Sale, 1990), very often at the same time as Phaneuf's audit. The request for the assessment, when performed by peer review, comes from the area itself. Ward staff are not identified by name in the report and remain anonymous. The report is fed back to them afterwards, and they are given the opportunity to meet with the assessors. The report will include the mean score of observed care, the assessors' overall impression, good points, points for improvement, comparisons with previous assessments and suggestions for change.

Criticisms of QUALPaCS include the fact that only a few patients have their care evaluated, and this might not be representative of the ward as a whole. There is also a possibility that a crisis situation in the ward may affect the care given during the observation period.

3. *Monitor* is a quality assurance package developed by Len Goldstone and Jean Ball (1983) from the American Rush Medicus System for use in the UK. In principle, it provides a quality of care index using a checklist approach, i.e. for the presence or absence of quality related, observable criteria. Since the first general nursing Monitor was published there have been different editions of Monitor developed for the various branches of nursing, e.g. Senior Monitor for Care of the Elderly, Junior Monitor for Paediatric nursing, Psychiatric Nursing Monitor, Cousin Monitor for the Community, and latterly A&E Monitor, followed by ICU Nursing Monitor (Thornton, Whitehead and Goldstone, 1992).

The authors of Monitor recommend an approach be made to the relevant Ethics committee, Trades unions and other interested parties before implementation; and that a steering group of ward sisters, nurse managers is set up to guide the assessors in the use of the documentation. The Unit staff should be educated about the use of Monitor and given a copy of the document so they are familiar with what is required before the audit is carried out.

As in all Monitors, the nursing process is audited, i.e. planning nursing care, meeting the patient's physical needs, meeting the patient's non-physical needs, and the evaluation of nursing care. Information is gathered from different sources, i.e. records, nurses, observation, inference and patients' relatives. The techniques used are non-participant observation, questionning of relatives, and analysis of records and inference.

The care of up to 30 patients would be audited using the tool as provided, covering nine aspects of care:

A. Procedures on admission 36 items
B. Introducing relatives to the ICU
   environment 16 items
C. Admission details 16 items
D. Progression to stability 46 items
E. Stability 124 items
F. Transport of the critically ill
   patient 20 items
G. Recovery 68 items
H. The dying patients and death 30 items
I. Transfer 17 items

There is also a section which allows for local criteria for review to be added.

Each section can be scored individually for each patient. As in other Monitors, the responses are Yes or No, or Not applicable. There is a score of one for yes and zero for no. From this a percentage of positive responses can be calculated from those applicable to give the unit an Index of quality achievement. The individual scores for each patient can also be calculated. The suggested desirable score is 70% or above.

The duration of assessment is said to be 2–3 hours per patient, and the suggested frequency of application is once a year or every six months.

Advantages of Monitor are that it is a ready-to-use package and takes into account aspects of care specific to the area for which it was designed. Criticisms of Monitor are that while it may identify areas for attention it is time consuming to use. The index score being identified as satisfactory at 70% in other Monitors has also been criticized because there are some aspects of care for which only 100% is adequate. In ICU Nursing Monitor the emphasis has been more on the qualitative results of the audit and less on the scoring, with no recommended satisfactory score.

4. *The Dynamic Standards Setting System (DySSSy)* was generated by Alison Kitson (1989) at the Royal College of Nursing, and is called the Dynamic Standards Setting System because those carrying out the care identify the quality problems in their area, set the standards to solve them, and through the review of their practice against the standards form action plans to improve. This approach can be used by all branches of nursing, including Intensive Care.

The method is based on the Donabedian (1966) model with *criteria* for the achievement of the standards described in terms of *structure, process* and *outcome*. National standards of care using this approach have been published by the specialist nursing forums at the Royal College of Nursing.

The core beliefs of DySSSy are that because the standards are written by nurses involved in practice, the standards are owned by them. This encourages nurses to review their practice and write standards directly relevant to their clinical area, unlike the quality assurance packages. It is central to the philosophy that all those in the clinical area feel involved. Because it is patient/client focused it is believed the standards must result in quality improvement for the patient with advances in practice. Standards set using the DySSSy approach aim to be practical and realistic, and in an area like ITU where nursing practice links so closely with that of other disciplines the principles are readily transferable to other disciplines and to multidisciplinary standards.

Principles to be considered when standards are being set are that they should be *desirable, observable, achievable* and *measurable*. For them to work it helps to remember that their criteria should RUMBA, i.e. be:

Relevant
Understandable
Measurable
Behaviourally stated
Achievable

Problems have arisen with nurses finding it difficult to word standards so they are measurable, resulting in disappointment and frustration. As in the writing of measurable goals in the nursing process it is essential that behavioural language is used (Waterman, 1992) so that each criterion only identifies one item in a specific way. Many of the difficulties experienced by groups initially can be overcome by having a facilitator experienced in the method to guide the group on the technicalities of standards writing, and then of audit.

To audit the standards the nurses who have written them devise an audit protocol specific to the standard, which identifies how the criteria are to be measured. Different types of criteria will need measuring in different ways as with Monitor, so a variety of methods to audit the standard will be required. These may be observation, documentation, questions to staff, or questions to patients and relatives. It will be important that whatever methods of measurement are chosen they are valid and reliable, that the sample is representative of the total population under review, and that the frequency of audits obtains the compromise of reviewing care without causing work that overloads the unit.

From the data collected at the audit the nurses can then identify areas of success, as well as areas where the standard was not reached. All audit being anonymous, individuals – whether patients or nurses – are not identified, but areas for improvement are. From this the action plan is derived.

This model is interesting because it measures outcomes whilst taking into account the causal factors in structure and process. It also incorporates the philosophies prevalent in much of the quality assurance literature from commerce, which expounds the importance of realizing the commitment of staff to quality through involvement in solving quality problems.

Outcome measurement
Luker (1981) suggested that evaluation of care research should focus on the process-outcome aspects, for then we will be able to identify those aspects of process which lead to favourable outcomes and those which do not. To look at outcomes in isolation from what care achieved them teaches us very little in terms of developing our nursing knowledge and expertise. Crow (1981) also identified that judging the effectiveness of nursing care involved "evaluation of the outcome of nursing in the light of all possible factors which contribute to care" (Crow, 1981, p. 495).

What are the positive outcomes of health care? They include:

☐ Possible improvement in Health state, sometimes known as health gain.

☐ Possible changes in knowledge, understanding and behaviour as a result of health education and counselling.

☐ Possible improvements in quality of life.

☐ Satisfaction with the care received.

The negative outcomes of care will be the reverse of these, and very often form the basis of negative indicators, e.g. pressure sores, infection rates, returns to theatre, complaints. Traditionally, negative indicators such as morbidity and mortality have been focused upon rather than quality of life issues. For purchasers of health care negative indicators still form the basis of many quality specifications. The reason being that it is easier to measure failure than it is to measure success (Maxwell, 1990).

However, with all forms of treatment it is now not sufficient to measure just the negative indicators. This is particularly so with expensive forms of health care like intensive care. The cost of health care has become a political issue in all parts of the world, and governments increasingly want to know what they are getting in terms of outcome for the money they are spending. A famous example of this is what has become known as the Oregon experiment (Honigsbaum, 1991), whereby decisions regarding what to offer on the state funded health programme were determined by taking into account the outcomes of treatments in relation to length of survival and quality of life.

The value of predicting outcomes is immediately apparent. This can only be done if they have first been evaluated using valid and reliable techniques, taking into account all the possible variables.

In intensive care the APACHE II (Acute Physiology and Chronic Health Evaluation) score (Knaus and Zimmerman, 1985) goes some way towards identifying the types of patient who will benefit from their intensive care treatment. The prognosis is deduced from the statistical analysis of comparable cohorts of patients backed up by clinical trials. The data on costs and benefits of treatment in the United Kingdom was identified by the King's Fund in 1989 as being deficient. However, as the statistical databases on the potential of different patient groups to benefit from particular combinations of treatment in intensive care increase worldwide, it should mean that those patients selected for intensive care and major interventions will be the ones who will benefit from it. This, in turn, will improve the outcome records of the units who work with this type of information.

Research

Research can contribute to choice of measures used, can serve as the background to standards and identify criteria which would be useful. It can also be used to identify the extent of problems in an area. Precise evaluation resulting in prediction over a population is only achieved through detailed research using valid and reliable techniques to collect data in a standardized way. It is the duty of

the researcher to use methods that make valid and reliable inferences about the effects of one set of variables on another. It is the responsibility of the nurse to ensure that if questions are identified as a result of other forms of evaluation there is some follow-up in terms of research.

Ashworth (1989) called for a systematic approach to identifying effectiveness, costs, criteria for use and levels of provision. Nursing is a large proportion of the costs and benefits of ITU, therefore there is a need to be rationally seeking out and systematically analysing information to use in effective decision-making regarding care interventions, policies and protocols. APACHE can be used to predict prognosis and possible choices of treatment. Nursing needs to evaluate process activities and research into them to ensure the best care given so that those admitted to ITU have minimal complications and greater benefit from ITU nursing.

However, nurses also need to measure outcomes of their care. Bowling (1991) highlighted the difficulties in this area. Outcome measures until recently have been based on a medical model, using survival up to five years, blood chemistry and other medical indices. Scales measuring quality of life are many, but they tend to focus on different aspects, whether it be level of function, physical well-being, psychological well-being or level of social well-being. Scales which have been combined to measure all these have had their validity and reliability questioned (Bowling, 1991).

These tools have also been criticized for their over prescriptiveness and that they only measure what professionals think patients ought to be feeling as opposed to what they actually feel. This is a problem with all highly structured quantitive research tools. The methods associated with qualitative research are therefore an important dimension to recognize in determining what the reality of a situation is for those experiencing it (Field and Morse, 1985). Hence in-depth interviews with just a few people can reveal a wealth of information if valid and reliable techniques of analysis are used.

Whilst health gain and quality of life are essential aspects of outcome measurement, other outcomes such as patient or relative knowledge, understanding and satisfaction are equally important in nursing. When trying to measure these outcomes it is important to remember that patients and their relatives experience health care (in intensive care as everywhere else) in a complex web of technical and expressive care.

The *Technical Care* relates to the procedures and investigations they undergo.

The *Expressive Care* relates to the interactions with health care staff (Zastowny *et al.*, 1989).

It has been shown that patients value the expressive part of their care to the extent it can effect their compliance with treatment and future interaction with the health care system (Zastowny *et al.*, 1989). The lay public is not usually able to make many judgements on the technical aspects of care. Indeed, no doubt they find it frightening in the intensive care environment, if they are conscious of their surroundings at all. The evaluation of the outcomes of expressive care in terms of understanding and satisfaction are therefore an area where nursing quality assurance and research can be beneficial.

However, before this leads nurses to issue patient or relative opinion questionnaires, it is advisable to look at the research.

The research

This section will look at some of the research related to evaluation of care in ITU, by looking at research of the quality assurance tools in the literature, and research of different aspects of care in relation to ITU, using the structure, process, outcome framework.

Research of quality assurance tools

Structure
Accreditation or organizational audit has not been in Britain long enough for the effects of it to be researched. However, research from Australia (Duckett, 1983), which reviewed its effect in 23 hospitals, suggests that it has the main effect on the organization of nursing, the physical facilities and safety, with a less marked effect on medical staff.

Process
The version of Monitor used in elderly care (i.e. Senior Monitor) was used by MacGuire (1991) to assess changes in the quality of care resulting from the introduction of primary nursing. Primary nurs-

ing was introduced into only one of the wards. The tool was used on three occasions a year apart before and after the change on the one ward. The Monitor scores showed that the quality of care had improved in all three wards. It was concluded that the process of using the tool made staff appraise their practice more critically, and that this rather than the introduction of primary nursing was what influenced the improvements in the quality of care.

Further research into QUALPaCS, Monitor and Senior Monitor (Tomalin *et al.*, 1992) assessed inter-rater reliability. Acceptable levels of inter-rater reliability were reached providing certain techniques were used to enhance reliability. These are discussed by Tomalin *et al.* (1992) and Redfern *et al.* (1993), who emphasize the importance of training and allowing enough time for discussion regarding areas of ambiguity in the tools prior to using them. It was also recommended that inter-rater reliability should be tested every time the raters or the setting changed. It is too early at the time of writing for research on ITU Monitor to be available. However, there are sufficient methodological similarities in all the versions of Monitor for this research to be relevant to ITU Monitor.

As to whether different types of tool can be correlated concerning results from an area, Ventura (1980) in the USA showed a low correlation between QUALPaCS and Phaneuf's audit. The reasons for this in that particular study were identified as:

☐ the differences in the tools themselves, and that they were measuring different things using different rating systems;

☐ there was low inter-rater reliability for QUAL-PaCS in the data used;

☐ the basic difference between retrospective and concurrent audit;

☐ the use of different data sources.

This highlights the importance of such issues as inter-rater reliability, and how results should be evaluated in the light of the methods of data collection.

Harvey (1991) evaluated the approaches to assessing the quality of care using the predetermined packages Monitor, QUALPaCS, Phaneuf and a patient satisfaction questionnaire 'What the patients think'. This research showed that the process of implementing a quality assurance tool is more important than the tool itself in determining how it is accepted by nurses. "A bottom-up approach which devolves ownership and control to practitioners was seen to result in the most positive outcomes for nursing staff" (p. 284).

The DySSSy system of practitioner-derived criteria was compared by Kitson *et al.* (1993) to expert-derived criteria. Locally-derived criteria and standards have been criticized for the amount of time it takes to set the standards, the doubt as to the reliability and validity of the criteria which result, and the audit tool. Two of the five wards achieved high levels of convergence with the experts, while the other three did not. Problems identified in the practitioner groups were broadly defined non-specific criteria which could not be measured, and therefore have no valid or reliable audit tool.

The wards in this study had inexperienced facilitators, and as the experts had an expert facilitator it was felt that the main finding of this study demonstrated the importance of the role of the facilitator. The authors also suggested the formulation of expert-derived core criteria which could be built up and used by staff as a basis for their own local work.

Outcome-structure-process evaluation

APACHE II has been used to evaluate the outcomes from 13 different Intensive Care Units in major American tertiary care hospitals (Knaus *et al.*, 1986). By using the APACHE scoring system it was possible to compare the actual and the predicted death rates, and identify what differences there were in structure and process factors to account for the differences that emerged. The differences in death rates from different centres varied remarkably, despite having similar technical facilities. The best outcomes were achieved by those centres where the units were well co-ordinated and staff communicated well with each other. The top ranked hospital in terms of successful outcomes had carefully designed protocols, a comprehensive nurse education system, clinical specialists with Masters degrees who oriented new staff, a high degree of doctor nurse communication and levels of mutual respect. The units who had high mortality rates lacked a comprehensive nursing organization,

staff education programme and there was poor communication between nurses and doctors.

This study demonstrates that:

☐ The way an intensive care unit is organized has major implications for the outcomes of care.

☐ By using such techniques as the APACHE system to control for the patient variables, it is possible to identify the influence of other variables on the outcomes.

☐ It highlights the importance of the links between structure, process and outcome.

Nursing evaluation, whether it be quality assurance or research, tends to focus on the link between process and outcome. An example of nursing research to evaluate the quality of patients' experience in intensive care is that by Ball (1992), who explored the nature of stressors identified by patients who had experienced intensive care. Using Neuman's classification of stressors as being Intrapersonal, Interpersonal and Extrapersonal as the areas for exploration, patients were interviewed after they had returned to the ward. The most frequently reported stressors were: feeling thirsty, helplessness, isolation/loneliness, real/unreal conflict, disorientation, room too hot, and frightening dreams. Hence the predominant stressors were identified as being intrapersonal. Several patients in the study felt emotionally labile, and expressed the need to see a nurse from intensive care after their return to the ward, so they could talk about their experiences to someone who would understand, rather than discuss it with the ward nurses or their relatives who they did not wish to alarm.

The tool devised for the research study, it was suggested, could be used as a quality assurance tool, and subsequently used to evaluate the effectiveness of changes in nursing practice that resulted from the research.

Some studies evaluate changes in practice and take into account cost-saving, thus indicating beneficial effects on management budgets. Such a study is that by Stromberg and Wahlgren (1988), who evaluated the introduction of in-line intravenous filters.

Questionnaires

Whilst it is unlikely that nurses in intensive care would consider giving their patients a questionnaire to complete because they are so ill, and their relatives so distressed that it would not be ethical to administer one, there will be occasions, such as that in the Ball (1992) study, when it is appropriate after the patient has left the unit and is back on the ward or may even be at home.

The methodological considerations to take into account before administering questionnaires to find out the opinions of patients or relatives become evident in a review of the research by French (1981), and are relevant over time. One of the main issues in any survey of opinions is to ensure a high response rate. Several factors can militate against patients responding to questionnaires. Patients can be too ill; they may have forgotten about the episode of care if they are questioned too long after it; they may not give truthful answers for fear it will affect their future treatment if they are critical; they may be influenced by the 'halo' effect in that they feel grateful for their care and do not want to appear critical; they may not understand the questions. All these issues should be considered when designing the questionnaire or interview schedule and making decisions about the timing of its distribution.

Some of these problems can be avoided by interviewing instead of giving self-completion questionnaires. The advantages of this are that patients often enjoy talking to a sympathetic and encouraging listener; the interviewer can ensure that they get a high response rate; and any questions that are hard to understand can be explained. However, it is time consuming and expensive. If the questions were open on the interview schedule then content analysis will also be time consuming.

How the survey is to be analysed should be considered early on in the deliberations for it, and support sought from experts at the pilot stage where uncertainty exists about its validity or reliability.

Practical nursing implications

Unit organization

All units exist to provide a service to their patients. The staff within the units want to give the highest standards of care possible. The literature and the research indicates that evaluation of practice is the key to knowing what level of care is being given in practice. The research by Knaus et al. (1986) demonstrates that the outcomes of care are inextricably linked to the way a unit is organized, how staff communicate, and how care is delivered within that framework. The unit therefore should have an organizational framework which facilitates good clinical care. The organizational audit programme standards contain all the standards for good practice outlined in the research as having a beneficial effect on clinical outcome, including well-defined protocols, and opportunities for communication. From this research it is also evident that the nursing should be organized so that the senior staff are trained in intensive care, and there are arrangements for all staff to up-date their knowledge, by attending continuing education events and studying for higher education.

The work by Schon (1983, 1991) indicates the importance of practice for learning and the vital role of reflection within that. The implication for this in practice is that opportunities should be enabled for institutionalized reflection to take place, such as case conferences and mentor systems.

Both the two main types of decision-making theory – the rationalist and the phenomenonological – have relevance for the evaluation of practice in intensive care nursing. In the situations where the nurses in a unit decide as a group on a policy or procedure relating to practice, they will use the rational approach, using rationale based on research to direct the actions selected. The evaluation as such will also fit into the infinitely rational processes of the nursing process, quality assurance or research.

However, in situations involving emergency treatment of an individual patient, where the patient's condition is rapidly changing, the phenomenological approach will be more appropriate. Evaluation afterwards by the individual nurse of his or her actions may be better facilitated by a mentor especially for those who are new to the unit or students to facilitate a positive learning exercise.

In situations where there has been a major event involving a lot of activity and many different individuals, there is the danger that afterwards some are left only partly understanding their own contribution to the whole event. As a result of this, the less experienced can be left haunted by their own inadequacies and misunderstandings. A short case meeting as soon as possible after this event for all those involved will allow feelings of inadequacy to be shared, but will enable important lessons to be learned, both by the team and individuals for the future.

Workload measurement

In the Knaus research the nurses in the better units were able to negotiate their workload according to the staffing. This is enabled if there is a recognized method of evaluating workload. There should be some method of measuring the workload generated by the patient dependency, so that the skill-mix required can be properly analysed and steps taken to ensure that it is correct. Ideally, the measurement will be on one of the bottom-up systems, so that the nurses working at the bedside who know the work required by their patients are the ones who in-put the data. This requires one of the computerized systems, for example, the FIP System.

Bottom-up approach

The structure of the unit should enhance the possibility for all staff to be involved in peer review of some sort. The 'bottom-up' approach has been shown to work (Harvey, 1991), whether one is using Monitor, QUALPaCS or DySSSy. This should be accompanied by good feed-back mechanisms, so staff can be aware of results and incorporate required actions into their practice.

The framework for evaluation

In determining a framework for evaluation of care, the Wilson model can be helpful. It helps by identifying the principal functions of the unit and how each is to be measured, whether or not the unit has a comprehensive quality assurance programme within which staff can participate, and how they fit into the overall scheme for evaluation of care.

Evaluation of care programme – Wilson model
If the principal functions of the unit are identified as follows, the quality assurance plan will be based on that:

☐ Assessment and planning

☐ Direct nursing care
☐ Patient education/psychological support of patients and relatives
☐ Staff/student education
☐ Maintaining a therapeutic environment
☐ Co-ordination of care.

Assessment and planning – can be evaluated by some form of documentation audit, but the routine evaluation of care by the bedside nurse will also have its place. Audit of the nursing notes can include not only the care plans and progress/evaluation notes but the charts as well. The audit can look at how well the notes are being completed, and how well the nursing process is being used; however, it can also be used as in Phaneuf's audit to look at the care given to patients during their stay. There are many areas which have devised their own audit tools to suit their own documentation and speciality. The effect of auditing documentation is usually to generate more interest in how care is documented, and ensures that the documentation itself is up-to-date with developments in care.

Direct nursing care – can be evaluated by use of one of the packages like Monitor or QUALPaCS. The auditors can be experts trained in the tool who are from another similar unit. This is peer review in its true sense. Other ways of measuring direct care include indicators such as pressure sores, infections and returns to theatre. Standards of care may have been written on some aspects of patient care such as tracheostomy care, or parenteral nutrition which will need to be audited.

Psychological support of patients and relatives – evaluation of this could include a standard about care of relatives and the audit of that by use of questionnaires following the patient's stay.

Staff/student education – may well be covered already by some form of education audit from the Colleges of Nursing.

Maintaining a therapeutic environment – could be monitored by equipment and environmental audits. The environment for care was identified by Florence Nightingale as being crucial to patients' well-being and potential recovery. It is no different today. Units should be clean and well maintained, and the same applies to the equipment in them.

Regular audit of the environment for domestic cleanliness and maintenance should be carried out. Routine maintenance of equipment is the best way to ensure it is always in working order, but this does not happen in a surprising number of places, and is something unit staff very often have to negotiate to achieve.

Coordination of care – organizational audit can be included in this. This would also include monitoring indicators in relation to staff such as sickness and absenteeism, study leave, and professional development.

The programme Wilson recommends should include information from four different sources of information:

P – patients
A – audits
I – indicators
X – outside experts

The programme above includes these for different principal functions. It has ensured that most aspects of the units' work are covered by some form of review. Wilson insists that units create their own quality assurance programme to suit their work in terms of their principal functions, and using data sources already in use in the unit for evaluation purposes. The indicators are something that again are individual to each area. If pressure sores are not a problem there may be something else which is, and which staff would feel is more worthwhile to gather data about.

The manager will need to keep records on indicators such as the number of incidents involving accidents, whether they be drug errors, or needlestick, and back injuries among staff, or patients falling out of bed. From these records, patterns can be identified and appropriate action taken to improve.

Information on any area of care about which there is concern can be collected in the form of statistics so that the extent of a problem can be identified and action taken to improve it. The very fact that statistics are being gathered on an issue indicates a willingness among staff to do something about it to improve the situation.

Opinion surveys should be used with due regard to the patient group, taking into account their illness and the distress of their relatives. Questionnaires should be used infrequently, and be short and to the point. Where possible, interviews should be carried out after the stay in ITU. This will have the added benefit for the patient of being visited by an ITU nurse to whom he or she can talk about unresolved anxieties.

CONCLUSIONS

As nursing progresses in the evaluation of care, and develops accurate measurements of structure, process and outcomes, so we enter a process that can only lead us towards better professional and accountable practice. It can only enhance the service we provide if action is constantly taken to make up in the areas identified as deficient.

CASE STUDIES

The two case studies selected demonstrate the importance of getting all parts of the system right, whether it be structure, process or outcome in ensuring good quality care, and how evaluation of care, whether it is through reflection on practice or formal audit, can feed into promoting improved practice and high quality care.

The importance of negotiation with other staff groups in identifying the best way forward to improve quality

Poor quality care often results from muddle and confusion over who should perform particular duties. In intensive care the overlap between what medical and nursing staff can do may lead to uncertainty about responsibility for certain areas of practice, which could place the nurse in an invidious position. Either nurses may be asked to perform a procedure which they feel incompetent to perform, or if they are competent, there may be doubt as to whether they would be covered legally for performing a procedure which is normally carried out by doctors in other clinical areas.

The staff in one ITU identified that they were persistently performing duties that some were more competent to carry out than others, and that there seemed to be a grey area as to whether the medical staff should perform them. At their Clinical Practice Group meeting the nurses identified and agreed which areas of practice were the problem in this regard. They then met with the Consultant to discuss the areas of responsibility for medical staff and the circumstances under which it would be appropriate for the nurses to perform particular procedures.

The parameters having been agreed, the extended role guidelines were drawn up identifying the criteria for patient selection, the competencies required by the nurses who would carry this out, and the training programmes for them. Those who were assessed as being competent had it identified in their personal professional portfolios in line with the Scope for Practice (1992). The procedures included extubation of particular patient groups, defibrillation, epidural top-ups, and alterations to identified ventilator settings.

The importance in this instance of discussion with senior medical staff was identifying the parameters for action by the staff groups involved. On other occasions it may be to seek expert advice, and to get agreement from several staff groups for a standard. For example, a standard on nutrition in ITU required consultation with dietitians, the nutrition nurse specialist, pharmacists and medical staff.

The heartaches and benefits of auditing standards by peer review

The staff in a combined CCU/ITU formed a standard setting group made up of five staff members of varying grades who were interested. They started by identifying the areas of practice which gave them concern and about which they would set standards. The first standard set concerned the management of chest pain in coronary care patients.

The aim of the standard was to reduce chest pain as quickly as possible. After much discussion the group agreed that the standard would state that pain would be controlled within 30 minutes. The full standard was agreed with the criteria for structure process and outcome. A pain assessment scale was agreed upon, and in the standard the nurse would document the level of pain on the observation chart at ten minute intervals after pain was identified for at least 30 minutes, or until it resolved. This had not been done in this particular unit before.

The standard and all it entailed was discussed with all staff on the unit before it was finalized. The audit protocol was agreed before the standard was implemented. Audit of the standard was to be mainly through patients' opinions and review of the documentation.

The standard was audited three months after its implementation. This meant that sufficient numbers of patients had been through the unit for a realistic appraisal of the standard to be made. The results were disappointing. 62% of patients said their pain was relieved within half an hour, and documentary evidence was found in only 46% of the notes. It was felt that nurses were treating patients' pain much of the time, but not documenting the pain scores. There was concern in the group as to whether it was realistic to relieve chest pain in all patients within 30 minutes. After further discussion it was agreed that they persist with the standard at 30 minutes. The action plan from this audit included further teaching sessions on pain assessment, its management and documentation.

The second audit of the standard after six months showed that 80% of patients stated they were pain free within 30 minutes, and it was evident in 66% of the nursing notes. The third audit after a further six months showed that although the nurses' documentation of the pain scores on the charts was variable in terms of time frequency from 10 to 15 to 30 minutes, that it was consistently documented and showed evidence of action being taken to relieve pain. All patients said they had their pain relieved within 30 minutes; 56.3% of patients had their pain relieved within 10 minutes.

At this stage it was decided the standard ought to be reviewed to incorporate changes such as improved timings, the latest research, and recent changes in medical protocols. This demonstrates the dynamic effects of evaluating care and the benefits it can have for patients and clinical practice.

The group has set other standards which are audited at regular intervals. They meet monthly and take minutes of their meetings which are displayed on the noticeboard in the coffee room, together with the latest standard being discussed, or the results of the most recent audit. This has resulted in others becoming interested and joining the meetings. Each group member takes responsibility for different standards. It has taken time to get used to carrying out audits and writing reports with action plans, but this is now done routinely and with interest.

Feedback to staff showing progress, comparing current results to previous audits and informing them of areas for action works eventually to encourage all concerned to work for continuous quality improvement.

STUDENT LEARNING QUESTIONS

1. What areas of care/procedures in your unit are carried out at present without formalized agreements as to who should perform them?
   Consider:
   - [ ] What knowledge and skills the staff who perform the procedure will need to have.
   - [ ] What circumstances would it be appropriate for nurses to perform the procedure, and what circumstances would it be more appropriate for a member of another discipline to do so?
   - [ ] Who will need to be approached to ensure that agreement is reached concerning multidisciplinary responsibilities, management support and vicarious liability?

2. In identifying a standard for good practice for an area of care in your unit, consider:
   - [ ] What the standard should be so that it is desirable and achievable.
   - [ ] What the criteria should be under the headings of Structure, Process and Outcome.
   - [ ] How you will audit the standard in terms of the methods used, the sample size and the frequency of audits.

3. If you wanted to ensure that care is effectively evaluated in your unit, consider:
   - [ ] How you would organize the nursing in the unit to ensure staff had sufficient support to reflect routinely on their practice.
   - [ ] Whether evaluation in the nursing process is being adequately utilized in your unit, and how you would improve it.
   - [ ] What methods of quality assurance you would use to ensure that care was evaluated effectively throughout the year in your unit; how you would distribute it through the year; and who would do it.
   - [ ] What area of practice has been identified in your unit as needing research? Has a literature search been done? What is the research question? What methods will be the most appropriate? What support are you going to need to carry it out?

KEY TERMS

Accreditation

The process of inspecting an organization according to explicit standards and awarding public recognition of excellence if the standards are met.

Audit

Systematic review of care whether concurrently or retrospectively.

Criterion

Specification of a desirable quality of a service.

Effectiveness

The extent to which outcomes, results or goals are achieved.

Evaluation

Judgement on the value of a process in terms of the outcomes achieved.

Expressive care

The interpersonal aspects of care.

Feedback

The process of communicating the results of audit in order to inform staff and management for further action.

Indicator

An aspect of performance which acts as a signal in the assessment of quality, e.g. complaints, pressure sores, number of patients treated.

Monitor

To watch, track, check or supervise. This relates often to quality control activities such as checking equipment before a procedure, or risk management checks of compliance with health and safety legislation.

Outcome

The results of health care for the patient/client/relative, including health status, well-being, knowledge, understanding and satisfaction.

Process

The actions undertaken (usually by health care staff) to deliver health care.

Quality assurance

The process by which a service continuously evaluates its performance against standards and takes action to improve.

Quality control

A process whereby items or products are checked against standards to identify whether or not they meet a standard.

Quality improvement

A process of working towards identified goals to improve the quality of service (very often as part of Total Quality Management).

Standard

A professionally agreed level of performance, which can be measured.

Structure

All aspects of the environment for care including resources such as buildings, equipment, staff, and organizational arrangements.

Technical care

The procedural aspects of care.

Total quality management

A system of management which involves the entire workforce in an organization working towards better quality of service to the customer.

FURTHER READING

Bowling, A. *Measuring Health: A review of Quality of Life Measurement Scales*. Milton Keynes: Open University Press, 1991.

Donabedian, A. *Explorations in Quality Assessment and Monitoring. Vol. 1: Definitions of Quality and Approaches to its Assessment*. Ann Arbor, MI: Health Administration Press, 1980.

Ellis, R., Whittington, D. *Quality Assurance in Health Care: A Handbook*. London: Edward Arnold, (Hodder & Stoughton), 1993.

Kitson, A., Hyndman, S., Harvey, G., Yerrell, P. *The Dynamic Standard Setting System (DySSSy): Quality Patient Care*. London: RCN, 1992.

McDowell, I., Newell, C. *Measuring Health: A Guide to Rating Scales and Questionnaires*. Oxford: Oxford University Press, 1987.

Sale, D. *Essentials of Nursing Management: Quality Assurance*. Basingstoke: MacMillan, 1990.

St. Leger, A. S., Schneiden, H., Walsworth-Bell, J. P. *Evaluating Health Services' Effectiveness*. Milton Keynes: Open University Press, 1992.

Wilson, C. R. M. *Strategies in Health Care Quality*. Toronto: WB Saunders, 1992.

REFERENCES

Ashworth, P. Editorial: Economics, effectiveness, evidence, ethics and education – five essentials for intensive care. *Intensive Care Nursing*. 1989; 5: 49–51.

Ball, C. A. Theory testing: Stressors in Intensive Care: a comparative survey. Unpublished MSc Dissertation, City University, London, and St. Bartholomew's College of Nursing, 1992.

Benner, P. *From Novice to Expert: Excellence and power in clinical nursing*. Menlo Park, CA: Addison-Wesley, 1984.

Bowling, A. *Measuring Health: A Review of Quality of Life Measurement Scales*. Milton Keynes: Open University Press, 1991.

Bradshaw, S. Phaneuf's Nursing Audit. In Ed. A. Pearson. *Nursing Quality Measurement: Quality Assurance methods for peer review*. Chichester: Wiley, 1987.

Crow, R. Research and the standards of nursing care: What is the relationship? *Journal of Advanced Nursing*. 1981; 6: 491–496.

Donabedian, A. Evaluating the quality of medical care. *Millbank Memorial Fund Quarterly*. 1966; 44(2): 166–206.

Duckett, S. J. Changing hospitals: the role of hospital accreditation. *Social Science Medicine*. 1983; 17(20): 1573–1579.

Field, P. A. Morse, J. M. *Nursing Research: The application of qualitative approaches*. London: Croom Helm, 1985.

French K. Methodological considerations in hospital patient opinion surveys. *International Journal of Nursing Studies*. 1981; 18: 7–32.

Goldstone, L. A., Ball, J. A., Collier, M. M. *Monitor: An index of the quality of care for acute medical and surgical wards*. Newcastle-upon-Tyne Polytechnic Products Ltd., 1983.

Guzzetta, C. E., Dossey, B. M. Nursing Diagnosis: Framework, process and problems. *Heart & Lung*. 1983; 12(3): 281–291.

Harbison, J. Clinical decision making in nursing. *Journal of Advanced Nursing*. 1991; 16: 404–407.

Harvey, G. An evaluation of approaches to assessing the quality of nursing care using (predetermined) quality assurance tools. *Journal of Advanced Nursing*. 1991; 16: 277–286.

HMSO. *Quality Assurance in Nursing: Report of a*

Working Group of National Nursing and Midwifery Consultative Committee. London: Scottish Home and Health Department, HMSO, 1988.

Honigsbaum, F. *Who shall live? Who shall die? – Oregon's Health Financing Proposals*. King's Fund College Papers, No. 4, 1991.

Hunt, J. M., Marks-Maran, D. *Nursing Care plans: The nursing process at work*. Chichester: Wiley, 1986.

King's Fund Panel. ICU in the United Kingdom. *Anaesthesia*. 1989; 44: 428–431.

King's Fund. *Organisational Audit (UK)*. London: King's Fund, 1991.

Kitson, A. *A Framework for Quality*. Harrow: Scutari, 1989.

Kitson, A., Harvey, G., Hyndman, S., Yerrell, P. A comparison of expert and practitioner-derived criteria for post-operative pain management. *Journal of Advanced Nursing*. 1993; 18: 218–232.

Knaus, A., Zimmerman, J. E. Prediction of Outcome from Intensive Care. *Clinics in Anaesthesiology*. 1985; 3: 811–829.

Knaus, W. A., Draper, E. A., Wagner, D. P., Zimmerman, J. E. An evaluation of outcome from intensive care in major medical centers. *Ann. Intern. Med.* 1986; 104: 410–418.

Lang, N. Issues in Quality Assurance in Nursing. *ANA Issues in Evaluative Research*. American Nursing Association, 1976.

Luker, K. A. An overview of evaluation research in nursing. *Journal of Advanced Nursing*. 1981; 6: 87–93.

MacGuire, G. Quality of care assessed: using the Senior Monitor index in three wards for the elderly before and after a change to primary nursing. *Journal of Advanced Nursing*, 1991; 16: 511–520.

Maxwell, R. J. Quality assessment in health. *British Journal of Medicine*. 1984; 288: 1470–1472.

Maxwell, R. J. What is health result? In Ed. N. Carle. *Managing for Health Result: Papers from a King's Fund International Seminar*. London: King's Fund, 1990.

Phaneuf, M. *Nursing Audit Self Regulation in Nursing Practice*. 2nd Ed. New York: Appleton-Century Crofts, 1976.

Pearson, A. (Ed.). *Nursing Quality Measurement: Quality Assurance Methods for Peer Review*. Chichester: Wiley, 1987.

Rainbow Pack – 5. Regional Consortium in Conjunction with Greenhalgue & Co. *Using information in managing the nursing resource*. Huddersfield: Charlesworth, 1991.

Redfern, S. J., Norman, I. J., Tomalin, D. A., Oliver, S. Assessing the Quality of Nursing Care. *Quality in Health Care* 2: 124–128.

Royal College of Nursing. *RCN Dynamic Standard Setting System (DySSSy)*. Harrow: Scutari, 1991.

Schon, D. *The Reflective Practitioner*. New York: Basic Books, 1983.

Schon, D. Educating the reflective practitioner: toward a new design for teaching and learning in the professions. San Francisco, CA: Jossey-Bass, 1991.

Stromberg, C., Wahlgren, J. Saving money with effective in-line filters. *Intensive Care Nursing*. 1989; 5: 109–113.

Thornton, J., Whitehead, T., Goldstone, L. A. ICU Nursing Monitor: An audit of the quality of nursing care for patients in Intensive Care Units. Loughton: Gale Centre Publications, 1992.

Tomalin, D. A., Redfern, S. J., Norman, I. J. Monitor and Senior Monitor: problems of administration and some proposed solutions. *Journal of Advanced Nursing*. 1992; 17(1): 72–82.

Tomalin, D. A., Oliver, S., Redfern, S. J., Norman, I. J. Inter-rater reliability of Monitor, Senior Monitor and QUALPaCS. *Journal of Advanced Nursing* 18: 1152–1158.

Ventura, M. R. Correlation between the quality patient care scale and the Phaneuf Audit. *International Journal of Nursing Studies*. 1980; 17: 155–162.

Waltz, C. F., Strickland, O. L., Lenz, E. R. *Measurement in Nursing Research*. 2nd Ed. Philadelphia: FA Davis Co, 1991.

Wandelt, M. A., Ager, J. W. *Quality Patient Care Scale*. New York: Appleton-Century Crofts, 1974.

Waterman, C. G. The problem with standards: a plea for a behavioural framework. *International Journal of Health Care Quality Assurance*. 1992; 5(3): 22–26.

Wiles, A. Quality of patient care scale. In Ed. A. Pearson. *Nursing Quality Measurement: Quality Assurance Methods for Peer Review*. Chichester: Wiley, 1987.

Wilson, C. R. M. *Hospital-wide Quality Assurance: Models for implementation and development*. Toronto: WB Saunders, 1987.

World Health Organisation. *Health for All by 2000*. New York: WHO, 1984.

Wright, D. An introduction to the evaluation of nursing care: a review of the literature. *Journal of Advanced Nursing*. 1984; 9: 457–467.

Zastowny, T. R., Roghmann, K. J., Cafferata, G. L. Patient satisfaction and the use of health services: Explorations in causality. *Medical Care*. 1989; 27(2): 705–723.

Section 3
THE FAMILY AND ASSOCIATED ISSUES

The major focus of this section is the family of the critically ill person. The chapters reflect the range and complexity of issues associated with care and the importance of more than one source of knowledge.

10

LIVING THROUGH A CRITICAL ILLNESS

The family perspective

Brian Millar

CHAPTER AIMS

- [ ] The purpose of this chapter is to present an overview of the significance of the increasing research into 'Family-centred nursing' in the critical care unit. In the chapter the relationship between the family, the social environment and the critical care unit will be examined, and evidence of how it is related to the ways in which the family regulates and orders its own inner life discussed. The literature relating to such issues as family stress and anxiety, family needs, nurse–family interactions, the environment and the family, and the role of the family in patient recovery (or death) will be explored.

- [ ] Attention will then be focused upon the challenges faced by critical care nurses and families. Suggestions will be made for meeting the needs of the family, and of the health care professionals.

- [ ] The chapter concludes with a summary of the key issues and suggestions for the future development of family nursing knowledge in the critical care unit.

INTRODUCTION

It has become increasingly obvious to nurses and others working in intensive care that a sudden critical illness may result in disadvantages not only for the patients but also for those closest to them. Furthermore, family's and social factors influence the patient's response to illness and its subsequent outcome (Kasl, 1986), and that a patient's family are a key resource in care and rehabilitation.

Critical care nurses are becoming concerned at the lack of information concerning the expectations, priorities, and assessments held by both the patient and the family, as well as the particular problems associated with everyday living during an acute illness episode (Millar, 1987; McIvor and Thompson, 1988; Coulter, 1989; Hayes, 1990). Problems faced by families of the critically ill are seldom the result of a single cause. It is also equally true that a family problem rarely has a single effect. The achievement of effective and ethical care during an acute critical illness event must lie in an increased awareness of and attention to the experiences, values, priorities and expectations of patients and their families.

A central premise of this chapter is that a family, through the course of its interactions with the Critical Care Unit staff, fashions fundamental and enduring assumptions about the world of critical care in which they find themselves. Critical care nurses are constantly attending patients and families who are experiencing a troubling situation. My emphasis is therefore upon 'working with' as opposed to 'working on' a family, which is consistent with the nursing profession's current belief in holistic practice.

Often when dealing with a critically ill patient, health professionals cling to an artificial distinction between the physical and the psychological. During a critical illness episode whilst the patient is experiencing a major physical insult, a family is living through a time of increased stress (Roberts, 1986). It is my hope that this chapter will help to identify a bridge between this artificial gulf that separates the needs of the patient from the needs of their family. Family are and continue to be a much undervalued and little used resource for care in the high tech domain of critical care nursing.

A central assumption of this chapter is that critical care nursing practice should be guided by theory (see Chapter 2). The application of nursing theories to the family as the unit of care appears to be superficial or, at best, incomplete. Among the major, recognized, nursing theorists there is a tendency to focus their assessments and interventions on individual patients as opposed to the family of the patient.

An increasing recognition of the value of collaboration between health care providers and a patient's family, points to the need for nurses working the critical care environment to review their practices. Communication and cooperation between health care providers and patients and their family are an urgent objective if we are to truly offer holistic care. It has been stated recently that in the future any hospital that does not have a family focus to its care will not survive. This sentiment must clearly be true for an environment such as the critical care unit.

THEORETICAL PERSPECTIVES AND THE FAMILY

During the past three decades, nursing in the United Kingdom has been in the midst of an exciting new era. Nurses have been developing and experimenting with nursing theories, and in addition advances

in nursing practice are now well established, for example, primary nursing in ITU (Chapter 2), Neuman's model in ITU (Chapter 3), and expansion of the nurses' role to include using complimentary therapies such as massage, reflexology and relaxation therapies. It has become possible, through the introduction of nursing development units, for nurses working in ITU to identify a significant role in the care of the critically ill. Discussion about the future of critical care units, and in particular the role and preparation of nurses who work in such environments, needs to be articulated and evaluated.

In the high tech world of critical care, the phenomena of interest to the nurse are concepts such as person, environment, health and nursing. Each of these concepts is clearly linked, and can be distinctly identified in the following three statements.

1. Critical care nursing is concerned with the standards and laws which regulate the life processes, well-being, and ideal functional levels of human beings who are seriously ill.
2. Critical care nursing concerns itself with the order of human behaviour in interaction with the environment during a critical life situation.
3. Critical care nursing has as its goal the identification and evaluation of the means by which positive changes in health status of the critically ill can be brought about (adapted from Gortner, 1980).

Generally, within nursing 'person' is referring to an individual. Family are seen as either a group of separate individuals identified in terms of their relationship with the ill person, or as an important though marginalized adjunct for the professionals (Friedman, 1981; Millar, 1987). Interest in and, indeed, recognition of the importance of the family has been acknowledged since the days of Nightingale. During the traumatic times of the Crimea, Nightingale recognized the importance of family needs, and worked tirelessly to support the wives and families of the soldiers. However, recently there has been a growing awareness of nurses' concern with the family as a whole, reflected in research into family needs and family stressors and the use of specific interventions with a critically ill person's spouse (Thompson and Cordle, 1988; Millar, 1987; Coulter, 1989). This growing body of literature provides a basis for modifying the critical care nurse paradigms to account for family phenomena, and to highlight the need for continued development of a body of family nursing science. In such a science the concepts become *family*, *family health*, *family environment*, and *nursing within the context of family* (Whall and Fawcett, 1991). Critical care nursing therefore becomes concerned with:

- [ ] the standards and laws which regulate *family* process, *family* well-being, and ideal functional levels of *families* in various states of critical illness;
- [ ] the order of *family* behaviour in interaction with the environment during a critical life situation;
- [ ] critical care nursing has as its goal the identification and evaluation of the means by which positive changes in *family* health status can be brought about (adapted from Whall and Fawcett, 1991).

Currently, the concept of individualized patient care has become central to a belief in what constitutes 'good' nursing practice. The importance of focusing upon the separate needs of the individual have been emphasized by Henderson (1982), and is frequently alluded to in the literature on nursing models (Pearson and Vaughan, 1986; Aggleton and Chalmers, 1986). There is also increasing support for the idea that individualized care equals quality care (see Monitor by Goldstone and Ball, 1983).

De La Cuesta (1983) claims the emphasis on individualized patient care can be traced back to nurses' dissatisfaction with Task Allocation. Claims such as these have, according to White (1989), serious implications for a profession which lays claim to its status through its altruistic concern for those in suffering, and the intimate nature of its work.

The introduction of primary nursing, which has increasingly gained in popular as well as political appeal, has been attributed by Reed (1992) as being partly due to the current political and ideological climate in the United Kingdom. An increasing emphasis upon individual responsibility and individual solutions to the problems within society, combined with an apparent reluctance to acknowledge a societal or community perspective, has been a major influence of political thinking throughout the 1980s.

Sociologists such as Bernardes (1989) report that there have been a number of alterations in our definition of family. Increasing numbers of one parent families, mixed race families and homosexual families have raised serious questions as to whether the family still exists. Whilst there is evidence of a decline in the traditional family household, there is no evidence that the traditional family values have changed. The health care team are increasingly finding themselves coming into contact with variations of the traditional family system. The result is often that they find themselves ill-equipped to deal with the complexities of a critically ill person's marital or personal relationship. It is not unknown for the critical care nurse to find herself becoming a gatekeeper, monitoring and controlling not only the number of visitors but also negotiating with visitors such that embarrassing situations do not or cannot arise.

John, a 38 year old accounts manager, was admitted with a diagnosis of chest pain; Myocardial infarction? A large number of people accompanied him to the unit. During an initial discussion with those present, Sheila identified herself as his ex-wife – they had been separated for some five years though never divorced. One of his daughters followed the nurse out of the relatives' room and asked if she could have a word in private. Her dad, she said, had a live-in girlfriend but her mother didn't know. She requested that the staff make sure that both women are not in the hospital at the same time.

Whilst the emphasis upon individualized patient care is pursued as a means of rehumanizing care and protecting nursing's claim to be a caring profession (Watson, 1988), it does create a potential dichotomy between humanism and the requirements of professionalism. Humanistic values as the basis for care are focused upon the respect and autonomy of the patient. In contrast, it is generally recognized that professionalism implies exclusive knowledge, practice and accountability, all of which views the patient and their family as passive recipients of care. An individualized practice philosophy may be interpreted as implying that one can dismiss the communal aspects of patient care. For example, systems theory argues that 'no man is an island' and that human lives can be viewed as a series of interrelated systems. There is strong support for the use of systems theory in the work of nurse theorists such as Rogers (1970), Parse (1993) and Neuman (1989). A system is defined as a set of interacting components which are interrelated and interdependent, and which function as a structured and bounded unit (Baker, 1973). Rogers (1970) states that each human being is an open system, in constant interaction with the environment. The health and well-being of each individual is therefore dependent in part upon the efficiency and effectiveness of the system operations that mediate the relationship with other systems. Examples of other systems within which a human system interacts include a network of relatives, family and friends, all of whom provide the support and communication systems during times of health or ill health, and extends to the organization within which the person works. Each of us as individual systems is, to a significant degree, interdependent on other people and integrated within the cultural, social and economic systems with which he or she interacts. If a person should experience a critical illness which necessitates their admission to a critical care unit, they find themselves becoming a part of an unknown set of open systems. At such a time both the patient and their family find themselves confronted with a need to integrate into a new and often threatening system.

Other theoretical perspectives which highlight the incongruence of individualism include symbolic interactionism (SI). Symbolic interactionists challenge the belief that people can be best understood at the level of the individual. SI focuses on the interactions which take place and how people construct their beliefs, their views and their identity (Dallos, 1991). A number of strategies have been developed to help a family learn to manage in the critical care environment. For these innovations to truly meet the holistic needs of the critically ill patient and the family, a profound change is required in the definition and image of health care professionals and organizations; an environment must be created within the critical care unit which favours empowerment of family and promotes patient/family participation. What is required is a transformation of the traditional 'patriarchal' approach which emphasizes power over, to one of power sharing through the development of new and innovative ways to share information.

Understanding family experiences in critical care

A major challenge for critical care nurses is to be able to describe, explain and ultimately predict the outcomes of family interactions in a critical care environment. Two key questions are How does what occurs in the critical care environment influence the critically ill patient's family? and What are the interventions and strategies by which nurses affect (positively or negatively) the outcomes of family interactions in the critical care environment?

These two questions serve to focus our research and theory building, and to determine how nurses in critical care units can ensure that the families whom they come into contact with, learn and grow from the experience, not suffer added traumas (Murgatroyd and Woolfe, 1985).

A serious illness and injury affects not only the patient but the family as well (Reed, 1992). The perceptions that a family may have about a serious illness or injury event can vary from family member to family member, and is influenced by their previous experiences, their coping strategies, the role that the patient fulfilled within the family (e.g. father, mother, child), and other factors.

Family stress theory can help to describe the effect of a stressor on a family. Families in the critical care unit experience an emotional response to the stress of a critical illness, and are often faced with the realization that they will have change forced upon them as well as the possibility of the loss of a family member (Hill, 1965).

The double ABCX model of family adjustment and adaptation describes the stressor event A interacting with B (the family's crisis meeting resources) and with C (the definition the family makes of the event) to produce X (the crisis) (McCubbin and Paterson, 1981; p. 141).

It is well recognized that a sudden critical illness in one family member impacts upon the entire family (Artinian, 1989; Molter, 1979; Leske,

1986). In the critical care unit, nurses come into contact with families experiencing a stressor (sudden admission with a life threatening injury or illness), which makes demands upon the family's resources for coping, and occurs in a strange environment where they have little control and often find themselves powerless to influence events. The combination of these three factors results in behaviours which may indicate a family in extreme crisis or one which is capable of handling the situation alone. The family's perception of the situation may be that it is a challenge. For example, if a doctor has painted a pretty grim chance for survival, the family may view the odds against survival as a challenge, or as a threat. They may see it as the worst possible situation they could be facing.

During this time of crisis, a family adapts to the situation by adjusting to the 'pile up' of previous and new stressors and strains (aA), by recalling their existing resources or by using new ones (bB), and by redefining their perception of the event (cC), they are able to cope with the shock of the event stressors.

At these times of stress, families are often faced with little or no time to prepare for the acuteness or the critical nature of the illness or injury. With the health care professional's attention being consumed by the needs of the critically ill patient, the family's attention becomes focused on the development of its perception of the situation, which clearly influences how they cope. Roberts (1986) has reported that, "a patient enters the critical care unit in a physiological crisis, the family, however, enter the critical care unit in a psychological crisis".

As a result, the family unit is prone to becoming disorganized through disruptions to its routines, roles and relationships. Using this framework, critical care nurses become more aware of the vulnerability the patient's family is experiencing, and to the importance of their relationships with the whole family in promoting positive recovery. Through strategies aimed at reducing the ambiguity and uncertainty about what is happening to their sick relative, such as providing time for communications, providing information about the treatments, prognosis and possible outcomes, families gain a shared understanding of events and can quickly muster their defences.

Assessment of the family's needs and providing a support group as well as developing collaborative protocols which include the family in the decision making process are additional interventions of value. It is important that nurses and health care staff in critical care areas do not simply view a family as dysfunctional because they are experiencing a crisis; what they need are sympathetic staff sensitive to their vulnerability and skilled at helping and supporting them towards a positive health experience.

As critical care nurses find themselves increasingly attending, for the most part, to families who are experiencing a difficult situation, it is important that the family are included in the patient's care plan. The focus of the interactions between the family and the critical care nurse is, therefore, dependent upon 'working with' rather than 'doing to' a family. Such an approach is seen as consistent with nursing's emphasis on holistic nursing practice.

A key assumption of this chapter is that if critical care nurses are to work in a therapeutic capacity with families, then it is essential that they systematically develop the knowledge upon which to base their practice. In doing so, it is important to reflect on their knowledge and to remain aware of the theoretical issues involved.

FAMILY EXPERIENCE OF CRITICAL CARE UNITS

The sudden onset of a life-threatening illness produces drastic changes in the lives of the patient and their family. Their day-to-day existence becomes constricted and focused upon disease, its treatment and its outcome. At such times, the stresses created by seeing a sick relation attached to tubes and highly technical machinery are accentuated by difficulties in communication between the patient, their family and the health care professionals.

A number of researchers describe the family experiences in the critical care unit as one which includes stress (Curtis, 1983; Breu and Dracup, 1978; Daley, 1984). Families often respond to a life-threatening situation with feelings of fear, anxiety and grief; however, this does not imply that they are incapable of participating in the decision-making process.

It is important to be aware that a critical illness extracts a severe toll from the patient, the family and society. The stress associated with being hospitalized during a critical illness is experienced by both the patient and the family.

High-tech and the family

Although the development of increasing high technology in medical care has resulted in the increased ability of intensive care medicine to prolong life, it has brought with it a growing concern with its dehumanizing effects. Families, when first confronted with the machinery, tubes and drains around their critically injured relative, can feel very insignificant and peripheral among the staff and equipment. Faced with the stress and anxiety of seeing their ill relative, many feel overcome with shock and frightened by such a highly technical setting.

Helplessness and hopelessness are common feelings experienced in this situation by a patient's family. As a consequence, they are left feeling devastated and depressed. Many families are so overwhelmed by the environment that they become passive or apathetic towards the conditions, and communications between themselves and the health care team become difficult. Loneliness is a major contributory factor, with long periods spent in the hospital waiting areas being the order to their days. Hours spent hoping and waiting for news, the opportunity to spend time near their critically injured relative, often leave them with a sense of despair at a time of great vulnerability. Families are very open to supportive and caring communications with the patient's nurse. Taking time to spend with a family conveys the feeling that someone cares about them.

It is important to be aware that, as Roberts states, "whilst the patient enters your unit in a physiological crisis, their family enters in a state of psychological crisis". A family's reactions to the crisis are often difficult to categorize. No two families respond in the same way; indeed, within a family individual members can and do react differently. Common behaviours both observed in interactions with families and reported in the literature include: an inability to concentrate and make de-cisions; an inability to absorb and utilize effectively communications between themselves and the health care team; fear; panic; demanding or irrational behaviour; aggressive and abusive behaviour; withdrawal and passivity.

Braulin, Rook and Sills (1982) reported that a family when confronted with a traumatic injury, experiences a number of stressors. For example, the suddenness of the onset; the smells, sounds and unpredictable critical care environment; unfamiliar professional staff; separation from their family member; the uncertainty of the prognosis with the very real possibility that the person might die; possible financial problems. At such times these stressors can elicit feelings such as fear, isolation, loneliness, being out of control, dependency, mistrust, loss, helplessness and hopelessness, and finally, guilt and anger.

The dilemma facing the critical care nurse is that her priority is to focus upon the needs of the trauma patient. The family in this situation is often left to deal with its stress alone.

Whilst the development of critical care units has gone some way towards its goal of caring for the critically ill patient, critical care units have created a unique threat to a family system and to each of the family members. At a time of great stress for both the patient and the family, a patient is deliberately separated from his or her family. The structure and visiting policies often mean families can only see their relative for short periods of time. Despite an increasing relaxation in the rigid enforcement of restricted visiting policies throughout the UK (Millar, Biley and Wilson, 1993), many families find themselves spending long periods alone or in the company of other families in the corridors or waiting areas attached to a critical care unit. It is interesting to speculate, as Sherizen and Paul have, as to why family waiting areas on many critical care units are so poor, and indeed so far away from the main critical care entrance. Sherizen and Paul suggest that a family waiting room which is some distance away from the main entrance to the critical care unit may indicate the health care professional's support for the view that 'out of sight is out of mind'. Whilst they clearly ignore factors such as the age of many hospitals, the fact that few hospitals have purpose built ITUs or indeed the lack of space in most units this does not detract from their important message. Families need to be continuously informed and interact with the health care professionals if they are to learn to trust them.

For a family the contact with a critical care unit is evaluated in terms of their contact with nurses and their perceptions of nursing practice. Increasingly, critical care nurses find themselves interacting with a family experiencing extreme stress or perhaps a 'crisis'. At such times, nurses are called upon to provide and coordinate the emotional support of the family or significant others.

Although critical care nurses are sensitive to the emotional needs of a critically ill patient's family, there is, nonetheless, often a lack of time spent supporting them. The importance of a family and their needs are rarely disputed; the priority, though, remains the critically ill patient.

Acknowledgement that families may face a crisis has led to the development of strategies for supporting a family through use of crisis theory (Cobb, Kaplan). By definition, 'crisis' care has been viewed as present orientated; this fails, however, to recognize that decisions concerning a family's well-being need to take account not only of the present implications, but also future outcomes. For a family confronted with a critically ill or injured person, crucial questions may include:

- [ ] What will the future bring?

- [ ] Will the patient recover?

- [ ] What kind of future will the patient have if he does recover?

- [ ] How will I cope if the patient dies?

The emotional and physical stresses associated with a critical illness and admission to a critical care unit have been reported by Aguilera and Messick (1976) to result in a situational crisis.

Having someone critically ill often means that families are separated for long periods of time, all of which limits a family's ability to assess the status of their relative (Breu and Dracup, 1978). Families find themselves dependent upon infrequent communications with the health care team, and short, stressful visits to the patient's bedside. This physical separation serves as a constant reminder to a family that the patient may die. Potential death of a

relative creates one of the major disruptions for a family, and often they enter a period of anticipatory grieving. Observations of the experience of family facing death in the critical care unit led Sherizen and Paul (1977) to suggest that the critical care unit environment places a major constraint upon a family's ability to face the death of their loved one.

Evidence that a family's experiences in the critical care unit cause them anxiety has been reported in a number of papers (Daley, 1984; Bouman, 1984; Curtis, 1983; Leske, 1986). Other authors (Caine, 1989; Epperson, 1977; Kuenzi and Fenton, 1975; Leske, 1986) have assumed that a family's experience is characterized by a crisis state. Only Epperson (1977), however, has identified a crisis reaction. From a study of 230 families, Epperson described six distinct phases in a family's experience prior to them reestablishing family homeostasis:

Eppersons six stages

1. High levels of anxiety
2. Denial
3. Anger
4. Remorse
5. Grief
6. Reconciliation

There are clearly similarities between the stages described by Epperson and those reported in the literature on death and dying by Kubler Ross (1981) and Murray Parkes (1968). What is interesting about Epperson's study is that it was conducted in a specialized emergency trauma centre, though it may not be representative of other critical care units.

Reports in clinical papers identify the fear of death or permanent disability of their relative as potential sources of stress (King and Gregor, 1985). Research in the coronary care environment has highlighted the fear of losing a partner or the reoccurrence of a myocardial infarction as stressors for the spouse of a patient (Bedsworth and Molen, 1982; Thompson and Cordle, 1988). A number of narrative accounts have claimed that a family experiences anxiety in the critical care unit (Bouman, 1984; Curtis, 1983; Caine, 1989; Millar, 1987). Research support for this assumption was not included. A more recent study of a family's experience (Rukholm *et al.*, 1991) in critical care did include assessment of State and Trait anxiety using the Spielberger State Trait Anxiety Inventory. Their results indicated that there was a significant relationship between family needs and situational anxiety.

Perceived needs of the family

Serious illness and injury affects not only the patient but also their family. The often life threatening events present as a major stressor for a family, and can lead to family crises (Epperson, 1977). Despite an increasing amount of evidence from the USA on the subject of needs, here in the UK the subject has received only minimal attention. The research literature which does exist can be divided into two categories; perceptions of the spouse (post death); and the family's perceptions of needs in the intensive care unit.

Spouse's perceptions of needs: The original research about families of critically ill patients focused upon the needs of grieving spouses (Hampe, 1975; Breu and Dracup, 1978). Both these studies aimed to discover if a grieving spouse could identify his or her own needs, and the relationship of nursing interventions to these needs.

Hampe (1975) interviewed 27 spouses during their partner's terminal illness. Hampe reported that the individuals in her study could identify their own needs. Eight needs were identified:

Hampe's eight needs

1. Being able to visit anytime.
2. Helping with the personal care of their partner.
3. Prompt attention to the physical and emotional needs of their partner.
4. Awareness of the partner's medical condition and daily progress reports by the nurses.
5. Awareness of the impending death.
6. Being able to talk about the impending death.
7. The comfort and support of family members.
8. Demonstrations by the health care team of friendliness and concern.

Of the spouses, 25 identified all eight of the needs; the other two reported five and seven of the

needs, respectively. Both studies reported that nursing interventions do influence whether or not the spouses' perceived that the needs were being met.

Gilks (1984), in a study of the needs and concerns of families of patients undergoing cardiac surgery, revealed that the surgery was significantly more stressful for the spouse than the patient. The spouses in the study highlighted waiting for the surgery as the most extreme stressor. Artinian (1989) explored the concerns of families experiencing a similar event to that of Gillis' group. Using a semi-structured interview with just five questions, families identified the following categories of concerns – feelings of fear and numbness about the events; concerns about their relationships with staff, usually related to staff insensitivity or staff members appearing too impersonal in their interactions with a family. Waiting was identified as a key concern, especially not knowing what the outcome of the surgery was and its potential effects on the patient and family in the future. With the current troubles faced by patients such as the uncertainty of the date of the surgery and, indeed, the not infrequent cancellations of planned surgery, the family's stress increases. Spouses in the research sample identified additional perceived strains such as added responsibility, demands on their time, fatigue, and increased telephone communications at home.

Family's perceptions of needs in critical care: Using an exploratory descriptive research design, Molter (1979) undertook to learn what were the perceived personal needs of family members of critically ill patients, how important the needs were to the family, and if the needs were being met, if so by whom. An inventory of 45 need statements developed by Molter was used to provide a structured interview guide. The sample of the study included 40 family members of critically ill patients in two large teaching hospitals. The needs were ranked in order of importance, importance by age of family member, and importance by social class. The ten most important needs identified were:

Ten most important needs

1. To feel there is hope.
2. To feel hospital personnel care about the patient.

3. To have the waiting room near the patient.
4. To be called at home about any changes in the patient's condition.
5. To know the prognosis.
6. To have questions answered honestly.
7. To know specific facts concerning the patient's progress.
8. To receive information about the patient once a day.
9. To have explanations given in understandable terms.
10. To see the patient frequently.

Demographic variables were reported to have no influence on the ten most important needs listed. Content validity of the Molter instrument has been tested by several researchers. Although the items appear comprehensive, a number of items have been identified as needing modification or deleting (Norris and Grove, 1986). Reliability of the Family Needs Inventory has been investigated and reported by Mathis (1984), Norris and Grove (1986), Leske (1986) and Rogers (1983).

Considerable evidence exists to support the importance of information and the need for hope as critical family needs. Several authors (Molter, 1979; Leske, 1986; Daley, 1984) have reported the importance of family needs using the Critical Care Family Needs Inventory. Daley (1984) used structured interviews within 72 hours of admission to the ITU to identify important needs of family members of 21 patients. In addition, she categorized the 46 need statements into six areas of need: personal needs; the need to decrease anxiety; the need for support and ventilation; the need for information; the need to be with the patient; and the need to be helpful.

The number of studies of family needs has increased steadily since the mid-1970s, the majority using the Critical Care Family Needs Inventory or modifications of it. In answer to the question 'What are the needs of families of critically ill patients?', a table of the ten most important is identified. Although there are some variations in the rank ordering of the need statements, the ten most important remain consistent. The needs identified were being met most frequently by other family members, with nurses being identified as the next major group.

Studies of family needs during the mid-1980s began to include both the families' perceptions of needs and the nurses, and to offer some comparison between the two groups (Norris and Grove, 1986; Forrester et al., 1990; Lynn-McHale and Bellinger, 1988). The results of such studies report some variations in the perceptions of need by the two groups. Specifically, families identified three needs as more important than the nurses did: to feel there is hope; to know about the hospital staff taking care of the patient; and to have questions answered honestly.

Mathis (1984) utilized the Molter 45 need statements to establish if there was a difference between the needs of those with an acute brain injury and those patients without. The sample included 26 family members of patients admitted to a large teaching hospital in the USA. Use of a Chi Square statistical test was applied to the needs statements to examine if there were differences in the frequency of identified needs between those reported by Molter (1979) and the families in this study. The author concludes that families of patients with an acute brain injury did experience differences in perception of personal needs. The results were reported as supporting the studies of Hampe (1975), Breu and Dracup (1979) and Molter (1979).

The implications of the studies of family needs for practice are often only tentative, since many of the research studies focus upon only one kind of patient sample or specific disease, thereby limiting the generalizability of the study. Leske (1986), in a integrative analysis of the American family needs studies, reports that the diversity of family member characteristics and patient demographics accumulated from the results of the large number of studies makes it possible to consider the wider applications of the findings for critical care interventions. From her analysis of the many studies reviewed, she concludes that there are primary family needs. These primary needs are those identified consistently in the nursing research as most important by the family members of a critically ill patient. A list of 15 most important needs have been identified, and are listed in Table 10.1.

These primary needs were identified from the results of 27 studies in which the Critical Care Family Needs Inventory was used. The results are

Table 10.1. Fifteen most important needs ($n = 950$) during a critical illness in family needs studies in the USA.

Need	Mean	SD
To have questions answered honestly	3.87	0.42
To be assured the best care possible is being given to the patient	3.85	0.42
To know the prognosis	3.84	0.46
To feel there is hope	3.81	0.44
To know specific facts about the patient's progress	3.78	0.45
To be called at home about changes in the patient's condition	3.75	0.62
To know how the patient is being treated medically	3.72	0.54
To feel hospital personnel care about the patient	3.72	0.59
To receive information about the patient daily	3.69	0.58
To have understandable explanations	3.68	0.60
To know exactly what is being done for the patient	3.68	0.60
To know why things were done for the patient	3.64	0.59
To see the patients frequently	3.59	0.65

also described in terms of three major categories: assurance, proximity, and information.

The need for *assurance* is emphasized by the families' reported need to have their questions answered honestly, and a feeling they reported of needing to be sure the best care possible is being given to their relative. It is important to a family that staff care about their relative, and in addition hope is a mechanism used by the family to help them define and understand the critical illness event (Sabo *et al.*, 1989). Providing assurance can help to reduce a family's stress, deflect a potential family crisis, and reduce the family's feelings of uncertainty (Mischel and Braden, 1988). All families report a need to be near to their relative. It is perhaps most significant during the first few days of the critical illness event. At this time the family feel a need to be close and to see the sick relative frequently. This closeness has been reported by family members to provide a source of comfort. Admission to a critical care unit should not mean that a family surrenders its involvement with or connection to a critically ill family member. Most

critical care units impose barriers which separate the family and the patient, and insist on restricting the interactions between family and patient. It is actions such as restricted or inconsistent visiting policies which serve to remind a family of their possible loss of a seriously ill relative. By allowing a family frequent access to their relative they are able to realistically appraise the situation and to validate the seriousness of the illness.

Of considerable importance is the need for information. Several information needs have been identified: for example, to know how the patient is being treated; to know exactly what is being done; information on the patient's progress. The desire to be kept informed is emphasized in a family's concern to have daily reports, and especially to be told about changes in the patient's progress. Although not always explicit in the research reports, a number of families are concerned about information being withheld from them. One point that is significant is for critical care nurses to remember that the seriousness of the situation often impedes a family's ability to both comprehend and to remember the information they are being given. Information may need to be repeated frequently and to all family members. Whilst the need for information is clearly very important, the process is two-way; often a family need the nurse to simply listen and provide a sympathetic ear.

The findings reflect increasing concern by critical care professionals for the families of critically ill patients. What is clearly needed over the next two decades is research to identify those interventions which support families and demonstrate the holistic caring commitment that the critically ill patient and his or her family deserve.

Family needs during a critical illness: the UK experience

Whilst it is true that most of the studies aimed at identifying family needs in a critical care unit are American in origin, a small number of researchers have investigated the issue in the United Kingdom. Many of the studies carried out in the USA adopted a quantitative research design. In contrast, the five UK studies included three quantitative research designs (Millar, 1987; McIvor and Thompson, 1988; Mongiardi *et al.*, 1987), one (Coulter, 1989) qualitative in design using grounded theory, and the other (Hayes, 1990) combines a quantitative and qualitative design. The purpose of this review is to summarize the findings and present some of the implications for practice and further research into families' needs during and after a critical illness event.

Millar (1987) investigated the needs of family members in intensive care units in South Wales. Three critical care units participated in the study, which used a semi-structured interview schedule developed by Molter and Daley. Thirty patients' relatives were approached to participate in the study; of these some 20 completed the interviews. Those who refused to take part included two who accompanied their relative in transfer from the hospital to another and therefore were unavailable, four who were too distressed by their visit to participate, and two who simply did not want to participate.

The families were asked to identify the importance of a list of needs ($n = 47$) statements, and in addition they were asked to indicate if the need was being met and by whom. A four point Likert scale ranged from not important to very important.

Descriptive statistics included means, modes, percentages and rank ordering of the responses. Field notes were kept of each interview, which lasted approximately 35 minutes (range 35 min through to 1.5 hours).

The ten most important needs were identified, and included the need to have questions answered honestly, and the need to feel that staff care about my relative as the joint most important.

The table of needs were also calculated to identify the most important category of needs (Daley, 1984). By far the most important categories were the need to have information and the need for relief of anxiety. These rankings compared well with those reported by Molter, Leske and Daley.

Limitations included the small sample size. In addition, three themes emerged from the field notes; the need for all the families to discuss the events prior to the admission to the critical care unit; the importance of being liked by the staff; and the need to be near and to be able to see their relative frequently. During some of the structured interviews the researcher was aware of fulfilling a cathartic and therapeutic role for the families which may clearly have influenced both the families' responses and the researchers' interpretation of the findings. The responses to the issue of who met the needs was poorly addressed, and proved impossible to analyse. This could have been due to a number of factors – for example, some family members were confused by the different health care staff who they met, others seemed afraid to be seen to be critical of the staff in case it influenced the care their sick relative received.

Recommendations for further research included increasing the sample size, using a qualitative as well as a quantitative approach, including staff in the assessment of perceived needs, and examining the factors which influence staff and family interactions in the critical care unit.

In a study of self-perceived needs of family members in ICUs, McIvor and Thompson (1988) found that the need for relief from anxiety was perceived as the most important category, followed by the need for information. McIvor and Thompson used Daley's six categories and 46 need statements in a questionnaire to collect data from 24 family members. Their results show similarity with those found by Millar (1987), and lend support to the conclusion that family members can identify their own needs. In common with the sample reported by Millar, the families in this study perceived the doctor as most appropriate for information concerning prognosis, diagnosis and treatments. Nurses in both studies were seen as the most appropriate for day-to-day information and progress reports.

Implications for practice reported included that it is important for nurses to be present when doctors interview families, strategies are needed to help nurses who are extremely busy to have the time to communicate with a patient's family. The importance of an accurate assessment for the provision of holistic nursing care was also stressed.

Limitations of the study included the inexperience of the two researchers, time constraints, and the small sample size. Despite this, the authors believe that nurses who have knowledge of the patient's needs will be in a stronger position to deliver the quality nursing care that critically ill patients and their families deserve.

In contrast, Mongiardi et al. (1987) reported on an exploratory study into the needs of partners of patients being cared for in a coronary care unit. The partners of 14 patients admitted to the CCU during May and June of 1985 were invited to participate in the study. A postal questionnaire was used to collect the data. Families were mailed the questionnaire two weeks post-discharge from hospital. A total of 15 relatives agreed to complete the study; unfortunately, owing to personal difficulties one person had to withdraw. Data from the 14 questionnaires included the usefulness of information and help they received on admission to the CCU. Information either given or needed dominates the data. Unfortunately, little information is provided on the design of the questionnaire, nor are the issues of validity or reliability addressed. Implications are noted with caution by the authors, who recognize the difficulties of evaluating what is given (in terms of information) and what is remembered. The issue of having difficulty in getting the information they wanted was identified, though no mention is made of how the information is given nor what types of language were used. Further research needs to include some structured interviews to help further clarify the important concerns about information identified by this small sample of relatives of CCU patients.

Coulter (1989) used grounded theory to explore the needs of family members of critically ill patients. A total of 11 personal interviews with a family member were undertaken 72 hours after admission to the unit. This time period was felt to be more appropriate in the experience of the interviewer, as families tended to be more anxious prior to this. Six themes emerged from the data: *the shock of admission to critical care with a critical illness; finding ways to cope with the situation; the need for information; the need for social support; satisfaction of personal needs;* and *retaining hope.*

The implications of this study were that relatives need a full and accurate explanation of their loved one's illness, they need information about their relative's progress with frequent updates, and finally, they need to feel they have ready access to the medical and nursing staff for information. The author suggests that greater emphasis needs to be given to improving communication and counselling skills of nurses in critical care units; a suggestion is also made for developing a specialist nurse to help support and meet a family's needs; families

need help to become involved in their relative's care; and finally, family assessment must be undertaken to develop appropriate interventions.

The final UK study is a report from Northern Ireland by Hayes (1990). While it is not clear what research design this study used, there are suggestions that it combined both the qualitative and quantitative approaches. Some mention is made of family interviews and of the needs statements developed by Molter, Daley and Leske. Particular attention is given in this study to the particular needs of specific patient/family groups. Given the political and troubled times in Belfast, the stresses and anxieties faced by both the nurse and a family member are highlighted. Similar findings to those already reported are described and discussed. Hayes concludes with a belief that holistic care in critical care requires an assessment of family needs and the development of intervention strategies to meet them.

The findings of these few UK studies represent an increasing awareness and concern by critical care nurses for their patient's families. Despite the limitations of the studies, it is evident that certain family needs are present during a patient's critical illness experience. With a family-focused and systematic approach to research on family needs, the next decade will surely reveal new data and lead to further innovations in critical care nurses' practice.

Who cares for the carers?
Caring for the critically ill patient and his or her family is often a source of profound moral conflict and personal suffering for nurses. Meeting the psychosocial needs of the patient and family in the critical care unit presents a constant reminder of the vulnerability that such units create. The continued expansion in the growth of knowledge and expertise in critical care nursing has served to increase the psychosocial concerns. The patients are now often sicker, older and undergoing more complex and invasive treatment regimes.

At such times the family of the ill patient looks to the nurse not only for information but also their emotional support and comfort. Over the past decade the literature has reported the increased attention given to the psychosocial needs of patients and their families. Of increasing concern, however, is the psychosocial needs of the primary care giver, the critical care nurse. The importance of identifying and meeting the needs of the critical nurse has been alluded to by Ball (1990) and Ashworth (1992). If we are to be successful in meeting the need for 'high tech/High Touch' care of our patients and their families, then nurse managers must be sensitive to the support needs of their staff.

Collaboration and outcomes of critical care

Traditionally, doctors have made the decisions concerning the care of the critically ill patient. It is widely recognized that the provision of high quality care for the critically ill cannot happen without the contributions of both nursing and medicine. The increasing costs of high tech medicine, an emphasis on value for money, a focus upon effectiveness and efficiency and increasing consumer questioning of the absolute power of the professionals to make decisions about their health has led to serious attempts to measure the outcomes of care.

Clearly, against such a background studies are needed to identify aspects of critical care that can demonstrate increased benefits for critically ill patients. Knaus et al. (1986) studied 5000 patients in 13 tertiary care centres in an attempt to predict mortality and morbidity rates. Data collection included use of the APACHE II severity of illness scale, the sophistication of the technology used, organizational structure, and the status of the hospital, e.g. teaching hospital or other. The results identified significant differences between predicted and actual patient death rates. Some of the units had better than predicted survival rates than could have been expected from the severity of illness data, whilst others recorded higher than predicted survival rates. The differences in the mortality predictions occurred for medical admissions alone, and when medical and surgical patients were combined.

Following this finding the data were further analysed, and suggested that the differences in mortality were not related to the patient's physiologic status, nor to the status of the hospital or the degree of sophisticated technology used. The differences, it would appear, were related to the degree of interaction and communication (collaboration) occurring between nursing and medicine. As a result of this examination, the researchers concluded that, "involvement and interaction of critical care personnel can influence the outcome of critically ill patients".

In an evaluation of nurse–physician collaboration in intensive care units, Maggs and Snoxall (1992), measured the impact of interdisciplinary collaboration upon patient outcomes and nurse satisfaction. Their study focused on the amount of interdisciplinary collaboration involved in deciding when to transfer a patient from the critical care unit to a less intense area. In addition, they assessed the satisfaction of the nurses and physicians with the decision-making process. Recognizing that the decision to transfer may be influenced by organizational or other constraints, the study included exploration of those transfer decisions where no other option existed. For example, increasing pressure on acute care beds means that decisions to transfer are based upon identifying the most stable for transfer, as their bed is needed for a new admission: clearly in this type of situation there are no alternatives.

A prospective descriptive design was used, and the study centre was a large university medical centre ICU. The unit had 17 beds and admitted all groups of critically ill patients. During January–July 1989, data was collected on the decision to transfer 286 consecutive patients from the ICU. The nursing sample included all of the 56 registered nurses on the unit and 31 medical residents who worked on the unit. Data collection instruments included a Decision about Transfer tool, which was designed specifically for the research and had a Likert scale graded from 1 (no collaboration) to (7 complete collaboration). From this study a critical care nurse's perceptions of the amount of interdisciplinary collaboration concerning the decision to transfer the patients from the ICU is positively associated with patient outcomes.

Limitations of the study include that it is unclear whether or not collaboration had the same meaning for the nurses and the medics, and that there is also some concern about the perceived importance of collaboration between the two groups. Despite these and other reported limitations from this study, important information has been identified, namely that collaboration is more important when there are alternative choices. Critical care units have often been described by practitioners as examples of interdisciplinary collaborative care in an acute care setting (Mechanic and Aitken, 1982). The results of this study suggest that collaboration can positively affect patient outcomes. The reported empirical association between collaborative practice and patient outcomes highlights the importance of continuing to study nurse–physician collaboration in critical care units.

Since our society has apparently accepted critical care units as an important system for care delivery, and in the future will probably increasingly continue to do so, it is imperative that we can identify aspects of such care delivery systems that positively influence patient/family outcomes. The provision of quality health care for the critically ill cannot occur without the contributions of both health care professionals and the patient/family. Increasing concerns related to such issues as value for money, effectiveness and efficiency, and the resolution of ethical dilemmas can only be resolved if the two groups (health care professionals and patients/families) work collaboratively. In addition, within nursing the increasing focus of attention on accountability and autonomy in practice means the time is right for innovative care delivery systems which enhance the critical care nurse's professional practice.

PRACTICAL NURSING IMPLICATIONS

Health care professionals and patient families in the critical care environment have a long history of conflicting relationships. The roots of this conflict are multifaceted, and enmeshed in social, economic and professional issues. Such a legacy serves to make cooperation difficult, though not impossible, to achieve. The barriers imposed by history need to be dismantled for critical care nurses, and for them to forge a new relationship with their patients/families. It is clear that such a relationship cannot be expected to simply 'happen'. What is required is a vision, an unswerving belief and commitment, and a giant leap of faith that cooperative care can dramatically improve patient care and provider satisfaction.

Over the past two decades, two concepts in nursing and health care have been identified as having a positive effect on patient/family care and provider satisfaction. The concepts are primary nursing and health care patient/family collaboration. Despite increasing widespread acclaim for primary nursing (Manley, 1991), a model of patient/family cooperation in a primary nursing setting remains elusive. Examples of collaboration between a primary nurse and a patient's family have been reported in some speciality units. However, in many critical units, nurses and patients/families work in a parallel fashion at best, and at worst in opposition. A mode of effective primary nurse–family cooperation remains to be evolved, defined, described and reproduced.

A family nursing philosophy for critical care nursing involves:

Care Partnerships		Collaboration
Open Visiting	FAMILY	Assessment Tool
Primary Nursing	NURSING	Family Support
Supportive Environment	PHILOSOPHY	Staff Development
Cooperation		Communication

Despite the increasing acknowledgement by critical care nurses that families are an integral part of their work, there is, nevertheless, a gap between what is espoused in the literature and what is evidenced in clinical practice. Closing the gap requires an understanding of the influences which prevent nurses from including a patient's family in their care programme. Some obvious factors are: a lack of time; rewards are for completing tasks, rarely for providing a family with support; many nurses believe themselves to be unqualified to provide family care; and finally, there is at present a lack of a nursing framework, specifically for the care of families.

Whilst nurses often present contradictory evidence in support of family-centred nursing practice, there are a number of potential benefits. For example, by encouraging the family to be present we can develop trust between a family and a nurse, obtain a more personalized view of the patient, develop effective communications with a family,

Table 10.2. Factors contributing to a family's concerns during a critical illness (evidence collated from the UK and USA literature).

Diagnosis related factors
Unsuccessful therapy
The need to use life saving technology
Uncertainty about the prognosis
Unpredictable relapse in the patient's recovery
Communicating with many specialists

Environmental factors
The lack of privacy in the critical care environment
Rigid hospital/ICU regulations
The technology attached to the patient
Inadequate rest facilities
Having limited access to the patient
Having to leave the unit frequently
Inadequate sleeping facilities

Personal factors
Role changes as result of the illness
Travelling to and from the hospital
Having to rely upon the good will of others
Feelings of guilt
Concerns about the future
Concerns about decisions and who makes them

Equipment-related factors
The use of ventilators
Sophisticated monitors
Numerous tubes and lines
Alarms and noise
Kidney dialysis machines

Social-related factors
Impersonalized environment
Being asked to provide very personal information
Restrictive visiting hours
Having to adapt to a hospital schedule
Problems in communicating with health professionals
Problems concerning information or the lack of it
A lack of social support

Table 10.3. Nursing interventions aimed at providing more control for a critically ill patient's family.

Contracting with a patient and his family the visiting hours.
Providing continuity of information through assigning a primary/family nurse.
Identifying times and the process of arranging to speak with the medical staff.
Providing a method of communication that is effective for the patient, family and ICU staff.
Developing mechanisms whereby the ICU team can be aware of the family needs.
Providing a suitable/comfortable family rest area.
Providing a choice of diversional activities that a family can choose from.
Encouraging the family to participate in the decisions about care.
Encouraging the family to become active in the caring process in whatever ways they perceive to be appropriate.
Developing a family care philosophy within the ITU.

and there is some evidence to support the belief that family visits can improve a patient's mental status.

In contrast, the negative effects of family involvement may include: a failure to promote trust between a family and a nurse; a family's presence has been reported to increase stress for the nurses; and emotional traumas caused by developing a close attachment to a patient's family. Some staff believe that a family's presence may also interfere with their ability to care for the patient.

Despite the evidence, it is the author's opinion that families are a much underused resource in patient care and recovery from a critical illness.

In response to the challenge to provide new ways of working with families, some suggestions follow.

A family nursing philosophy

A philosophy of care states the unit's values with regard to a family's nursing. As stated earlier, the family is seen as an open system in constant interaction with its environment. Since admission to a critical care unit is described as a major source of family disruption and stress, the nurse's role is to support a family unit's integrity. A number of nursing frameworks support the systems view, (Rogers, Parse and Newman). Rosemary Parse's (1993) theory of human becoming offers critical care nurses a framework for organizing their knowledge about the family–universe–health interrelationship. Parse believes that "human beings cannot be reduced, they are more than and different from the sum of the parts". Human beings are characterized by patterns of relating. This framework provides a means for assessing where a family are in their understanding of the patient's critical illness. Questions that a nurse might ask a family include, How did they feel when first told of the relative's situation? What concerns them most at the present time? What is helpful to them? A family assessment tool could be structured around the family's perception of the event, their concerns, their goals and the resources they have or need to meet them.

Family needs

A number of studies have been reported which use the Critical Care Family Needs Inventory (Molter, 1979). Information and communication were identified as major family concerns. Loos and Bell (1990) report a family interviewing technique which involves the use of circular questioning techniques developed by Tomm (1985). Examples of such questions include: Who best understands the doctor's explanations? How is your understanding different from your mother's? If you wanted to ask for more information, who could you ask? If you asked for more information, what would be most helpful? (see Loos and Bell, 1990, p. 49).

Family support groups

The value of family support groups has been reported. Such a group is usually led by a senior nurse from within the ITU, with many reports citing the need to be an effective communicator, and committed to a philosophy of family care.

The primary purpose of a family support group is to meet families' needs for support in whatever ways they find appropriate. Its goals are to provide emotional support, information, and to clarify information about the care of their relative. The intended outcome is to contribute to a family's ability to mobilize their resources for coping with the situation. Sabo et al. (1989) identified the following perceived benefits from a family support group:

- ☐ reduced anxiety;
- ☐ improved communications;
- ☐ family satisfaction.

The evidence on the value of support groups is, however, contradictory, and though some evidence exists of their potential benefits, there is no real evidence that such a group is the most beneficial or indeed cost-effective means for supporting the family of a critically ill patient (Sabo et al., 1989; Halm, 1990).

Staff development

The need for continuing education programmes for staff is an ongoing and increasing concern. With the current emphasis on individualized care, staff find themselves with little knowledge and few skills for helping and supporting a family group. What is needed are specific programmes to help staff explore the values and influences on their interactions with a patient's family.

Reflecting as a group on the value systems within the unit can help staff to identify what strengths they have for helping a family as well as identifying potential weaknesses. Role models and mentors provide a useful and effective strategy for helping new staff to acquire the knowledge and skills needed to provide family-centred nursing in practice.

Essential skills needed for overcoming barriers to successful nurse–family interactions include attention to such issues as lack of time, families as a source of stress, lack of insight into the dynamics of nurse–family relationships, poor interaction style, and nurses making premature value judgements about a family.

The development of a trusting relationship takes time, which in a busy critical care unit is at a premium. However, critical care nurses should consider a number of strategies to help them improve their relationships with a family. Family relationships need to be seen as important, and the nurse needs to create time for supporting and communicating with a patient's family. Some units have introduced a 15 minute family–nurse communication slot into their routine. Families know that at certain times of the day the nurse caring for their relative will be available to meet with them. The interactions are best carried out at the patient's bedside; families need to see their relative frequently, and find time away from the patient stressful. By introducing planned and systematic family interactions they will take less time. Families knowing they have planned time with a nurse will save their questions for the time allocated. They may also help to address the issue of a family asking individual questions throughout the day. Nurses will need to remember, however, that communication needs to be simple, short and often. Families under stress have difficulty comprehending the large volumes of information given and in retrieving it.

Perceptions of a family as a stressor

Surrounded by the strange environment and staff, a family's fears, anger, mistrust, helplessness and lack of control can combine with the uncertainty about their relative's future to create the worst kind of behaviour in individuals who would otherwise be understanding and likeable. Although a number of researchers have reported nurses' concerns and feelings towards families in critical care, one study (by Logan, 1987) perhaps illustrates many of the problems. Logan interviewed critical care nurses about their interactions with the families of critically ill patients. Although the study was undertaken in the USA, from experience and through communications with nurses in the UK similar findings could be expected. Logan reported on families that nurses found easy to get on with, and on those that were exactly the opposite.

Her results indicated that a sample of nurses interviewed found the following to result in poor family communications:

- [ ] A family who were physically or emotionally abusive.
- [ ] A family who are known or perceived to be abusers, either of drugs or alcohol.
- [ ] When large numbers of family are present at the same time.
- [ ] When no one in the family speaks English.
- [ ] When family members are perceived by the nurses to be 'uneducated'.

In contrast, 'good' families were:

- [ ] Friendly towards the staff.
- [ ] Concerned about the patient.
- [ ] Inquisitive, but patient.
- [ ] Appreciative.

- [ ] Showed their anxiety.
- [ ] Were educated or intelligent.

These findings have been reported by Millar (1989) as very similar to Stockwell's experience when researching the unpopular patient. Making quick judgements about a family based upon their appearance or behaviour may seriously damage critical care nurse–family relationships. To achieve success in family–nurse interrelationships, critical care nurses need to avoid acting in haste. Whilst none of us can ever truly stop making judgements about others, nurses can resist the temptation to act prematurely on such reactions.

The essential prerequisites for successful nurse–family relationships includes being sensitive to the emotional traumas a family is experiencing, being aware of and responding to their increased vulnerability at a time of crisis, effective communications skills including the important skill of active listening, and communicating respect to a family.

CONCLUSIONS

Critical care nurses find themselves increasingly coming into contact with families struggling to come to terms with a life-threatening event. At such times critical care nurses are in a unique position to support a family which finds itself incredibly vulnerable to the potential loss of a loved one. Identification of important needs and research aimed at developing our understanding of the families concerns at such times provides the basis for developing appropriate interventions. As the 1980s have been a period of increased awareness of the needs of families, so it is hoped the 1990s will be recognized as the period when critical care nurses developed their research to focus on interventions and the identification of the significant contribution that all critical nurses make to the health and well-being of a critically ill patient and his or her family.

Cooperative relationships, although positive and progressive, are not easily created. They require nurses and families to examine their inner feelings. Families and nurses need to communicate openly and to confront their conflicts directly. Change brings with it anxiety, uncertainty and frustration. It is often seen as easier to continue with 'outdated' practices. Cooperation is a conscious, learned behaviour that needs constant nurturing, reinforcing and reflection, if the promise of cooperative care is to be realized by both critical care nurses and the patient's family. According to Peters (1983), "Developing a vision is a messy, artistic process. Living it convincingly is a passionate one way beyond any doubt".

CASE STUDIES

Case study one

John is a 50 year old bank manager. He has just undergone a triple coronary artery bypass graft operation and has been admitted to the unit straight from theatre. You are assigned to care for him and during the report you are informed his family are in the hospital and are very anxious. His wife and two daughters have been told that this surgery was the only answer to John's unstable angina. The family are still shocked by the surgeon's bluntness, "without this treatment your husband will not live". John was still asking how could this be happening; he had not been ill before this.

Case study two

Mary is a 24 year old single mother. She had recently separated from her boyfriend and has left her two year old son with friends for an evening out on the town. She accepted a lift from some people she met at the pub and on the way home they were involved in a head on collision with another car. Mary had not used the seat-belt and had been projected through the windscreen landing some 20 feet from the crashed cars. She is unconscious, has multiple fractures, needs ventilator support and is cardiovascularly unstable. Her parents arrive at the same time as the ex-boyfriend.

STUDENT LEARNING QUESTIONS

The following questions are presented to help you reflect on the content of this chapter:

1. What factors in the critical care environment may influence nurse–family interactions?

2. Think of a family with which you felt comfortable at work. Identify what factors about the family helped you to relate to them.

3. Now think of a family with whom you had some difficulty relating to at work. Can you identify the factors which influenced this situation?

4. Is family assessment part of your unit's practice? What form could/does this assessment take and is it comprehensive?

5. How do you feel when you first meet a patient's family?

6. What interventions can you identify to help a family during a situational crisis such as the sudden admission to ITU of a critically injured or ill relative?

7. What impact does a critical illness or injury have on the family?

8. How can family–nurse communications be improved during times of family crisis?

KEY TERMS

Family

With society rapidly differentiating the traditional conception of a family is experiencing some profound changes in its structure. In this chapter the broadest possible definition is used. The family is a group of individuals closely related by blood, marriage or friendship ties (nuclear family, cohabiting couple, single parent, blended families, etc.) characterized by a continuum of stability, commitment, mutual decision making, and shared goals. Each family member is a composite of interacting variables that affect individual and family health. The family as an open system interfaces with the environment (Berkey and Hanson, 1991).

Family Nursing

There are at least two approaches to family nursing: *family-centred nursing*, and *family nursing*. The more traditional family-centred nursing regards the family as a critical background or context for the individual. Here the individual remains the focus of concern. The second approach, described by Leaghy and Wright (1984), as family systems nursing, views the family as the central focus of inquiry and the client of nursing.

FURTHER READING

Leaghy, M., Wright, L. *Families and Life-threatening Illness*. Pennsylvania: Springhouse, 1984.

Lunsberry, C., Richards E. Family nursing practice: paradigm perspectives and diagnostic approaches. *Advances in Nursing Science*. 1992; 15(2): 66–75.

Berkey, K., Hanson, S. *Pocket guide to Family Assessment and Intervention: Mosby Year Book*. Philadelphia: C V Mosby, 1991.

Dallos, R. *Family Belief Systems: Therapy and Change*. Milton Keynes: Open University Press, 1991.

Whall, A., Fawcett, J. *Family Theory Development in Nursing: State of the science and art*. Philadelphia: FA Davis, 1991.

Miller, J., Janosick, E. *Family Focused Care*. New York: McGraw Hill, 1980.

Gillis, C., Highley, B., Roberts, B., Martinson, I. *Toward a Science of Family Nursing*. Menlo Park, CA: Addison Wesley, 1989.

Hudak, C., Gallo, B., Benz, J. *Critical Care Nursing: A Holistic Approach*. 5th ed. Philadelphia: JB Lippincott, 1990.

Friedman, M. *Family Nursing: Theory and Practice. 3rd Edition*. Norwalk, Connecticut: Appleton and Lange, 1992.

Koka, K. J. *Living with life threatening illness*. New York: Lexington Books, 1993.

REFERENCES

Aggleton, P., Chalmers, H. *Nursing Models and the Nursing Process*. Basingstoke: MacMillan, 1986.

Artinian, N. Family member perception of a cardiac surgery event. *Focus on Critical Care*. 1989; 16: 301–308.

Ashworth, P. Nursing is not just the tasks nurses do. *Intensive and Critical Care Nursing*. 1992; 8(3): 129.

Auguilera, D., Messick, J. L. *Crisis Intervention* 5th. ed. St Louis, Toronto: CV Mosby, 1986.

Baker, F. *Organisational Systems: General systems approaches to complex organisations*. Homewood, Illinois. Richard D. Irwin Inc, 1973.

Ball, C. Humanity in intensive care. *Intensive Care Nursing*. 1990; 6(1): 12–16.

Bedsworth, J. A., Molen, M. T. Psychological stress in the spouses of patients with myocardial infarction. *Heart and Lung*. 1982; 11: 450–456.

Bernardes, J. Whose family? A note on the changing sociological construct of the family. *Sociological Review*. 1989; 36: 267–272.

Braulin, J., Rook, J., Sills, G. Families in crisis: the impact of trauma. *Critical Care Quarterly*. 1982; 2: 248–254.

Breu, C., Dracup, K. Helping the spouses of critically ill patients. *American Journal of Nursing*. 1978; 78: 50–53.

Bouman, C. Identifying priority concerns of families of ICU patients. *Dimensions of Critical Care Nursing*. 1984; 3: 313–319.

Caine, R. Families in crisis: Making the critical difference. *Focus on Critical Care*. 1989; 16: 184–189.

Caplin, M., Sexton, D. Stresses experienced by spouses of patients in a coronary care unit with myocardial infarction. *Focus on Critical Care*. 1988; 15(5): 31–40.

Chartier, L., Coutu-Wakulczyk, G. Families in ICU: their needs and anxiety level. *Intensive Care Nursing*. 1988; 5: 11–18.

Clifford C. Patients, relatives and nurses in a technological environment. *Intensive Care Nursing*. 1986; 2: 67–72.

Coulter, M. The needs of family members of patients in Intensive Care Units. *Intensive Care Nursing*. 1989; 5: 4–10.

Continenza, K. Who cares for the care givers? *Focus on Critical Care*. 1989; 16(6): 435–443.

Curtis, N. M. *Caring for families during the 'unknown' period*. DCCN 1983: 2: 238–244.

Daley, L. The perceived immediate needs of families with relatives in the intensive care setting. *Heart & Lung*. 1984; 13: 231–237.

Davenport, Y. The waiting period prior to cardiac surgery – when complicated by sudden cancellation. *Intensive Care Nursing*. 1991; 7: 105–113.

Davies, J. Visiting acutely ill patients; a literature review. *Intensive Care Nursing*. 1987; 2: 163–165.

De La Cuesta, C. The nursing process from development to implementation. *Journal of Advanced Nursing*. 1983; 8(5): 365–371.

Dunkel, J. Eisendrath, S. Families in ICU: Their effects on the staff. *Heart & Lung*. 1983; 12(3): 258–261.

Dyer, I. Meeting the needs of visitors – a practical approach. *Intensive Care Nursing*. 1991; 7: 135–147.

Epperson, M. Families in sudden crisis: process and interventions in a critical care centre. *Social Work in Health Care*. 1977; 2(3): 265–273.

Forrester, D., Murphy, P., Price, D., Monaghan, J. Critical care family needs: nurse-family member confederate pairs. *Heart & Lung*. 1990; 19(b): 655–661.

Friedman, M. *Family Nursing –Theory and Assessment*. Norwalk, CT: Appleton-Century-Croft, 1981.

Gardener, D., Stewart, N. Staff involvement with families of patients in critical care units. *Heart & Lung*. 1978; 7: 105–110.

Gilks, C. Reducing family stress during and after coron-ary bypass surgery. *Nursing Clinics of North America*. 1984; 19: 103–112.

Goldstone, L. A., Ball, J. A. Monitor: an index of nursing care for acute medical and surgical wards. Newcastle-upon-Tyne Polytechnic Products Ltd., 1983.

Hampe, S. The needs of the grieving spouse in a hospital setting. *Nursing Research*. 1975; 24(2): 113–120.

Hayes, E. Needs of family members of critically ill patients – a Northern Ireland perspective. *Intensive Care Nursing*. 1990; 6: 25–29.

Henderson, V. The nursing process – is the title right? *Journal of Advanced Nursing*. 1982; 7(2): 103–109.

Hill, R. Generic features of families under stress. In: H. Parad (ed.). *Crisis Intervention Selected Readings*. New York. Family Service Assoc., 1965.

Hylton Rushton, C. Care Giver suffering in critical care nursing. *Heart & Lung*. 1992; 21(3): 303–306.

Jacono, J., Hicks, G., Antonioni, G., O'Brien, K. Comparison of perceived needs of family members between registered nurses and family members of critically ill patients in intensive care and neonatal intensive care units. *Heart & Lung*. 1990; 19(1): 72–78.

Kasl, D. The measurement of grief. *Hospice Journal*. 1986; 2(4): 21–36.

King, S., Gregor, F. Stress and coping in families of the critically ill. *Critical Care Nurse*. 1985; 5(4): 48–51.

Knaus, W. A., Draper, E. A., Wagner, D. P., Zimmerman, J. E. An evaluation of outcome from intensive care in major medical centres. *Annals Intern Med*. 1986; 104: 410–418.

Kubler Ross, E. *Living with Death and Dying*. New York: Macmillan, 1981.

Kuenzi, S. H., Fenton, M. V. Crisis intervention in acute care areas. *American Journal of Nursing*. 1975; 75: 830–834.

Leavitt, M. Nursing and family focused care. *Nursing Clinics of North America*. 1984; 19(1): 83–87.

Lees, F., Bell, J. Circular questions: A family interviewing strategy. *Dimensions in Critical Care Nursing*. 1990; 9: 46–53.

Leske, J. Needs of relatives of critically ill patients: A follow up. *Heart & Lung*. 1986; 15: 189–193.

Liddle, K. Reaching out . . . To meet the needs of relatives in intensive care units. *Intensive Care Nursing*. 1988; 4: 146–159.

Logan, N. Nurses' perceptions of caring for families of the critically ill. Masters Nursing Thesis, University of California, San Francisco, 1987.

Lynn-McHale, D., Bellinger, A. Need satisfaction levels of family members of critically ill patients and accuracy of nurses perceptions. *Heart & Lung*. 1988; 17(4): 447–453.

Maggs, C., Snoxall, S. *A survey of the literature on outcomes and recommendations to the Department of*

Health. Unpublished report. 1992, Maggs Research Associates.

Manley, K., Constable, P. Intensive disagreement . . . total patient care . . . primary nursing . . . in an intensive care unit. *Nursing Times*. 1991; 87(4): 66–67.

Mathis, M. Personal needs of family members of critically ill patients with and without brain injury. *Journal of Neurosurgical Nursing*. 1984; 16: 36–44.

McCubbin, H., Paterson, J. *Systematic assessment of family stress and coping*. St. Paul M. N. University of Minnesota School of Home Economics, 1981.

McIvor, D., Thompson, F. The self perceived needs of family members with a relative in the intensive care unit. *Intensive Care Nursing*. 1988; 4: 139–145.

Mechanic, D., Aitken, L. H. A cooperative agenda for medicine and nursing. *Massachussets Nurse*. 1982; 51(12): 5–6.

Millar, B. A study to describe the needs of families whose relative is critically ill in a general intensive care unit. (Unpublished Masters in Nursing dissertation). University of Wales Cardiff, 1987.

Millar, B. Family centred care in the ICU. *Nursing Times*. 1988.

Millar, B. Relatives: critical support in critical care. *N. Times*. 1989; 85(16): 31–33.

Millar, B. Caring and the family in the critical care unit. *Surgical Nurse*. 1991; 4(5): 4–9.

Mikhail, J. Developing a family assessment and intervention protocol. *Critical Care Nurse*. 1989; 3: 114–118.

Millar, B., Biley, F., Wilson, A. Issues in intensive care visiting. *Intensive and Critical Care Nursing*. 1993; 9(2): 75–81.

Mischel, M., Braden, C. Finding meaning: Antecedents of uncertainty in illness. *Nursing Research*. 1988; 37: 98–103.

Molter, N. Needs of relatives of critically ill patients. *Heart & Lung* 1979; 8: 332–339.

Mongiardi, F., Payman, B., Hawthorn, P. The needs of relatives of patients admitted to the coronary care unit. *Intensive Care Nursing*. 1987; 3: 67–70.

Murgatroyd, S., Woolfe, R. *Helping Families in Distress*. London: Harper & Row, 1985.

Murphy, P., Forrester, A., Price D., Monaghan, J. Empathy of intensive care nurses and critical care family needs assessment. *Heart & Lung*. 1992; 21(1): 25–29.

Murray-Parkes, C. *Bereavement. Studies of grief in adult life*. London: Penguin, 1968.

Neuman, B. *The Neuman Systems Model* 2nd ed. Appleton Lange, 1989.

Norris, L., Grove, S. Investigation of selected psycho-social needs of family members of critically ill adult patients. *Heart & Lung*. 1986; 15: 194–199.

O'Keeffe, B., Gillis, C. Family care in the coronary care unit: An Analysis of clinical nurse specialist intervention. *Heart & Lung*. 1988; 17(2): 191–198.

Olsen, E. The impact of serious illness on the family system. *Postgraduate Medicine*. 1970; 47: 169–174.

Parse, R. A theory of human becoming. *Parse International Interest Group Newsletter*. 1993.

Pearson, A., Vaughan, B. *Nursing Models for Practice*. 1986, London: Heinemann.

Peters, T. *In Search of Excellence*. 1983, London: Harper and Row.

Reed, J. Individualised patient care: some implications. *Journal of Clinical Nursing*. 1992; 1(1): 7–12.

Roberts, S. *Behavioural Concepts and the Critically Ill* 2nd ed. Norwalk: Appleton-Century-Crofts, 1986.

Robinson, C., Thorne, S. Strengthening family interference. *Journal of Advanced Nursing*. 1984; 9: 597–602.

Rogers, C. Needs of relatives of cardiac surgery patients during the critical care phase. *Focus on Critical Care*. 1983; 10: 50–55.

Rogers, M. *An introduction to the Theoretical Basis of Nursing*. Philadelphia: FA Davis, 1970.

Rukholm, E., Bailey, P., Coutu-Wakulczyk, G., Bruce Bailey, W. Needs and anxiety levels in relatives of intensive care unit patients. *Journal of Advanced Nursing*. 1991; 16: 920–928.

Sabo, K., Kraay, C., Rudy, E. *et al*. ICU family support group sessions. Family members perceived benefits. *Applied Nursing Research*. 1989; 2: 82–89.

Sherizen, S., Paul, L. Dying in a hospital ICU: The social significance for the family of the patient. *Omega*. 1977; 8(1): 29–40.

Simpson, T. Needs and concerns of families of critically ill adults. *Focus on Critical Care*. 1977; 16: 388–397.

Stillwell, B. The importance of visiting needs as perceived by family members of patients in intensive care units. *Heart & Lung*. 1984; 13(3): 238–242.

Thompson, D., Cordle, C. Support of wives of myocardial patients. *Journal of Advanced Nursing*. 1988; 31: 223–228.

Tomm, K. Circular interviewing: a multifaceted clinical tool. In: Campbell, D., Draper, R. (eds.). *Applications of Systemic Family Therapy: The Milan Approach*. Grune & Stratton, 1985.

Watson, J. *Nursing Human Science and Human Care: A theory of Nursing*. New York: National League for Nursing, 1988.

White, S. Collaboration benefits critically ill patients. *Focus on AACN: Focus on Critical Care*. 1989; 16(4): p. 325.

11
SPIRITUAL CARE IN THE INTENSIVE CARE UNIT
Rebecca Lesley Carter

CHAPTER AIMS

☐ To stimulate critical thought and discussion regarding the spiritual care of patients.

☐ To provide the reader with a general overview of spiritual care within the intensive care unit.

☐ To review relevant literature and research concerning the spiritual care of patients – necessarily general in nature due to the deficit of specific writings pertaining to the ICU.

☐ To briefly consider some of the meanings of spirituality.

☐ To suggest a framework (the use of the nursing process) with which nurses can approach the spiritual care of patients within the ICU, and to look at the assessment, planning, implementation and evaluation of spiritual needs.

☐ To convey to the reader that spiritual care is inherent within caring for the patient holistically and that communication is a vital component in such care.

☐ To outline that spiritual care is not a narrow field confined to facilitating religious rituals, but is open to patients of all spiritual and religious persuasions (including atheists, agnostics and humanists).

☐ To show that spiritual care is within the capabilities of most nurses and need not be something to be feared, but advocates the necessity for support groups for nurses, so as to provide a forum for the discussion of spiritual issues in the ICU.

INTRODUCTION

The spiritual care of patients is often seen by nurses as the responsibility of the hospital chaplain, and is often linked with death and dying, e.g. the administration of the last rites by a Catholic priest. This chapter aims to broaden the arena of spiritual care to include the non-religious perspective within the intensive care unit. It does not seek to proselytize any one religion, but proposes that all religious/ spiritual faiths are equally important.

Spiritual care is seen as inherent in the holistic care of patients, and various sources of literature are reviewed which support this. Spirituality is acknowledged as being complex in nature, and is something that the nurse will address as an ongoing issue when caring for patients. It is not something that can be 'cured' or, like a wound, dressed once a day/week and forgotten the rest of the time. The patients' spirituality may alter during their experience of critical illness, and the nurse must be alert to signs of spiritual distress, spiritual growth, etc.

Although spirituality itself is very individual to each patient, the care need not be complex, e.g. it may involve sitting and holding a patient's hand, playing a particular piece of significant music to the patient, or even reading poetry. Communication skills such as listening and the use of touch are seen as important interpersonal skills in the administration of spiritual care. Observation and listening skills are seen as the key to helping nurses determine spiritual needs. These needs should be verified with the patient if possible so that appropriate care may be planned.

There are numerous expressions of spirituality patients may use, both religious and secular. The nurse in ICU needs to be alert at all times to these expressions. These may be wide-ranging, such as the use of facial expression or statements of fear or anxiety. Constraints to spiritual care such as a lack of time, low priority over physiological and psychological care and nurses' own fears are discussed. The nurse does not have to share the same spirituality as the patient for the care to be of benefit.

It can be approached by the use of the nursing process – assessment, planning, implementation and evaluation. Spiritual issues may arise at any time, especially as the nurse–patient relationship deepens, or at critical periods in the patient's illness, therefore it is ongoing and is continually evaluated. Relatives are acknowledged as an important part of the spiritual care process, and their help and views may be of great value to the nurse in helping a patient spiritually. The nurse may also find herself addressing spiritual needs of the relatives themselves as they struggle to determine meaning in the patient's critical illness.

A support group for nurses working in ICU and involved in spiritual care is advocated. This group may provide a useful opportunity for the discussion of fears and feelings regarding all aspects of spiritual care. The education of nurses concerning spirituality is seen as important, and should include a wider perspective apart from specific religions. However, it is acknowledged that spiritual care is difficult to teach formally and much confidence comes with experience, and this will only be achieved if nurses recognize the need for, and start providing for, the spiritual care of patients.

LITERATURE REVIEW

What is meant by spirituality?

Interpretations of the meaning of spirituality vary widely. It is a concept that receives little universal consensus (Carson, 1989). Words, as Burnard (1990) points out, "mean what people want them to mean". Carson (1989) concurs with this stating that spirituality holds a different meaning for different people.

Despite this, attempts have been made to define spirituality religiously, humanistically and philosophically. Kreidler (1978), in a survey of the nursing literature, found that in most cases spirituality was used synonymously with institutionalized religion. Bunston (1987) reports that a religious definition of spirituality could be "a personal closeness to God".

However, some literature published more recently than 1978 has attempted to provide a broader understanding of spirituality. It is, as Colliton (1981) indicates, more encompassing than just equating it with religion. It needs to be redefined away from its synonymity with religion to include a wider perspective of man's search for meaning (Dickinson, 1975). Burnard (1990) explains that formalized religion is perhaps an avenue for the expression of spirituality – but it does not equal religion. Bhuddists, Hindus, atheists and agnostics, for example, have spiritual needs which are not necessarily Christian orientated.

A humanistic definition may include the need for man to search for meaning in life, to find answers to ultimate questions about, for example, illness and death (Burnard, 1990; Colliton, 1981; Cosh, 1988; Highfield and Cason, 1983; Simsen, 1985). Cosh (1988) includes in a definition the "desire to contemplate those things which lie beyond our control but which affect us" (p. 102).

A number of authors (Conrad, 1985; Reed, 1987; Simsen, 1985) incorporate a reference to the transcendental concept. This involves recognition that something may lie "beyond temporal and spatial boundaries" (Reed, 1987). O'Brien (1982) proposes a definition which could be appropriate and applicable to any perspective of spirituality, whether from a Christian, atheistic, humanistic or philosophical angle; spirituality is "that which inspires in one the desire to transcend the realm of the material" (O'Brien, 1982, p. 88).

What is clear is that spirituality is not a concrete and easily definable entity. It holds a personal meaning for each individual. As Carson (1989) indicates, it is "multidimensional and complex". It interacts, influences and is influenced by the physical, psychosocial and emotional aspects of a person (Labun, 1988; Conrad, 1985). Perhaps because of its subjective and personal nature, it is an area of interest and inquiry within nursing which is equivocal.

Should spirituality be a part of nursing care?

Spirituality, although perhaps at present not a prominent element in patient care, is an area which needs addressing if nursing is to take on board the concept of holistic health care. A number of nursing authors (Brallier, 1978; Bunston, 1987; Burnard, 1988; Byrne, 1985; Cosh, 1988; Ellerhorst-Ryan, 1985; Fish and Shelly, 1983; Labun, 1988; O'Brien, 1982; Uys, 1980; Yura and Walsh, 1983) feel that spirituality is an important component of holistic care. A patient's wholeness and integrity is dependent upon the health of the physical, psychosocial and spiritual aspects of the person. Distress in any one of these domains will have an effect on the others (Stallwood and Stall, 1975). Although they may be viewed as distinct, they are interrelated (O'Brien, 1982). Nurses frequently divide these domains of a patient into 'prioritised parts' (Fish and Shelly, 1983), and often forget the spiritual domain altogether (Dettmore, 1984). Yet to ignore spirituality may be classified as an "act of omission" (Burnard, 1988).

Some models of nursing, for example those conceived by theorists such as Peplau, Johnson, Orem, King, Roy and Rogers, have a holistic perception of man as an underlying philosophy. Prominent spokespersons within the nursing profession focus on a holistic approach to nursing care. Peplau (1952), in reviewing the nurse–patient relationship, perceives that during the identification phase (the second out of four phases, which the nurse–patient relationship proceeds through), the nurse attempts to understand the meaning of a patient's

interpersonal situation. Travelbee (1971) ascertains that nurses assist individual families and communities to find meaning in the experiences of illness and suffering – surely also a spiritual task. Spirituality has been described as 'wholeness', implying that nurses should maintain the unity of the patient. Acknowledging that holistic care encompasses spirituality, ideally it could be incorporated into the patient's care plan through the use of one such model (Bunston, 1987).

What other evidence is there for a need to provide spiritual care for patients?

Curtin and Flaherty (1982) argue that nurses have an ethical responsibility to provide spiritual care. Society is increasingly becoming more multicultural, and therefore it is necessary for nurses to be aware of their patients' differing customs and beliefs (Bell, 1987). Indeed, the UKCC Code of Professional Conduct (1992) 6th Statement supports this: "Take account of the customs, values and spiritual beliefs of patients/clients".

Sampson (1982) and Soeken and Carson (1986) report that the ICN Code of Nursing Ethics (1973) puts an obligation on nurses to provide spiritual care. Codes of conduct therefore regard spirituality to be important.

How do patients express spirituality and spiritual needs?

Since this is how nurses can assess that patients require care in this area, expression of spiritual needs can be divided into the religious and the secular. Commencing with religious expression, O'Brien (1982) indicates that spiritual needs are influenced by a person's particular religious affiliation or culture. It is therefore important to assess each patient individually as needs, beliefs, practices, etc. will vary accordingly.

Often, a hospitalized patient with a particular religious affiliation will enquire about available services within the hospital, perhaps requesting that their routine of taking communion is sustained (Fish and Shelly, 1983; Sodestrom and Martinson, 1987; Labun, 1988). Other patients may ask directly to see a hospital chaplain, or their own priest, rabbi, etc. (Sodestrom and Martinson, 1987; Labun 1988). A nurse might notice a patient quietly reading a Bible/religious book (Sodestrom and Martinson, 1987; Reed, 1987) and "underlining passages that hold special meaning" (Conrad, 1985). This was the case Conrad (1985) found specifically when looking at terminal care patients.

Linked with religion, many patients express a spiritual need through statements of life questions such as Why did God let this happen?, Why me? (Fish and Shelly, 1983; McGilloway and Donnelly, 1977; Ryan, 1984; Cosh, 1988), showing they may be angry with God (Simsen, 1986). Also, patients may express a "lack of will to live" because "life has no meaning" (Forbis, 1988). Although they appear to relate more to death and dying in the literature (e.g. Byrne, 1985), life questions such as these could be asked by a patient suffering from any condition.

Patients may express spiritual needs in a way that can relate to either a religious or a secular perspective, such as the use of facial expression or statements indicating fear, anxiety, doubt, depression or despair (Byrne, 1985; Labun, 1988; McGilloway and Myco, 1985). Ryan (1984) acknowledges that patients may not be so overt in their expression of spiritual pain, for example, and may direct this pain "inward" causing an increase in anxiety and associated symptoms such as vomiting. Focusing specifically on dying patients (but which may be relevant to any patient), Conrad (1985) cites four categories of spiritual needs, drawn from Highfield and Cason (1983):

1. Search for meaning.
2. Sense of forgiveness.
3. Hope.
4. Love.

It is thought that the search for meaning in life and meaning in illness, suffering and death are important (Burnard, 1986; Dickinson, 1975; Frankl, 1962). Man is thought to be attempting to find answers to the ultimate questions of life (Highfield and Cason, 1983). A sense of forgiveness is important for a lot of people who may, if they are religious, seek confession as a means of overcoming

the guilt they feel (Shelly, 1983; Rambo, 1984; Conrad, 1985). The need for hope is seen as one major spiritual need requiring attention (Bunston, 1987). The need for love is seen as important also. The patient needs to feel he or she is loved and wanted, but also to give love and feel a relatedness to others, family, deity or God (Conrad, 1985; Bunston, 1987).

The search for meaning in life need not necessarily be equated with religion but can be looked upon as spiritual because, as Burnard (1988) states, it "concerns the very heart of human life".

Another avenue for the expression of spiritual needs which nurses should be aware of is that of creative expression. This, too, can apply equally to a religious or a secular expression of need. Connell (1989), again referring specifically to the terminally ill, feels that creative expression helps patients spiritually. Patients may express spiritual needs through the channels of art, music, writing and poetry, for example. This is a good way of communicating feelings, experiences, anxieties, etc. (Labun, 1988), although perhaps not so for all patients. Again, it is a matter of individual choice.

Lastly, when considering how patients may express themselves spiritually, it is important to recognize that many patients may find it difficult to "articulate their spiritual needs and problems in hospital surroundings" (Cosh, 1988). Some patients may take offence at enquiring nurses probing about their spiritual/religious beliefs (Neuberger, 1987). Nurses therefore have to be alert to those patients for whom spirituality is not something they wish to share.

How may the nurse help to meet the spiritual needs of patients?

After considering how patients might express spirituality and spiritual needs, it is apt to consider how the nurse may help to meet these needs and provide spiritual care for patients.

Important in this process is firstly the assessment of spiritual needs. Labun (1988) advocates that the use of the nursing process should include a spiritual assessment of the patient. However, there are a number of methods of obtaining such information. Stoll (1979) published a formal tool. This is quite a specific and detailed assessment tool, and would possibly be very time consuming to use, perhaps also because of the terminology used, but there is no research available to determine if this is the case. Stoll (1979) explains that it is the nurse's responsibility to fully inform the patient before such an assessment is undertaken to explain why the information is required. Stoll (1979) believes the nurse should inform the patient thus: "to increase our knowledge of your sources of strength so that we may offer you the best possible care" (p. 1577).

O'Brien (1982) and Colliton (1981) have similarly proposed the use of an assessment tool, but the same criticisms are perhaps also valid for these tools. O'Brien (1982) acknowledges the length and detail of the tool and feels that it is perhaps more useful to research. It is perhaps also too Christian to be helpful in a wider spiritual assessment.

The tool is somewhat complex, and it would be difficult to categorize patient behaviours as many of the categories and defining characteristics overlap. As nurses, should we and can we do an assessment to this degree of comprehensiveness for every patient?

On a more informal basis, Peterson and Nelson (1987) suggest there is much in the patient's environment to give nurses cues about a patient's spirituality. Such cues include religious books, music, photographs, crucifixes and other religious objects. These cues, however, would not be present with atheistic, agnostic and other non-believers, which is not addressed, therefore assessment via this method is made more difficult. But it does not mean that nurses should ignore spirituality here altogether. Cues can also be gained from relationships between the patient, family and friends, and from casual conversations both with them and with the nurse over time (Peterson and Nelson, 1987). Labun (1988) and Byrne (1985) advocate the use of more generalized questions regarding the meaning of life, death, illness, etc. Sampson (1982) argues that although spiritual needs might be identified and spiritual care planned and provided, the evaluation of the effectiveness of such care might be difficult to assess. Overall, the practical assessment of spiritual needs is perhaps not as simple as is advocated on paper.

After assessment when considering intervention, Hubert (1963) acknowledges that many nurses

stop at the identification of a patient's religious affiliation and possibly the organization of particular dietary needs. Has spiritual care progressed since then? The writings of more contemporary authors suggest not. It is important to remember that there is no one right approach to the provision of spiritual care (Carson, 1989; Shelly, 1982; Burnard, 1986). Much is dependent upon the patient, nurse and their relationship (Colliton, 1981; Simsen, 1988). The use of self, incorporating factors such as attitude (Uys, 1980; Bunston, 1987; Dickinson, 1975), touch (Colliton, 1981; McGilloway and Myco, 1985), talking (Shelly, 1982; Burnard, 1988), listening (Shelly, 1982; Dugan, 1987; Neuberger, 1987; Forbis, 1988; Conrad, 1985; McGilloway and Myco, 1985), empathy (Dickinson, 1975; Shelly, 1982) and support (Shelly, 1982) is an oft quoted way of fulfilling spiritual care. Also deemed important are flexibility, patience, honesty, trust, humility and hope (Colliton, 1981).

Other interventions identified in the literature include mobilizing resources such as referral to the clergy when appropriate (Conrad, 1985; Burnard, 1988), the use of scripture and prayer (Shelly, 1982; Conrad, 1985; Connell, 1989; Forbis, 1988) and the inclusion of music therapy, visual arts, poetry, etc. What is evident is the lack of published research undertaken into the provision of spiritual care.

Why is the arena of spiritual care neglected by nurses?

It is important to consider if and why the arena of spiritual care is neglected by nurses. One oft quoted reason is the lack of time nurses have to cater for these needs (Bunston, 1987; Forbis, 1988; McGilloway and Myco, 1985). Fish and Shelly (1983) expand on this to suggest that the number of nursing staff and the dependency level of the patient may contribute to this lack of time. It is not acknowledged that spiritual care can be carried out when attending to other, perhaps physical patient needs.

Low priority over physical and psychological care (Soeken and Carson, 1986; McGilloway and Myco, 1985), perhaps because of increased secularization, is another reason suggested. Forbis (1988) feels nurses omit this aspect of care because they find it difficult to identify problems and needs. This leads to the topic of nurse education. It is reported by many authors (Forbis, 1988; Highfield and Cason, 1983; Soeken and Carson, 1986; Cosh, 1988) that nurses' education focuses on only the superficial aspects of spirituality, to do with religious rites and rituals, and omits to delve deeper into spirituality in general. To add to this there is a scarcity of nursing literature which addresses spirituality (Labun, 1988; O'Brien, 1982; Morrison, 1989): perhaps because, as Morrison (1989) acknowledges, it is not only patients but nurses too who have difficulty in articulating spiritual concerns. Teachers may also have difficulty instructing students on this aspect of patient care.

Some authors (Brallier, 1978; Stallwood and Stall, 1981; Dickinson, 1975; Fish and Shelly, 1983; Hubert, 1963; Soeken and Carson, 1986; Simsen, 1988) feel that many nurses refer any spiritual problems conveniently to the hospital chaplain or patient's own spiritual leader, especially as there is a lack of clear distinction between the role of the nurse and the clergy in giving spiritual care.

Other suggested reasons include the nurses' own spiritual vulnerability, not having clarified for him or herself exactly what personal meaning spirituality holds (Colliton, 1981; Burnard, 1988; Dettmore, 1984; McGilloway and Myco, 1985). Henderson and Nite (1978), cited in McGilloway and Myco (1985), suggest that the more comfortable nurses are with their own spirituality, the easier it would be to discuss spiritual questions with patients. Fish and Shelly (1983) put forward the proposal that because of the nature of nursing work, often leaving the nurse mentally and physically exhausted, this can have a limiting effect on the ability to perceive spiritual needs. They also suggest that peer support is needed, and is often not overtly available. All these factors can have a limiting effect on the nurses' ability to provide spiritual care.

RESEARCH

Is there any research to suggest that patients value spiritual care?

There is a small amount of published American research which illustrates that spirituality is used as a coping strategy in times of ill-health across the lifespan.

Miller (1983) undertook a qualitative study to assess the coping strategies of 56 chronically ill adults with a variety of diseases. Results showed the second most frequently used strategy was gaining strength from one's spiritual life. Strength came from prayer, feeling God's love, meditation, receiving love and support from others and a life review.

Baldree et al. (1982) and O'Brien (1982) separately undertook research with dialysis patients. Baldree et al. (1982) found that among 35 haemodialysis patients, coping methods identified were, in rank order:

1. hope

and

2. trust in God and prayer.

O'Brien (1982) interviewed 126 chronic dialysis patients and only 26.2% responded that religious beliefs were never relevant in their adjustment to the illness.

In researching 114 hospitalized adolescents, Silber and Reilly (1985) reported that adolescents felt intensified spiritual and religious concerns during severe illness. The greater the severity of the illness, the greater was the level of spiritual change and concern, regardless of sex and race.

Simsen (1986) conducted 45 interviews (semi-structured), including five in-depth interviews, to assess if patients brought spiritual resources to the experience of illness and hospitalization, and also to determine if patients experience spiritual needs during this time. Results showed that medical and surgical patients have spiritual needs and also spiritual resources. Personal aspects of faith were found to be important. Simsen (1988) reporting on her research repeated that patients had "a constant need to make sense of their circumstances, to find meaning in the events of their day, their relationships and their life".

In a book on spiritual care by Fish and Shelly (1983), two studies carried out on patients' spiritual needs are cited. Both were carried out in the United States, the first in 1969 by Hess; 109 hospitalized patients were interviewed and their spiritual needs identified. These needs were present to some degree in most cases. Identified needs included prayer, an awareness of God's presence, meaning and purpose in life, death and suffering. Expression of faith was achieved by reading the Bible, Holy Communion and attending services. Spiritual counselling was preferred by the hospital chaplain or appropriate spiritual leader, with nurses being identified as helpers.

The second study, conducted by Martin (1976), surveyed 90 adults in two general hospitals by means of a 34-item questionnaire and an interview. The findings bore a similarity to those of Hess (1969). Again, clergymen were preferred over nurses for spiritual counselling, but help from nurses was also appreciated. Identified spiritual needs included in rank order of importance to the patient:

---

1. Relief from fear of death.
2. Visit from clergyman.
3. Prayer.
4. Knowledge of God's presence.
5. Purpose and meaning in life.
6. Expression of caring and support from another person.
7. Sacraments, e.g. Communion.

Spirituality has been shown as a significant human experience during terminal illness by authors such as Reed (1987), Kemp (1984) and Sodestrom and Martinson (1987). In research carried out by Sodestrom and Martinson, data collected indicated that cancer patients used a variety of resource people and spiritual activities to help them cope. Patients reported their most frequently used coping strategy was personal prayer and asking others to pray for them. Almost half the patients used nurses and resources for spiritual needs and for assistance with spiritual activities.

These research findings emphasize the need for nurses to incorporate assessment and support of spiritual coping strategies into their daily nursing care. However, it is also important to remember, as Hess (1969) indicates, that the nurse should be sensitive to the patient who does not see spiritual care as part of the nurse's role, and also to the patient who desires no help from nurses at all.

Do nurses recognize a need for spiritual care of patients?

Research, again carried out in the United States, by Chadwick (1973) looked at hospital nurses representing all three shifts. Results showed that nurses were aware of the presence of spiritual needs only in some of their patients, but that 75% of nurses reported that they would not find reading the Bible or praying with a patient troublesome. However, this begs the question, would these nurses feel comfortable discussing or talking about spirituality to patients in general, i.e. with patients who did not have a Christian faith, and were perhaps atheists, agnostics or had a humanistic outlook on life?

Soeken and Carson (1986) conducted research to examine if there was a correlation between the personal spiritual well-being of qualified and student nurses and their attitudes towards providing spiritual care. They used the spiritual well-being scale, developed by Ellison and Paloutzian, to elicit the nurse's personal, religious and existential welfare, and also another instrument, the Health Professional Spiritual Role (HPSR) Scale, developed by Soeken and Carson, to find out the role of the nurse in providing spiritual care for patients. Results showed that both for existential and religious well-being, the nurses displayed a positive correlation between personal spiritual well-being and attitude towards providing spiritual care. The relationship was not significantly different when qualified and senior students were analysed separately.

A study to determine if nurses were aware of patients' spiritual needs and problems was undertaken by Highfield and Cason (1983). Of 100 oncology nurses surveyed, 35 responded. Results showed these nurses to be competent in the identification of spiritual needs which related directly to God or pertained to a particular religious belief, which shows a somewhat narrow ability. Furthermore, what is clearly shown is that most of these nurses equated a large number of signs of spiritual health within the domain of psychosocial health. Only those signs relating directly to religious beliefs and practices were designated as belonging to the spiritual category. Therefore, are spiritual needs being misdiagnosed and treated within the psychosocial dimension? What about the patients who do not follow a particular religion; is spiritual care being neglected altogether or slotted into the psychosocial domain?

Sodestrom and Martinson (1987) asked nurses to identify their patients' religion, spiritual beliefs and use of spiritual resource people. 44% of nurses correctly identified their patients' religion. The rest simply did not know. 64% felt nurses did not identify patients' spiritual coping strategies well, and it is not surprising since it is difficult to do if you do not know about your patients' spirituality. A small minority (four nurses), however, incorporated a spiritual assessment as part of their daily nursing care. What is interesting is the fact that nurses felt there was a need to increase their knowledge regarding spiritual assessment of patients and spiritual coping strategies.

Martin (1976) in their research asked patients how they envisaged nurses might help them to meet spiritual needs. The response that occurred most frequently was one that involved the nurse listening to patients: 77% agreed that by listening, a nurse helped a patient spiritually.

Boutell and Bozett (1991) undertook a study to determine the extent to which nurses assessed patients' spiritual needs. Findings showed that they most frequently assessed for fears, sources of strength and feelings of hope. Least frequently assessed were meaning in suffering and transcendence.

Nurses aged 50–59 and psychiatric nurses were more likely than other nurses to assess the spiritual realm. Availability of time and patient acuity were major factors which influenced assessment. Data and information was most frequently obtained through observation and discussion with patients.

It appears that patient acuity hampered spiritual care in that physiological concerns were found to be a priority above spiritual care. The more acutely ill the patient, the less likely the nurse was to carry out a spiritual assessment, i.e. nurses in critical care settings were least likely to do so. This has implications for the patient whereby the acutely/ critically ill patient may desperately want/need spiritual ministry and is yet unable to communicate this to the nurse.

Time of day was found to be a factor in that spiritual needs were more commonly expressed by patients and nurses during late evening and night when patients perceived nurses' time was more plentiful. However, this may not be appropriate to ICU environments, where 24-hour care is often required and daytime care may not differ significantly from night-time care.

The researcher felt that age of the nurse was significant. It was postulated that as nurses grow older, spiritual needs of patients may come into focus more than for younger nurses, as the older nurse experiences the death of her own parents, and as their own death and mortality approaches. The research also found that in-service education and continuing education programmes concerning spirituality are needed.

In 1980, Piles in the USA, carried out a descriptive research study to assess the extent of the teaching of spiritual care in 98 nursing schools. Findings from the questionnaire showed that spirituality was addressed as part of holistic care and more deeply investigated as part of the psychosocial nature of man. The conclusion demonstrated the need for nurse educators to gain a greater awareness of the spiritual dimension. Nurse education concerning spirituality appears to be confined mainly to talk/discussion with the hospital clergy. There are isolated examples of specific courses concerning spirituality and nursing care in America which have proved to be extremely popular (Carson and Gerardi, 1987; Ellis, 1986; Shelly, 1982).

Nurses who work with the critically ill may find in-service education courses on the importance of metaphysical and supernatural dimensions of the human experience to nursing practice of special benefit.

Sodestrom and Martinson (1987) in their research found nurses identified lack of time as a reason for the omission of spirituality from their nursing care.

PRACTICAL NURSING IMPLICATIONS

It may appear to many people that nursing has become centred around technology and techniques.

A glance at the array of current journal titles supports this, many focusing upon so-called 'high-tech' specialities. There are numerous articles examining particularly biological needs and to a lesser extent psychosocial needs, but a dearth examining spirituality, and even less when considering spiritual care in the intensive care unit. Indeed, in an intensive care environment, familiarity with technological equipment is a vital role for the competent nurse, but it is essential not to lose sight of the less 'high-tech' nursing roles, one of which is to attempt to meet the spiritual needs of the critically ill patient. It is not solely in an intensive care environment that spiritual care may be relegated near to the bottom of nursing priorities. Secularization has permeated throughout hospital and institutional care, and until recently, 'disease' was perhaps considered more important than person.

Considering a critical care situation, it may be easy to neglect the mind and soul in caring for an acutely ill, unconscious patient. Dame Catherine Hall, addressing an international intensive care conference in London in 1982, said, ". . . whilst technology plays an important part in intensive care nursing, the nurse must always be concerned with the patient as a whole person, with his need for total care – physical, social, psychological and . . . spiritual." (McGilloway and Myco, 1985, p. 130).

The nurse must not become so lost amongst the technology and equipment that she becomes unable to communicate on human terms. For it is this communication which is a vital component in spiritual care from a religious to humanistic perspective. Physiological needs are more easily quantifiable, whereas spiritual needs are subjectively assessed and ideally benefit from patient verification. This is not always easy, especially if the patient is unconscious or ventilated. Spiritual ministry requires that the nurse communicates openness, a willingness to listen and to use themselves as a tool to help meet spiritual needs when a patient exhibits distress. It is often in a critical care situation that a person may feel a previously subconscious spiritual need. Anyone surrounded by a plethora of 'high-tech' equipment, experiencing a life-threatening disease may lose their sense of belonging, may question the meaning of life, may question their relationship with significant others (including their God). These feelings can apply equally to patients of a religious

or humanistic persuasion. They may feel vulnerable and alone, and be brought abruptly to the realization of their own mortality. This, coupled with the separation from, for example, a religious ritual which may have been highly significant for an individual's faith, may further intensify spiritual needs in such a crisis situation.

There are many issues which may appear to impinge upon spiritual care in an intensive care unit. The time factor involved, lack of space due to necessary equipment, noise levels, anxious relatives, emergency situations, lack of privacy, to name but a few. Some nurses may feel spiritual concerns too private to explore, but other personal habits are enquired after without hesitation. These constraints should not be a barrier to an awareness of spiritual needs, although nurses may rightly question where they begin to deal with such issues under such circumstances.

Patients are admitted to intensive care from a number of places such as the Accident & Emergency department, as a transfer from another hospital ward, even from another hospital. Also, they may be admitted electively and in an emergency from the operating theatre. Some patients the nurse may have met prior to admission to the unit, others, such as crisis admissions, perhaps not. How can nurses address issues of spirituality with such a diverse and complex range of patients? Some suggestions are considered in the next section, but it is necessary first to look at four fundamental spiritual needs proposed by McGilloway and Myco (1985).

The first of these needs is the need to determine meaning in illness/suffering and in life in general. The threat of imminent death may propel the patient abruptly into thinking about the meaning of the world and his place in it. Considering pain and suffering, often acutely felt in critically ill patients, solace and strength to cope with the pain may be found from a spiritual faith or belief – not necessarily religious in origin. Some patients may view pain as a revelatory experience. However, the need to find meaning in suffering and pain is problematical for all patients whatever their spirituality.

The second need is concerned with love – both the need to love and to be loved, to experience a sense of belonging. The threat of death may increase the patient's need to feel loved and hence may rely heavily on family, friends and even staff to aid the fulfilment of this need. The third spiritual need to be considered is hope. Hope for the future is evident perhaps in aspirations concerning an afterlife or in an unfailing belief that the critical situation will pass.

Often, patients express the need to make peace, both with themselves, with family and friends with whom they may have had misunderstandings, and also with their God. This is explicit within the fourth need – the need to feel self-worth. Self-worth is enhanced if a patient is shown dignity and respect. Dignity is achieved when a nurse considers the patient as an individual, with unique needs and as a unique spirit. A depersonalized approach may have been the case when intensive care units were first operationalized, but nowadays great care is taken by nurses to ensure patients are treated as holistic human beings instead of as a challenge to medical science.

THE PROCESS OF SPIRITUAL CARE

Spiritual needs in intensive care can be approached in the same systematic way that nurses may approach biopsychosocial needs. The nursing process, i.e. Assessment, Planning, Implementation and Evaluation, can be used to guide and address spiritual care issues. This approach is only one way but is considered below.

Assessment

Within the realm of assessment, the nurse is using all possible senses to assimilate any expressions of spirituality a patient may exhibit, to also determine what clues to a patient's spirituality, level of spiritual distress (if any) are evident. From the assessment a nurse can then formulate a nursing diagnosis in relation to spiritual care.

How might a nurse working in intensive care recognize clues related to a patient's spirituality? Assessment is partly dependent upon how/from where the patient is admitted to the intensive care unit. There may already have been an assessment carried out if the patient is admitted from another ward, in which case the nurse can build upon this.

Conversely, the nurse may have no prior information regarding a patient's spirituality. If the patient is conscious, they may express verbally a desire to see their spiritual leader. They may ask for information concerning hospital services. The relatives may also ask for the above on a patient's behalf, particularly if he or she is unconscious, knowing that the patient may find comfort in such provision. The nurse should be observant of any religious artifacts within the patient's environment, such as a holy cross, a Bible, religious clothing, religious jewellery, and be receptive to requests for a particular diet on religious grounds. It is important to respect these artifacts, but care should also be exercized so as not to read too much into their meaning without first clarifying their meaning with the patient.

The nurse should observe whether the patient receives any religious get well cards and assess whether the patient uses any personal photographs, artworks or music to help keep spirits up. These latter examples may also be applicable to patients who view life from a humanist angle.

The nurse, when enquiring (either from the patient if conscious or relatives/friends if unconscious) about spirituality, should determine whether the patient has a particular faith or belief system rather than a specific religion. In this way, spirituality is opened up for wider consideration and may encompass a humanistic/atheistic/agnostic perspective. If not, the nurse is in danger of provoking the patient into admitting to a particular religion when in fact they have none, but do have for example, a particular humanistic belief system which is equally important and relevant to that individual patient. It is possible, however, to enquire whether the patient has any concept of a God, or whether he or she has any particular sources of strength and hope, e.g. significant others.

It is possible to assess spirituality by determining whether the patient or the patient's relatives are showing any signs of spiritual distress. This may be defined as

"The state in which the individual experiences or is at risk of experiencing a disturbance in his belief or value system that is his source of strength and hope". (Carpenito, 1983, p. 415).

Examples of defining characteristics include:

1. The expression of concern with the meaning of life or suffering.
2. Questions such as Why me? Why did God let this happen?
3. Questioning beliefs or the meaning/significance of relationships.
4. A straightforward plea for spiritual help of some description.
5. The questioning of medical treatment on religious/moral/ethical grounds.
6. Alternating behaviour/mood swings – although not especially a sign of spiritual distress, it may be an indication of inner conflict and needs investigating further.

It is important to verify with the patient or relatives if possible any spiritual assessment and diagnosis reached, as otherwise interpretation is only based on the nurse's perception of the patient's situation, and incorrectly interpreted spiritual concerns could lead to ineffective nursing care.

Nursing diagnoses in relation to spirituality relevant to a critical care situation may include:

1. "Potential spiritual distress related to disruption of normal religious practices because of hospitalisation" (Carson, 1989).
2. Spiritual distress due to a broken relationship with a significant other.
3. Potential spiritual distress related to confronting the unknown.
4. Potential spiritual distress related to separation from a support system in a potentially life threatening situation.

In the case of (1) and (4), faith may slide and spiritual problems arise which need nursing intervention.

It is imperative to approach the assessment of spiritual needs with acceptance and sensitivity. It is helpful to share with the patient, relatives or friends the rationale for seeking information concerning spiritual matters. The nurse should explain that it will enable enhanced care to be given to the patient. As the nurse–patient relationship develops, deeper and more meaningful spiritual concerns may be unearthed than an initial assessment allows for.

Planning

Once an assessment has been made and a nursing diagnosis formulated, planning should be carried out to identify how spiritual needs can be met. This stage should be conducted with the patient if conscious and able, if not, with family/friends or appropriate spiritual leader. Planning may even have to be carried out by the nurse alone. The ideal situation is for the nurse and patient together to formulate mutual goals. During this stage goals for care are established and outcome criteria ascertained. The overall aim is to minimize the spiritual distress. Outcome criteria examples include:

☐ To facilitate the continuation of spiritual practices.

☐ To increase feelings of spiritual peace.

☐ To provide rest and comfort.

☐ To find positive meaning in existence and in the present life situation.

☐ To decrease feelings of guilt and anxiety.

☐ To feel able to 'mend' broken relationships with family, significant others or God.

Outcome criteria and goals need to be considered so that provision can be properly made and appropriate interventions carried out.

Nursing interventions in spiritual care

The intensive care unit is, by necessity, a clinical area which focuses largely on the medical model as a means of intervention and patient management. The result upon the individual psyche may be an adverse one if not adequately catered for. There are a number of ways in which nurses can minister spiritual care to both patients and relatives in ICU. Apart from referring a patient to a specific spiritual leader or facilitating religious rituals, what avenues are open for a nurse to give spiritual care?

One important factor is the use of interpersonal skills (see also Pearce, Chapter 16). All nurses in ICU, whatever their spiritual persuasion, can use these skills to help spiritually any patient of likewise any spiritual persuasion. How can this be achieved?

Listening is an important interpersonal skill which can be utilized and was identified by patients in some of the research. Along with listening, counselling may be a valuable skill to help patients/relatives cope with spiritual distress. Listening, for example, may help the nurse in ICU discover how a patient deals with his own death. This requires 'active listening', to be open to what the patient is saying, conversely to be alert to what the patient does not say, to listen out for signs of depression and sorrow, e.g. tears of despair, sighs of resignation. The nurse should acknowledge what a dying patient in ICU has to teach others and express this to the patient and family. Nurses can learn much from dying patients that may help them care spiritually for others. The nurse in a critical care situation should worry less about say the 'wrong' thing than about being able to communicate caring.

Another avenue for communicating caring is the use of touch. The nurses' touch and caring is a holistic nursing intervention and there are known to be degrees of touch. Touch, however, should be used with caution as some patients may interpret it as invasive. In ministering to a patient's spiritual needs through the use of touch, the nurse is entering into a patient's 'intimate zone' – essential if a patient is, for instance, unconscious. The duration of touch is significant (especially for the unconscious patient), as moderate to long durations encourage the patient's fullest integration of sensory input. The location of touch is important as this conveys positive messages regarding body image. The frequency and generous use of touch can be a major influence in increasing a patient's self-esteem. Touch in ICU should not only be confined to patients but should also encompass the family. Nurses should touch members of the family when appropriate, e.g. when they are distressed and likewise encourage them in turn to touch the patient. Relatives in ICU are surrounded by unfamiliar equipment likely to be in an unfamiliar situation, and are also subjected to emotional and spiritual distress. Non-verbal communication in the way of touch is just as supportive to the family as to the patient. It is necessary to remember that with an unconscious patient, it is impossible to know the exact level of sensory input which is being registered by the patient – but the nurse and family must believe that total sensory awareness is possible.

There are many reasons why communication between nurses and patients is thought to be effective in acute nursing care situations, some being, for example, staff shortages, pressure of workloads, language barriers. The intensive care unit, as well as these general constraints, poses its own nurse–patient communication barrier. It is not easy to communicate with an unresponsive, unconscious patient. Conversations are necessarily one-sided. This communication problem may also be felt by relatives. However, it is essential to remember the presence of a spirit within the body. The presence of a spirit may be a contentious issue if a patient is known to be brain dead and is being kept alive by positive pressure ventilation. Regardless of this, the nurse should apply the same spiritual care to such a patient as to any other, for it is not known whether the spirit remains with the body under such circumstances.

The nurse, in allowing for catharsis and also showing compassion and empathy, is helping a patient spiritually.

Carson (1989) lists five elements involved in spiritual care.

1. Listening.
2. Empathy.
3. Vulnerability.
4. Humility.
5. Commitment.

In considering vulnerability the nurse has to leave behind the image of professionalism. This may be especially difficult in the intensive care environment where nurses may deliberately hide behind the wall of professionalism to cope with the everyday reality of life and death crisis situations. Keeping up a professional barrier between nurse and patient will not allow a nurse to minister spiritually to a patient. This professional barrier introduces a sense of 'distance' between the nurse and patient, and will not allow for the closeness necessary for beneficial spiritual care. Often, nurses may be unsure of their own reactions in such a situation; however, if a patient and a nurse are to grow spiritually then the removal of the nurse–patient barrier is a prerequisite.

Humility allows a nurse to accept both themselves and their patients for what they are. Commitment involves being available for a patient or the patient's relatives for as long as support is required. It is a full-time commitment and must not be entered into on a part-time basis as the patient will not receive the full benefit of the nurse's spiritual care. The nurse must share in the patient's/family's hopes, fears, anger, sadness, etc., and must not suddenly withdraw when times are difficult.

Another avenue a nurse may have open is one of being an advocate for the patient's spiritual beliefs. There are many occasions when medical treatments may not be consistent with a patient's spiritual beliefs. One such occasion may be when a patient needs an urgent blood transfusion but is also a Jehovah's witness. The nurse may be required to represent the patient's views to medical staff. Nurses are often faced with a dilemma when a patient refuses much needed medical treatment on spiritual grounds. This conflict of the nurse's own spiritual beliefs with that of the patients may lead to 'spiritual dissonance'. It may be helpful in this situation for the nurse to learn more about the patient's specific beliefs, to read about them if possible, or perhaps talk to members of the patient's family or even the patient's spiritual leader, to increase their understanding of why a particular medical treatment is not desired.

Alternative approaches to spirituality apart from religious interventions may be helpful. Such non-religious interventions can include poetry, music, massage and aromatherapy. An unconscious patient may benefit spiritually from hearing a tape recording of, for example, meaningful music or perhaps poetry readings. Coinciding with touch, massage may be appropriate in some cases.

Privacy is an important factor in spiritual care, something that is perhaps scarce in an intensive care environment as there are often constant interruptions from doctors, nurses, physiotherapists, technicians, cleaners, etc. Sensitivity and discretion are necessary on the nurses' part and the tactful use of screens may be helpful. It is, however, acknowledged that complete privacy is difficult in an intensive care unit.

Another difficulty due to the environment is posed by the multitude of various lines attached to the patient, e.g. CVP, arterial lines, catheters and drains. These lines must restrict free movement for both the patient and the nurse and therefore impinge on certain aspects of spiritual care, e.g. participation in religious rituals such as facing Mecca to pray.

Looking specifically at religious interventions, the nurse must realize that barrier nursing in an intensive care unit does not mean a barrier, for example, to the patient receiving holy sacraments. Every effort should be made to facilitate this aspect of spiritual care if the patient or his relatives desire it. The nurse should be available to read from the scriptures, pray with/for the patient if requested to by the patient or relatives, and liaise with appropriate chaplain or spiritual leader. One spiritual intervention which may be highly significant to the intensive care situation is the facilitation of forgiveness between a patient and their significant others, or perhaps the facilitation of reconciliation. Often patients may tell the nurse of an argument between themselves and a member of their family and how they wish the situation could be reconciled. It may be up to the nurse (if the patient wishes) to perhaps ring the relative on behalf of the patient and facilitate a meeting.

If a patient is religious in everyday life, attending church regularly, the interruption to this posed by a critical illness may mean that spiritual problems arise and spiritual distress ensues. The nursing staff have a responsibility spiritually to help the patient maintain rituals important to their faith. It should be noted, however, that before playing a cassette recording of religious music or a religious service, etc. to an unconscious patient, it is critical to give an explanation in case the patient misconstrues the motive and feels all is lost and death is near (McGilloway and Myco, 1985).

Detailed spiritual/religious needs should be documented within the care plan and not simply stated as, for example, Jew, Hindu, Muslim. This explains nothing about the patient's personal religious or spiritual perspective. It needs to be expanded upon, and if the patient is unable to, perhaps relatives may be brought in to help clarify the situation and to help plan appropriate spiritual care (see Chapter 18).

It is a difficult task for the nurse to keep abreast

of the multitude of religious and spiritual beliefs and practices. A patient's reaction to a life threatening situation may well be influenced by their religious and spiritual beliefs, which in turn influences their coping abilities. The nurse must learn to help mobilize this form of assistance for the patient.

It is imperative to support the patient's personal spiritual beliefs even if they are at odds with the nurses'. Spiritual beliefs are extremely varied, and provide comfort dependent upon their meaningfulness to the patient. Indoctrination or attempting to alter a patient's beliefs shows indignity, disrespect and can lead to extreme spiritual distress for the patient.

Evaluation

The evaluation of the effectiveness of interventions employed to meet patients' spiritual needs is perhaps the hardest step of the process. There are no quantifiable criteria on which to base judgements. It is not possible to monitor or take a reading from a machine with spirituality as it is with, for example, central venous pressure. However, the nurse can still attempt an evaluation by using observational and listening skills with both the patient and relatives. The nurse can clarify how patients are feeling spiritually by determining whether they continue to express distress about their condition, about the meaning of life, etc. The nurse can determine whether qualities indicative of spiritual well-being are being demonstrated. If a patient is found to be still experiencing spiritual distress, then the process should be repeated commencing with a reassessment of spiritual well-being. The process is an ongoing one, and evaluation is carried out constantly. It is even more difficult to perhaps evaluate spiritual care when the patient has been transferred to another hospital ward. The nurse may never know that the patient is experiencing inner peace, spiritual security, renewed faith, etc. brought about by the experience of critical care. This may not occur immediately, but often long after discharge from the intensive care unit. It may be necessary to involve patients' relatives in the evaluation process to gain their views on the patients' spiritual state, especially if they have been involved in the spiritual care process.

Relatives and spiritual care in the intensive care unit

As well as assessing and meeting the spiritual needs of the patient in intensive care, the assessment and meeting of spiritual needs of relatives may also be a top priority. In thinking along the lines that a therapeutic relationship between a nurse and patient is beneficial, such a relationship between the nurse and patients' relatives may also be beneficial. Out of this relationship the relatives may be better able to provide support for the patient. Family cohesion and integration may help the patient spiritually by conveying to him or her a sense of belonging.

Intensive care units are placed where relatives are often found sitting, watching, feeling completely helpless in the face of the distress or death of a loved one. Relatives are often scared in the intensive care environment, afraid to touch lest they disturb some vital equipment. Whilst often it is difficult for relatives to become involved in much of the physical nursing care, relatives may be of particular value in aiding the nurse to provide spiritual care for the patient. It is important to impress upon relatives that no matter how busy nurses appear to be, they are always open to requests for information, and that nurses do have the time to talk about the relatives' fears, concerns and perhaps issues pertaining to their own spiritual well-being.

One momentous time for both patient and relatives is when the patient has recovered sufficiently to be able to be moved to another ward in the hospital. Feelings of fear may flow over the patient and relatives alike as he or she is moved from a 'secure' environment to what he envisages as a less secure one. A thorough handover should be given to the ward nurse to enable her to carry on with all aspects of the patient's spiritual care which has been assessed, planned, implemented and evaluated in the intensive care unit to date.

Relatives of patients in intensive care find themselves in unfamiliar situations subjected to emotional and spiritual distress. They may easily reach breaking point and vent pent up feelings of, for example, anger or frustration upon the staff, the patient or their God. The nurse can help by listening and by counselling. Some patients may have numerous relatives and friends which comprise a spiritual support system for the patient. It may be necessary to limit visits to short and frequent visits suitably spaced to enable all who need to to visit.

Preparation for practice

It is often felt by many nursing authors (Highfield and Cason, 1983; Forbis, 1988; Cosh, 1988) that there is a lack of formal education regarding spirituality. Education often focuses on superficial aspects of spirituality, or focuses solely on religious considerations. It has been reported to stop at a talk from a member of the clergy or at a list of practical considerations for a particular religious faith, e.g. Jewish, Jehovah's Witness, etc. It can be questioned if a talk given by a hospital chaplain and a list of religious practical considerations pertinent to nursing care, although perhaps informative and necessary, is adequate preparation for the spiritual care of humanists, atheists and other non-religious patients. It may be slotted into the psychosocial domain by some educators, and is therefore lost. Perhaps some nurse teachers, along with nurses themselves, find difficulty in articulating their thoughts about spirituality. Some question whether spirituality can be taught formally. It could possibly be approached experientially on the ICU course, but must include a perspective apart from the context of death and dying.

The nurses in ICU could start a resource pack and collect information concerning spiritual care, e.g. journal articles, newspaper cuttings or any other information gained whilst caring for a particular patient, and filed for future reference.

Ongoing support for nurses

To enable nurses in the ICU to care for patients spiritually, a support group may be useful as a forum for allowing nurses to air their fears and problems in this area. It may allow for discussion about particular religious/spiritual issues and help to clarify situations. It could, for example, help nurses come to terms with issues such as the refusal of blood transfusions. It may also allow the nurse to perhaps start to explore his or her own spirituality and to feel more comfortable in addressing such needs in patients. Such a group may provide the peer support needed, as identified by Fish and Shelly (1983).

Support may come from four sources.

1. The hospital chaplain
2. Nursing colleagues outside the Intensive Care Unit.
3. Friends/family outside nursing.
4. Solitary, individual coping methods, e.g. time for reflection.

A pre-arranged but informal support group may fulfil the needs of those nurses who may find it quite difficult to actively go and seek support. Perhaps it may be necessary to call in someone from outside as the group facilitator or, in other circumstances, a member of staff working in the ICU may be the appropriate person; it is, however, the responsibility of the individual unit to decide on their own personal needs and to determine the best method of fulfilling them.

SUMMARY

This chapter has considered spiritual care to be inherent within the holistic care of patients in the intensive care unit. It is acknowledged that an individual's spirituality is complex and not easily definable, meaning different things to different people. A patient's spirituality is not to be judged by the nurse, rather it is to be assessed and care planned accordingly. The nurse in the intensive care unit is in a prime position, due to the nature of the relationship, to assist patients to use their spiritual beliefs as a coping strategy in times of critical illness.

Literature and research pertaining to spirituality and spiritual care has been reviewed, of necessity general in nature as literature specifically orientated to ICU is scarce. Literature concerned with whether spirituality should be part of nursing care has been considered. Some of the many different expressions of spirituality and spiritual needs have been explored briefly, and consideration given to avenues open for the nurse to minister spiritual care. A number of constraints to the provision of spiritual care have been identified.

The critical care situation and practical nursing implications relevant to spiritual care have been briefly examined. Four fundamental spiritual needs have been considered. The nursing process – Assessment, Planning, Implementation and Evaluation – has been used as a framework to guide spiritual care of ICU patients. The importance of communication has been stressed, and is a vital component of beneficial spiritual care. The necessity for a broad approach to spiritual matters has been emphasized so as not to equate spirituality with religion, thereby including for example humanists and atheist perspectives within the realm of spiritual care. The term 'spiritual distress' has been examined briefly, and a few examples of nursing diagnoses in relation to spirituality included.

Nursing interventions relevant to spiritual care in the intensive care unit both religious and secular have been proposed. Interpersonal skills such as listening, the portrayal of empathy, vulnerability, humility and commitment have been exemplified as useful skills in such care. The communication of spiritual caring by the use of touch has also been considered. The conflict which may occur between a nurse's spirituality and that of her patient's has

been highlighted. Some examples of alternative approaches to spiritual care apart from religious interventions have been proposed alongside the traditional religious ministration. It has been acknowledged that the evaluation of spiritual care is perhaps the hardest step of the process due to its subjective and qualitative nature.

The spiritual care of relatives and their role in supporting a patient in the intensive care unit has been briefly explored. Finally, the importance of adequate preparation in spiritual care for nurses has been highlighted. This should include a specific consideration of spirituality within the intensive care course and not solely addressed within the psychosocial domain. It should not be narrowly focused on religious care, but encompass a wider perspective and provision made for experiential learning. It should also include opportunity for the nurse to examine his or her own particular spiritual beliefs and fears, and explore further the whole arena of spiritual care within a safe and partially structured environment.

The reader may not agree with all that is written, but its purpose has been to perhaps stimulate thought and discussion regarding spirituality and the intensive care unit.

KEY TERMS

Catharsis

The process of releasing repressed emotions.

Deity

Of Divine Nature.

Existential

Having Existence or a 'State of Being'.

Humanistic

Pertaining to ethical views as opposed to religious views.

Metaphysical

An ultimate abstract principle concerned with the ultimate nature of being and knowing.

Secular

Not ecclesiastical.

Secularization

A departure from religious influence on life.

Spiritual dissonance

The incompatibility between one spiritual belief and another. For example between the nurse's own spiritual belief and that of the patients.

FURTHER READING

Carson, V. B. *Spiritual Dimensions of Nursing Practice*. Philadelphia: W.B. Saunders, 1989.

McGilloway, O., Myco, F. (Eds.). *Nursing and Spiritual Care*. London: Harper & Row, 1985.

Neuberger, J. *Caring for Dying People of Different Faiths*. Lisa Sainsbury Foundation Series, 1987.

Sampson, C. *The Neglected Ethic: Religious and Cultural Factors in the Care of Patients*. Maidenhead: McGraw-Hill, 1982.

Burnard, P. Learning to care for the spirit. *Nursing Standard*. 1990; 4(18) 38–39.

REFERENCES

Books

Bannister, D., Fransella, F. *The Psychology of Personal Constructs*. 2nd Ed. London: Penguin Books, 1980.

Burnard, P., Chapman, C. *Professional and Ethical Issues In Nursing*. Chichester: Wiley, 1988.

Carpenito, L. J. *Nursing Diagnosis. Application to Clinical Practice*. J.B. Lippincott, 1983.

Carson, V. B. *Spiritual Dimensions of Nursing Practice*. Philadelphia: W. B. Saunders, 1989.

Chadwick, R. *Awareness and preparedness of nurses to meet spiritual needs*. In Eds. S. Fish, J. Shelly. *Spiritual Care – The Nurse's Role*. Illinois: Intervarsity Press, 1983, 177–178.

Colliton, M. *The Spiritual Dimension of Nursing*. In Eds. I.L. Beland, J.Y. Passos. *Clinical Nursing Pathophysiological and Psychosocial Approaches*. 4th Ed. London: Collier MacMillan, 1981.

Cosh, R. In Eds. Tiffany, Webb. *Oncology for nurses and health care professionals*, 2nd Ed. *Care and Support*. Vol. 2. London: Harper & Row, 1988, pp. 102–118.

Curtin, L., Flaherty, M. J. *Nursing Ethics: Theories and Pragmatics*. Englewood-Cliffs, NJ: Prentice-Hall, 1982.

Fish, S., Shelly, J. *Spiritual Care – The Nurse's Role*. IL 1983, Intervarsity Press.

Frankl, V. *Man's Search for Meaning – An Introduction To Logotherapy*. London: Hodder & Stoughton, 1962.

Glaser, B. G., Strauss, A. L. *Awareness of Dying*. New York: Aldine Publications, 1966.

Hess, J. *Spiritual Needs Survey*. In Eds. S. Fish, J. Shelly. *Spiritual Care – The Nurse's Role*. IL: Intervarsity Press, 1983.

International Council of Nurses. *Code for Nurses, Ethical Concepts Applied to Nurses*. Mexico: ICN, 1973.

Martin, *Spiritual needs of patients' study*. In Eds. S. Fish, J. Shelly. *Spiritual Care – The Nurses's Role*. IL: Intervarsity Press, 1983.

McGilloway, O., Myco, F. (Eds.). *Nursing and Spiritual Care*. London: Harper & Row, 1985.

Neuberger, J. *Caring for Dying People of Different Faiths*. Lisa Sainsbury Foundation Series, 1987.

O'Brien, M. E. *The need for spiritual integrity*. In Eds. H. Yura, M. B. Walsh. *Human Needs 2 and the Nursing Process*. Norwalk, CT: Appleton-Century-Crofts, 1982, pp. 85–115.

Peplau, H. E. *Interpersonal Relations in Nursing*. Putnam & Sons, 1952.

Rambo, B. J. *Adaptation Nursing – Assessment and Intervention*. Philadelphia: W. B. Saunders, 1984.

Sampson, C. *The Neglected Ethic: Religious and Cultural Factors in the Care of Patients*. London: McGraw-Hill, 1982.

Stallwood, J., Stall, R. *Spiritual dimensions of nursing practice*. In Eds. I. Beland, J. Passos. *Clinical Nursing*, 3rd Ed. Part C, Chapter 19. New York: MacMillan, 1981.

Travelbee, J. *Interpersonal Aspects of Nursing*. 2nd ed. F.A. Davis, 1971.

UKCC. *Code of Professional Conduct for the Nurse, Midwife and Health Visitor*. London: UKCC, 1992.

Yura, H., Walsh, M. B. (Eds.). *Human Needs and the Nursing Process*. Appleton-Century-Crofts, 1982.

Periodicals

Baldree, K. S. *et al*. Stress identification and coping patterns in patients on haemodialysis. *Nursing Research*. 1982; 31: 109–111.

Bell, R. Understanding patients' beliefs. *Nursing*. 1987; 16: 681–682.

Boutell, K., Bozett, F. Nurses' assessment of patients spirituality, continuing education implications. *The Journal of Continuing Education in Nursing*. 1991; 21(4): 172–176.

Brallier, L. W. The nurse as holistic health practitioner. Expanding the role again. *Nursing Clinics of North America*. 1978; 13(4): December, 643–655.

Bunston, L. *The Spiritual Needs and Resources of the Hospitalised Depressed Psychiatric Patient*. Unpublished M.N. Thesis, University of Wales College of Medicine, 1987.

Burnard, P. Picking up the pieces. *Nursing Times*. 1986; 82(17): 37–39.

Burnard, P. Spiritual distress and the nursing response: Theoretical considerations and counselling skills. *Journal of Advanced Nursing*. 1987; 12: 377–382.

Burnard, P. Searching for meaning. *Nursing Times*. 1988; 84(37): 34–36.

Burnard, P. Learning to care for the spirit. *Nursing Standard*. 1990; 4(18): 38–39.

Byrne, M. (Sr.) A zest for life. *Journal of Gerontological Nursing*. 1985; 11(4): 30–33.

Carson, V., Gerardi, R. 1987: Cited in Bunston (1987).

Connell, H. Promoting creative expression. *Nursing Times*. 1989; 85(15): 52–54.

Conrad, N. L. Spiritual support for the dying. *Nursing Clinics of North America*. 1985; 20(2): 415–425.

Dettmore, D. Spiritual care; remembering your patient's forgotten needs. *Nursing*. 1984; 10: 46.

Dickinson, C. The search for spiritual meaning. *American Journal of Nursing*. 1975; 75(10): 1789–1793.

Dugan, D. O. Death and dying: emotional, spiritual and ethical support for patients and families. *Journal of Psychosocial Nursing and Mental Health Services*. 1987; 25(7).

Ellerhorst-Ryan, J. Selecting an instrument to measure spiritual distress. *Oncology Nursing Forum*. 1985; 12(2).

Ellis, C. Course prepares nurses to meet patient's spiritual needs, St. Joseph's Hospital, Houston. *Health Progress*. 1986; 67(3): 76–77.

Forbis, P.A. Meeting patients' spiritual needs. *Geriatric Nursing*. 1988; 158–159.

Highfield, M. F., Cason, C. Spiritual needs of patients: Are they recognised? *Cancer Nursing*. 1983; (3): 187–192.

Hubert, M. (Sr.) Spiritual care for every patient. *Journal of Nursing Education*. 1963; 12(2): 9–11, 29–31.

Kemp, J. T. Learning from clients, counselling the frail and dying elderly. (1984). Cited in Reed, P. G. Spirituality and well-being in terminally ill hospitalised adults. *Research in Nursing and Health*. 1987; 10: 335–344.

Kreidler, M. C. (1978). Cited in Labun, E. Spiritual care: An element in nursing care planning. *Journal of Advanced Nursing*. 1988; 13: 314–320.

Labun, E. Spiritual care: An element in nursing care planning. *Journal of Advanced Nursing*. 1988; 13: 314–320.

McGilloway, O., Donnelly, L. Religion and patient care: The functionalist approach. *Journal of Advanced Nursing*. 1977; 2: 3–13.

Miller, J. Hope doesn't necessarily spring eternal. *American Journal of Nursing*. 1983; January, 23–25.

Morrison, R. Spiritual health care and the nurse. *Nursing Standard*. 1989; 20 December; 4(13/14): 28–29.

Peterson, E. A., Nelson, K. How to meet your clients' spiritual needs. *Journal of Psychosocial Nursing and Mental Health Services*. 1987; 25(5): 34–39.

Piles, C. (1980). Cited in Brittain, J., Boozer, J. Spiritual care integration into a collegiate nursing curriculum. *Journal of Nursing Education*. 1987; 26(4): 155–160.

Reed, P. G. Spirituality and well-being in terminally ill hospitalised adults. *Research in Nursing and Health*. 1987; 10: 335–344.

Ryan, J. The neglected crisis. *American Journal of Nursing*. 1984; October: 1257–1258.

Shelly, J. A. (1982/83). Cited in Bunston, L. *The Spiritual Needs and Resources of The Hospitalised Depressed Psychiatric Patient*. Unpublished M.N. Thesis, University of Wales College of Medicine, 1987.

Silber, T. J., Reilly, M. (Sr.) *Spiritual and Religious Concerns of the Hospitalised Adolescent*. Cited in Soeken, K. L., Carson, V. J. (1987).

Simsen, B. *Spiritual needs and Resources in Illness and Hospitalisation*. Unpublished M.Sc. Thesis, University of Manchester, 1985.

Simsen, B. The spiritual dimension. *Nursing Times*. 1986, 26 November; 41–42.

Simsen, B. Spiritual care, nursing the spirit. *Nursing Times*. 1988, 14 September; 84(37): 31–33.

Sodestrom, K., Martinson, I. Patients spiritual coping strategies: A study of nurse and patient perspectives. *Oncology Nursing Forum*. 1987; 14(2): 41–45.

Soeken, K. L., Carson, V. J. Study measures nurses' attitudes about providing spiritual care. *Health Progress*. 1986; 67(3): 52–55.

Soeken, K. L., Carson, V. J. Responding to the spiritual needs of the chronically ill. *Nursing Clinics of North America*. 1986, September; 22(5): 603–611.

Stoll, R. I. Guidelines for spiritual assessment. *American Journal of Nursing*. 1979; 79(9): 1574–1577.

Uys, L. R. Towards the development of an operational definition of the concept 'therapeutic use of self'. *International Journal of Nursing Studies*. 1980; 17.

12
DEATH AND DYING IN CRITICAL CARE

David Thompson

CHAPTER AIMS

The aim of this chapter is to relate how nurses can help the patient in the critical care setting achieve a good death by providing skills and compassionate personal care for the dying and their loved ones. Specifically, it will examine three aspects:

☐ To briefly review the literature concerning: the dying person, the needs and concerns of the dying patient, and the process of grief and loss.

☐ To briefly review the available research concerning: nurses' attitudes towards death and dying, communication with the dying, care of the dying, and care of the family.

☐ To describe in some detail the practical nursing implications, based on the earlier reviews, for: meeting the needs of the dying patient, meeting the needs of the family, and meeting the needs of the nurses.

☐ Finally, there will be a short summary of the main points of the chapter.

INTRODUCTION

The purpose of critical care units is to reduce mortality and morbidity. Much of this is achieved by the application of life-sustaining medical technology. However, despite dramatic medical advances and increasingly sophisticated technologies, patients will inevitably die in these units.

Caring for those patients facing death is not an easy task. Although death may be anticipated, the magnitude of the impact and its ramifications can never be accurately predicted.

THE LITERATURE

Throughout time people have been concerned with questions regarding life and death. Philosophers, historians, theologians, poets and scientists, among others, have attempted to understand. The only thing certain in life is death, but there are many uncertainties as to why, when, where and how.

Death is the permanent cessation of all vital functions, the end of human life, an event and a state. *Dying* is a process of coming to an end: the final act of living.

The dying person

Most of the literature concerning death and dying in contemporary societies emanates from the United States. A brief review of the seminal work of Glaser and Strauss (1965, 1968) and Kubler-Ross (1970) is pertinent.

The concept of a dying trajectory was offered by Glaser and Strauss (1965, 1968) to refer to the pattern of death. Glaser and Strauss distinguish between 'quick' and 'slow' dying trajectories. Generally, deaths which occur over a short span are easier for hospital staff (but not for the family) to cope with than slow deaths, unless they are unexpected. These quick deaths most commonly occur in critical care situations.

In most cultures, young adults, especially young parents, have the highest social worth, and their deaths are accounted the greatest social loss (Glaser and Strauss, 1968). Typically, in critical care units, patients are relatively young.

Kubler-Ross (1970) described a series of stages through which people pass in response to their dying:

1. *Denial and isolation*   This stage is typically the initial reaction to the diagnosis of a terminal illness. It is the initial defence mechanism used to deal with news of impending death.
2. *Anger*   This stage involves feelings of anger, rage and resentment as the dying person attempts to answer the question, 'Why me?'
3. *Bargaining*   This stage involves an attempt to postpone the inevitable by asking that death be delayed in return for a particular promise.
4. *Depression*   This stage is marked by two types of depression: reactive depression, resulting from losses that are experienced as a part of the illness, and preparatory depression, which anticipates impending losses, such as separation from the family.
5. *Acceptance*   This stage is marked by a degree of quiet expectation. Kubler-Ross (1970) stated that provided patients have had enough time (i.e. not a sudden, unexpected death) and have been helped in working through the previously described stages, they will complete this stage.

Kubler-Ross was careful to make clear that dying patients do not always progress through these stages precisely in the order she described. She pointed out that these stages will last for different periods of time and will replace each other or exist at times side by side. Weisman (1974) and Pattison (1977) have challenged the accuracy and utility of stages of dying for guiding care. Instead, they offer discernible phases in the process of dying. For example, Pattison describes three common clinical phases of the dying process:

1. The *acute crisis phase*, which is triggered by the crisis of knowing that death is approaching, and marked by anxiety and a sense of threat to one's self.
2. The *chronic living-dying phase*, which is usually the longest and is typified by a variety of fears as well as grief for the many losses that occur as a part of the dying process.
3. The *terminal phase*, which is characterized by an increased withdrawal into one's self and an increased acceptance of the anticipated death.

Although these frameworks are helpful in understanding the changing emotional state of the dying person, it is crucial to respond to each person as an individual.

Needs and concerns of the dying patient

The dying process is unique to each individual, although there are needs and concerns commonly experienced by dying persons (Cook and Oltjenbruns, 1989):

☐ *Pain*   Pain is the most commonly experienced symptom of terminally ill patients. To assure as high a quality of life as possible effective pain control is necessary.

☐ *Body image*   Altered body image may occur as a result of such changes as loss of weight, body functions, or body parts.

☐ *Fear*   Dying persons often experience a wide variety of fears, especially of pain or suffering, isolation or abandonment, indignity, rejection, and the unknown.

☐ *Grief*   The dying person often grieves in anticipation of the death itself and the end of life.

☐ *Awareness*   Glaser and Strauss (1965) identified four contexts in the awareness of dying:

1. *Closed awareness*: the patient does not know they are dying but the staff (and possibly family) know it.
2. *Suspected awareness*: the patient does not know, but suspects, that they are dying. The staff and family do know it.
3. *Mutual pretence*: the patient, staff and family know the patient is dying but there is tacit agreement to act as if this were not so.
4. *Open awareness*: the patient, staff and family know that the patient is dying and act as if they do.

Authors such as Kubler-Ross (1970) and Hinton (1972) believe that dying patients should be informed of their terminal condition for both moral and practical reasons, although it is clear that most patients become aware they are dying even if they are not told (Glaser and Strauss, 1965, 1968; Kubler-Ross, 1970; Hinton, 1972). Those who do not wish to know of their impending death seem to turn a deaf ear (Kubler-Ross, 1970).

☐ *Withdrawal*   Withdrawal is often experienced by the dying person and those in their social environment. There are three main contributory factors (Charmaz, 1980):

1. Environmental conditions (such as the distance between the hospital and home) that interfere with communication between the dying person and family.
2. Withdrawal by the dying person because of factors such as pain and unconsciousness.
3. Social avoidance of the dying person because factors such as fear of death and uncertainty as to how to interact with the dying.

☐ *Control and independence*   The need for retaining some degree of control in their life can be crucial to a dying person's well-being. Closely related to the desire to retain a sense of control is the desire to remain as independent as possible.

☐ *Meaning*   There is often a need to find meaning in one's life.

☐ *Hope*   Hope is a powerful force and the one thing that usually persists throughout the dying process (Kubler-Ross, 1970). Without hope life is meaningless.

Many factors affect the dying process, including the person's developmental stage and ethnic or cultural background.

Dying patients may worry about the future for their families and be concerned about how they will cope. The experience of dying also has an impact on families, and may serve as a cohesive force in some families and a disruptive force in others. Generally, families who have responded to stresses or crises as a unified force in the past will offer each other strength and support, whereas for those who have strained relationships, the dying experience may promote further strain. Dying persons occasionally use the experience to manipulate and control the behaviour of members of the family.

Grief and loss

There is a variety of theoretical perspectives that provide insight into the grief process. For example, Bowlby (1980) provides a framework for understanding separation and loss which is closely linked to his theory of attachment. He explains that humans have an instinctive need to form strong attachments to others. Separation due, for example, to death, elicits various behaviours (such as crying or clinging), indicating that an attachment bond existed.

A variety of authors, including Engel (1964), Bowlby (1980) and Parkes (1986), have categorized the grief process in stages. For example, Engel (1964) categorized three separate stages:

1. *Shock and disbelief*   Immediately after the loss there is complete confusion. The family may be stunned and unable to accept or comprehend their loss, particularly if it was unexpected.
2. *Developing awareness*   The stage of shock and disbelief is relatively short, and the loss gradually becomes a reality. Each family member, in their own way, will experience pain, anguish, sadness, anger and even denial. The family may feel helpless and hopeless, and members may blame themselves for the death and suffer guilt.

Anger may be directed at the loved one for dying, or at the staff for failure to save the victim's life.

3. *Restitution and recovery* This stage begins after the family leaves the hospital. Funerals and religious beliefs help the family accept the reality of their loss and they begin to cope with the absence of the loved one. Feelings of guilt and idealization gradually disappear as detachment occurs and intellectual reasoning takes over.

Bowlby (1980) described the overall grief experience as progressing through four stages:

1. Numbing.
2. Yearning.
3. Disorganization.
4. Reorganization.

Parkes (1986), on the other hand, categorized five stages of grief:

1. Alarm.
2. Searching (for the lost person).
3. Mitigation, or finding sources of comfort.
4. Anger and guilt.
5. Gaining a new identity, or adjustment to loss.

Although the stages differ in number and terminology, there are essentially many similarities in these authors' descriptions. Nevertheless, these stages are not clear-cut, and may have varying lengths and manifestations according to the individual and the circumstances surrounding death. The strength of the attachment, the dependency of the bereaved on the deceased, the age of those who die, and the circumstances of their illness and death affect the emotional response.

Persons who fear the death of a loved one often begin the process of grieving before any loss actually occurs, a phenomenon known as anticipatory grief (Lindemann, 1944).

The acute reactions to loss include an initial period of shock followed by intense emotional pangs of grief. Lindemann identified the following symptoms of normal grief:

☐ Somatic distress (e.g. feelings of tightness in the throat).
☐ Preoccupation with the image of the deceased.
☐ Guilt.
☐ Hostile reactions.
☐ Loss of patterns of conduct.

He defines pathognomonic grief as an exaggeration or persistence of these symptoms. Raphael (1977) has suggested that 30% of those who are bereaved may develop maladaptive or pathological grief, indicated by such actions as retaining all of the deceased's possessions as if in readiness for use.

According to Parkes (1986), the pain of grief is perhaps the price paid for love, the cost of commitment. The duration and intensity of grief varies considerably. Although Lindemann stated that 4–6 weeks was adequate time for recovery, the most intense feelings typically begin to diminish within six months to two years, and many people experience grief-related feelings for a much longer time.

The intensity of the grief reaction may be increased periodically, for example on occasions such as birthdays and anniversaries, particularly of the date of the death.

It is well known that bereavement can cause increased morbidity (Maddison and Viola, 1968; Lundin, 1984a) and mortality (Parkes *et al.*, 1969; Jones, 1987), especially during the first years after loss.

THE RESEARCH

It is pertinent to briefly review the available research concerning nurses' attitudes towards death and dying; communication with the dying; care of the dying; and care of the family.

Attitudes towards death and dying

Since nurses are a product of their culture they are likely to share similar attitudes and beliefs towards death and dying.

The pioneering research work of Glaser and Strauss (1965, 1968), and of Quint (1967) presented a depressing picture of the care of dying patients in general hospitals. They found that health workers withdrew from the dying patient and changed the subject or terminated conversation in which patients hinted of or talked openly about death and dying.

The difficulties encountered by the dying may be exacerbated by the failure of nurses and others to deal adequately with their own reactions to death and dying. It has been suggested that personal fear of death is related to anxiety about dealing with dying among health care professionals (Glaser and Strauss, 1965). For example, a significant number of nurses in Gow's (1982) study reported that they were incapacitated from helping dying patients by their own fear of death. The first experience of nursing a dying patient seems to be especially important (Quint, 1967).

Various other studies have shown that nurses suffer from feelings of helplessness, inadequacy and depression when dealing with the dying (Quint, 1967; Murphy, 1986). Interestingly, Stoller (1980) found that uneasiness associated with interactions with dying persons increased with nursing experience.

Clearly, nurses must confront and reconcile their own fear of death before they can help others meet death and dying. Improving the first experience of nursing a dying patient through better support and advice is an obvious and essential step towards enabling nurses to cope.

A number of studies report more favourable, less fearful and less avoiding attitudes towards death and dying as a result of a variety of educational strategies dealing with death and dying (Murray, 1974; Ross, 1978; Bugen, 1980; Miles, 1980; Field, 1986). For example, Hurtig and Stewin (1990) recently reported a study examining the effect of death education and experience on nursing students' attitudes towards death. The sample comprised 76 diploma nursing students who had had no clinical experience. These students were roughly equally divided into three groups. The researchers found that the group who received an experiential programme of death education was more positive towards death and dying than the groups who received either the didactic or placebo programmes.

Communication with the dying

The literature emphasizes that effective communication influences the quality of the experience of dying. Both verbal and non-verbal communications are important in interactions with patients,

and with dying patients in particular the non-verbal channel may be crucial. Field (1989a) stresses that nurses should be able to recognize non-verbal signs of distress, a willingness to listen, and information seeking, as well as to control their own signals to the patient.

Patients tend to assume a passive role; they do not want to appear to be a nuisance or to be ignorant, and hence are reluctant to ask questions or express concerns. Nurses may find it difficult to broach the subject of dying. Unfortunately, nurses may use 'distancing tactics' to remove themselves from patients' and relatives' emotional suffering as a way of coping with the stress of the situation. These distancing tactics include false reassurance and selected inattention to communication about psychosocial concerns (Maguire, 1985).

Nimocks *et al.* (1987) identify 'communicational apprehension' as an important factor inhibiting conversation with the dying. This may be due to social sources, such as the disclosure norms which are practised in a particular unit, or individual sources, such as the attitudes of nurses or their poor communication skills.

The two main ways to rectify the problem of deficient communication skills are education and guided experience. Although formal didactic teaching may be beneficial, experiential learning is reported to be more appropriate (Durlak, 1978).

In most hospital settings, including critical care units, communications with patients and families have improved considerably since the early findings of Glaser and Strauss and others. A recent study (Seale, 1991) examined communication and awareness about death. It reported the perceptions of relatives, hospital doctors, general practitioners and nurses who knew of 639 adults dying in England in 1987. The findings from professionals suggest a general preference for openness about illness and death, provided that bad news is broken slowly, in a context of support, while recognizing that not everyone wishes to know all. Seale noted that doctors' and nurses' openness about communicating with the dying and their families has increased in the past three decades, partly influenced by the hospice movement. However, he also added that situations of 'closed awareness', and situations where patients were left to guess the likely outcome for themselves, were still quite common in 1987.

Based on his research, Field (1989a) made a number of recommendations, including the adoption of a clear policy of disclosure of the diagnosis and prognosis of terminal conditions. He also recommended that there should be full communication of information about the terminally ill, joint decision making about their care, and full co-operation in the implementation of such care.

Care of the dying

In critical care units patients are likely to be young and acutely ill, their stay is short, 'recovery' and 'success' the norm, and turnover rapid. The dying patient if often unconscious and maintained on an aggressive treatment regime with life support systems, and although these units typically have a high nurse–patient ratio, and the nurses are invariably trained and specialized, the focus of nursing work is still generally of a medico-technical nature rather than of a psychosocial one. In these settings, the dying patient is generally viewed as an anomaly (Field, 1989a).

The mode of organization of nursing care is an important factor. For example, in critical care units where primary nursing or individualized patient care is practised, nurses are more likely to develop an attachment to their patient, thus facilitating a therapeutic relationship. The research work of Field (1989a) is important here. Amongst other studies, he reported on one in a coronary care unit which used patient allocation as the basis for organizing care. Field (1989b) noted that in this unit, patient allocation facilitated close and continuing contact between nurses and their patients, thereby increasing the chance that emotional involvement would develop. In his study of nurses' reported experiences about nursing people dying in this unit, and their attitudes to such work, Field (1989c) found that nurses did not report any severe coping difficulties associated with their nursing care of dying patients. Their most severe difficulties were those relating to telling relatives about a patient's death.

Field noted that the elements within the unit's ethos and organization associated with this positive coping included the high staff–patient ratio, low staff turnover, good relationships among staff, and a policy of open and honest communication.

Care of the family

Care of the dying patient is incomplete unless there is care of the family. Families may respond with despair and disbelief on hearing that there is nothing more that can be done for their loved one.

Nursing care to meet the needs of family members may enable the family to adapt and enhance their ability to support their critically ill relative. They can provide comfort and encouragement to the dying person and a sense of warmth to the environment.

Molter (1979) identified 45 needs of relatives of critically ill patients. The ten highest ranked ones were:

1. Hope.
2. Caring hospital personnel.
3. A waiting room near the patient.
4. Frequent telephone calls at home about changes in the patient's condition.
5. Knowing the patient's condition.
6. Receiving honest answers to questions.
7. Knowing specific details concerning the patient's progress.
8. Receiving updated information about the patient each day.
9. Receiving explanations which can be understood.
10. Frequent visits with the patient.

Spouses, in particular, may experience intense feelings of loss due to the perceived threat of their partner's death. Hampe (1975) has identified eight needs that are acutely felt by the spouse going through the stages of anticipatory grief:

1. To be with the dying person.
2. To be helpful to the dying person.
3. For assurance of the comfort of the dying person.
4. To be informed of the dying person's condition.
5. To be informed of the impending death.
6. To ventilate emotions.
7. For comfort and support of family members.

8. For acceptance, support, and comfort from health professionals.

These needs are confirmed in a study by Breu and Dracup (1978), who also identified a ninth need – the relief from anxiety. These authors consolidated these nine needs into five basic needs of grieving spouses:

1. Relief of initial anxiety.
2. Information.
3. Time with the patient.
4. Need to help the patient.
5. Support and expression of feelings.

Daley (1984) added a sixth need – to meet personal needs.

The family's primary needs are to be informed of their relative's condition, for the information to be as honest as possible, to be able to speak with the doctor, and to know that the relative is receiving the best possible care.

PRACTICAL NURSING IMPLICATIONS

Critical care units are still largely dominated by medical intervention and the use of a range of increasingly sophisticated technologies. Often, the nurses' work involves tending the machines that monitor the patients' condition or assisting them to maintain their vital functions. Thus, these units are geared to preserving life, and the death of a patient is often perceived to be a failure on the part of the staff. Those who die in these units generally end their lives attached to all manner of life-prolonging apparatus, and often death occurs following intensive heroic activity by the staff (Benoliel, 1988).

A major problem in critical care units is that of the ethics of decisions regarding treatment; whether to prolong life by the use of invasive and often distressing measures or to stop or withhold treatment. The doctor's priority may be to sustain life at all cost, whereas the nurse's may be to enable the patient to die with dignity. Such serious issues often pose personal and professional dilemmas.

A problem in some critical care settings, notably coronary care units, is that nurses may have initially tried to convince patients that they are *not* dying. Nurses may then have difficulty in reconciling their care which was planned for the predicted recovery, with care planned for the actual death.

Factors such as the type of person dying, and the type of dying trajectory, have implications for the nurse. For example, the death of a young person is, in most cases, harder to accept than the death of the elderly. Obviously, the loss is greater for the survivors if the death of a relative or friend means that their way of life must change drastically, such as a person with children who loses a partner whose earnings were the family's sole means of support.

There may be difficulty in establishing whether a patient is likely to die and, if so, in estimating when death is likely to occur (Field, 1989a).

Slow dying is more common and more problematic for staff. It is this type of dying trajectory in particular which generates the various problems associated with awareness and disclosure of dying. In slow dying the person is on a lingering downward trajectory with symptoms often becoming worse and harder to manage. In some instances, patients are moved off the critical care unit to die in a ward side room. This clearly interferes with the nurse–patient relationship and affects the needs of the patient and family.

Although most dying people express resentment, fear or sorrow over the major changes that are forced on their lives by their progressive debilitation, some view dying as an achievement.

The prime function of the nurse is to give patients and their families the help they need with the activities of living, to help them maintain their independence as long as possible, and to make it possible for patients to have what they consider a good death, and to minimize any pain or discomfort associated with the dying process.

Each nurse must assess and work with the patient and family to help them cope realistically with death (Hampe, 1975). The price of this involvement is sometimes very high.

Meeting the needs of the dying patient

To help a person die well is to support that person's sense of self-respect, dignity, control and choice until the final moment of life. Achieving this entails skilled and compassionate care designed to promote comfort and control suffering.

Although patient care cannot be separated into neat compartments, it will be considered under the following headings.

Attending to physical needs

Meeting the physical needs of the dying patient generally includes interventions that prevent debilitation and provide comfort.

Controlling pain and discomfort

The primary symptom found in the dying is pain. Thus, the aim is to keep the patient free from pain and discomfort yet not dull their consciousness or ability to communicate. This is usually achieved by pharmacological measures, essentially using opiates, but other methods of pain relief should form an integral part of the nurse's repertoire. These methods include being with the patient, using therapeutic touch, promoting comfort through careful body positioning, and using relaxation and distraction techniques.

The patient needs to have the opportunity and means to exert control over pain (for example, in using a syringe drive) and participate in its assessment and evaluation.

Providing nourishment

With progressive weakness the physical effort of eating or drinking may prove too great for the dying patient. Nausea and vomiting may interfere with adequate food consumption. Poor nutrition leads to exhaustion, infection and other complications such as the development of pressure sores, therefore parenteral nutrition may be indicated.

If the swallowing reflex is present, offering sips of water at frequent intervals is helpful. The patient who can eat and drink may need small amounts of nutritious food and drink, and advice can be sought from the dietician.

Maintaining elimination

Some patients may be incontinent of urine and faeces, whereas others may have retention of urine and constipation, all of which cause discomfort and embarrassment. Certain drugs may indirectly cause these effects. A sense of helplessness and loss of dignity may occur, for example, in a patient who requires the insertion of a urinary catheter.

Attending to hygiene

Attention to personal hygiene is important, not only to keep the dying patient clean, feel refreshed, well groomed and free of unpleasant odours, but to maintain the patient's sense of dignity.

Careful sponging may promote relaxation as well as cleanliness. Mouth care, including removal of secretions and lubrication, is particularly important.

Open lesions my be a source of offensive odours as dead tissue and bacterial growth accumulate within the wound. Wound care is needed to not only minimize the risk of infection and further tissue damage, but to prevent unsightliness and embarrassment for the patient and others.

Men may require assistance with shaving. Women may have their morale boosted by attention from the hospital hairdresser or beautician. The involvement of relatives in the provision of such care helps reduce their sense of helplessness and increase their sense of worth.

Promoting rest and sleep

Patients who are dying often have problems sleeping and resting. Features such as monitors and alarm systems which characterize critical care units are not conducive to the promotion of rest and sleep. Indeed, many patients, especially those who fear they are dying, are frightened to sleep. The nurse needs to consider the appropriateness of observations and interventions which are likely to interfere with the achievement of adequate rest and sleep. Coordination is necessary to minimize disruption of the patient. Planning specific rest periods, communicating them to the family as well as other staff, and adhering to them, as well as maintaining sleep-promoting rituals, such as hot milky drinks at night-time, are measures that facilitate rest and sleep.

Modifying the environment

Having familiar objects, such as photographs of loved ones, in view can help to make the patient feel more comfortable and secure.

Attention should be paid to lighting, temperature, ventilation and especially noise. Many dying patients are placed in a side room and the nurse needs to consider the appropriateness of this and its impact upon the patient and family, as well as other patients. It is often difficult to strike a balance between the intended aims of achieving privacy, peace and quiet, and the potential for isolation, fear and abandonment.

Encouraging close relatives and friends to visit is important to avoid loneliness. Kastenbaum (1981) claims that one of the greatest concerns among people who are dying is that they will be left alone. The nurse needs to respond to individual situations; some families may find it too distressing to spend a lot of time with the patients, whereas others do not want to leave the bedside. Family members may require reassurance that when they choose to go the patient will not be left alone.

Involving the family in the patient's care

An important role of nurses is to share their skills and knowledge with family members and help them to relieve pain and discomfort, and to encourage their participation in the care of the patient.

There is no substitute for the presence of the family at the bedside of dying persons when they want them there. Family members often appreciate helping with the patient's care and should be made to feel welcome and reassured that they are not in the way.

Responding to emotional needs

The dying patient is likely to require emotional support more than at any other time. Patients' feelings of helplessness may cause them to depend upon others to provide them with a sense of safety, security, love and worth. Patients who have previously occupied the dominant role in the family may find that their relationships with other member are significantly altered. They may find they can only be themself with the nurse or a relative stranger. The nurse can help the patient and family by understanding common fears, facilitating communication, and helping them accept reality.

Understanding common fears

There are many fears associated with the process of dying. Common fears include pain, abandonment, loss of control, loss of dignity, dependence, body image changes and financial worries. Patients may feel that their fears and concerns are trivial or unwarranted. Nurses can help patients by being open and uncritical, reassuring them that such fears are common and encouraging them to be expressed so that they can be dealt with.

Facilitating communication

Open communication between the nurse, the patient and the family can help individuals to cope and deal with the reality of the issues concerning death. The mode of organizing and delivering nursing care is an important consideration; primary nursing is the mode most likely to facilitate a strong nurse–patient relationship and continuity of care, and hence good communication. Important points to remember in establishing an atmosphere conducive to good communication are listening, patience and honesty. Field (1992) suggests that three main skills are required. First, nurses need to maintain their self-composure and convey a feeling of being at ease with the patient when discussing the patient's concerns. Adopting a relaxed stance, sitting at the same level as the patient, maintaining eye contact and using touch to convey concern and support demonstrate the nurse's availability and willingness to listen to the patient. Second, patients' feelings and anxieties may be explored through the skills of listening and being still, the use of 'minimal prompts' and the technique of 'reflecting back' to them what they have said. Field warns nurses against saying that they understand the patient's feelings and concerns as this not only devalues and trivializes them, but is untrue: although nurses may feel empathy they cannot fully appreciate what the patient is experiencing. Third, nurses need to more directly seek out patients' concerns and to answer practical questions or refer them to other sources.

Effective communication means that the nurse makes time available to be with the patient and family, and that all members of the health care team adopt a similar approach and are fully aware of what is going on through regular exchange of information. This reduces the likelihood of staff conveying conflicting information to the patient and family.

Accepting reality

Sometimes patients may prolong dying while awaiting a sign that others are prepared to accept the loss: a phenomenon described as 'waiting for permission' to die. For the family, especially the patient's partner, letting go can be a devastating experience. Many are afraid that it will be interpreted as giving up or demonstrating that they no longer care. This is, of course, *one* view of the process: other people may take a different one.

Meeting spiritual needs

Death sometimes shakes but also strengthens a person's faith, particularly if they have had time to think about the impending death. Some patients look forward to their death, believing that it will be followed by great reward and peace for having lived a good and faithful life. Others may believe that death may involve some form of punishment, or that when life ends so does all form of existence.

Hinton (1972) found that dying patients who had a firm religious faith were the most free from anxiety. Those who maintained that they had no religious beliefs also appeared calm during their last illness. The patients who showed most anxiety were those who were uncertain and wavering in their belief in and practice of a religious faith.

Many dying patients find great comfort in the support they receive from their religious faiths. The spiritual needs of the dying include a search for meaning, a sense of forgiveness and a need for love and hope. The patient should not be left to die without meaning, and feeling guilt-ridden, hopeless and lonely.

In a multicultural society patients may be of many religious and ethnic backgrounds. For practising Christians, the clergy has a vital role as a friend and confidant who will discuss with the dying person their hopes and fears, their plans for their families, the fact that they are dying and the consequences of their death. The hospital chaplain's job includes comforting relatives as well as caring for patients, and also a willingness to care for staff.

The nurse should become informed regarding the religious and cultural background of the dying patient.

Meeting the needs of the family

While many patients will have been well up until the moment of the crisis, such as heart attack or accident, that brought them to the critical care unit, other patients will arrive just as ill, yet quite aware and prepared for death. However, even if patients come to terms with death and are ready to relinquish life, those around them may not reach that point at the same time.

News of impending death is best communicated to the family group rather than to an individual member and should be done in a setting of privacy where the family can behave naturally and without restraint of public display (Engel, 1964).

The death, or impending death, of a family member usually increases the emotional dependency of other members upon each other. The family is usually a source of comfort, support and sympathy for all of its members.

Ideally, the bereaved individual should feel that someone has a personal interest in their welfare and that there is someone available to whom they can talk freely and who will not consider it an imposition. The bereaved should be encouraged to express their emotions through talking, crying and venting their hostility and feelings of guilt. Their responses need to be accepted without criticism or shock (Hampe, 1975).

Relatives who have been presented with an optimistic outlook will need extra support, and feelings of guilt may need to be worked through by relatives and the nurse together. For example, if the patient has been unconscious for a long time, the survivors may feel guilty when relief is the dominant emotion they feel.

Euphemisms such as 'passed away' or 'no longer with us' are often used to describe and avoid the use of the word 'dead' or 'died'. Whatever approach is used, once death has occurred this needs to be conveyed unambiguously to the family so that they can begin the process of grieving. Relatives may wish to see the dead person. The nurse should prepare them as to what to expect; this experience may help the relatives in accepting the reality of the death. Family members and close friends should not be rushed to leave, but rather encouraged to say their private goodbyes. They should be given a telephone number in case they have any queries.

The nurse may wish to contact them to enquire as to how they are coping, and to offer them an opportunity to meet to discuss it.

Practical issues, such as dealing with the deceased's personal property and the death certificate, need to be handled with tact and sensitivity. It may be more appropriate to give such information to a more distant relative. Certainly, such information should be unambiguous, provided in a written form, and include a contact name and telephone number.

A particularly distressing event for the family may be when they are requested to give permission for a *post-mortem*. They may feel guilty about refusing permission because it hinders the advancement of medical science.

Worden (1983) points out that there are certain tasks which must be accomplished before a loved one can adjust to a bereavement:

- ☐ To accept the reality of the loss.
- ☐ To experience the pain of grief.
- ☐ To adjust to an environment in which the deceased is missing.
- ☐ To withdraw emotional energy and reinvest it in another relationship.

Efforts to help the bereaved should encourage the expression of normal grief – the resolution of grief – and should discourage the development of pathological, abnormal, or persistent grief.

To plan interventions for helping grieving persons help themselves an accurate assessment of their grief is required. Raphael (1983) suggests the following assessments of the bereaved that yield information but also facilitate the expression of emotion and promote the grieving process:

1. *Tell me a little about the death. What happened?* These questions give the griever permission to talk about the death while providing information about the nature and circumstances of the death. At the same time, the griever's feelings, ability to talk about the death and stresses related to it can be evaluated.
2. *Tell me about (name the deceased) and about your lives together?* This opening allows the nurse to evaluate the relationship, particularly with regards to its quality and the interactions associated with it. It also provides the opportunity to determine whether there is any denial of the loss, and whether the griever speaks of the loss in realistic terms.
3. *What has been happening since the death? How have things been with your family and friends?* This question provides the opportunity to explore patterns of family and social support that the bereaved perceive to be available. It also provides the opportunity to assess other crises that may affect the grieving process.
4. *Have you been through any other bad times recently or when you were younger?* This offers the opportunity to explore past and present experiences, and opens the way to help the bereaved identify successful ways of coping.

People need to grieve in their own way, and to be reassured that the common physical reactions are normal and will pass, however painful.

The experience of dying may serve as a cohesive force in some families and a disruptive force in others. In general, families who have responded to stresses or crises as a unified force in the past will offer each other strength and support.

Making a will

In the busy atmosphere of a patient dying, often suddenly and unexpectedly, it is easy to overlook the availability of a will. The nurse may be asked about the advisability of making a will and should encourage the dying patient to do so.

Organ donation

Body organs and tissues, such as the kidneys, heart, liver, pancreas, corneas, may be donated by the patient for availability for transplants. Donor cards are in common use and cover the requirements of the Anatomy Act 1984. The bereaved family may decide to donate the patient's organs, in which case the next of kin would have to grant permission.

Nurses may find that they are involved in discussing such matters with the patient or family, and therefore they must be sensitive, compassionate and articulate. Particular care must be taken to ensure that these individuals are not coerced into agreeing to organ donations or made to feel guilty for refusing.

Most critical care units have access to a person such as an Organ Transplant Coordinator, whose expertise is invaluable.

Meeting the needs of nurses

Caring for the critically ill and dying is a major stressor for nurses (Caldwell and Weiner, 1981). Stress sources include workload, organizational support, home-work conflict, dealing with patients and relatives, and role confidence and competence.

In critical care units a factor most commonly referred to as causing stress for nurses is lack of support in dealing with death and dying. In a recent study, Cooper and Mitchell (1990) assessed stressors associated with nursing the critically ill and dying. They investigated 117 nurses from a number of coronary care, cancer and other hospital units, together with hospice nurses. They found that hospital nurses dealing with death and dying were significantly more job dissatisfied than hospice nurses. However, hospice nurses were significantly more anxious and showed more signs of psychosomatic complaints.

The sources of stress include coping with a patient's awareness of their forthcoming death, death trajectory and the special nature and importance of the, often final, relationship between the nurse and the patient (Cooper and Mitchell, 1990).

Vachon (1987) believes that emotional involvement with the dying is an important source of stress for nurses, and that is may interfere with their personal lives. Vachon (1978) suggests five ways of improving coping skills for staff working with the dying:

1. The encouragement of personal insight to understand and acknowledge one's own limits.
2. A healthy balance between work and outside life.
3. The promotion of a team approach to care.
4. An ongoing support system within work and outside work.

5. For those working in isolation, continuing guidance and support, from peers and superiors.

Better training and preparation may help, but a system of social and psychological support for nurses is an important corollary to individualized patient care (Field, 1989c).

It is important for nurses and doctors working in critical care units to have regular opportunities to discuss issues of death and dying. Other health professionals and specialists, such as a chaplain, psychologist or social worker, may be involved. 'Death meetings' are sometimes used as a forum to discuss, plan or evaluate the care of a dying patient, or to carry out a '*post-mortem*' on the care of a patient who has recently died. Such meetings might occasionally include recently bereaved relatives.

Nurses who have cared for a dying patient for a lengthy duration are likely to require support and some respite from this stressful situation. Primary nursing, for example, can provoke stress and isolation in the nurse. Nurses might feel that they are expected to shoulder the burden of responsibility for a particular dying patient and become isolated and reluctant to seek help. There needs to be an opportunity, therefore, to discuss and reflect on such issues at the end of each shift.

SUMMARY

This chapter has sought to describe the responses that can be observed when working with the dying patient and their family, and the needs and concerns of the patient and family. The chapter has also sought to discuss the research pertaining to nurses' attitudes towards death and dying, communication with the dying, and the care of the dying patient and family, as well as suggesting appropriate nursing interventions in caring for them. Finally, the chapter has sought to briefly address nurses' reactions to working with dying patients, and the support of nurses caring for them.

Critical care units are geared to preserving life, and thus for many nurses and doctors who practice in these settings, the meaning of death is a failure. Yet at times, the inevitability of death must be acknowledged in the critical care unit. The provision of good quality nursing care so that the person dies comfortably and retains dignity demands a variety of attributes, not least of which include skill, knowledge, sensitivity and compassion. However, there is a real danger that the care of the dying might be delegated to the most junior or least qualified nurse while the more senior nurse handles what is often, but erroneously, considered to be the more complicated or 'technical' aspects of nursing care.

Nurses' attitudes and communication skills, the mode of organization of nursing care and the support networks for nurses, are fundamentally important factors which affect the quality of care the dying patient and family receive.

It is important to listen and be sensitive to the patient's and family's feelings and concerns about dying, and include them in discussions and decisions about care. It is also important to recognize that caring for the dying patient and family is a major stressor for nurses. Though education and experience may be helpful, a system of social and psychological support is also necessary.

Some important issues, such as the ethical justification for terminating or withholding treatment and discontinuing life support, definitions of death and the impact of Acquired Immune Deficiency Syndrome (AIDS), present serious dilemmas, and have implications for the nursing care of the dying. These issues, however, are beyond the scope of this chapter.

Care of the dying patient and their family can present the critical care nurse with one of the greatest challenges, and whilst it is certainly not easy, it is invariably one of the most rewarding aspects of nursing.

ACKNOWLEDGEMENT

Grateful thanks are extended to Rose Webster, Clinical Nurse Specialist, Coronary Care Unit, Leicester General Hospital, for her helpful comments.

CASE STUDIES

Case study one

James White is a 63 year old retired teacher who had a kidney transplant three years ago. He and his wife are well known to the critical care unit. Over the past few months James's renal failure has progressively worsened and he has been re-admitted to the unit. Initially, he and his family were optimistic and planning for the future. However, despite dialysis and drug therapy, James has significantly deteriorated and the nurses feel that the prospect of James's death needs to be discussed. After consultation with other members of the health care team, the primary nurse discusses this with James and his wife. It transpires that James recognizes that he has not been this ill before and has been talking about dying to his wife, even though she has been discouraging this. Now, although upset, she feels more able to discuss the subject and hopes that she can be a source of support for her husband. The control of pain and discomfort are identified as nursing priorities, and Mrs White is encouraged to become involved in the physical care of her husband. She values the honest approach of the staff, but still holds out hope for recovery. James, although initially angry at the prospect of dying and later somewhat depressed and withdrawn, now appears calm and to appreciate the close contact with his family. He feels reassured that he and his wife have made provisional plans for her future. James eventually becomes unconscious and dies with his family around him. The nurses feel that they have helped James and his family through a difficult time.

Case study two

Bill Jones, a 38 year old factory worker, has been admitted to a critical care unit after complaining of chest pain whilst at work. On admission he appears cheerful, reporting that his pain has almost gone. The nurse admitting him telephones his wife Pam at home to tell her what has happened, reassuring her that he seems better. Pam says that she will visit after picking up their two young children from school. Half an hour later Bill suffers a cardiac arrest and resuscitation attempts prove unsuccessful. The nurse is very upset, feeling guilty at not reporting the potential seriousness of Bill's condition and advising his wife to visit sooner. Unable to contact Pam, the nurse worries about what to tell her when she arrives. When Pam does arrive with the children, the senior nurse asks her into the office whilst a colleague looks after the children. The senior nurse informs Pam of her husband's death. She is distraught and angry at not being told how poorly he was.

Pam becomes more subdued and seems to want to talk about her husband and their life together. She admits to feeling guilty about an argument she and Bill had that morning, and is sorry that she could not say goodbye to him. Later, her parents arrive to take her and the children home. They are given the unit telephone number and encouraged to ring at any time. The staff meet at the end of the shift to discuss events. The nurse who admitted Bill expresses gratitude to the senior nurse for support and for speaking to his wife. All the staff seem to benefit from talking things through prior to going home.

STUDENT LEARNING QUESTIONS

1. As the senior nurse on duty at the time of Bill Jones' death, how would you have broached the subject of his death to his wife, Pam?

2. What would you have said and done to support the nurse who had been caring for Bill?

3. After the initial shock of her husband's death, Pam wanted to talk about him and their life together. How would you have facilitated this?

4. As James's primary nurse, what would have been your strategy for discussing his deteriorating condition and bleak outlook with him and his wife?

5. Mrs White knew that her husband was dying and wanted to be involved in his care. What were her needs likely to have been and, as a primary nurse, how would you have ensured that they were met?

KEY TERMS

Anticipatory grief

Grief experienced prior to the death of a loved one.

Bereavement

State of being that results from a significant loss.

Death

Permanent cessation of all vital functions, the end of human life.

Dying

Process of coming to an end; the final act of living.

Grief

Outcome of being bereaved.

Loss

State of being deprived of or being without a valued object.

Mourning

Social prescription for way in which one is expected to show one's grief.

FURTHER READING

Cook, A. S., Oltjenbruns, K. A. *Dying and Grieving: Lifespan and Family Perspectives.* New York: Holt, Rinehart and Winston, 1989.

Field, D. *Nursing the Dying.* London: Tavistock/Routledge, 1989.

Jackson, I. Bereavement follow-up service in intensive care. *Intensive and Critical Care Nursing.* 1992; 8: 163–168.

Stroebe, M. S., Stroebe, W., Hansson, R. O. (Eds.). *Handbook of Bereavement.* Cambridge: Cambridge University Press, 1993.

REFERENCES

Books

Bowlby, J. *Attachment and Loss: Loss, Sadness and Depression. Vol. III.* New York: Basic Books, 1980.

Charmaz, K. *The Social Reality of Death.* Menlo Park, CA: Addison-Wesley, 1980.

Cook, A. S., Oltjenbruns, K. A. *Dying and Grieving: Lifespan and Family Perspectives.* New York: Holt, Rinehart and Winston, 1989.

Field, D. *Nursing the Dying.* London: Tavistock/Routledge, 1989a.

Glaser, B. G., Strauss, A. L. *Awareness of Dying.* Chicago, IL: Aldine Press, 1965.

Glaser, B. G., Strauss, A. L. *Time for Dying.* Chicago, IL: Aldine Press, 1968.

Gow, K. M. *How Nurses' Emotions Affect Patient Care.* New York: Springer-Verlag, 1982.

Hinton, J. *Dying.* Harmondsworth: Pelican, 1972.

Kastenbaum, R. *Death, Society and Human Experience.* St. Louis, MI: C V Mosby, 1981.

Kubler-Ross, E. *On Death and Dying.* London: Tavistock, 1970.

Parkes, C. M. *Bereavement: Studies of Grief in Adult Life.* Harmondsworth: Penguin, 1986.

Pattison, E. M. *The Experience of Dying.* Englewood Cliffs, NJ: Prentice-Hall, 1977.

Quint, J. *The Nurse and the Dying Patient.* New York: Macmillan, 1967.

Raphael, B. *The Anatomy of Bereavement.* New York: Basic Books, 1983.

Vachon, M. C. S. *Occupational Stress in Caring for the Critically Ill, the Dying, and the Bereaved.* Washington, DC: Hemisphere, 1987.

Weisman, A. D. *The Realization of Death: a Guide for Psychological Autopsy.* New York: J. Aronson, 1974.

Worden, J. W. *Grief Counselling and Grief Therapy.* London: Tavistock, 1983.

Chapters in Edited Books

Benoliel, J. Q. Institutional dying: a convergence of cultural values, terminology, and social organization. In Eds. H. Wass, F. M. Berardo, R. A. Neimeyer. *Dying: Facing the Facts.* Washington, DC: Hemisphere, 1988, pp 159–184.

Periodicals

Breu, C., Dracup, K. Helping the spouses of critically ill patients. *American Journal of Nursing.* 1978: 78: 51–53.

Bugen, L. A. Coping: effects of death education. *Omega.* 1980; 11: 175–183.

Caldwell, T., Weiner, M.F. Stresses and coping in ICU nursing. *General Hospital Psychiatry.* 1981; 3: 119–127.

Cooper, C. L., Mitchell, S. Nursing the critically ill and dying. *Human Relations.* 1990; 43: 297–311.

Daley, L. The perceived immediate needs of families with relatives in the intensive care setting. *Heart & Lung.* 1984; 13: 231–237.

Durlak, J. A. Comparison between experiential and didactic methods of death education. *Omega*. 1978; 9: 57–66.

Engel, G. L. Grief and grieving. *American Journal of Nursing*. 1964; 64: 93–98.

Field, D. Formal teaching about death and dying in UK nursing schools. *Nurse Education Today*. 1986; 6: 270–276.

Field, D. Emotional involvement with the dying in a coronary care unit. *Nursing Times*. Occasional Paper. 1989b; 85(13): 46–48.

Field, D. Nurses' accounts of nursing the terminally ill on a coronary care unit. *Intensive Care Nursing*. 1989c; 5: 114–122.

Field, D. Communicating with dying patients in coronary care units. *Intensive & Critical Care Nursing*. 1992; 8: 24–32

Hampe, S. O. Needs of the grieving spouse in a hospital setting. *Nursing Research*. 1975; 24: 113–120.

Hurtig, W. A., Stewin, L. The effect of death education and experience on nursing students' attitude towards death. *Journal of Advanced Nursing*. 1990; 15: 29–34.

Jones, D. R. Heart disease mortality following widowhood: some results from the OPCS longitudinal study. *Journal of Psychosomatic Research*. 1987; 32: 325–333.

Lindemann, E. Symptomatology and management of acute grief. *American Journal of Psychiatry*. 1944; 101: 141–148.

Lundin, T. Morbidity following sudden and unexpected bereavement. *British Journal of Psychiatry*. 1984a; 144: 84–88.

Lundin, T. Long-term outcome of bereavement. *British Journal of Psychiatry*. 1984b; 145: 424–428.

Maddison, D. C., Viola, A. The health of widows in the year following bereavement. *Journal of Psychosomatic Research*. 1968; 12: 297–306.

Maguire, P. Barriers to psychological care of the dying. *British Medical Journal*. 1985; 291: 1711–1713.

Miles, M. S. The effects of a course on death and grief on nurses' attitudes towards dying patients and death. *Death Education*. 1980; 4: 245–260.

Molter, N. C. Needs of relatives of critically ill patients: a descriptive study. *Heart & Lung*. 1979; 8: 332–339.

Murphy, P. A. Reduction in nurses' death anxiety following a death awareness workshop. *Journal of Continuing Education in Nursing*. 1986; 17: 115–118.

Murray, P. Death education and its effect on the death anxiety level of nurses. *Psychological Reports*. 1974; 35: 1250.

Nimocks, M. J. A., Webb, L., Connell, J .R. Communication and the terminally ill: a theoretical model. *Death Studies*. 1987; 11: 323–344.

Parkes, C. M., Benjamin, B., Fitzgerald, R. G. Broken heart: a statistical study of increased mortality among widowers. *British Medical Journal*. 1969; 1: 740–743.

Raphael, B. Preventative intervention with the recently bereaved. *Archives of General Psychiatry*. 1977; 34: 1450–1454.

Ross, C. Nurses' personal death concerns and responses to dying-patient statements. *Nursing Research*. 1978; 27: 64–68.

Seale, C. Communication and awareness about death: a study of a random sample of dying people. *Social Science and Medicine*. 1991; 32: 943–952.

Stoller, E. Impact of death-related fears on attitudes of nurses in a hospital work setting. *Omega*. 1980; 11: 85–95.

Vachon, M. Motivation and stress experienced by staff working with the terminally ill. *Death Education*. 1978; 2: 113–122.

13
ETHICAL ASPECTS OF CRITICAL CARE

Cei Tuxill

CHAPTER AIMS

The aims of this chapter fall into two main sections: those concerned with a more general introduction to the nature of ethical inquiry, and those concerned with the application of ethics in health care, in particular in the field of critical care nursing.

The first section, 'The Literature and Research', has as its aims:

☐ to introduce the main content and typical processes and procedures of ethical inquiry;

☐ to explore the difficulties in, and some methods of, identifying an ethical issue or problem;

☐ to consider some typical forms of moral reasoning;

☐ to examine three principal types of moral theory.

The second section, 'Practical Nursing Implications' has as its aims:

☐ to examine applied ethics, bioethics and, in particular, nursing ethics;

☐ to identify four possible principles of nursing ethics and their implications;

☐ to examine some of the moral dilemmas that occur in critical care ethics.

THE MAIN ISSUES

The main issues dealt with in this chapter concern, in the first section, the nature of ethical inquiry and decision-making in terms of a fairly constant range of subject matter and of methods. One issue is the importance, and sometimes the difficulty, of accurately identifying moral problems, and some of the features by which they may be recognized are suggested. Some common types of moral argument are considered, and a model for approaching moral dilemmas is explored. This section concludes with a brief look at three types of moral theory: absolutist type theories; consequentialist or utilitarian ones; and those based on human flourishing and the human virtues.

The second section moves into the field of applied ethics, in particular health care, and identifies nursing ethics as a key contributor to the development of ethical models for health care. Four principles of nursing ethics are proposed, respect for autonomy, non-maleficence, beneficence and justice, and their implications in practice for critical care nursing briefly explored. Consent and paternalism are identified as two of the main moral concerns which occur in the application of these principles. Finally, some of the key moral problems facing the critical care nurse are noted, and those centering around two key areas are explored further: decisions about initiating intensive therapy and, crucially, that group of dilemmas associated with decisions about withdrawing life-sustaining treatment. In this context, the morality of suicide is an important issue which is considered, together with the usefulness of the distinction between 'ordinary' and 'extraordinary' methods of treatment and the problems of judging 'quality of life'.

THE LITERATURE AND RESEARCH

The meaning of ethics

One way in which to approach the attempt to elucidate the nature and distinctive practice of ethics and ethical inquiry is to divide what might well prove an unwieldy and confusing enterprise into more manageable parts. These will inevitably overlap, and the division will to some extent be artificial, but may perhaps give some structure to the discussion which follows. I propose, then, to begin by looking at ethics in general, both in terms of what might be called its content or subject matter, and in terms of the characteristic methods by which it approaches this content. The discussion will move next to the question of identifying the characteristic features of a moral issue or problem and the importance of accurate and sensitive identification and classification. From there it will progress to an examination of the nature of moral reasoning, and will survey, briefly, some models which have been proposed for dealing with moral dilemmas and disputes, in the form of strategies for decision-making and of substantial moral theories.

The subject matter of ethics

Accounts of the content of ethics tend to overlap with general descriptions of its processes and purposes. The first and most obvious point to make is that ethics is a branch of philosophy, and its major concern is to apply the methods of philosophical inquiry, whatever they may turn out to be, to the realm of mortality, whatever, in turn, that may turn

out to contain. Raphael (1981), for example, categorizes moral philosophy as "philosophical inquiry about norms and values, about ideas of right and wrong, good and bad, what should and should not be done" (p. 8). This gives us an indication of some at least of the content of ethics, incorporating both ideas, 'right and wrong', standards, 'norms and values' and behaviour, 'what should and what should not be done'. This dual concern with both ideas or beliefs and action is essential. He goes on to describe the main purpose of moral philosophy, "as practised in the Western world", as being the critical evaluation of assumption and argument. Every society, and every cultural group (and health care practitioners would count as a cultural group for these purposes), he claims, tends to accept without question a number of beliefs: questioning these does not happen just 'out of the blue' but is often due to a conflict between old and new beliefs. This latter is an important point, that ethical inquiry is not some merely theoretical and self-generating activity, carried on for its own sake by unworldly academics, or at least, should not be only that, but is a response to the real world and its events and vicissitudes. In a specifically health care context, Jameton (1984) argues, in general terms, that the eruption of ethical problems is a symptom of crisis, reflecting sharpened feelings of frustration, chaos and loss of control (p. 2), and, more specifically, that the rapid increase in studies of ethics in the health sciences can be traced to the burgeoning uncertainty, distress and dilemmas arising in clinical practice (p. 57).

One of the key areas of which this is true, it can be argued with some conviction, is critical care where developments in technology, in particular, have thrown previous certainties and values into disarray, not least by making possible achievements which had previously been regarded as beyond human control and so raising the question of whether, when and how these new powers should be deployed. This process has challenged far more fundamental and general beliefs in a way that, as Curtin and Flaherty (1981) recognize, is characteristic of moral problems. The answers to, in fact the very existence of, these problems have far reaching effects, not just on the immediate topic, but on our perceptions of human beings, their relations to one another, to society and to the world itself. Further attempts at definition add detail, both to the content and to the characteristic methods and concerns of ethics. Grassian (1981), for example, claims that what distinguishes ethics, that is the philosophical study of morality, whose content he lists as "right conduct, moral obligation, moral character, moral responsibility social justice and the nature of the good life" (p. 3) is its "generality, systematic nature and above all its attempts to prove its claims through arguments" (p. 3) and adds, as a characteristic concern of moral inquiry, the attempt to unify divergent moral beliefs and judgements about particular questions and issues, to arrive at general underlying moral principles. This is amplified by Teichman and Evans (1991), who include in the list of topics with which ethics is concerned: the justification of moral codes; motivation, in particular altruism and selfishness; moral principles; happiness; justice; courage and, in a general way, human states which are regarded as valuable and desirable or valueless and undesirable (pp. 2–3). Jameton (1984) summarizes this by describing philosophers as being interested in discovering, analysing, challenging and systematizing the principles, concepts and reasoning underlying our daily choices and conduct. One method of systematization is to seek to distinguish various forms or levels of inquiry. Jameton suggests, therefore, that the study of ethics can be roughly divided into three levels: exploring the central and basic values which we hold and which have some claim on us, the conventional values; exploring values and principles in a deeper way, finding the more fundamental principles which underlie specific conventional ones, which involves the development of concepts like 'respect for persons', 'justice', 'rights' and of general and unified theories; and exploring the more general methods and definitions used in the first two levels, that is meta-ethics, the study of the study of ethics itself. This division into levels is paralleled by a number of other theorists in a variety of ways. Beauchamp and Childress (1983) provide a more substantial version of this distinction in their account of the difference between rules and principles; principles, they claim, are more general and fundamental than moral rules (e.g. 'do not lie') and serve as their foundation and source of justification; theories, in turn, are bodies of principles which are more or less systematically related (p. 5).

For Billington (1988), similarly, principles are concerned with the overriding aims of human behaviour, rules with the application of those aims in daily situations.

Seedhouse (1988) proposes a stratification based on distinct though cognate criteria which can be seen as a route or trajectory through a moral issue; 'dramatic ethics', immediate, difficult hard choices and dilemmas; persisting ethics, continuing, underlying issues; general ethics', how we should live and how we should act. This is echoed by McNaughton's (1988) division into three 'branches' of ethics; practical ethics, the study of particular moral problems; moral theory, the attempt to develop a theory of morals which will give a general method of answering moral problems; and questions about the nature and structure of moral thought, meta-ethics.

The final general point to be made about ethics, one which has already been shadowed in the discussion so far, is that it is an intensely practical activity, not simply in the previously noted sense of being a response to conflict and uncertainty, but in the more immediate sense of being inherently designed to guide conduct or practice (Singer, 1979, p. 2). One does ethics properly, Finnis (1983) asserts, only if one is questioning and reflecting so as to be able to act. This connection with action is built into the definition of ethics. Ethical examination implies, as Pierce (1989) maintains, the use of reasoned, logical argumentation to arrive at judgements about what to do, what to value and what virtues to cultivate. Ethics, then, has as its subject matter a particular and comprehensive area of human life, encompassing both reflection, belief and behaviour, involving values, principles and standards, including the widest and most fundamental choices about one's own personality and character. It has as its method the systematic questioning and analysing of this content with the aim in part being the achieving of generality and consistency, but also, vitally, the guiding of conduct and practice.

Two more particular questions, however, present themselves at this juncture, given that we have a general overview of the nature and process of ethical inquiry: how do we recognize particular ethical problems and issues when they present themselves and distinguish them reliably from other kinds of problem, particularly technical or factual ones and, once we have done so, how specifically do we go about tackling them; what are the characteristic modes of ethical reasoning? These two questions are necessarily interdependent, in that one of the reasons for which it is so important that ethical problems should be identified is precisely in order that inappropriate methods should not be used, since the results of such a misapplication of technique can be disastrous.

The recognition of a moral dilemma

Though it may appear obvious that most people can and do recognize moral issues, dilemmas, principles and judgements when they appear, it is neither obvious nor uncontentious how they do so. It is, nevertheless, important that an attempt should be made to arrive at some framework within which such a recognition can be structured and through which it might be rendered more reliable and accurate, perhaps more so in the field of bioethics or health care ethics than elsewhere. One reason for this is that the danger of confusing moral issues with practical, medical or technical ones is very real, as is the temptation to do so. One possible explanation for the strength of this temptation lies in the nature of moral argument and judgement itself, and precisely in those features in which it differs from scientific or technical practices and procedures, its apparent uncertainty and ambiguity. Unlike, in ideal at least, scientific, technical and medical problems and solutions, ethical questions are not amenable to empirical investigation, scientific methods of analysis and firm resolution.

It is this, the nature of moral thinking and its difference from scientific modes of thought and inquiry, which is the reason why the accurate recognition of moral issues is crucial. To attempt to apply the methods of the physical, or even the social, sciences and to seek the same type of answers is to court confusion and frustration. It is this attempt to apply inappropriate methods that leads to much of the impatience and bafflement that seem to accompany moral problems, and to the complaint that 'there are no answers' often with the apparently explanatory rider that 'it's all a matter of individual opinion or feeling, anyway'.

A further reason for the importance of moral recognition is that once an issue is identified, the location of decision making itself alters; the question of who has the right to, and the responsibility for, making and contributing to decisions becomes contentious and, itself, an ethical issue. Indeed, some of the most intractable moral dilemmas in health care are precisely those which focus on the rights of various individuals to make the final decision.

A number of writers have advanced suggestions, of variable degrees of specificity, for the recognition or definition of a moral issue; these typically tend to refer to the content of such issues. In some cases, they identify particular locations or causes of moral problems, and in others, the kinds of puzzlement or disagreement that are involved. Billington (1988), for example, puts forward as characteristic of moral issues: that no-one can avoid them; that they involve other people; that they matter, in that they affect the lives and self-esteem and happiness of others; that there can never be a final and definitive solution; that they necessarily involve choice; that they aim to discover the right form of action, and that, ironically, while there is no definitive answer, action is unavoidable. Jameton (1984), in turn, gives a four-point account of the nature of moral issues: issues involving important social values and norms, for example respect for life, independence, love; issues which involve conscience, and arouse feelings such as guilt, shame, self-esteem; issues to which we respond by using such words as 'right', 'wrong', 'good', 'bad', 'should', 'ought'; issues that appear unusually complex, frustrating, irresoluble or difficult. Beauchamp and Childress (1983) offer a categorization in terms of moral concerns as those that are accepted as supreme or overriding, which are universalizable and which involve human welfare. It is possible to extract from these accounts some typical or persisting symptoms by which the presence of a moral dilemma may be diagnosed: it will involve a certain content, including such established principles as respect for life, or the rights of individuals or such notions as happiness or welfare; it will employ a certain characteristic vocabulary, that of 'good', 'bad', 'ought', 'right', or the vocabulary of certain character traits, 'courage', 'kindness', 'meanness' or 'honesty'; the issue will appear particularly important, imperative, and demanding and will involve characteristic emotions such as guilt, shame and remorse; the decision will not be allowed to stand on its own, but will have wide reaching implications for other areas of conduct and debate; finally, it will be directly and unavoidably connected with action.

Jameton (1984) goes further, to provide a more detailed categorization of moral issues into: moral uncertainty; moral dilemmas and moral distress. Moral uncertainty arises when we are unsure which principle or value applies or, even, what the moral problem is: a moral dilemma comes about when one or more moral principles conflict; moral distress occurs when we are clear about the right thing to do but are prevented by restraints of one sort or another from doing it. The notion of a moral dilemma seems to be one that attracts much attention from commentators, perhaps because it can appear to be the most puzzling and painful of moral experiences. Mitchell (1990) categorizes it as that situation in which two things taken for granted ethically collide and doing one precludes the possibility of doing the other. She emphasizes that not every ethical issue is a moral dilemma and provides, as an illuminating example of a typical moral dilemma that might occur in the critical care setting, a situation in which a nurse believes that it would be 'torturing' a child to engage in various painful interventions when the child will be permanently ventilator-dependent and in a near vegetative state, whereas the mother thinks this would be 'caring' for the child and that everything possible should be done. In Mitchell's example, the dilemma belongs to the senior nurse who sympathizes with both. But it also illustrates not only some of the typical features of a moral dilemma, but also how, particularly in health care settings, these can take the form of a dispute between different interested individuals. There is the disagreement over the meaning of certain highly charged emotion and value laden words; a conflict about what ought to be done between two, or more, participants in the form of a dispute about who is the best, or who has the right, to decide; a conflict of loyalties when two people's interests or welfare conflict and, a feature endemic to moral disputes in the field of critical care, there is an apparent contradiction between quality of life and sanctity of life.

Rushton (1988) also identifies settings in which moral dilemmas may be a product of a conflict of loyalties: to oneself; to colleagues and other members of the health care team; to the profession itself; to patients and their families; to the employing institution and even to society. It would seem, indeed, that a conflict of loyalties is one of the most common forms that a moral dilemma can take in the health care setting.

Pierce (1989) extends the notion of ethical dilemmas as a conflict between participants by identifying typical areas in which ethical dilemmas can occur: nurse-patient interactions, where, for example, a patient may refuse treatment which the nurse thinks necessary or beneficial; nurse-colleague interactions, where colleagues are incompetent or fail to treat patients with respect; nurse-institution interactions, where the admission, placement or discharge of patients is at issue or conditions are unsafe. Critical care settings, in particular, would appear to be fertile ground for the growth of moral dilemmas; as Uustal (1990) points out, involvement with people who are critically ill makes nurses vulnerable to a conflict of values and confronts them with a myriad of ethical dilemmas.

Forms of moral reasoning

Once a moral dilemma has been identified the problem then arises of how to tackle it. Is there a set of techniques or procedures which are particularly appropriate to and effective in the handling and solution of moral dilemmas?

In one sense, it is true that moral philosophy, unlike the sciences and social sciences, has no methods and techniques, whether for discovering information, testing hypotheses or establishing and verifying conclusions that are peculiarly and exclusively its own. The processes and procedures are largely those of everyday discussion and argument rather than of some esoteric and unfamiliar systems. One type of comment that is frequently made in the literature, therefore, is the negative one of specifying, more or less forcefully, what moral argument is not, primarily that it is not scientific, empirical, factual, a matter of observation and the amassing of factual information but neither is it a matter of 'common sense', intuition or emotion.

Curtin and Flaherty (1981), for example, claim that ethical problems cannot be resolved by an appeal to empirical data and are inherently perplexing. Fitzpatrick (1988) notes the peculiarly intractable nature of ethical issues, in their guise as philosophical ones, in particular that they are not resoluble by the application of standard procedures yielding definite and generally accepted solutions and unamenable to solution by common sense or the special sciences. Jameton (1984) characterizes this as, in general, the difference between normative and descriptive issues. Fowler (1990) notes that ethical decision making is always decision-making under conditions of uncertainty; ethical questions cannot be settled by acquiring all the facts, since they are questions of value not of fact.

There are, despite this, some forms of argument which appear with particular frequency in the equipment of moral philosophy. One such, very general but distinctive, approach and the one which, in particular, tends to give philosophy its unsavoury reputation for avoiding rather than tackling problems, can be referred to as the 'socratic' method (and perhaps goes some way to explain why Socrates was put to death, since it is very annoying for those on whom it is practised). This is the method which, rather than seeking to establish judgements or principles, confines itself to questioning and analysing them, letting their proposer discover in the course of the interrogation the insufficiency or contradictions in her beliefs (Grassian, 1981). Another method might be called 'testing to destruction'; this involves seeking to uncover the more general principle which is implied by, or supports, a particular moral judgement and then testing this against either imaginary or real life examples, anticipating that this will produce results repugnant to ordinary moral intuition or even common sense. If, for example, it is argued that a particular patient is no longer to be respected as a person and may, therefore, have her life support discontinued on the grounds that she lacks reason, communication and self-consciousness, the general principle is extracted, 'beings which lack those qualities are not to be respected' and is then tested against, the case of, for example, very young children or the severely mentally ill or impaired and the possibility of terminating their lives. A further familiar form of argument is the 'slippery slope';

roughly that if a principle is broken in one case, even though this particular instance is morally acceptable, there will be no barrier to its being broken in others which are not acceptable. For example, that if we allow the 'passive' voluntary euthanasia of the terminally ill and severely pain-ridden we will end by accepting the forcible killing of all people over the age of 70. There has been considerable dispute over this particular tactic (see Williams, 1985; and Lamb, 1988), but nonetheless, there do seem to be areas, in particular those of respect for human life and dignity, where it does have a firm purchase.

Some writers suggest more detailed strategies with which to approach moral dilemmas or disputes, usually in the form of a series of structured and ordered steps. One example of such a framework is Seedhouse's (1988) 'ethical grid'. This operates as a series of 'layers' which correspond to the four different sets of elements which make up comprehensive ethical deliberation (p. 127). These move outwards from a central 'blue' layer incorporating the core rationale of the idea of health (equal respect for persons, autonomy, needs and wants), through a 'red' layer, which focuses on duties and motives (promise keeping, truth telling, minimizing harm, beneficence) and corresponds to deontological theories of ethics, followed by a 'green' layer incorporating aspects of consequentialist ethics (individual good, social good) to the final, outer 'black' layer which deals with 'external' considerations.

Other approaches tend to focus more on steps in the decision making process than on content or actual values. Typically these tend to include the following stages:

Steps in the decision making process

1. Identify the problem.
2. Identify how you feel about it.
3. Identify the patient's values (significantly, this stage is often bypassed).
4. Identify the ethical principles involved and order them.
5. Determine the relevant factual information.
6. Identify who will be involved in the decision making.
7. Identify the values of the decision makers.

8. Examine and categorize the alternatives.
9. Rank order the various alternatives.
10. Decide upon a course of action.
11. Evaluate your action in relation to the current and possible future ethical dilemma's.

(Based on work by Uustal, 1990, and others.)

These are useful and reassuring formulae with which to approach what frequently appear to be confusing and intractable areas of professional practice. One of the difficulties with such approaches is, however, that far from being the neutral frameworks which they might at first sight appear they contain within themselves the very moral problems which they are designed to solve. Step one, for example, the identification of a moral problem is, as earlier sections have argued, itself morally loaded. What might be in general a routine procedure, blood transfusion, for example, becomes morally fraught when the intended recipient is a Jehovah's Witness. Examining possible alternatives cannot be, in such settings, a factual matter, since some outcomes will be ruled out even from initial consideration because of the moral repugnance they inspire even though they are practically perfectly possible. Identifying the decision makers is a matter of deciding on rights and duties rather than of simply picking out the facts. Determining the relevant factual information is similarly loaded, since what is to be counted as relevant is itself a matter for moral consideration. To take, for example, the ethnic origins, the religious affiliations or, even, the age of a patient as relevant to a decision about his or her treatment could, in most situations, be seen as morally wrong. Finally, the requirement to choose the alternative outcome which breaks the fewest moral principles or values or which produces the least harm or the most benefit for the patient throws into sharp focus one of the central sources of moral conflict, the operation of very distinct and, in application quite often contradictory, modes of thinking about moral matters, frequently categorized as the difference between absolutist, or deontological, moral theories and consequentialist ones.

Most commentaries (see, for example, Beauchamp and Childress (1983); Teichman and Evans (1991); Fitzpatrick (1988), Garrett *et al.* (1989)) divide ethical theories into two main types: absolutist or deontological theories and consequentialist or utilitarian theories. More recently, though, a third has become prominent, particularly in health care ethics, 'virtue-based' ethics focusing on human flourishing. Deontological theories are typified by a strategy for dealing with ethical issues which involves deploying against them an array of morally pre-coded concepts such as absolute values, duties, principles or rights. Various foundations are proposed for these; the will of God, human nature, nature itself, reason or the nature of morality itself. Moral principles might include: 'respect for persons'; 'do not kill'; 'do not lie'; 'do not break promises'. Rights would include such human or natural rights as the right to life, dignity, respect, freedom, autonomy and privacy. Garrett *et al.* (1989) characterize deontological ethics as those which determine the rightness or wrongness of an action in terms of certain formal properties which it possesses, such as duty, justice or respect for autonomy, independent of its consequences.

For consequentialist theories, in contrast, the focus is on the results of the action rather than the action itself, on states of affairs and their goodness and badness rather than on actions and their rightness and wrongness. Consequentialist modes of reasoning do not have recourse to prior notions such as rights, duties and principles; they refer only to consequences. For the classical Utilitarianism of Bentham (1948) and Mill (1962), the only consequence of moral significance is happiness; the good action is that which has the consequence of making as many people as happy as possible (Teichman and Evans, 1991). Later utilitarians have modified this, either to include a plurality of 'goods' such as friendship and beauty (Moore, 1959) or knowledge or, because of difficulties with the concept of happiness, into 'preference' utilitarianism in which that action is good that satisfies as many people's preferences as possible. The basic principle remains the same, however; actions are judged not in terms of their intrinsic character or by comparison with some absolute rule, but solely by their results.

Both types of theory generate problems in application. Deontological theories can, indeed, be seen as paradigmatic sources of the classical moral dilemma when two principles, rights or values conflict. Utilitarian theories either seem to demand actions which are repugnant to intuitive moral consciousness, sacrificing justice or the rights of individuals to the general interest, or to be unable to take account of the special relationships to individuals that are created by promises, duties, roles and responsibilities. One version of utilitarianism, rule or restricted utilitarianism, does go some way to remedying this by applying the test of utility to rules rather than particular actions, and so restoring most principles, values and obligations to the moral vocabulary.

It is not difficult to see, however, how in particular situations the application of these two theories can generate moral problems, when absolute rights or rules come into intractable conflict with happiness and welfare.

A third type of theory has recently been advocated, in particular in health care ethics, neo-Aristotelianism (Hursthouse, 1987) or virtue ethics, the ethics of human flourishing. Fitzpatrick (1988), for example, defines morality as a matter of human flourishing, as does Seedhouse (1988), who identifies as truly immoral the deliberate restriction of human potential and defines "the system with the goal of the fullest possible individual human flourishing" as "the most moral system of care" (p. 89). This pattern of moral thought focuses on those features of the human being which are regarded as most typical and most valuable, and judges actions by whether they tend to promote or inhibit them, using the language of virtues and vices to do so.

PRACTICAL NURSING IMPLICATIONS

This section will be 'practical' in the sense of seeking to apply the concepts, methods and theories explored in the previous section to the moral problems and issues that occur in the actual practice of nursing, particularly in the field of critical care. It will start with a brief account of bioethics as a branch of applied ethics, and then move on to look at nursing ethics as a distinct and independent area within the wider field, with its own principles and key values, which will be identified and discussed. Finally, there will be an attempt to identify and examine some of those moral problems and

dilemmas which occur most frequently and crucially in critical care nursing.

Applied ethics, bioethics and nursing ethics

Beauchamp and Childress (1988) identify bioethics as one type of applied ethics, the application of general principles and rules to the problems of therapeutic practice, health care delivery and medical and biological research. A note of caution needs to be struck, here, however, in the form of a reminder that bioethics itself developed as a field of study partly because traditional principles and values failed to provide solutions to or, even, effective ways of considering, new problems in the field of health care such as those, in particular, created by new technology (Jameton, 1984), a factor of considerable importance in critical care nursing where ventilators, transplant techniques and other high technology interventions have generated new and increasingly difficult dilemmas.

Within the wider field of applied ethics, nursing ethics occupies a unique and important place. Nursing is of its nature, intrinsically and not merely incidentally a 'moral art' (Curtin and Flaherty, 1981, p. 8); since there exists a body of nursing practice which is specific and distinct from medical practice there are distinctive ethical problems which arise in nursing which differ significantly from medical ones (Fitzpatrick, 1988, p. x). This is to do, in part, with the nature of nursing as 'care', in part with the role of the nurse as 'patient advocate'. Jameton (1984) goes so far as to state that "nursing is the morally central health care profession. Philosophies of nursing, not medicine, should determine the image of health care and its future direction" (p. xvi). Other commentators emphasize the moral nature of nursing and the distinct nature of the ethics of caring as forming the characteristic role and purpose of the nurse (e.g. Fowler, 1990; Uustal, 1990; Levine, 1989), and identify as one of the nurse's main functions to attend and relate to a person in such a way as to protect them from "being reduced to the moral status of an object" (Fowler, 1990), a danger which is particularly acute in technologically sophisticated medicine (Braine and Lesser, 1988).

Given the aims, values and purposes inherent in the practice of nursing, in particular the nurses's role as 'patient advocate' and the types of moral problem and decision to which it typically gives rise, certain principles and concepts stand out as peculiarly cogent, appropriate and important. Particularly central are the principles of autonomy, non-maleficence, beneficence and justice (Beauchamp and Childress, 1988; Jameton, 1984; Jennet, 1986; Seedhouse, 1988); to these can be added truthfulness, fidelity and confidentiality. Together with these, in a sense giving practical and formal shape to them, goes the notion of patient rights. The overarching general principle, which forms the foundation and justification for the particular requirements and formulations, is that of 'respect for persons'.

Autonomy

Respect for the principle of autonomy entails that patients should be treated as rational, deliberating, thinking agents with values, preferences and purposes of their own, whose wishes, choices and priorities should be respected. In practice, this requires that patients should be provided with the opportunity and the environment necessary to enable them to make their own decisions; in particular, they must be given whatever information is necessary for informed choice in a manner which they can understand and, crucially, they must be protected from the various forms of coercion and undue influence which may operate. In critical care, because of the intimidating nature of the setting and, frequently, the extreme state and needs of the patient, this is a particularly acute requirement and will entail positive efforts to enhance independence rather than merely care to avoid influence and pressure, since sufficient of this will be provided by the unfamiliarity and oppressiveness of the environment itself. Autonomy means, in particular, that one of the key aims of nursing care must be to protect, enhance and, where necessary and possible, restore the autonomy and independence of patients, and that consequently one of the most serious wrongs that carers can perpetrate is to engage in practices which deprive the individuals in their care of independence or maturity or which encourage dependence and subjection (Seedhouse, 1988). Respect for autonomy, together with non-maleficence, is the principle that powers the

requirement of informed consent and is part of the foundation for the rule of truth telling or veracity.

One of the major difficulties confronting this principle in practice is posed by patients who might be regarded as, to a greater or lesser degree, incompetent to make choices. This is a particularly troubling issue in critical care nursing with its preponderance of highly dependent and severely ill patients, the high proportion of unconscious patients, the presence of high levels of stress, fear and anxiety and the possibility of psychological disturbance (Hinds, 1987). In this context, one of the most difficult dilemmas is posed by the question of who has the right to decide for the non-competent patient and on what basis such decisions should be made.

It is clear, also, that the principle of respect for autonomy can, in practice, conflict with other key principles in particular non-maleficence and beneficence, and in so doing can generate some of the most intractable dilemmas experienced in critical care nursing.

Non-maleficence

The principle of non-maleficence requires, in its simplest form, that the nurse should do no harm, or, in a wider interpretation, that she should prevent or remove already existing harm. One of the issues here is the definition of 'harm', which can be as narrow and specific as physical injury or as wide and general as damage to reputation or peace of mind (Beauchamp and Childress, 1988), with the psychological harms such as fear, anxiety, humiliation, invasion of privacy, loss of independence, occupying a central place. In part, at least, harm must be subjectively defined; what to a nurse may seem innocuous and routine may seem to a patient harmful and degrading. In such instances, the safest rule would seem to be that the patient's perception of harm must be given priority or at the very minimum, be treated seriously. Because there is such a wide range of possible harms, the principle of non-maleficence can give rise to a number of specific rules which in some interpretations can be seen as forming the core of morality and which would include: 'do not kill'; 'do not cause pain'; 'do not disable'; 'do not deprive of freedom' (Beauchamp and Childress, 1988). In intensive care nursing, however, it would seem impossible to refrain from harm in this absolute sense. An ICU, for example can be an extremely dangerous environment (Jennet, 1986; Hinds, 1987), with treatment frequently involving invasive and often painful procedures. The principle of non-maleficence therefore has to operate in the shape of 'proportionality'; the balancing of unavoidable harms against the possible benefit of given procedures to the patient; here a more utilitarian style of moral reasoning might be appropriate, though limited by the restraints of rights and autonomy. The wider interpretation of non-maleficence in the shape of injunctions to prevent or remedy harms can give rise to some of the most difficult of moral dilemmas for the nurse; the conflict of loyalties which can arise when surrogate decision makers appear to be requesting procedures which appear to be harmful (because fruitless and disproportionate, perhaps) or, even more acutely, when colleagues or members of the care team seem to be engaging in or requiring interventions which are harmful, incompetent or lacking in respect for the patient. Such dilemmas can be particularly difficult for the nurse, both because of her close involvement with the patient and family and because of her position in the team with reference to medical personnel.

Consider, for example, the following situation:

Mary was a 30 year old mother of five children. She was admitted 24 hours earlier following a serious road traffic accident. She is unconscious; all the signs are that she is brain dead; her neurological signs are indicating raised intracranial pressure and she has decerebrate movements to painful stimuli. The medical team continue to be aggressive in their treatments, though admit the prognosis is not good. Her husband is shocked by the magnitude of what has happened and is being comforted by the elderly parents of Mary. His children, all under 10 years of age, are being cared for by friends.

Beneficence

There will be occasions, almost inevitably, when the requirement to refrain from or prevent harm will come into conflict with autonomy, when, for example, patients refuse treatment which the nurse considers necessary. It is, however, the principle of beneficence, the requirement to 'do good' which can come most starkly into conflict with autonomy. This can be the case particularly in nursing, since the role requires that moral obligations to others cannot be fulfilled merely by refraining from harming or interfering with them; in the nature of the profession there is a positive commitment to benefit others, to contribute to and enhance the welfare of patients. The major problem posed in such a setting by the principle of beneficence is the temptation it poses of paternalism, of promoting the well-being of patients without their consent or, even, contrary to their known and expressed wishes. The most obvious examples of this occur with the decision of a patient to refuse, or request the termination of, treatment which is essential to her life, in effect a request to be allowed, or even assisted, to die. The point frequently seen as being at issue here (and it is perhaps an example of the temptation to disguise moral issues as technical ones) is the competence of the patient to make such a decision, since 'weak' paternalism (Feinberg, 1971) may be justified when the conduct is substantially non-voluntary or where the capacity for rational reflection is substantially impaired (Benjamin and Curtis, 1981). Though this distinction between 'weak' and 'strong' paternalism may be theoretically unexceptionable, its application in practice is less certain if only because of the 'slippery' nature of the concept of 'competence' itself. We do, for example, tend to apply it in practice to identify the patient who refuses necessary treatment, but not to the one who accepts highly risky interventions, and we frequently get caught in the double bind of either using the concept to make a general assessment of an individual's ability to take decisions – in which case we may in fact overlook areas in which she is perfectly competent and which may include the decision in question – or of restricting it to particular decisions when it is more likely to equate to agreement with the decisions of the care-giver. The best or safest assumption, on both rule utilitarian and 'respect for persons' grounds would seem to be to assume that an adult is competent in a particular area, unless there is clear evidence to the contrary (Garrett et al., 1989). For the competent patient, however, who is properly informed and who understands the consequences of any decision, it would seem that the principle of autonomy has to take precedence over those of non-maleficence and beneficence, though the former would seem to have stronger claims to consideration. This does not, however, mean that all competent requests to die must necessarily be acceded to; only that refusal cannot be justified in terms solely of the patient's own good.

A requirement posed by both autonomy, in the particular shape of anti-paternalism, and by non-maleficence is that of informed consent. There are, clearly, considerable difficulties with the application of this in critical care in terms both of the nature of the patient and of the environment, with its complex technology and procedures. Even with conscious and competent patients, the question of the nature and extent of the information necessary to make an informed decision is problematic. A broad standard might be available in the shape of a combination of the 'prudent person' and 'subjective substantial disclosure' requirements (Garrett *et al.*, 1989), that is all the information that a prudent person would want before making the decision plus anything that would be relevant to that particular individual – factors which would be material to or would change his or her decision. It is the latter part of this, the information relevant to a particular person rather than the more general standard of prudence, which is likely to call on the nurse with her, usually, more detailed and intimate contact with particular patients and their relatives and their feelings, wishes and values.

Garrett *et al.* (1989) set as the 'prudent person' standard:

1. The diagnosis.
2. The nature and purpose of the treatment.
3. The known risks and consequences of the treatment.
4. The benefits with the likelihood of their occurring.
5. Alternative treatments with the relevant (2) and (3) information.
6. The prognosis for no treatment.
7. All costs, including the amount and duration of pain and the social and lifestyle costs.

Justice

The principle of justice raises, in particular in critical care, problems of both micro- and macro-allocation. In terms of macro-allocation, it is not unacceptable to ask whether there should be ICUs and associated interventions at all. Certainly, from a utilitarian point of view the argument could be put that the huge resources such interventions consume could be used more productively within the health service to provide a greater balance of net welfare, happiness or preference-satisfaction. If, however, a case is made for critical care in its 'rescue' function (Jennet, 1986) and its unique ability to save life then, in consistency, the priority of life over other welfare values ought to be reflected in micro-allocation decisions within critical care. Micro-allocation issues of justice occur most dramatically in the admission and selection of patients for intensive care, and the criteria by which this is performed. Distributive justice is the most important form of justice operating in such allocations (Seedhouse, 1988), with the general requirement that individuals should be treated equally unless there is a relevant difference between them to justify differential treatment, and the identification of 'need' as the main morally relevant difference (Jameton, 1984). Within critical care, however, the requirement to distribute resources according to need serves to pose rather than to resolve one of the key dilemmas, sometimes seen as the conflict between the sanctity of life and the quality of life. There is also the question of compensatory justice; should those to whom nature or the human animal has dealt an unfair blow receive priority over those whose need is, or could be considered to be, a product of their own conduct or lifestyle?

Against this background it is possible to identify a set of moral dilemmas which occur with particular frequency and acuteness in critical care nursing, and which raise fundamental issues about human life, personhood, dignity, suffering and death (McCann, 1990). These seem to gather under a number of broad headings: admission and initial treatment decisions; decisions about life and death – withdrawing support, requests to die, quality of life decisions, irreversibly comatose patients, permanently ventilator-dependent patients, incompetent patients, in particular children, and surrogate decision makers. Of these most attention seems to be given to decisions to withdraw treatment, surrogate decisions for incompetent patients and quality of life decisions.

Ethical issues in critical care

Admissions to critical care

One of the ethical dilemmas seen as being particularly acute for nurses in critical care is that of 'inappropriate admissions' (Fowler, 1990, p. 432). It is in this context that Jennet's (1986) distinction between two levels of decision making is pertinent; on the one hand, strategic decisions about which conditions it is appropriate to monitor and treat and, on the other, tactical decisions about individual patients and the initiation of intensive therapy (p. 6). One of the possible dangers here is the substitution of one level for the other, allowing information at the strategic level to determine choices at the tactical level, and so failing to treat each individual case on its merits. Jennet provides a clear and statistically supported account of those categories of patient unlikely to benefit from intensive therapy, in particular the patient with multiple organ failure or advanced chronic progressive illness, who requires painful interventions and whose quality of life is likely to be unacceptable, where intensive care may merely prolong the process of dying (p. 86). He makes the point that inappropriate initiations of intensive therapy are wrong, from the moral as well as the economic, perspective (p. 76). Such strategic statistical information does not, however, provide an answer to decisions about individual patients, even though it might furnish part of the information on which such an answer might be based; to allow it to do so would, in effect, be an abdication of moral responsibility. It is, however, at the tactical level that the nurse's involvement is likely to be most important. One patient, for example, might have multiple system failures and a very poor prognosis and need painful and invasive interventions but the few days or, even, hours that intensive therapy might secure him or her might be all that is needed finally to put her affairs in order and achieve something approaching a good death; another might have a good prognosis

for survival and require few and limited interventions but find her subsequent quality of life unacceptable. Information about categories of disease and success rates here will be of limited use, if only because criteria of what is to be counted as 'success' are different in each case.

While the principle of distributive justice, allocation of benefits and burdens according to need, may provide a broad framework for decision making in this area, and does at least rule out morally irrelevant considerations, it does not help with the more particular question of what is to count as a 'need' and which needs, in situations of scarcity, are to be seen as having priority. In the case of life sustaining treatment it is possible here to apply to Harris' (1985) guideline, that, whatever its quality or duration, we do individuals the same injustice when we deprive them of a life they wish to continue, since we deprive them of the same good: the rest of their life, (p. 89). "Each person's desire to stay alive should be regarded as of the same importance and as deserving the same respect as that of anyone else, irrespective of the quality of their life or its expected duration" (p. 101). Harris makes appeal, however, to the 'fair innings' criterion only in those cases where it is impossible to save all of a number of lives. (The argument here being that though the same injustice is done to both individuals who are denied continued life, an additional injustice is done to someone who has not had a 'fair innings'). But even in those instances in which resource constraints do not force the making of invidious choices, the use of critical care facilities in particular situations may still be morally problematic (Hinds, 1987, p. 2); where they involve loss of dignity and fruitless suffering to the patient and to relatives, justice and charity may require us to refrain from using them (Campbell and Collinson, 1988, p. xii). There will, however, be cases in which the appropriateness of treatment cannot be established prior to its inception and a 'trial' of treatment is needed (Jennet, 1986). It is in this context that the claim that there is no moral distinction between not commencing and withdrawing treatment comes into question. ". . . the distinction between failing to initiate and stopping treatment – that is withholding *versus* withdrawing treatment – is not itself of moral importance. A justification that is adequate for not commencing a treatment is also sufficient for ceasing it". President's commission for the Study of Ethical Issues in Biomedical and Behavioural Research, report *Deciding to Forego Life-sustaining Treatment* (1983). The claim that there is no moral difference between them would seem to fail to acknowledge some of the critical distinctions between the two kinds of decision, as well as to overlook the different contexts in which they might occur. For nursing staff in particular, a decision to withdraw treatment cannot, save in the most abstract and bloodless sense, be regarded as morally the same as a decision not to initiate it; decisions to stop treatment require qualities of courage, clear-sighted compassion and integrity to a degree that is absent from decisions not to start it, and it is only from an unrealistically detached and Olympian viewpoint that these can be regarded as morally irrelevant (Jennet, 1986, p. 90). Not only this, but, decisions to withdraw treatment made in the context of 'trial', where the outcome is known to be uncertain are different from such decisions in cases where there has been a full commitment to, and the hope of, a successful outcome. In the second case there occur not only issues of trust and implicit contract, together treatment with emotional involvement with the patient and relatives, but, however inappropriately, feelings of failure and defeat, which make the decision more difficult.

It is in this, second, context that decisions to withdraw treatment, particularly when the treatment is, as it almost always is in critical care, life-sustaining, raise and typify some of the most intractable and controversial problems in critical care nursing: matters of life and death; 'active' and 'passive' 'euthanasia'; incompetent patients and surrogate decision makers.

Matters of life and death

The growth and deployment of new technology in the critical care field has meant that the definition and determination of life and death are now matters of decision and judgement rather than of the observation and recognition of natural fact; it has also to be suggested that 'mere' life, in its biological or organic sense, is now less unquestionably an ultimate or intrinsic good, since it can be maintained with none of the accompaniments with which previously it was inextricably associated and which give it its value. It is more possible, in the age of ventilators and PVS, to suggest that it is not life itself which is valuable but those states which it makes possible, consciousness, experience, thoughts and feelings (Nagel, 1979). It follows that questions about the quality of life and the choice of death become more than abstract. In this context, it is helpful to structure discussions about withdrawing treatment in terms of categories of patient; competent patients or patients who have executed an 'advanced directive'; patients who were once competent but are not now and who have not executed an 'advance directive'; patients who are not now, and who have never been, competent, (Stanley *et al.*, 1989). Each category raises different moral issues, of consent, surrogate decision making and quality of life.

With reference to the first category in particular, but with implications for all three, a key debate which must underlie and precede discussion of decisions to withhold and withdraw treatment is that concerning the morality of suicide. If suicide is defined as categorically wrong then many of the other discussions are vitiated before they have even begun. It is possible to argue, indeed, that the distinction between suicide and euthanasia is one of detail and degree; by gradually altering details, as Campbell and Collinson (1988) show, it is possible to move almost imperceptibly from a case which is clearly one of suicide to one which is clearly euthanasia (p. xi). The initial question must be whether or not suicide is necessarily and intrinsically wrong. Campbell and Collinson set out clearly the roots of the general moral unease that suicide occasions and which, for many people, make it a special kind of moral wrong (p. xvii); it denies the value of life itself and so threatens us in a particular fundamental way. But it would seem that, in the context of modern medical technology, suicide now rather makes explicit what such technology has already suggested than initiates it. There are, however, further and more particular standards by which suicide might be regarded as morally wrong: it can be seen as "yielding to despair ... giving up or giving in" making it a "reprehensible and shameful act" (Campbell and Collinson, p. 25), or as poor-spiritedness, arrogance, despair, a denial of the virtues of fortitude and courage (Braine, 1988, p. 61). Not all acts of suicide, however, necessarily display these features, and those which did not, which might in fact display qualities of courage, compassion, fortitude and altruism would not, by these criteria, be wrong. Unless we adopt, for whatever reason, the view that all life is supremely valuable it would seem impossible to condemn without qualification all acts of suicide (Garrett *et al.*, 1989) some might be, not simply morally permissible, but honourable, positively right and commendable, even sensitive, dignified and altruistic (Campbell and Collinson, 1988, p. 116). If some acts of suicide are to be regarded as morally right, what then are the implications of this for the nurse?

One of the questions is whether or not the distinction between 'active' and 'passive' suicide has any moral weight here; a tentative answer would seem to be that, while it carries no weight in terms of the morality of the decision from the agent's point of view, it does have implications for the morality of the various kinds of assistance that might be called for. The case of 'passive' suicide, refusing life-saving or life-sustaining treatment, seems the more clear cut (though there are ambiguities, particularly in the context of critical care, as to what is, in practice, to count as 'passive' and what as 'active'). The paramount consideration here is the right of the competent patient to refuse treatment, whatever the consequences of that refusal might be. Far from its being the case that the carer has an obligation to interfere or, even, that such interference would be morally permissible, it would appear that, since it would amount to the coercive imposition on the patient of treatment that she had refused, interference would be morally wrong.

The more difficult problem is that of 'active' suicide; while an individual may have the right to refuse treatment, even though that refusal may be considered to be wrong, does she have the right actively to kill herself? It is possible to argue that, given the identical intention, the means of its realization are morally insignificant and that active suicide can be as morally right (or, indeed as morally wrong) as passive, (this has been argued by a number of writers with reference to 'active' and 'passive' euthanasia and the arguments are transferable. See, for example, Campbell and Collinson, 1988), but this does not necessarily carry with it the right to be assisted or, even, not prevented (Garrett *et al.*, 1989). If suicide, whether active or passive, is

seen merely as simply morally permissible or allowable, as not wrong, then it does not seem to carry with it a negative right not to be interfered with. If, however, it is seen as the right to seek a good death (Campbell and Collinson, 1988), even as a component of the endeavour to live a good life, then there would seem to be, at the least, an obligation of non-interference. A great deal hangs, here, on whether suicide in general, or in particular instances, is seen as merely not wrong or as a right; if it is seen as a right then it generates a duty of non-prevention. Even though it might be agreed that there is a right to non-interference, could there, also, exist a right to positive assistance? One approach to this question would be to argue that in the case of those who are incapable of killing themselves without it, to deny assistance is to offend against the principle of justice, since it is to discriminate, in an area of great importance, on irrelevant grounds, on the mere possession of the physical capacity to perform a particular action. So on the basis of justice, rather than the right to suicide, those who are incapable of killing themselves without assistance are entitled to help if it is the case that those who are so capable are entitled not to be prevented. Even in the case of those who are not incapable and who do not, therefore, acquire an entitlement to assistance it could be argued that help would in certain cases be permissible if the suicide is itself regarded as permissible, and could be seen as an act of compassion and care, if not of obligation. This would be to respect the principles of justice and autonomy as well as not offending, necessarily, against those of non-maleficence and beneficence, since in such instances death is not necessarily a 'harm' or continued life a 'benefit'. Some of the most difficult decisions in practice, however, are those in which 'harm' and 'benefit', not simply to the patient but to others, are in dispute. If the carer sincerely believes that death in a particular instance is not a benefit to the patient but a harm, then while on the grounds of autonomy, given that the decision is a competent and informed one, the prohibition against interference remains, the provision of assistance no longer becomes permissible or a matter of compassion or care, let alone an obligation, since though individuals might have the right to harm themselves this does not make it right to help them to do so

(Campbell and Collinson, 1988, p. 165). If the harm is significantly to others, who are entitled not to be harmed, then even the prohibition on interference comes into question since preventing one individual harming others does not offend against the principle of non-paternalism.

The slippery slope argument does, however, seem to have some purchase here: in the case of National Socialist Germany (Lamb, 1988) there is empirical evidence for the dangers involved. It has to be recognized, nonetheless, that refusing to allow or assist a particular patient to die because of the fear of slippery slope effects has to be seen as an example of preferring the general good to that of the individual patient; in the health care context, particularly for the nurse in the role as patient advocate, this is a problematic and difficult choice.

Surrogate decision making and the incompetent patient

Although some of the moral characteristics of 'euthanasia' are encompassed by the discussion and decisions about suicide, with the question of 'assistance' being the morally distinguishing feature, this parallel holds less securely in the case of the patient who is deemed to be incompetent to make such decisions, since here issues of surrogate decision making come into focus. The question is less distinct and, in theory at least, less fraught with difficulty in those cases where the patient has, when competent, made a 'living will' or provided for a 'durable power of attorney'. Though such instruments have no legal standing in the UK, nevertheless the principle of respect for autonomy would seem to require that such requests should be treated exactly as would the expressed will of the patient when competent and, therefore, adhered to with the same provisos and safeguards, even though the carer may not think them actually to be in the patient's best interests; to override them would be no less an act of paternalism than overriding the wishes of a competent patient.

The case is different, however, with the last two categories of patient in Stanley et al's (1989) classification: those who have been competent but are now incompetent and have left no statement of intention and those who are not, and never have

been, competent. There are two questions here: what should be the basis of judgement and who should be the person to decide? In these instances there are broadly three principles of choice: the 'rational person' principle, where what is chosen is what a rational and informed individual in similar circumstances would have chosen; the 'substituted judgement' principle, where what is preferred is what the individual would have chosen, even though this might be neither rational nor, in the narrow sense, in her best interests, and the 'best interests' principle, where the choice is of what is best in the judgement of the carers for the particular individual, ignoring the interests of others, even if the patient would have given them weight or even preferred them to his or her own (see Jameton, 1984, and Garrett et al., 1989, for slightly different versions of these options). Non-paternalism dictates that, of these, it is 'substituted judgement' that should form the basis of decision making, that is what the patient herself, with her preferences, values, affections and irrationalities would have chosen even if that entails sacrificing her interest to that of others. With this as the basis of judgement the nurse has a vital role to play, since she is the person in the care team most likely to know the patient and her significant others. The question of who should decide on the patient's behalf is based, by these criteria, not primarily on who has the patient's best interests at heart, but who is in the best position to judge what the patient would have chosen in the circumstances, who knows the patient best, with the greatest understanding of and sympathy for her views. Surrogate decision makers will usually, but not necessarily, be relatives, on the grounds that they are usually in the best position to know, and to act in accordance, with the patient's values, (Garrett et al., 1989). Problems arise when two surrogates disagree, when there is conflict between the interests of the patient and the surrogate, or when what the patient desired when competent is at odds with the decision and desires of the surrogate. Organ donation is probably one of the most difficult of these cases, when the patient has expressed a wish that his or her organs should be taken for donation and the relatives reject this option. It is easy to say that the wishes of the patient should be respected, difficult to do in the face of the grief and genuine reluctance of relatives. Here it might be that respect for autonomy in the form of the wishes of the patient is to be outweighed by the requirement not to do harm; where the harm is to someone other than the patient, prevention of it is not an instance of paternalism but the weighing of the distress of the living against the wishes of the dead.

In the case of the patient who has never been competent the matter is different; here substituted judgement is not possible and the criterion must be 'best interests'. It is this which makes neo-natal intensive care such an acute locus of moral problems; decisions have a potentially tremendous effect on patients and their families over a long time span while the patient is not able to express any views and has no personality or history on which to base decisions. Such factors present carers with the classic dilemma: is there an infant so ill, premature or defective that it should not be treated but should be allowed to die? (Jameton, 1984, p. 245). Jameton suggests that in borderline cases decisions should be based on the potential to obtain the basic elements of a worthwhile human life, the potential for loving relationships with other humans; the likelihood of survival to adulthood and the possibilities of developing a concept of the self. One of the most difficult problems is that of a conflict between the interest of the parents and those of the child, both instances in which the parents want the child treated when the carers deem this to be ineffective and harmful, and those in which parents do not want the child treated, even though the professional carers regard it as having the potential for a worthwhile life. The easy and obvious answer is that the interests of the child should have priority; in the latter type of case, however, the interest of the child are so inextricably dependent on those of the parents that parental rejection has to be counted as one of the important, though by no means decisive, factors in the assessment of the child's possibilities of attaining a worthwhile life.

It is in the treatment of non-competent patients that the distinction between 'ordinary' and 'extraordinary' treatment might be thought to have most substance, since in other cases the patient's wishes as to treatment will cover most decisions about its deployment. If we accept that not everything should be done, every procedure utilized, however painful and finally ineffective, to prolong life of every kind, does the distinction between forms of treatment provide a guide to the 'cut off' point? The problem is to discover why the distinction should carry moral significance and whether it can actually be applied in a value-neutral and objective manner. Part of the answer would seem to be that whether or not a treatment is counted as 'extraordinary' is not a feature of the treatment itself but a function of the state and prospects of the particular patient; its moral significance, similarly, lies not in the intrinsic features of the procedure but in a judgement of proportionality, of pain and indignity against possible benefit. If the means required for the preservation of life involve great pain or severe mutilation and promise no genuine benefit then they are to be regarded as 'extraordinary', so that, for example, artificial life support is, of itself, neither 'ordinary' or 'extraordinary' but is one or the other depending on the condition of the patient (Fitzpatrick, 1988, p. 218). Even nutrition and hydration, when they involve painful and invasive procedures, are not equal to normal food and drink, but can become 'extraordinary' in relation to certain patients whose quality of life is judged to be extremely poor and not capable of improvement (Garrett et al., 1989).

Judgements of 'quality of life' are frequently called for in critical care; in the case of the competent or 'living will' patient, the patient's own assessment of worthwhile quality must have priority, though this can be the source of some of the most severe moral distress for the carer. Consider, for example, Buehler's (1990) comment: "withdrawing treatment is in many ways the ultimate ethical dilemma, particularly where it is the clear preference of the patient in question and when we ourselves disagree with that decision" (p. 465). In the case of the incompetent patient with no prior directive or the never competent, Garrett et al. (1989) suggest as a minimum the ability to interact with other human beings in even the simplest way (p. 134).

CONCLUSION

This chapter has offered a general introduction to ethics and some of the main ethical theories and their application in the field of critical care nursing.

The four principles, of autonomy, non-maleficence, beneficence and justice, have been identified, and their implications for the practice of nursing considered. Finally, some of the most frequent locations of ethical dilemmas in critical care nursing – the selection of patients for treatment and the issues surrounding 'euthanasia' or decisions to withdraw or withhold life-sustaining treatment – have been briefly explored, together with the distinction between 'ordinary' and 'extraordinary' measures and the concept of 'quality of life'.

CASE STUDIES

Case study one

Ann Evans is a 52 year old woman admitted to the critical care unit following a road traffic accident in which she apparently lost control of her car on a sharp curve while driving at high speed on a dangerous road late at night. She has suffered severe damage to the spinal cord. She is at the moment only intermittently conscious, though it is expected that a return to full consciousness should occur fairly soon. Should she survive the initial trauma she will almost certainly be completely paralysed and will need constant care and assistance in every activity of living. When the appropriate people are contacted it is discovered that Ms Evans is a successful and well respected novelist whose sixth novel has recently been shortlisted for the Booker prize and that she lives alone, having separated from her partner ten months ago, and has no immediate family. It also turns out that she has lodged a 'living will' with her G.P. which states that should she find herself in a situation of helplessness and permanent dependence and in need of permanent artificial intervention to maintain life she does not wish such intervention to be initiated or maintained. Her friends substantiate and support this view and request that life-support should be withdrawn and that she should be allowed to die with dignity.

Case study two

Albert Price is admitted to the critical care unit after being brought in to hospital by the police after having been discovered unconscious in an isolated section of the local moors by a motorist who had been searching for her dog, which had escaped from the car as she was driving through the area late at night. It is discovered that he has taken a large number of paracetamol accompanied by almost a whole bottle of Scotch. Inquiries reveal that Mr Price was admitted two weeks previously following a similar suicide attempt involving car exhaust fumes which was discovered only by chance when thieves broke into his garage. The police officer who brought him in informs the sister in charge of the unit that Mr Price is about to be prosecuted on charges involving child abuse and sexual assault, and that the national papers will be publishing details of the case in the next few days. It is evident that if he is immediately ventilated and an antidote to the paracetamol administered there is a possibility that he will recover, though his overall prognosis is poor and the possibility of liver damage acute.

STUDENT LEARNING QUESTIONS

Case study one

1. Should Ms Evans's status as a novelist and the imminence of her inclusion on the Booker short list have any relevance to the decision about her treatment? Would it?

2. Should the fact that she apparently has no dependents influence this decision?

3. Does she have a right to decide the conditions under which she wishes to be allowed to die? Is there a right to die?

4. Is there any morally significant difference in this case between withholding or withdrawing life-sustaining treatment and, for example, administering a fatal injection?

5. Who has the right to decide whether Ms Evans should be allowed to die or not?

Case study two

1. Does the fact that Mr Price has made two apparently serious attempts at suicide, which were prevented only by accident, have any bearing on the decision whether to initiate life-support or not?

2. Should the circumstances of his alleged offence, together with a strong presumption that he is guilty, have any relevance to the decision? Is this a matter of justice?

3. Do the reasons for his decision to end his own life have any bearing on the decision?

4. Does the almost certain possibility that, if he recovers, his future is going to be one of serious unhappiness, loss of liberty and humiliation have any bearing? Is this a 'quality of life' decision?

5. Would it be necessary to determine whether or not Mr Price has any relatives or dependents before making a decision?

General questions

Reflecting on what you have read, consider the following questions in the context of your practice.

Identify common 'ethical' dilemmas which you face in your unit.

How are ethical dilemmas dealt with on your unit?

Who is involved and why?

What are the problems you face when an ethical dilemma occurs?

KEY TERMS

Absolutism

That group of moral theories which maintains that morality is a matter of the recognition of, and adherence to, pre-existing moral rules, principles and values. Typically, they deploy the language of principles, duties, rights and absolute values, and the decision making process within them is to identify correctly the nature of the action in question: does it infringe a moral rule or principle (is it, for example, a lie); does it involve a failure of duty or an infringement of rights; is it unjust? Once the formal properties of the action are identified then recourse can be made to the relevant moral absolutes to decide on its rightness or wrongness without reference to its consequences.

Altruism

That set of motives for action which is concerned with the well-being and good of others, either particular individuals or humankind in general, rather than that of the agent and which values benevolence as the primary moral motivation.

Aristotelianism/neo-Aristotelianism

That group of theories which takes as its basic value human flourishing and the development of human potential. The focus is on those aspects of human nature which are seen as most essential and valuable, notably the capacity for rationality and social existence, from which are derived a set of human characteristics such as courage, cowardice, generosity and meanness, in terms of which actions are judged. The vocabulary is that of the 'virtues' and 'vices', and conduct is judged in terms of whether it displays or is likely to foster or inhibit these.

Egotism

That set of motives for action which takes as primary and over-riding the good and well-being of the agent, considering that of others only insofar as it contributes to this. That ethical theory which claims that this is the proper foundation for morality.

Health care ethics/bioethics

The application of moral theories, rules and concepts in the field of health care but, crucially, also the testing, modification and sometimes rejection, of these in the light of the dilemmas and practice of health care and the generation of new values and perspectives as a result.

Moral dilemma

The particularly acute form of a moral problem in which, because two moral rules or values conflict and only one can be respected, or two incompatible rights operate, the choice is between two conflicting and legitimate demands and whatever is chosen will be morally undesirable.

Rights

Those legitimate moral claims of the individual which derive solely from her status as a human being or person which generate duties in others and which cannot be justifiably over-ridden by the demands or welfare of other individuals, the general good or well-being or considerations of efficiency or economics. Either 'negative' rights: the rights to be left alone, not to be prevented or interfered with; or 'positive' rights: rights to assistance or provision. Typically, in health care the rights to privacy, life, autonomy and respect and, contentiously, the right to die.

Principles

Those more fundamental and universal values or ideals, for example respect for persons, from which particular rules are derived and which serve as their justification and foundation.

Rules

Particular moral requirements which translate into practice, or are applications of, more general and comprehensive principles or values. Sometimes when the presence of two or more moral rules in a situation generates a moral dilemma a choice can be made by applying to the moral principle from which the rules are generated.

Utilitarianism

The set of moral theories which judges the morality of an action in terms of its consequences, in its classical form, in terms of the happiness or misery of the individuals affected. At its simplest, that those actions which produce a surplus of happiness over pain, or the least possible amount of unhappiness, are morally right and those which do the reverse are wrong.

Virtues

Those human characteristics which are morally valued and, in the Aristotelian scheme of things, ought to be cultivated for their contribution to human flourishing and in terms of which the morality of actions is judged.

FURTHER READING

Campbell, R., Collinson, D. *Ending Lives*. Oxford: Blackwell, 1988.

Braine, D., Lesser, H. *Ethics, Technology and Medicine*. Aldershot: Avebury, 1988.

Jameton, A. *Nursing Practice: The Ethical Issues*. Englewood Cliffs, NJ: Prentice-Hall, 1984.

Evans, D. (ed.). *Why Should We Care?* Basingstoke: Macmillan, 1990.

Brown, J. M. *et al. Challenges in Caring: Explorations in Nursing and Ethics*. London: Chapman & Hall, 1992.

REFERENCES

Books

Beauchamp, T., Childress, J. *Principles of Biomedical Ethics*. Oxford: Oxford University Press, 1983.

Beauchamp, T., Walters, L. (Eds.). *Contemporary Issues in Bioethics*. Belmont, CA: Wadsworth, 1982.

Benjamin, M., Curtis, J. *Ethics in Nursing*. Oxford: Oxford University Press, 1981.

Bentham, J. *Utilitarianism*. Ed. W. Harrison. Oxford: Blackwell, 1948.

Billington, R. *Living Philosophy*. London: Routledge, 1988.

Braine, D., Lesser, H. (Eds.). *Ethics, Technology and Medicine*. Aldershot: Avebury, 1988.

Collinson, D. *Ending Lives*. Oxford: Blackwell, 1988.

Curtin, L., Flaherty, M. J. *Nursing Ethics: Theories and Pragmatics*. Englewood Cliffs, NJ: Prentice Hall, 1981.

Dworkin, G. *The Theory and Practice of Autonomy*. Cambridge: Cambridge University Press, 1988.

Finnis, J. *Fundamental Ethics*. Oxford: Oxford University Press, 1983.

Fitzpatrick, F. J. *Ethics in Nursing Practice: Basic Principles and their Application*. The Linacre Centre, 1988.

Garrett, T. M., Baillie, H. W., Garrett, R. M. *Health Care Ethics: Principles and Problems*. Englewood Cliffs, NJ: Prentice-Hall, 1989.

Grassian, V. *Moral Reasoning*. Englewood Cliffs, NJ: Prentice-Hall, 1981.

Harris, J. *The Value of Life*. London: Routledge and Kegan Paul, 1985.

Hinds, C. J. *Intensive Care: a Course Textbook*. London: Baillière-Tindall, 1987.

Hursthouse, R. *Beginning Lives*. Oxford: Blackwell, 1987.

Jameton, A. *Nursing Practice: The Ethical Issues*. Englewood Cliffs, NJ: Prentice-Hall, 1984.

Jennet, B. *High Technology Medicine: Benefits and Burdens*. Oxford: Oxford University Press, 1986.

Lockwood, M. (Ed.). *Moral Dilemmas in Modern Medicine*. Oxford: Oxford University Press, 1985.

McNaughton, D. *Moral Vision: an Introduction to Ethics*. Oxford: Blackwell, 1988.

Mill, J. S. *Utilitarianism*. Ed. M. Warnock. London: Fontana, 1962.

Moore, G. E. *Principia Ethics*. Cambridge: Cambridge University Press, 1959.

Nagel, T. *Mortal Questions*. Cambridge: Cambridge University Press, 1979.

Raphael, D. D. *Moral Philosophy*. Oxford: Oxford University Press, 1981.

Seedhouse, D. *Ethics: The Heart of Health Care*. Chichester: Wiley, 1988.

Singer, P. *Practical Ethics*. Cambridge: Cambridge University Press, 1979.

Teichman, J., Evans, K. C. *Philosophy: A Beginner's Guide*. Oxford: Blackwell, 1991.

Periodicals

Braine, D. Human Life; its secular sacrosanctness. In Eds. D. Braine, H. Lesser. *Ethics, Technology and Medicine*. Aldershot: Avebury, 1988.

Buehler, D. A. Informed consent and the elderly. *Critical Care Nursing Clinics of North America*. 1990; 2(3): 75–78.

Feinberg, J. Legal paternalism. *Canadian Journal of Philosophy*. 1971; 1(1): (Cited in Dworkin, G. 1988).

Fowler, M. Reflections on ethical consultations in critical care settings. *Critical Care Nursing Clinics of North America*. 1990; 12(3).

Lamb, D. Down the slippery slope. In Eds. D. Braine, H.

Lesser. *Ethics Technology and Medicine*. Aldershot: Avebury, 1988.

Levine, M. A. Ration or rescue: the elderly patient in critical care. *Critical Care Nursing Quarterly*. 1989; 12(1).

McCann, J. M. P. Ethics in critical care nursing. *Critical Care Nursing Clinics of North America*. 1990; 2(1).

Mitchell, C. Ethical dilemmas in critical care. *Critical Care Nursing Clinics of North America*. 1990; 2(3).

Nagel, T. Death. In T. Nagel *Mortal Questions*. Cambridge; Cambridge University Press.

Novack, J. An ethical decision making model for the neonatal intensive care unit. *The Journal of Neonatal and Perinatal Nursing*. 1988; 1(3).

Pierce, S. F. The critical care nurse: an ethicist by trade. *Critical Care Nursing Quarterly*. 1989; 12(3).

Rushton, C. H. Ethical decision making in critical care. *Paediatric Nursing*. 1988; 15(5).

Stanley, J. M. *et al*. The Appleton Consensus: suggested international guidelines for decisions to forego medical treatment. *Journal of Medical Ethics*. 1989; 15(3).

Uustal, D. Enhancing Your Ethical Reasoning. *Critical Care Nursing Clinics of North America*. 1990; 2(3).

Williams, B. Which slopes are slippery? In Ed. M. Lockwood. *Moral Dilemmas in Modern Medicine*. Oxford: Oxford University Press, 1985.

Section 4
PSYCHO-SOCIAL ASPECTS OF CRITICAL CARE NURSING

This section emphasizes the contributions to our knowledge which are derived from other disciplines. The chapters provide an insight into how we can draw on these areas to develop further our understanding of the care we deliver to critically ill individuals.

14
PSYCHOLOGICAL ASPECTS OF CARE

Paul Morrison

CHAPTER AIMS

☐ To provide an overview of the potential application of psychology in critical care nursing.

☐ To encourage the reader to think about the issues raised in the chapter, and consider how these issues may influence the work of the nurse.

☐ To suggest ways in which psychology can help to promote better quality care.

INTRODUCTION

In this chapter the role of psychology in the critical care unit will be explored. The scope of psychology is enormous, so here we have limited the chapter to issues which I feel are particularly relevant and which reflect my own orientation towards applied social psychology.

THE CRITICAL CARE ENVIRONMENT

The purpose of the critical care unit is to provide life-saving interventions using specialist technology and treatments. One of the problems of being looked after in ICU is that the technology becomes the focus of staff's attention and the patient is often seen as a secondary consideration. This frequently happens in any health care environment where sophisticated technology such as ventilators, haemodialysis machinery, and other diagnostic and treatment machinery is involved (Canter, 1984). Operating theatres and busy out-patient clinics are other examples which highlight the emphasis on the procedure or the staff timetables while treating the 'person' receiving the professional care as a non-person. While there may be several reasons for this technology orientated practice, the most likely explanation is that professional staff perceive loca-

tions within the hospital or care environment as having a special function which requires particular modes of behaviour.

The nurse who works in the ICU environment therefore must behave in a way which conforms to the expected norms for that social environment, even if this means ignoring the people he or she is caring for. This is not to advocate that ICU nurses should ignore the sophisticated technology at their service. Far from it. Patients and their relatives need to be sure that the nurse knows how to use the available technology and how to act appropriately and promptly to significant changes in the pattern of technological observations or machine malfunctions. The ability to *observe*, *assess* and *act* are primary functions of the ICU nurse. However, it is important that nurses remember they are looking after people, and attempt to establish a link between personal and technological aspects of the work.

One of the problems which workers and indeed patients and their relatives face in a high technology environment is the fear of the unknown and the constant awareness that things may change in an instant. This uncertainty causes a lot of anxiety in nurses, patients and their families. People cope with this anxiety in different ways. Some nurses, for example, may come to rely totally on the machinery to provide all relevant information about their patients. Others may shy away from the technological side of things and rely on other nurses to use the information which this technology provides. In general, however, nurses should have the opportunity to become familiar with the technology at their disposal, and to learn how it works and how to utilize it to best advantage. Patients and relatives may find all the technology bewildering and experience 'crushing vulnerability' (Morrison, 1992).

The way in which the nurse deals with the patient attached to machinery is particularly important here. I remember as a visiting tutor to one ward an instance when an elderly patient's cardiac monitor became dislodged and her heartbeat did not show up on the monitor. The nurse came into the room and promptly reminded the patient that she was still alive! She then reattached the monitor and told the elderly lady how useless the machine was. Such action can hardly be said to be reassuring for patients or their relatives. Great care and skill is needed to help the patient and his or her relatives to be less anxious about the technology and the strange and frightening environment at a time of illness and great uncertainty.

The ICU environment can also be a source of great stress for the people who work there. Some aspects of the role of the ICU nurse are particularly stress inducing; breaking bad news to relatives, helping recently bereaved friends and families, approaching families with a view to seeking permission for organ donations (see Stoeckle, 1990). These require special communication skills (see Chapters 15, 16). As a general rule in our culture, we tend to shy away from these sorts of situations in the hope that someone else will do the necessary deed and save us the anxiety and embarrassment of getting it wrong. It is not always recognized that those nurses who always seem to be good at dealing with these scenes derive a lot out of them because they can help relatives and family members to achieve something positive by being there for them, spending time with them, and letting them know that they 'care'.

It is important, too, that a nurse should never be placed in a position where he or she is utterly unable to cope with a difficult situation, though all of us have had to deal with new and difficult situations at some point during training and when staffing. I have heard of one instance where a student was left to look after a mother and her child who was on the point of death. No student or

qualified nurse should be left in a situation so painfully outside her clinical ability.

The ICU nurse often has to cope with aspects of nursing work which the general nurse meets only infrequently. Unexpected deaths or traumatic injuries to children, or which involve people of a similar age to the ICU nurse, can elicit feelings of shock and vulnerability which have to be coped with. The difficulties of the role may in part be counter-balanced by the great sense of achievement and satisfaction which follows the successful rehabilitation of individual patients who make a good recovery. These successes cannot negate the huge burden which the ICU nurse must sustain.

Other special considerations of the role may be in coping with anxious relatives (Chen, 1990) and difficult families when life-saving machinery has to be switched off, or dealing with cases of child battering, assault and other types of abuse. All of these issues raise very important ethical questions for the nurse, but in addition they will influence the nurse's reactions to the individuals involved in these situations and affect the relationships with patients and their relatives. Sometimes conflict between nursing staff or nursing and other professional staff can be the direct result of one individual reacting to a particular traumatic situation. Hence the importance of effective communication within the immediate nursing team and with other professional colleagues like doctors, social workers, psychologists and the clergy.

It is clear that the ICU environment is particularly demanding for patients and their families and for the individual nurses and other staff that work there. An understanding of some important aspects of psychology can help nurses fulfil their role more effectively, and in doing so help the patients and relatives to cope with their experiences.

SOME POINTERS FROM ENVIRONMENTAL PSYCHOLOGY

Environmental psychology focuses on the interaction between a person and his or her environment (Canter and Craig, 1981). The relationship between the physical environment and the social environment is complex (Altman, 1975). Environmental psychologists have attempted to examine the relationship between design features and the ethos of therapy which is claimed to exist in a wide range of therapeutic settings. Canter and Canter (1979) described five models of therapeutic environment, normalization, custodial, enhancement, medical and individual growth models, with ICU assuming the framework of the medical model. In all of these, however, the link between the physical environment and the social milieu is critical.

Hospitals are very particular types of environments, and research has shown how the hospital environment can influence the ways in which people in hospitals behave and interact (Canter, 1984). But it is interesting to note that the design and layout of hospital wards in general, and ICU in particular, is often determined more by the requirements of the nursing, medical and paramedical staff than patient needs. However, there are several factors which planners, designers and workers should take heed of in their attempts to ensure that ICU environments are indeed therapeutic. This is highlighted in one study of post-operative recovery in surgery (Ulrich, 1984) in an American context.

Ulrich examined the recovery records of surgical patients in an attempt to see if being in a room with a natural view influenced recovery in patients undergoing cholecystectomy. He noted that 23 patients allocated to rooms with a window looking out onto a natural scene of trees and plants had shorter post-operative stays, received fewer negative evaluations in the nursing notes, and received fewer analgesics when compared with a matched sample of 23 patients in identical rooms with windows facing a brick wall. We don't actually know why this discrepancy exists, and more research is obviously needed. However, it does highlight the need to take account of the role of the physical hospital environment if it influences the well-being of the patients.

There is a growing awareness of the influence of work environment, including issues such as the architecture, layout, acoustics and lighting, on professional activities (Canter, 1984). In one study into the ways in which nurses evaluate their working environments, Kenny and Canter (1981) examined directly the role of the physical environment in nursing practice. They noted that there was a 'spatial' dimension to the provision of nursing care. Care could be administered at very close quarters, for example while performing a dressing procedure, but care could also be given at varying distances from the patient; patients may find that

having the nurse in view, and therefore accessible could be a source of comfort and indirect care.

However, although there is a growing awareness and appreciation of the important relationship between hospital design and human behaviour (Reizenstein, 1982), there is a notable lack of studies which refer specifically to ICU, so care must be taken before general recommendations and policy decisions may be made. Nevertheless, the available research shows that the physical environment can and does help to shape the psychological environment in all health care settings. In a recent review of studies which examined the role of the physical environment on patient care, Williams (1988) described a number of research studies which examined the influence of design, space, sound, light, colour, temperature and the weather on patients. All of these considerations will also influence patients in ICU. Williams (1988) acknowledged the huge debt owed to Florence Nightingale for providing an impetus for hospital designers and practitioners through her desire to ensure that hospitals should do the patients no harm. Adequate ventilation, cleanliness and hygiene facilities and infection control gradually became the order of the day.

More recent attempts to design facilities 'around' the patient have often been done with minimal patient participation (Kenny and Canter, 1981), and the resulting emphasis in design has been the activities of the staff. In one study of nurses working in an intensive care setting, circular or semicircular designs were perceived by nurses to be more desirable than the more traditional rectangular or other design types (Macdonald *et al.*, 1981). Williams (1988) rightly points out, however, that there is no empirical evidence supporting the view that the nurses' perceptions have any direct effect on patient care. More research is needed to clarify the situation before design and nursing policy initiatives may be developed, although Reizenstein (1982) noted the failure of hospital designers to utilize the research that is available and accessible.

Sensory deprivation

A number of studies have shown how alterations in the hospital environment have affected the psychological reactions and well-being of patients. Suedfeld (1980), for example, referred to a series of studies in which some form of 'iatrogenic immobilization' took place. Typically, the patients reacted to immobilization which resulted from orthopaedic surgery, prolonged bed rest and post-operative recovery from surgery such as heart surgery by reporting false sensory sensations, frequent nightmares, depression and heightened anxiety. In some cases, these psychological reactions, exhibited as changes in the ways in which the patient thinks, feels and behaves, have been referred to as the 'ICU syndrome' (McKegney, 1966).

Glen (1991) highlighted many of the stressors in the intensive care environment which may invade the patients perceptual world. The constant assault on the patient by medical and nursing staff, as well as the noise of the environment, can disturb the rest and sleep patterns which are so vital for recovery. The unconscious ICU patient is in a difficult position. On the one hand, he or she needs to rest, but also needs to have contact with other human beings. The nurse must aim therefore at ensuring that environmental noise is minimized, but also that the unconscious patient is not ignored. Glen (1991) has emphasized the importance of 'touch' and 'verbal communication' as ways of making sure that the patient's isolation is minimized. This may be particularly important for patients who are ventilated (Smith, 1989), and where the modes of communication may vary (Easton, 1988).

Distance zones

Psychologists also study how close people get when they talk to each other. The study of how people use space or distances in normal social interactions with others is known as 'proxemics'. Hall (1966) described four zones which characterize most types of interaction. These were: intimate distance (0–18 inches), personal distance (1.5–4 feet), social distance (4–12 feet) and public distance (12 feet and more). It is assumed that the distances which people keep between each other tell us something about the type of relationship which they have. While this may apply in general, in hospital, and particularly in places like ICU and the operating theatre, these social norms are often given scant consideration.

It is quite common for a total stranger (nurse) to touch, lift or wash patients who are unable to do these things for themselves. In one study of 76 hospitalized patients, Allekian (1973) assessed patients' responses to intrusion into their personal space. She found that patients experienced anxiety when hospital staff entered the patients' immediate territory, but showed indifference when personnel intruded on the patients' more intimate 'personal space'. In other words, a nurse coming into the patient's room to remove a drip stand was more anxiety provoking than the same nurse administering a form of treatment to a personal area of the body (Allekian, 1973). It is likely that the special situation of the hospital has caused a change in the way in which social norms operate. Nevertheless, many aspects of the nurse's work can be a source of acute embarrassment for some people from different cultures (see Helman, 1990). Nurses must not assume that their powerful position allows them to dismiss some of the common social norms.

SOCIAL PERCEPTION AND CLINICAL JUDGMENTS

Nurses in ICU are constantly perceiving others and making judgements about their patients, but the basis for these observations and judgements is often unclear. Some judgements about patients can be made in a straightforward manner and pose no special problems for the nurse or the patient; the patient in pyrexial, anaemic or dehydrated. The criteria for these sorts of judgements may be validated by referring to the objective criteria. Other types of judgements which the nurse makes about patients are less clear cut; the patient is confused, uncooperative, demanding or drunk. These sorts of judgements can lead to the inappropriate labelling of patients, and can lead to the imposition of sanctions on individual patients (Jeffrey, 1979; Stockwell, 1972). The psychological theory of attribution may help us to understand how these sorts of judgements are made in clinical settings.

Attribution theory

Attribution theory deals with the ways in which people attribute *causes* to their own behaviour and the behaviour of other people in a social context. People generally try to understand *why* they acted in a certain way under certain conditions by attributing their behaviour to *personal* or *environmental* factors. The theoretical foundations can be found in the work of Fritz Heider (1958) and the approach is phenomenologically grounded. Heider emphasized the importance of conscious experience within his approach as follows:

> "Our concern will be with 'surface' matters, the events that occur in every day life on a conscious level, rather than with the unconscious processes studied by psychoanalysis in 'depth' psychology" (p. 1).

Heider (1958) claimed that this common sense or naïve psychology had great relevance for the scientific study of interpersonal relationships because it attempted to explore peoples' perceptions about the world in their own terms, and legitimized these personal accounts as data deserving of scientific scrutiny. Later influential developments in the theory can be found in the work of Jones and Davis (1965) and Kelley (1982). Jones and Davis (1965) emphasized the attribution of internal motivations, and were concerned with how people infer lasting characteristics about others from their behaviour. Kelley (1972), on the other hand, focused on the perceived cause of an event or course of action.

The attribution theory approach has been successfully applied to a range of social problems (Graham and Folkes, 1990), including attempts to reduce interpersonal conflict (Baron, 1985), promoting an understanding of the reactions of people to the victims of serious crimes such as rape (Kanekar, Pinto and Mazumdar, 1985), in the field of marital difficulties (Holtzworth-Munroe and Jacobson, 1985), and learning difficulties (Wilson and Linville, 1982). Attribution theory has also been employed in studies of helping behaviour which has direct relevance here.

The emotional component of our attributions must be considered. Weiner (1986) emphasized the mediating role that affect has on helping. When a nurse perceives a person in need of help, he or she *attributes* the cause of this distress to internal or external factors. Where an internal or controllable cause has been attributed the observer may feel anger or disgust and refuse to give help or help the person in a very half-hearted fashion. A good example here might be the critically ill RTA patient who drove while under the influence of alcohol, injuring himself and perhaps fatally injuring innocent bystanders. In this instance, the nurse's feelings of anger or disgust evoke an internal cause for the behaviour of the patient who drove the vehicle and as a consequence the nurse is reluctant to care

for the patient in a comprehensive manner. On the other hand, if external or uncontrollable causes of the distress have been attributed, then the observer may feel sympathy and concern, and be more likely to help. Innocent victims of crime or road traffic accidents typically elicit feelings of sorrow and sympathy as a response in professional carers. A number of empirical studies offer support for this general theory (Barnes, Ickes and Kidd, 1979; Meyer and Mulherin, 1980), though none of these focused on professional staff who are paid to care (Campbell, 1985).

Attribution theory is one psychological approach which can influence the clinical judgements which nurses make about patients and their families. The attribution theory model of helping (Weiner, 1986) may prove to be particularly helpful in understanding how nurses care for particular patients. In another study exploring the relationships between nurses and patients, Morrison (1992) noted that nurses reacted with strong emotional feelings to the hopeless, helpless and most vulnerable patients. In so doing they may well have attributed external or uncontrollable causes of the distress or illness. Feelings of sympathy or concern for these patients tend to coincide with a greater likelihood that help, and high quality care, was given to the patient. The nurses really wanted to help and do their best for patients. This brief application of attribution theory could be usefully explored in further studies into the field of professional helping and caring and to examine the ways in which clinical judgements about patients and relatives are made and validated. Some examples of the types of covert attributions and labelling which carers apply to particular patient groups may be found elsewhere (see Jeffrey, 1979; Kelly and May, 1982).

THE INSTITUTIONAL PATIENT ROLE AND HELPLESSNESS

Many patients in ICU have little say in what they can do or what is done for them by the nurses and doctors looking after them. They are passive and unquestioning. They have surrendered their independence to the institutional care system, and are often not able to do much about their circumstances. They are seeking expert help. Their families too may often become dependent on the staff.

This process has been described as learned helplessness (Seligman, 1975; Clifford, 1985) and can have serious consequences:

> "Institutional systems are all too often insensitive to their inhabitants' need for control over important events. The usual doctor–patient relationship is not designed to provide the patient with a sense of control. The doctor knows all, and usually tells little; the patient is expected to sit back 'patiently' and rely on professional help. While such extreme dependency may be helpful to certain patients in some circumstances, a greater degree of control would help others . . . This loss of control may further weaken a physically sick person and cause death." (Seligman, 1975, pp. 182–183).

It is important, therefore, whenever possible to attempt to ensure that patients and their relatives maintain some degree of *control* over what is happening in the ICU. This is easier said than done, especially when a patient is not fully conscious. Nevertheless, the nurse should always ask patients to cooperate with their instructions and keep patients and relatives well informed. This will enable them to keep a sense of control over what is happening, and help to prepare them for difficult decisions about the future. Professional groups may inadvertently tend to promote dependence in patients and their relatives.

The theory of learned helplessness has also been linked with attribution theory which we mentioned earlier. Abramson *et al.* (1978) noted that the impact of helplessness on humans could be understood in terms of the attributions people make about their own lives and immediate circumstances. This further supports the potential of attribution theory for research into the work of nurses and other professional carers, and understanding the world of the patient and their families in the ICU.

We mentioned earlier that helpless or hopeless patients elicited very strong caring responses in the nursing staff looking after them (Morrison, 1992). Helplessness or hopelessness may provide a powerful stimulus for the carers to respond in a particular way. There is, however, a danger that nurses and doctors may actively foster this type of learned helplessness, a point openly acknowledged by some nurses. Patients and their families are often encour-

aged to be excessively compliant and unquestioning in their approach to the staff and treatment. Those who do ask questions or are in any way deviant or who try to maintain some measure of control over what is happening to them, run the risk of becoming unpopular and being 'sanctioned' by the staff (Stockwell, 1972; Lorber, 1975).

Doctors and nurses are part of the institutional environment so they too have an important role to play and contribute to the process of learned helplessness. Paradoxically, doctors and nurses must promote independence in their patients if recovery and health are to be achieved, or the patients and their families are to achieve some degree of control over their lives at this point of crisis. The likely outcomes of the system of care for the short stay patients and those who require long stay care is probably quite different. It should be borne in mind that hospitalized care can be misguided and paternalistic (Gadow, 1980).

THE PROBLEM OF PAIN

Pain is an unpleasant aspect of life which we usually try to avoid. As we develop we learn about the experience of pain, how to cope with it and where to seek help. Many of our important life experiences involve learning to deal with our own pain or the pain of close relatives and friends at times of traumatic injury, bereavement, childbirth, loss, acute and chronic illness. People usually learn to cope with painful experiences without professional help. However, pain is often the important stimulus which leads people to seek out medical advice (Zborowski, 1969), for pain is synonymous with ill-ness and poses a tremendous problem for professional carers including nurses. The management of pain in ICU poses additional problems for the nurse.

To care effectively, nurses need to utilize the findings of research into pain in the daily practice of nursing (Wilson-Barnett and Batehup, 1988). While there are many different facets to pain research which could enhance nursing practice, the emphasis here is on some psychological aspects of pain. In particular, the way in which the nurse perceives another person's pain is highlighted, since this is a continuous and critically important part of the nurses' role in effective pain management.

The need to question common assumptions

It is commonly assumed that pain is always the result of disease or injury, and that the level of pain is directly influenced by the level of disability or injury. Both assumptions are incorrect (Burns, 1991). Pain can and does occur even when there is no apparent physiological cause, as is the case in phantom pain. The origin of this type of pain may be referred to as 'psychological', but it is still a very real experience for the patient. The degree of pain experienced by an individual is not always directly related to the level of injury or disease sustained. Some patients arrive in casualty uncomplaining after sustaining serious injuries, while others demand immediate pain relief for what seem on the face of it to be fairly trivial injuries. In ICU the situation is often complicated by the inability of the patient to express him or herself.

Nurses and patients are also prone to making incorrect assumptions about pain and pain experiences. Nurses often assume that patients will tell them when they are in pain, that analgesia will always eliminate patient's pain, or that patients react similarly to the same type of operation, injury or procedure. While patients or their relatives, on the other hand, may assume that the nurse knows about the pain which the patient is experiencing, that the nurses are too busy dealing with more deserving and demanding patients, or that pain is an inevitable and inescapable part of being in hospital. As nurses we must learn to question the assumptions about patients with respect to their pain and pain management. Nurses are in close proximity to the patients in their care, and this position provides the nurse with a great opportunity to assess patients carefully. Conscientious assessment of patients' pain is the first step towards rapid and effective pain relief. The nurse must take the lead here and question his or her own assumptions. This requires self-awareness. Because of their vulnerable position, patients and their relatives are much less likely to challenge the social norms which exist in hospital environments.

Individual responses and the meaning of pain

In dealing with patients in pain it is important to note straight away that individuals respond differently to their experience of pain. Psychology can help us be aware of the individual way in which we respond to and make sense of our experiences. In one classic study, Beecher (1956) found that the need for analgesia was related to the *personal meanings* which individuals attached to their injuries and pain. Soldiers injured in the battlefield were found to have a much higher threshold for pain than civilians with comparable injuries. The civilians required greater quantities of pain killing drugs than the soldiers. The need for surgery in both of these cases signified different things to the people concerned. For soldiers, injury, surgery and pain meant that they could escape and survive, but for civilians, it meant a catastrophic interruption to their daily life pattern.

The precise nature of the pain, too, will also have significance for the patient. Acute pain can be devastating, but it may also be short lived and quickly forgotten about. It can lead to a temporary interruption in a person's home and work life, it can be anxiety provoking and frightening. Acute pain can also be the first sign of a serious and long-term illness. In contrast, chronic pain may signify loss of work, the breakup of interpersonal relationships, handicap and severe disability, loss of self-esteem, crushing vulnerability, impending death (Kleinman, 1988). The nurse must therefore pay close attention to the individual patient if he or she is to develop a clear understanding of the psychological significance of pain for each individual.

In the ICU nurses may also have to deal with relatives who 'watch over' the patient in pain knowing that they can do nothing to ease the pain which the patient is experiencing. This can be particularly painful for relatives, and can lead to feelings of hopelessness and guilt in relatives – helping those people is an aspect of the work which is often overlooked.

Pain and culture

There is also some research evidence which demonstrates the influence of culture on our perceptions and experiences of pain. Culture plays an important role in the development of a person's psychological make up. People learn how to think, feel, and behave in a manner which is acceptable for his or her social group through socialization; and it appears that socialization is also partly responsible for teaching us how to respond to pain. One of the most famous studies exploring the relationship between pain and culture was carried out by Zborowski (1952). He observed and interviewed four different cultural groups (members of Irish, Jewish, Italian and Old American stock) in an attempt to explore how these groups responded to pain. The Italian and Jewish groups were found to have a very low tolerance to pain, and demonstrated a very emotional and expressive response to pain. They demanded rapid pain relief and were uninhibited in their reactions.

In contrast, the Old American group were much more reserved in the way they reacted to their pain. They described their pain to the carers in an unemotional manner, they preferred to be alone when they experienced severe pain and refrained from tears except when they were alone. The Irish patients were reluctant to discuss their pain with anyone, but admitted to family and friends that they did suffer. Both the Irish and the Old American patients assumed the sick role and conformed to the stereotype image of a cooperative patient (Segall, 1976). Similar results have been noted in several different studies (McMahon and Miller, 1978). (See also Chapter 18).

Anxiety and pain

Anxiety also influences the experience of pain. Pain can be heightened by anxiety (Niven, 1989), especially at times of stress such as the onset of illness, unforeseen trauma or hospitalization. A number of studies have examined the relationship between anxiety and pain. In one study of women giving birth (Connolly *et al.*, 1978), personality profiles and pain and anxiety levels were monitored during the birth. While anxiety and pain levels were raised throughout the birth generally, the pain and anxiety levels of those women who were classified as having 'anxious-depressive' personalities was raised significantly higher. Following a review of a number of studies examining the relationship between anxiety and pain, Sternbach (1968) noted a consistent relationship between high levels of pain and high levels of anxiety.

Furthermore, the physical environment of the hospital can influence patients' experiences of pain. Wainright (1985) noted that the well established link between anxiety and pain may be understood more fully by setting it within the hospital environment. He argues that environmental factors may elicit or reduce anxiety and in so doing, heighten or lessen patients' experiences of pain.

The nurse therefore has an important role to play in helping the patient to cope with his or her anxiety. Helping the patient to cope successfully with anxiety will have a direct effect on the level of pain experienced by the patient. There is now a considerable body of research available which demonstrates the positive effects of providing supportive information to patients (Devine and Cook, 1983) which can be applied to nursing practice.

Attribution theory and pain

The attribution theory discussed earlier can also help here in developing and understanding of patients' pain, and is worth reinforcing here. As nurses we must take stock of the way in which we attribute characteristics to patients in our care in the ICU, or more generally. A patient in hospital for a hernia repair may meet with a much more sympathetic response from the nurse than a similar patient with cirrhosis of the liver. In the first case, the illness and pain associated with it are attributed by the nurse to environmental factors – the hernia is the result of an occupational hazard. In the second case, the nurse may attribute the cause of the liver cirrhosis to the patient. The illness has been brought on by the patient by drinking alcohol at a dangerously high level. In both cases, the response of the nurse to the patient's pain and discomfort, or indeed to his family, may vary greatly. The process of attribution is one which we are constantly engaged in, so great care is needed to prevent us from ignoring the needs of particular patients in pain. We must attempt to explore the nature of our own attributions about patients and their life circumstances. Sometimes nurses may be prone to a 'blaming the victim' attitude, which may result in the patient and his or her family being stigmatized. It is important to remember that many sick people are the unfortunate victims of serious illness and accidents.

Promoting effective pain management

A knowledge of some of the psychological factors which can influence the patient's experience of pain and the nurse's assessment of pain can help the nurse to achieve a higher level of effective pain management. This knowledge can be just as effective in eliminating the 'routine' approach to administering analgesia to patients who do not require it, as the 'unintentional neglect' of patients who need frequent analgesia. An awareness of some of the psychological processes which can affect pain experiences will help the nurse to develop a clearer understanding of 'particular patients' and what an illness, operation or pain actually 'means' for them in their daily existence. There is a critical need therefore to spend a time with the patient and really listen to the patient and observe the patient's movements. Moreover, this is all part of the process of 'assessment of pain' in which the nurse plays a significant role.

The nurse's role in providing information to the patient and his or her family will help to reduce anxiety and pain. Research, shows however, that professional carers are not good at communicating clearly and effectively with patients (Ley, 1988), so a more studied approach to providing information will prove more successful. Ley has suggested several practical techniques for improving the information giving strategies employed by health care professionals such as avoiding the use of jargon, giving specific instructions, organizing the material into a coherent package and reinforcing verbal information with written material. Nurses in ICU could use these and other techniques to improve patients' understanding and memory for information, compliance and overall satisfaction with the services provided. Although a great deal of research into the phenomenon of pain has been carried out, much of this new knowledge about pain has not been utilized in day-to-day nursing practice (Sofaer, 1985).

STRESS AND ANXIETY IN PATIENTS, RELATIVES AND STAFF

Patient stress

The ICU is a source of stress for many patients. The sources of stress are varied and include sleep disturbances, flashing lights and sounds associated with technology, visitors and noise, the lack of privacy. Turner et al. (1990) carried out a survey of 100 patients discharged from the ICU to explore their perceptions of the ICU experience. The sample of patients selected for the study included people from a wide range of racial, religious, occupational and educational groups. In addition, most of these patients were diagnosed as having asthma,

pneumonia, trauma and adult respiratory distress syndrome. The respondents in general felt that atmosphere within the unit was friendly or relaxed (94% of patients). However, the most frequently mentioned unpleasant experiences were: arterial blood gas sampling (48%) and tracheal suctioning (30 of the 68 ventilated patients). Other factors which worried patients during their time in ICU included pain, noise, family worries, frustration hunger, alarms, and so on. A small number (6%) of patients expressed a dislike for ward rounds and discussions at the bedside. Relatives who observe painful procedures or 'watch' the life-saving technology monitoring their loved ones or who have to cope with distressing news are likely to find these factors anxiety provoking and stressful, too (Mongiardi, Payman and Hawthorn, 1987).

Staff stress

Working as a nurse in ICU can be stressful (Hay and Oken, 1972). Smith (1991) wrote about the cost of caring in critical care areas, and identified some of the major stressors in this particular environment. These included the technology which played an important role in monitoring and maintaining patients, stressful issues which were related to the job such as workload, dealing with death and dying, coping with relatives, staff shortages and inter-staff disagreements.

The important thing from a psychological perspective is to recognize that people respond to these stressors in different ways. Some nurses seem to respond to certain forms of stress as a 'challenge', while others find that it quickly becomes too much and can't cope. This is not to suggest that those who find it hard to cope are at fault – there are real problems of funding, staffing, training, and so on, which must be addressed by service managers. The differences in perception, however, do highlight the fact that stress is perceived on an individual basis as the mismatch between what a person has to do and his or her ability to do it.

In addition, we should also recognize the fact that many of the issues which practising nurses perceive as stressful may also be sources of stress to patients and their families, and in some instances even more so. The use of technology is a good example. As nurses learn about the technology and become more familiar with it, they should spare a thought for the patients and families at the bedside who might benefit from a little time and thoughtful explanation.

How should nurses set about dealing with the stresses and strains of their role in ICU? A number of things can be done. Smith (1991) suggested that the first thing we must do is to *recognize* some of the tell-tale signs that indicate stress. Then several strategies can be initiated to help people to overcome the stress, and these include regular group meetings which are properly facilitated, sufficient and experienced staff, interdisciplinary group meetings, continuing education and training, as well as relaxation programmes. These changes to the working patterns of nurses and other staff in ICU entail a change in attitude if they are to be put into practice.

Some specialized ICU areas are recognized as being particularly stressful for staff and relatives. The paediatric (LaMontagne and Pawlak, 1990) and neonatal areas of ICU, for example, highlight the 'crushing vulnerability' (Morrison, 1992) which parents (and indeed nursing staff who also have children) must experience in these units. While some possible suggestions for coping with these experiences have been mentioned, we should also acknowledge the positive contribution which individual nurses can make to the atmosphere and climate of these units. Wilson (1989) wrote:

"... it is clear that a compassionate and understanding atmosphere will do much to alleviate stress and to prevent the chronic maladaptive responses outlined earlier, which will lead to a deterioration in the standards of care and hence increasingly poor staff morale. Just as low morale is contagious, the same is true of a congenial atmosphere allowing all staff to adapt constructively to the stresses which form an integral part of their daily work." (p. 368).

GROUPS AND TEAMWORK

Although the ICU is a place of stress it can also be seen as a place in which nurses can achieve a great deal of job satisfaction. In ICU nurses have the opportunity to become very technically and interpersonally skilled. To be able to help a person make a speedy and satisfactory recovery after major surgery or traumatic injury can be very fulfilling

and rewarding. In ICU the hierarchy within and across professional boundaries often becomes rather blurred, and this can help to promote effective communication and establish a sense of teamwork and togetherness which helps people to cope with the difficult and demanding situations which arise in the ICU. The positive aspects of this role help to negate the considerable stresses and strains which the staff have to cope with.

In a professional context, groups (Huczynski and Buchanan, 1991) also shape and maintain particular modes of thinking, feeling and behaving which go to make up the organizational culture, so it is appropriate to look in a little more detail at some issues which influence work groups. Although an important area of social psychology, it has not been extensively researched. This is due in part to the lack of interest in social psychological issues until the last 25 years or so, and because 'tight' experimental studies are difficult to set up. Recent interest has focused on studying 'naturalistic' settings.

Groups consist of two or more persons engaged in social interaction who have some stable, structured relationship with one another, are interdependent, share common goals, and perceive that they are, in fact, part of a group (Baron and Byrne, 1987). The American sociologists R.F. Bales (1950) noted that in groups: "... each member receives some impression or perception of each other member distinct enough so that he can ... give some reaction to each of the others as an individual person ..." (Bales, 1950).

Social groups have a number of important characteristics which help us to understand how they operate. Some form of social interaction between group members is common, and some form of interdependence between the members of the group is acknowledged. If the group is to function it must be relatively stable, and the members of the groups must share some common goals which justify its existence. When people interact in a social group effective relations tend to develop – group members express a like or dislike for other members of the group. Finally, all these factors together tend to generate a perception of 'belonging' amongst the individual members of the group.

There are, of course, different types of groups, but the main types of groups which we commonly participate in include: family groups, friendship groups and work groups. The work group is of interest here. It is notable that even within the larger group of ICU staff, all of whom share the common goal of helping patients to recover, that subgroups are established. We have the nurses, the doctors, the physiotherapists, and so on, but all of these subgroups are dependent upon each other to ensure that the larger group of health care staff is effective and promotes their common goals. This interdependence raises questions about motivation (see Coombs, 1991), conflict, management, leadership, organized structure and bureaucracy within the health care system which the organizational psychologist studies in depth (Hucyznski and Buchanan, 1991).

The social scientist Erving Goffman, who studied people in hospitals and other institutions, discussed the role of 'teams' and 'teamwork' (Goffman, 1971). He argued, however, that teamwork within profession groups was one of the strategies which helped them to engage in 'impression management' and to foster a particular perception of the professional group which outsiders such as patients, relatives and visitor acquire. He wrote:

"A team, then, may be defined as a set of individuals whose intimate cooperation is required if a given projected definition of the situation is to be maintained. A team is a grouping, but it is a grouping not in relation to a social structure or social organization but rather in relation to an interaction or series of interactions in which the relevant definition of the situation is maintained . . . Since we all participate on teams we must all carry within ourselves something of the sweet guilt of conspirators. And since each team is engaged in maintaining the stability of some definitions of the situation, concealing or playing down certain facts in order to do this, we can expect the performer to live out his conspiratorial career in some furtiveness" (p. 108).

Group morale

The morale of the group can influence the quality of the care provided to patients. Revans (1964) investigated the morale in hospitals and the possible causes and effects of morale on working patterns. Revans noted that in hospitals where morale was high, patients were discharged more rapidly and the mortality rate was lower than in a hospital with a low morale. Staff turnover and absenteeism were taken as indicators of the level of morale. In situations of low morale, the accident rate was found to rise. In the 1964 study the main problems were not ones of policy or value system, although this may be different today, of course. Although this study was completed some time ago and focused on general issues, the findings are probably still relevant today and could be applied to the ICU. Consider the following issues which emerged in the Revans study: the ward sisters felt that the doctors did not pay enough attention to their advice; the students did not feel that the ward sisters credited them with any ability; the sisters often felt that the senior nurses were not interested in their problems, and their junior staff felt the same way about the sisters; the patients felt that no-one listened to them. It was suggested that the poor exchange of information was created by anxiety, and also increased the anxiety which staff experience.

In another study, Menzies (1970) alleged that the nature of nursing work is anxiety-provoking, and elicited very powerful emotions in staff such as pain, compassion, love, guilt, fear, disgust, anger, resentment and envy. The nurse has to deal with these emotional responses in some way to be able to work. According to Menzies, relationships between staff are also important sources of conflict. The status of the nurse within the total care system, frustrations about teaching and learning, the allocation of priorities, the sense of personal responsibility are all anxiety provoking. Some defences are necessary for survival, and Menzies suggested the following strategies were commonly used: work assignment rather than patient assignment; emphasis on the importance of procedures as opposed to people; a marked tendency to curtail the intensity of the nurse–patient relationship; adhering to routine to reduce the need for decision making; and maintaining a rigid hierarchy which removes responsibility from any one person. Although Menzies' research was completed some time ago, many of the processes which she described can be found in any modern hospital setting or environment.

The influence of the organizational culture

People who work together in groups are usually part of a larger organizational structure. Organizations such as hospitals and schools have their own culture (Pettigrew, 1983). Schein (1984) described the organizational culture as:

> "... the pattern of basic assumptions that a given group has invented, discovered, or developed in learning to cope with its problems of external adaptation and internal integration, and that have worked well enough to be considered valid, and, therefore, to be taught to new members as the correct way to perceive, think, and feel in relation to those problems" (p. 3).

In hospital workers, and perhaps nurses in particular, some of the following ways of thinking and feeling can be readily identified: being taught not to get involved; refraining from expressing emotions; being subordinate and uncritical of the *status quo*. These and other similar assumptions are part of the culture of nursing, and have an important role to play in maintaining practice rituals as well as patterns of thinking, feeling and behaving which convey much about the institutional setting and the way in which care is managed. Think about the following example for a moment.

The physical care of patients has become unfashionable because of its low status in the organizational system. The general devaluation of physical care minimizes trained nurses' opportunities for caring for patients in a full personal sense, since the basic physical care skill offers a bridge for developing closer psychological relationships with patients (Morrison, 1992; Morrison and Bauer, 1993). This may be less true in ICU environments where the qualified staffing ratios tend to be higher, but it is nevertheless important to note the trend, particularly because of the technology orientation in ICUs (Sinclair, 1988). However, the introduction of schemes of care such as primary nursing (Giovanetti, 1986; MacGuire, 1989a,b) may help to redress this imbalance.

In addition, Sathe (1983) described the profound influence which the organizational culture may have on different aspects of organizational life, such as communication, cooperation, commitment, decision-making and implementation of decisions. He pointed up some of the problems of having a predominantly culture driven organization, and stated that if: "... culture guides behaviour in inappropriate ways, we have efficiency but not effectiveness" (Sathe, 1983, p. 10).

Nichols (1985) also suggested that a hospital culture, which emphasized technology and cure, tended to provide poor quality and insensitive psychological care to patients and their immediate relatives. If this situation is to be remedied, then enormous changes in the structure and fabric of the organizational culture of most institutions is needed. However, changing organizational cultures is time-consuming and difficult, and should be done in a progressive and step-by-step manner (Cope, 1984). Promoting change through administrative decrees is often unsuccessful because the established values within the organizational culture have a powerful influence of daily activity (Sofer, 1955). Positive changes in practice must be planned for and achieved in an evolutionary way.

Furthermore, the culture of the organization can also affect patients, and can lead to a heightened feeling of vulnerability in patients and their families. Zaner (1982) asked:

> "What, after all, can it mean 'to care' in that commonly accepted term "health care"? Stripped of rituals, guises and disguises, what is called health care most often goes on among strangers, in settings which seem structured more to encourage than to ameliorate strangeness: the large, highly bureaucratized, technologised and impersonal urban health centers. In these, it is as common as coffee to find one's treasured privacy and integrity compromised and assaulted and even one's confidential condition at the daily disposal of anonymous people and databanks" (p. 42).

While Goffman (1968) described a process where the patient is treated like a non-person as follows:

> "... the wonderful brand of 'non-person treatment' found in the medical world, whereby the patient is greeted with what passes as civility, and said farewell to in the same fashion, with everything in between going on as if the patient weren't there as a social person at all, but only as a possession someone has left behind" (p. 298).

Great care and skill are needed to ensure that patients or relatives do not experience this 'non-person treatment' in the critical care environment.

Conformity and compliance

Another aspect of working in a group that needs to be mentioned here is the way in which members of the group conform to group norms and comply with instructions from more senior members of the group. In one study, Hofling *et al.* (1966) explored the nurse/doctor relationship. They tried to establish how willing nurses would be to follow instructions from a doctor which contravene professional practice, and set up a small experimental study to do so. The study was carried out in a hospital context. Nurses received a phone call from a doctor in 'psychiatry' asking the nurse to give a particular patient a drug named 'Astroten' which could be found in the drug cupboard. The bottle in which the drug was kept indicated that the maximum dose to be administered was 10 mg. After checking that the drug was in the cupboard, the nurse was then instructed to give the patient a dose of 20 mg. As part of the experimental setup, a real doctor (experimentor's assistant) was posted nearby and who intervened before the nurse took any dangerous action. He then told her about the experiment. It is clear that the drug should not be given; however, 21 out of 22 nurses poured out the medication and were willing to give it!

Why did the nurses obey the instructions of a bogus doctor? There are several psychological explanations for why this happens. First, people tend to obey instructions from those they *perceive* to have power over them, even though this may not be the case. Second, by following instructions unthinkingly it is possible to transfer the responsibility for any actions taken – the nurses were just carrying out the doctor's instructions. Third, people in authority often have visible signs of status and power such as uniforms, or as in the study by Hofling (1966), 'doctor' titles, badges, and so on, and are seen as people who can be trusted. All this highlights the need for nurses to be independent and reflect carefully on their work. Obviously, there must be times when you have to depend on other members of the team, but that should not hide the need to nurse a patient in a thoughtful and professional manner.

THE CONSUMER

We should not forget that the patients and their families are the consumers of the services provided in the critical care environment. As nurses we have a responsibility to ensure that the care which these people receive is of the highest possible standard. We should not, therefore, neglect the apparently 'simple' things which can create a very positive impression for the consumer and help to provide quality care.

Privacy for patients and their relatives is an aspect of care which has been identified as an important consumer consideration. Even in ICU, the fact that a nurse makes an attempt to ensure that unconscious patients are covered, treated with dignity and are afforded the privacy they deserve can make a great difference to families and friends of critically ill people. Professional staff, however, may feel that their needs for organizational proficiency and effectiveness may be compromised if too much attention is paid to these sorts of issues. Screens can cause a lot of clutter and minimize opportunities for observation. The availability of a soundproof payphone (see Raphael, 1974) is well appreciated by people in hospital, and is an important consumer consideration which managers must heed. The ability to exchange information which is understandable (Ley, 1988) and relevant for patients and family members, and which is provided in a sensitive and caring way, is also another important issue which all professionals working in an ICU setting must achieve. The added costs of producing such 'extras' may be a constant thorn in the managers' side, and therefore seen as of less importance in these times of fiscal constraint.

The hotel services for patients and their relatives also need evaluating, for these apparently unimportant facets of hospital life can come to be seen as 'symbolic' to patients and their families. If scant attention is paid to the fact that sanitary and hygiene conditions are poor, then people can infer from these poor conditions that they as individuals are of little consequence and unworthy of psychological care (Morrison, 1992).

SUMMARY

In this chapter we have highlighted some important aspects of psychology which have a direct bearing on critical care nursing. We have examined a number of issues related to the critical care environment, social perception and attribution theory in particular, anxiety, stress and pain and work groups. Throughout we have used some of the research studies which have been completed in these areas, and used this information to highlight issues and concerns which will enable the critical care nurse to develop a deeper understanding of the role of psychology in practice.

CASE STUDIES

Case study one

Stuart is 18 years old. He fell 40 feet while out climbing in Snowdonia with his friend. He had to be air lifted to hospital. When he arrived at hospital he was unconscious. After a series of investigations he was transferred to the ICU in a very agitated state. His parents were informed that he had fallen and were asked to come to the ICU. When the relatives arrived, Stuart's mother became hysterical.

Case study two

An alcoholic patient is admitted to the unit after jumping from the second floor of a multi-storey car park and sustaining severe facial injuries which require reconstructive surgery. She looks unkempt and smells of alcohol. She has no known next of kin. The unit is full and very busy.

STUDENT LEARNING QUESTIONS

1. What factors may influence the attributions which you make about these patients?
2. What can you do to help Stuart's parents deal with their personal tragedy?
3. How can you alter the ICU environment to promote better care and management?

KEY TERMS

Attribution

The process through which we infer the causes of peoples' behaviour and acquire knowledge about their stable traits and attitudes.

Conformity

Going along with what other people do and think because of group or peer pressure.

Impression management

Presenting oneself in a most favourable light to other people.

Learned helplessness

An acquired sense of loss of any control over the environment so that the person gives up trying.

Organizational culture

The values that are found within an institution setting which influence education and working practices.

Personal space

The zone around each person into which most people are not supposed to intrude.

Sensory deprivation

Reduced stimulation to the sense organs which leads to disorientation in time and space, unclear thinking and hallucinations.

Social groups

Two or more people who interact, share a common goal, are independent and who recognize the close relationship between themselves.

Social perception

The process through which we learn to know and understand other people in the social world.

Stress

Defined as (1) a psychological and physiological response in demanding situation; (2) a stimulus which requires an uncommon response; (3) a cognitive appraisal of the demands placed on the individual and their ability to cope with these demands.

FURTHER READING

Baron, R. A., Byrne, D. *Social Psychology*. 5th ed. Boston: Allyn and Bacon, 1987.

Gleitman, H. *Basic Psychology*. 3rd ed. New York: W.W. Norton, 1992.

Huczynski, A., Buchanan, D. *Organizational Behaviour*. London: Prentice Hall, 1991.

Kleinman, A. *The Illness Narratives: Suffering, Healing and the Human Condition*. New York: Basic Books, 1988.

Skevington, S. (Ed.). *Understanding Nurses: The Social Psychology of Nursing*. Chichester: Wiley, 1984.

REFERENCES

Abramson, L. Y., Seligman, M. E. P., Teasdale, J. D. Learned helplessnes in humans: critique and reformulation *Journal of Abnormal Psychology*. 1978; 87: 49–74.

Allekian, C. Intrusions of territory and personal space: an anxiety-inducing factor for hospitalised persons – an exploratory study. *Nursing Research*. 1973; 22(3): 236–241.

Altman, I. *The Environment and Social Behaviour*. Monterey, CA: Brookes/Cole, 1975.

Bales, R. F. *Interaction process analysis: A method for the study of small groups*. Reading, Mass: Addison-Wesley, 1950.

Barnes, R. D., Ickes, W. J., Kidd, R. F. Effects of the perceived intentionality and stability of another's dependency on helping behaviour. *Personality and Social Psychology Bulletin*. 1979; 5: 367–372.

Beecher, H. K. Relationship of significance of wound to pain experienced. *Journal of the American Medical Association*. 1956; 161: 1609–1613.

Burns, R. B. *Essential Psychology: For Students and Professionals in the Health and Social Services*, 2nd Ed. London: Kluwer, 1991.

Campbell, A. *Paid to Care: The Limits of Professionalism in Pastoral Care*. London: SPCK, 1985.

Canter, D. The environment context of nursing: looking beyond the ward. In: Ed. S. Skevington. *Understanding Nurses: the Social Psychology of Nursing*. Chichester: Wiley, 1984; 167–183.

Canter, D., Canter, S. (Eds.). *Designing for Therapeutic Environments: A Review of Research*. Wiley: Chichester, 1979.

Canter, D. V., Craig, K. H. Environmental psychology. *Journal of Environmental Psychology*. 1981; 1: 1–11.

Chen, Y. Psychological and social support systems in intensive and critical care. *Intensive Care Nursing*. 1990; 6: 59–66.

Clifford, C. Helplessness: a concept applied to nursing practice. *Intensive Care Nursing*. 1985; 1: 19–24.

Connolly, A. M., Pancheri, P., Lucchetti, L. *et al.* Clinical psychoneuroendocrinology in reproduction. In: Eds. L. Carenza, P. Pancheri, L. Zichella. *Clinical Psychoneuroendocrinology in Reproduction*. New York: Academic Press, 1978.

Coombs, M. Motivational strategies for intensive care nurses. *Intensive Care Nursing*. 1991; 7: 114–119.

Cope, D. Changing health care organisations. In: Ed. S. Skevington. *Understanding Nurses: the Social Psychology of Nursing*. Chichester: Wiley, 1984; pp. 149–166.

Devine, E. C., Cook, T. D. A meta-analytical analysis of effects of psychoeducational interventions on length of postsurgical hospital stay. *Nursing Research*. 1983; 32(5): 267–274.

Easton, J. Alternative communication for patients in intensive care. *Intensive Care Nursing*. 1988; 14: 47–55.

Gadow, S. Existential advocacy: philosophical foundation of nursing. In: Eds. S. F. Spicker, S. Gadow. *Nursing: Images and Ideals: Opening Dialogue with the Humanities*. New York: Springer, 1980; pp. 79–101.

Giovannetti, P. Evaluation of primary nursing. In: Eds. H. H. Weilty, J. J. Fitzpatrick, R. L. Taunton. *Annual Review of Nursing Research*. New York: Springer, 1986; pp. 127–151.

Glen, A. Psychological aspects of critical care. *Surgical Nurse*. 1991; 4(3): 15–17.

Goffman, E. *Asylums: Essays on the Social Situation of Mental Patients and Other Inmates*. Harmondsworth: Penguin, 1968.

Goffman, E. *The Presentation of Self in Everyday Life*. Harmondsworth: Penguin, 1971.

Graham, S., Foulkes, V. S. (Eds.). *Attribution Theory: Application to Achievement, Mental Health and Interpersonal Conflict*. London: Laurence Earl Books, 1990.

Hall, E. T. *The hidden dimension*. Garden City, New York: Doubleday, 1966.

Hay, D. Oken, D. The psychological stresses of intensive care unit nursing. *Psychosomatic Medicine*. 1972; 34(2): 109–118.

Heider, F. *The Psychology of Interpersonal Relations*. New York: Wiley, 1958.

Helman, C. *Culture Health and Illness. An Introduction for Health Professionals*. London: Butterworth/Heinemann, 1990.

Hofling, C. K., Brotzman, E., Dalrymple, S., Graves, N., Pierce, C. M. An experimental study in nurse–physician relationships. *Journal of Nervous and Mental Disease*. 1966; 143–171.

Holzworth-Munroe, A., Jacobson, N. S. Causal attributions of married couples: When do they search for causes? *Journal of Personality and Social Psychology*. 1985; 48: 1398–1412.

Huczynksi, A., Buchanan, D. *Organizational Behaviour*. London: Prentice Hall, 1991.

Jeffrey, R. Normal rubbish: deviant patients in casualty departments. *Sociology of Health and Illness*. 1979; 1(1): 90–107.

Jones, E. E., Davies, K. C. From acts to dispositions: the attribution process in persa perception. In: Ed. L. Berkowitz. *Advances in Experimental Social Psychology, Vol. 2*. New York: Academic Press, 1965.

Kanekar, S., Pinto, N. J. P., Mazumdar, D. Causal and moral responsibility of victims of rape and robbery. *Journal of Applied Social Psychology*. 1985; 15: 622–637.

Kelly, M. P., May, P. Good and bad patients: a review of the literature and a theoretical critique. *Journal of Advanced Nursing*. 1982; 7: 147–156.

Kenny, C., Canter, D. A facet structure for nurses' evaluations of ward design. *Journal of Occupational Psychology*. 1981; 54: 93–108.

Kleinman, A. *The Illness Narratives: Suffering, Healing and the Human Condition*. New York: Basic Books, 1988.

LaMontagne, L. L., Pawlak, R. Stress and coping of parents of children in a paediatric intensive care unit. *Heart & Lung*, 1990; 19(4): 416–421.

Ley, P. *Communicating with Patients: Improving Communication, Satisfaction and Compliance*. London: Chapman and Hall, 1988.

Lorber, J. Good patients and problem patients: conformity and deviance in a general hospital. *Journal of Health and Social Behaviour*. 1975; 16(2): 213–225.

Macdonald, M. R., Schentag, J. J., Ackerman, W. B., Walsh, M. A. ICU nurses rate their work places. *Hospitals*. 1981; 55(2):115, 116, 118.

MacGuire, J. An approach to evaluating the introduction of primary nursing in an acute medical unit for the elderly – I. Principles and practice. *International Journal of Nursing Studies*. 1989a; 26(3): 243–251.

MacGuire, J. An approach to evaluating the introduction of primary nursing in an acute medical unit for the elderly – II. Operationalising the principles. *International Journal of Nursing Studies*. 1989b; 26(3): 253–260.

McKegney, F. P. The intensive care syndrome. *Connecticut Medicine*. 1966; 30: 633–636.

McMahon, M. A., Miller, P. Pain Response: The Influence of Psycho-Social-Cultural Factors. *Nursing Forum*. 1978; 17(1): 59–71.

Menzies, I. E. P. *The Functioning of Social Systems as a Defence Against Anxiety*. Centre for Applied Social Research, Tavistock Institute of Human Relations, London, 1970.

Meyer, J. P., Mulherin, A. From attribution to helping: an analysis of the mediating effects of affect and expectancy. *Journal of Personality and Social Psychology*. 1980; 39(2): 201–210.

Mongiardi, F., Payman, B., Hawthorn, P. J. The needs of relatives of patients admitted to the coronary care unit. *Intensive Care Nursing*. 1987; 3: 67–70.

Morrison, P. *Professional Caring in Practice. A Psychological Analysis*. Aldershot: Avebury, 1992.

Morrison, P., Bauer, I. A Clinical application of the multiple sorting technique. *International Journal of Nursing Studies*. 1993; 30(6): 511–518.

Nichols, K. Psychological care by nurses, paramedical and medical staff: essential developments for general hospitals. *British Journal of Medical Psychology*. 1985; 58: 231–240.

Niven, N. *Health Psychology: An Introduction for Nurses and Other Health Care Professionals*. Edinburgh: Churchill Livingstone, 1989.

Pettigrew, A. M. On studying organisational cultures. In: Ed. J. van Mananen. *Qualitative methodology*. London: Sage, 1983.

Raphael, W. *Just an ordinary patient: A preliminary survey of opinions on psychiatric units in general hospitals.* London: King's Fund, 1974.

Reizenstein, J. E. Hospital design and human behaviour: a review of recent literature. In: Eds. A. Baum, J. E. Singer. *Advances in Environmental Psychology: Vol 4. Environment and Health.* Hillsdale, NJ: Lawrence Erlbaum, 1982.

Revans, R. W. *Standards of Morale: Cause and Effect in Hospital.* London: Oxford University Press, (Nuffield Provincial Hospital Trust), 1964.

Sathe, V. Implications of corporate culture: a manager's guide to action. *Organisational Dynamics.* 1983; 12(13): 5–23.

Schein, E. Coming to a new awareness of organisational culture. *Sloan Management Review.* 1984; 25(2): 3–16.

Segall, A. The sick role concept: understanding illness behaviour. *Journal of Health and Social Behaviour.* 1976; 17: 163–170.

Seligman, M. E. P. *Helplessness: On Depression, Development and Death.* San Francisco: Freeman, 1975.

Sinclair, V. High technology in critical care. *Focus on Critical Care.* 1988; 15(4): 36–41.

Smith, K.M. Critical care: the cost of caring. *Surgical Nurse.* 1991; 4(3): 10–13.

Smith, S. A. Extended body image in the ventilated patient. *Intensive Care Nursing.* 1989; 5: 31–38.

Sofaer, B. Pain management through nurse education. In: Ed. L. A. Copp, *Perspectives on Pain.* Edinburgh: Churchill Livingstone, 1985.

Sofer, C. Reactions to administrative change. *Human Relations.* 1955; 8: 291–316.

Sternbach, R. A. *Pain: A Psychophysiological Analysis.* New York: Academic Press, 1968.

Stockwell, F. *The Unpopular Patient.* London: RCN, 1972.

Stoeckle, M. L. Attitudes of critical care nurses toward organ donation. *Dimensions of Critical Care Nursing.* 1990; 9(6): 354–361.

Suedfeld, P. *Restricted Environmental Stimulation: Research and Clinical Applications.* New York: Wiley, 1980.

Turner, J. S., Briggs, S. J., Springhorn, H. E., Potgieter, P. D. Patients' recollection of intensive care unit experience. *Critical Care Medicine.* 1990; 18(9): 966–968.

Ulrich, R. S. View through a window may influence recovery from surgery. *Science.* 1984; 224: 420–421.

Wainright, P. The impact of hospital architecture on the patient in pain. In: Ed. L. A. Copp. *Perspectives on pain.* Edinburgh: Churchill Livingstone, 1985.

Weiner, B. *An Attribution Theory of Motivation and Emotion.* New York: Springer, 1986.

Williams, M. A. The physical environment and patient care. *Annual Review of Nursing Research.* 1988; 6(3): 61–84.

Wilson, J. R. A. Stress related to neonatal intensive care nursing. *Midwives Chronicles & Nursing Notes.* 1989, November; 366–368.

Wilson, T. D., Linville, P. W. Improving the academic performance of college freshmen: Attribution therapy revisited. *Journal of Personality and Social Psychology.* 1982; 42: 367–376.

Wilson-Barnett, J., Batehup, L. *Patient Problems: A Research Base for Nursing Care.* London: Scutari, 1988.

Zaner, R. M. Chance and morality: the dialysis phenomenon. In: Ed. V. Kestenbaum. *The Humanity of the Ill: Phenomenological Perspectives.* Knoxville: University of Tennessee Press, 1982; pp. 39–68.

Zborowski, M. Cultural Components in Response to Pain. *Journal of Social Issues.* 1952; 8(4): 16–30.

Zborowski, M. *People in Pain.* San Francisco, CA: Jossey-Bass, 1969.

15
TECHNOLOGY AND THE NURSING DILEMMA
A sociological analysis of modernism and post-modernism in intensive care units
Evelyn P. Parsons

CHAPTER AIMS

This chapter will explore the sociological significance of technology and complementary modes of healing in the context of current debates about modernism and post-modernism. It will begin with a review of the significance of the Enlightenment and the Cartesian revolution in replacing religion by science as the dominant cultural paradigm. A dominance, reflected in the medical model, that has lasted nearly two centuries. It will discuss the development of both positive and negative perspectives on modern industrial society, technology and scientific medicine. The main theme will be the paradox in modern society where the positive benefits and power of technology is being offset by the costs, in terms of dehumanization and threats to individual autonomy and creativity. This ambivalence is well illustrated in the ITU: the ITU owes its very development to advances in technology and growing specialization in medicine, but there is an increasing recognition of the 'double-edged sword'.

SOCIOLOGY: PERSPECTIVES ON TECHNOLOGY

Introduction

The Intensive Care Unit (ITU), whether neonatal, medical, surgical or coronary, is a specialist unit for the treatment of patients with acute life threatening conditions. It is very different from the normal hospital setting; it is crowded with health care workers and technology. Each bedside, or cot area, is set up with complex technical equipment necessary for the continuous monitoring of the patient's physical condition, and the atmosphere is dominated by equipment noises, bleeps, alarms and visual displays on monitors. Strauss *et al.* (1985)

describe the ITU as an environment that is 'machine rich' where nursing is the "monitoring of machine medical work." (p. 59).

The response to critical illness in the 1960s was to save life by the application of scientific medicine and, where appropriate, high technology. In subsequent decades individual life trajectories, both geriatric and newborn, have been renegotiated. In the ITU at Brighton recently, a 93 year old patient was given a new battery for her pacemaker (Cooper, 1992) whilst in Nottingham staff were nursing a 10 oz. baby (*Independent*, 13 June 1992). But many ITUs, in their initial enthusiasm, failed to address the social and psychological needs of the staff, patients and families. The life-span may have been extended, but the issue of the quality of that life and those around them was often overlooked. Life was prolonged by high technology, but at what cost?

The paradox of modern society: technology offers gains in terms of length of life, but is it at the cost of the quality of that life?

There has been evidence of a growing tide of informal responses to developments in technology. Definitions of health are increasingly seen to include a combination of physical, social, psychological and spiritual dimensions. This holistic well-being, it is argued, can be achieved by means other than, or in addition to, traditional medical intervention. Does this informal response herald a significant erosion in the scientific paradigm and a return to a situation where other healers are seen as legitimate? Have the roots of scientific medicine been sufficiently trimmed that one can talk about the emergence of a post-modern culture in ITU? Have informal changes in practice been reflected in more formal changes in philosophy? These are some of the issues that will be addressed in this chapter, beginning in the next section with an exploration of different theoretical perspectives sociologists have developed about science and technology.

Do you think it can be argued that science and medicine are no longer supreme in explaining and treating illness?

The scientific paradigm: optimism in the face of technology

The role of the sociologist is to generate knowledge and understanding about human society and the everyday world in which we live. Sociology emerged as a recognized discipline at the beginning of the 19th century. Saint-Simon (1760–1825) set out to establish a 'social physiology', or a 'science of society', out of the critical and revolutionary philosophies of the 18th century European Enlightenment. He believed that the only way to construct an ordered and stable society was to let scientists become the new religious leaders and fill the moral vacuum left by the churches' failure to demonstrate their spiritual power.

These ideas were developed by Auguste Comte (1798–1857), who aimed to create a naturalistic, positivistic science capable of both explaining society's past and predicting its future. His theory, 'The Law Of Human Progress', likened society to a giant biological organism which increased in complexity as it developed through well-defined stages. Social order was maintained by religion (seen as the 'social cement') and the interdependency created by specialization in the division of labour.

Early sociologists, such as Saint-Simon, Comte and Durkheim (1858–1917), wanted to see the creation of a modern, secular, industrial society rooted in rational scientific technology. Their perspective inevitably reflected the influence of the Enlightenment which offered 'man' the prospect of greater control over the negative forces of nature by recognizing the centrality of a 'value free' science. The discovery that smallpox could be prevented by simple inoculation was only one, amongst a range of scientific innovations, which seemed to roll back the frontiers. Scientific medicine promised extensive benefits, far in excess of those offered by religion. Scientists, inventors and doctors were seen as the new 'priests' whose knowledge, based on facts, observations and experimentation was supreme. The positive portrayal of science, technology and scientific medicine, offered by the Enlightenment and early sociologists, became the dominant paradigm. This is reflected by Durkheim:

"Science is the great novelty of our century, and for all those who experience it as such, scientific culture seems to form the basis of all culture." (Durkheim, 1977, p. 12).

---

1. Can you think of areas of life that were once seen to be the domain of the church that have now come under the control of the scientist or the doctor?
2. Can you think of examples where sickness is now being treated using means other than, or in addition to, traditional medicine?

However, this ready paradigm shift within Western culture was not just rooted in the Enlightenment and the perceived failure of the church to offer immediate solutions to ultimate questions about life and death, pain and suffering. The seeds of change were sown some 100 years earlier with the Cartesian revolution. The impact of the 17th century philosopher Rene Descartes is still being felt today. His theory that the mind and body were separate entities had far-reaching implications. The church had always contended that the body and soul were one, and if the human body was not preserved intact the soul could not ascend to heaven; this led to an inevitable embargo on any human dissection. The acceptance of a distinction between the body and the mind acted as a major liberating force. Descartes opened the way for the development of a medical science that could be orientated towards the physiology of the human machine, leaving questions of the mind and soul to philosophers and theologians. This emancipation laid the foundations for the emergence of the 'clinical gaze' and a scientifically dominated, physically orientated medicine. Figlio (1977) describes the subsequent growth of laboratory science as removing any mystery which had surrounded the human body and its functioning. The body was portrayed as a series of interrelated parts and illness as a mechanical failure which could be remedied by technical intervention. By the beginning of the 20th century the magical and religious had been superceded by a scientific medicine which offered the framework for explaining the meaning of life, and gave the promise of intervention when that life was threatened.

The 20th century has seen the rise of scientific

medicine at the expense of religion. Science and medicine claim to be more effective in explaining the meaning of life and healing sickness.

The preeminence of science and scientific medicine has been widely criticized, and it is the nature and extent of these challenges, aimed at restoring a plurality of knowledge and a holistic approach to health and illness, that will be discussed next.

The scientific paradigm challenged : pessimism in the face of technology

For Giddens (1990), living in the modern world is more like being "aboard a careering juggernaut than being in a carefully controlled and well-driven car" (p. 53). He asks the question: why are we living in a runaway world so different from the one the Enlightenment anticipated? Toffler (1980), in similar vein, says that technology, instead of being seen as the engine of progress, is increasingly being portrayed as the juggernaut that destroys the freedom of the individual.

The uncritical, enthusiastic representation of science and technology by early sociologists was not perpetuated by Karl Marx (1818–1883) and Max Weber (1864–1920). They recognized the inevitability of progress and the new opportunities offered by modern industrial society, but they retained a pessimism about its qualitative nature. For Marx, the capitalist mode of production called for increasing complexity in the division of labour which, combined with exploitation of the work force, meant that human beings were estranged, or alienated, not only in the workplace but in their social relationships, and eventually in themselves.

Marx argued that technology created strains in social relationships.

Weber, like Durkheim, acknowledged the all-pervasive nature of science:

> "Science in the name of "intellectual integrity", has come forward with the claim of representing the only possible form of a reasoned view of the world . . ." (Weber, 1970, p. 355).

But he recognized there was a price to pay; any benefits had to be weighed against the costs. In his social theory, Weber identified 'rationality' (the process of making things calculable and predictable) as a key feature of modernity. He argued that material progress was inevitable, and could only be sustained by the expansion of bureaucracies and increasing rationalization. Bureaucracies were those stable, administrative hierarchies, regulated by a system of rules, where social action was routinized and predictable. His ambivalence was evident: these developments offered both the promise of liberation and the threat of imprisonment. There was the ultimate paradox: the potential freedom from the irrational, repressive traditions of pre-industrial society would only lead to a greater incarceration in the 'iron-cage' of bureaucracy and rationalism, which threatened to dehumanize relationships and crush individual creativity, personal values and autonomy:

"Bureaucracy is busy fabricating a shell of bondage which men will perhaps be forced to inhabit some day, as powerless as the fellahs of ancient Egypt . . . how can one possibly save any remnants of individualistic freedom?" (Weber, 1978, p. 1403).

Weber predicted that the world would become secular, materialistic and instrumental, dominated by scientific and technological rationality, against which there was no defence. There would be an inevitable 'disenchantment' and the world would become a place which lacked meaning and mystery. Advanced technology might make society economically more comfortable, but people would find their lives empty and spiritually bleak. The rational world might be more orderly and reliable, but it would certainly not be more meaningful.

Weber argued that the price to pay for modern technology outweighed any advantages. The modern world would be cold, calculating and unfulfilling.

This pessimism and disenchantment with modern society was reflected by other writers. For Tonnies (1957) the rise of industrialism and the city meant the loss of a 'Gemeinschaft' type of community that gave individuals emotional cohesion, meaningful relationships and a sense of belonging. Relationships in modern society were characteristically 'Gesellschaft' in nature, that is impersonal, calculative and contractual.

Tonnies argued that the modern world brought with it a loss of community.

The Frankfurt School, represented by critical social theorists such as Horkheimer, Adorno, Marcuse and, more recently, Habermas, held a similar pessimism. They wrote of feelings of utter hopelessness in the face of the unstoppable movement of science and technology:

"The chaotic and frightening aspect of contemporary technological civilisation has its origins. . . . in the fact that technology has assumed a specific position in modern society, which stands in a highly disrupted relationship to the needs of human beings. . . . Technology has not only taken bodily possession of the human being but also spiritual possession." (Frankfurt Institute, 1973, pp. 94–95).

They identified certain key features of modern mass society: impersonality, conformity and the quantification of the qualitative. The domination of science and technology had created a phenomenon called 'scientism': the ideology that there was only one pure, true form of knowledge which was not open to criticism. They called for science to be subject to critical reflection from other disciplines:

". . . it is naïve and bigoted to think and speak only the language of science . . ." (Horkheimer, 1972, p. 183).

"The facts of science and science itself are but segments of the life process . . . (Horkheimer, 1972, p. 159).

In the drive for greater rationality, scientific and philosophical reason had been segregated: there was a need to combine 'the fact' and 'the value', the theoretical and the practical; the only way forward lay in synthesis. The incorporation of the social into the scientific called for a recognition that there was not one, absolutely preeminent form of knowledge that could supplant the validity of other forms:

". . . science although it can and must illuminate cannot finally settle questions of practical morality. . . ." (Keat, 1981, p. 21).

The Western world is dominated by technology and fails to take account of the personal and social dimension.

They argued that Western society had become crippled because of the unique preeminence it had given to the development of modern science and 'technical reason'. Other world cultures developed empirical knowledge, but they had retained a critical humanistic element in terms of philosophical and theological reflection; the fatal dichotomy had not been made between the mind and the body. The Frankfurt School welcomed the rise, in the late 1960s, of new radical movements which challenged the *status quo* by focusing on issues such as human rights, ecology, equal opportunities and the quality of life.

This pessimism about the repressive nature of modern industrial society has been developed more recently by other social theorists into a specific critique of modern medicine. They have combined two charges: first, medical expertise has become increasingly specialized and technocratic; second, there has been a progressive medicalization of everyday life. Illich (1976) argues that human beings have lost control over their destiny because of their dependence, fostered over several generations, on 'licentious technology':

"Awe-inspiring medical technology has combined with egalitarian rhetoric to create the impression that contemporary medicine is highly effective." (Illich, 1976, p. 22).

Medicine has created a dependency by undermining people's natural capacities to respond to the experiences of everyday life such as birth, death, pain, fear and suffering. This dependency, Illich argues, is not founded on any evidence of achievement. Contrary to current conventional wisdom, medical services have not played an important role in curing diseases; in fact, the damage they have done to the health of individuals and

populations is very significant. He talks about the "increasing and irreparable damage" (Illich, 1976, p. 270) that accompanies technology and industrial expansion, and specifically the iatrogenic damage in medicine:

"Iatrogenesis is clinical when pain, sickness and death result from medical care; it is social when health policies reinforce an industrial organisation that generates ill-health; it is cultural when medically sponsored behaviour and delusions restrict the vital autonomy of people. . . ." (Illich, 1977b, p. 271).

An advanced industrial society is 'sick-making' because it disables people, and the only solution lies in retreating to small-scale, intimate communities which are not dominated by bureaucracies, scientific expertise and technology. He claims that the public is disenchanted with the 'monster of technology', and that a society which can reduce professional intervention to a minimum will provide the best conditions for health.

Illich argues that modern medicine induces more disease than it cures.

The effectiveness of scientific medicine in combating disease has also been challenged by McKeown (1979). He concluded that over 60% of the decrease in mortality between 1850 and 1970 was due to a reduction in infectious disease, and the majority of that decrease had come before biomedical treatment was available. He makes a similar claim for the decrease in measles, scarlet fever, pneumonia, bronchitis and whooping cough: all were in decline before the introduction of effective treatment by drugs and vaccines. Improvements in health, he contends, have not come from medical intervention but from better nutrition, cleaner water and improved sanitation. Individuals need to recognize that they will remain healthy if three basic requirements are met:

- [ ] they are adequately fed;
- [ ] they are protected from a wide range of environmental hazards;
- [ ] they do not depart radically from the seven basic rules for health: do not smoke; sleep for seven hours; eat breakfast; keep weight down;

drink moderately; exercise daily; do not eat between meals.

Kennedy (1983), in his series of Reith Lectures entitled 'Unmasking Medicine', warns that we must guard against a mentality which conceives of medical care only in terms of technology and science. He calls not for an abandonment, but a 'curb' of medicine that is dependent upon even more complex technology. His view is that the nature of modern medicine makes its positively deleterious to health:

> "Modern medicine has taken the wrong path. An inappropriate form of medicine has been created. . . . We have all been willing participants in allowing the creation of a myth, because it seemed to serve our interest to believe that health could be achieved, illness can be vanquished and death postponed until further notice." (Kennedy, 1983, p. 25).

For Kennedy, science has destroyed our faith in religion; reason has challenged our trust in magic and new 'magicians' have appeared "wrapped in the cloak of science and reason" (p. 25). It is the dominance of the medical model of health, portraying health as a product of medical care, that he finds unacceptable. The power of this paradigm has meant that a psychosocial model of health, which takes account of the individual as a whole person in their contextual setting has been successfully 'elbowed out'.

Like Weber before, these writers were seeing technology in medicine not as offering the 'discourse of hope', but rather the dehumanizing imperative that ignores the human situation and crushes individual autonomy. The only solution they saw lay in what Kleiman (1978) calls a 'paradigm shift' with an integration of the biomedical and the 'ethnomedical'. This new approach would take account of cultural diversity, alternative modes of healing and recognize that health was about social, psychological, cultural and spiritual issues.

Writers who are critical about modern medicine see the only solution to lie in widening the scope of medicine and taking into account other methods of healing.

The next section will put these very different perspectives about modern medicine and technology in the context of current debates about modernism and post-modernism.

MODERNISM AND POST-MODERNISM

Modernism: the grand design

In 1665 the editor of the first volume of the Philosophical Transactions of the Royal Society exhorted his readers to "contribute what they can to the Grand Design of improving Natural Knowledge" (Royal Society, 1963). This 'Grand Design' was seen in terms of scientific understanding and technical mastery that would move the world on to a new phase, or stage, in its progressive development. It has been argued that the grand theories, sometimes referred to as 'meta-narratives', developed in the 18th and 19th centuries, were the inevitable result of the failure of religion to provide order and meaning in the face of social crisis. They offered a new framework to explain the world and the meaning of life using Post-Christian language. One common thread in these meta-narratives was an overarching storyline of ceaseless progress and the discovery of universal truths about nature, humanity and society.

Modern theories about society are referred to as Post-Christian because they do not explain the meaning of life in Christian terms, but see inevitable progress for humanity in terms of man's own scientific success.

A good example of a grand narrative is seen in the writings of the early founding fathers of sociology. Their theories, rooted in evolutionary concepts, traced the unilinear progress of society through well defined stages from simple organizations to those with increasing complexity. They described a single historical time-scale along which every society was deemed to be moving, albeit at different speeds, towards the positive goal of modernity. The nature of these theories has been widely debated, but there is agreement on one thing: modernity or modernism has arrived in

Western society. Giddens (1990) identifies it as a way of life and organization that emerged in Europe around the 17th century. Although writers stress different features of modern society, there are certain core themes that distinguish traditionally-based societies from their modern counterpart. Modern society, with its rapid changes in the economic, technological, political and cultural spheres, has seen the gradual disappearance of traditional sources of identity in terms of the community, the extended and nuclear family and religion. There are three hallmarks of modernity: first, the pace of change, especially technological change; second, the scope of those changes; third, the nature of modern institutions (Giddens, 1990).

Hobsbawm (1962) describes the Industrial Revolution as having taken off the 'shackles' of productive power and radically altered, not only the location of production, but its very nature. The predominant productive unit had been the family who controlled the whole process of production. The Industrial Revolution changed all that: production became machine- and factory-centred with its ensuing increase in the division of labour. Production changed and so did social relationships, no longer based on custom and common rights they were renegotiated on the basis of the 'cash-nexus' which was impersonal and contractual. Capitalism called for rational action that would maximize profits, and it is on this basis that the bureaucratic organization was arguably seen to be the most efficient.

The division of labour that developed in manufacturing was parallelled by a similar division and specialization in knowledge and the professions. It was the Enlightenment, with its new scientific framework, that provided the impetus to segregate knowledge into specific specialized disciplines. Science and scientific medicine created its own specialist language and body of knowledge that became increasingly inaccessible to the lay person. Fagerhaugh et al. (1980) recognized the parallel and yet interactive nature of technological innovation and medical specialization:

> "Medical specialisation leads to technological innovation; then as given technology is used, physicians and industrial designers collaborate to improve it. As it is refined, it leads to ever more sophisticated specialisation and

associated work and Procedures." (Fagerhaugh et al., 1980, p. 666).

Modernism, then, is characterized by a secular value system which places science and the language of science central, together with a highly sophisticated division of labour and differentiation of knowledge. This specialization has led to an effective closure of the professions and the creation of a dominance and distance that is perpetuated by an ever increasing knowledge gap. The overarching scientific storyline claims to hold the keys to absolute truth refusing to allow critical appraisal from other disciplines.

Modernism sees science as central and its theories as 'the truth'

Post-modernism: pluralism and synthesis

The very term 'post-modernism' implies a stage in the progression of society beyond modernism. The term was adopted in the 1960s to describe what was seen as a distinctive cultural change in society. In place of the overarching scientific story line, with its stress on the virtues of scientific and technical knowledge, competing claims to knowledge were emerging together with a growing demand that science and scientific medicine should not hold a privileged place and be exempt from pragmatic and piecemeal judgements beyond the scientific community. Lyotard (1985) described the post-modern movement as an attack on elitism and the grand narrative, an attack that was rooted in a growing scepticism of any absolute, universal claim to 'the truth'. In place of a single rationality, or legitimation, the post-modern perspective offers plurality, diversity and fragmentation. It heralds a loss of unity and certainty of knowledge, and signals an erosion of previously rigid boundaries as a new synthesis develops between academic disciplines. Eagleton (1987) talks about the laid-back pluralism and fragmentation of post-modernism:

> "Science and philosophy must jettison their grandiose metaphysical claims and view themselves more modestly as just another set of narratives." (Eagleton, 1987).

For Crook, Pakulski and Waters (1992) this is

the 'gloss fading' on the grand design and the writing 'being on the wall' for the monumental edifice of organized science as it becomes just a constituent part of a much greater whole. They predict that categorical distinctions between the technical and the social, the fact and the value will begin to disappear and the only issue at stake is:

"... the manner in which science will dissolve into and transform other discourses." (Crook, Pakulski and Waters, 1992, p. 218).

Post-modernism does not see science as supreme but takes account of a number of different explanations for life.

The current debates over whether post-modernism as such has arrived or, as Giddens (1990) contends, is just beginning as one sees the contours of a new era are not highly relevant. What is significant is that the traditional conflict between man and nature and the mechanistic segregation between mind and body is being replaced by a new order which recognizes the importance of symbiosis and synthesis. An era where traditional values and scientific bigotism is being challenged and health, it is argued, consists of more than freedom from a medical diagnosis.

Post-modernism questions the fact that science and scientific medicine can offer all the answers.

This analysis of modernism and post-modernism is important as a theoretical framework to address the key question: is there any evidence to suggest that the transition to post-modernism, highlighted at a societal level is being reflected in nursing, and in particular in the ITU?

MODERNISM AND POST-MODERNISM: TECHNOLOGY, NURSING AND THE ITU

Introduction

The language of post-modernism is synthesis, heterogeneity, fragmentation and plurality. One distinguishing feature of the new era is a growing scepticism of any absolute, universal claim to truth with science, and scientific medicine no longer holding a privileged place but being subject to appraisal by outside disciplines. Is there any evidence to indicate that the predominant medical model has been significantly challenged and the language of science and technology is being replaced? Are other modes of healing and humanistic philosophies of nursing being recognized, or do patients and nurses alike experience feelings of powerlessness and helplessness in the face of bureaucracy and technology, as some sociologists predicted? Have relationships become alienated and dehumanized and individual autonomy and creativity threatened by the growing tide of technology? It is the paradoxical relationship between technology and nursing that will be explored in the next section.

The paradox of technology: is nursing an art or a science?

The nursing literature reveals an uneasy tension between two very different perceptions of nursing. The first, often portrayed as being 'traditional', focuses on the affective role of the nurse. It emphasizes the importance of meeting the emotional needs of the patient by establishing a caring relationship. Mason (1985) argues that nursing, unlike medicine, is based "on the use of self to listen, teach, guide, support and be there". This 'art' of nursing draws heavily on the concept of intuition, something Carnevale (1991) describes as the act of knowing without the use of rational processes.

The second philosophy emphasizes the 'scientific' nature of nursing, the need to acquire a systematic body of knowledge and a high level of technical competence. Heidt (1981) argues that the history of health care has reflected a decreasing interest in the bedside manner and human contact and a growing dependence on drugs, instrumentation and technological advances. This philosophy is rooted in the assumption that the technical and mechanical aspects of nursing are 'real work' and more in keeping with an aspiring profession anxious to disengage itself from the assumption that nursing is an extension of the female role and dependent upon a woman's natural capacity to be intuitive. It is argued that nurses in practice favour this approach (Buckenham and McGrath, 1983; Melia, 1987; Smith and Redfern, 1989). They see their main function as assisting and supporting the doctor, and define 'real nursing' as the technical and medical aspects of their job. They feel their primary allegiance is to the professional health team rather than the patient, and basic nursing care is seen as low status, uninteresting, a job that can be done by anyone.

An Apparent Role Tension in Nursing: The nurse as emotional and caring vs. the nurse as technically competent. Do you think that the two roles can co-exist?

This divergence in philosophy is well illustrated in the ITU: its origins are attributed to two different eras, according to the writer's perspective. For some it is described as a phenomenon of the 1950s and 1960s with the development of technology, in particular the iron lung: "the concept of intensive therapy has developed since the early 1950s following the poliomyelitic epidemic when patients required respiratory assistance." (Stanton, 1991, p. 230). For others it is historically located in terms of nursing process rather than technology. Fairman (1992), for example, traces its origins back to the last century when Louisa May Alcott wrote about 'holding her watch' wherever the sickest and most helpless were. She sees this as the start of the principle of separating the 'recovery' patients from the 'helpless'. Similarly, Florence Nightingale wrote in 1852: "It is valuable to have one place in the hospital where post-operative and other patients needing close attention can be watched." Is the ITU a locale defined by its concentration of 'high tech' equipment, or is it a process defined by the nature of its nursing? This difference over the historical roots of the ITU is a reflection, not only of very different perspectives, but an inherent ambivalence about the role of the nurse and the essence of nursing. Is nursing about technical competence or therapeutic relationships?

The changing face of nursing

The last 25 years has seen a distinct change in nursing as a profession. The impetus has come from four main areas. First, the development of an academic body of research and theory. Nursing historically has been described, together with teaching and social work, as one of the 'semi' or 'lower' professions. It has been evident over the past few decades that there has been a strong move, from within, to establish its professional claims more securely. Hofoss (1986) delineates stages in the process of profession-building, one being 'educational improvement'. The development of a research-based body of theory and knowledge, that can not only inform practice, but be incorporated into an academic training programme, has been witnessed in nursing. Second, the women's movement that has challenged the traditional gender typification of the nurse. Third, the rapid expansion of medico-scientific technology. Fourth, the growth of consumerism, with its calls for greater patient autonomy.

FOUR changes in Nursing:

1. The development of an academic body of research and theory.
2. The influence of feminism.
3. The growth of technology.
4. The growth of consumerism.

These forces may, on the surface, appear to be inter-related in their calls for greater professionalization in nursing, but a closer analysis reveals that there are potential inbuilt contradictions. It is these tensions, in particular the paradox between technology and humanistic interventions in nursing, that will be explored in the context of the wider debate about post-modernism. 'High-tech' is increasingly being used to save lives, and yet there is a growing acknowledgement that health is about more than physiological fitness. The use of technology may reinforce the scientific, professional face of nursing and fulfil certain feminist demands, but this development has been paralleled by an incorporation into nursing theory of a psychosocial dimension. In addition, nursing research is demonstrating that the dehumanizing effects of technology can be countered by effective interventions, and that patients now judge the quality of nursing, not by its technical competence but by its emotional style, preferring to be treated with warmth, kindness and sensitivity (Smith, 1992). Do the changes that have taken place in nursing over the past 25 years indicate that there has been a significant challenge to the dominant mechanistic, medical paradigm of modernism?

Which of the four changes do you think has been the most influential?

The technological imperative

Fuchs (1968), an economist, was one of the early writers to identify an issue that has become increasingly significant: what can be done in terms of health care may not necessarily coincide with what should be done. Technical manipulation may not take account of human values:

> "The problem, as I see it, is that the physician's approach to medical care and health is dominated by what may be called a "technological imperative". In other words, medical traditional emphasises giving the best care that is technically possible; the only legitimate and explicitly recognised constraint is the state of the art." (Fuchs, 1968, p. 192).

Crawshaw (1983) refers to the same phenomenon as 'the technical fix', warning that "scientific therapeutic zeal has become a new, dangerous, iatrogenic disease" (p. 1859) that needs to be controlled before it distorts our humanity.

High technology has become synonymous with the ITU, and has created a situation where the central focus can easily become human needs that are machine measurable, visible and readily recordable. Fairman (1992), in her historical review, notes that as the number of ITUs multiplied in the 1960s and 1970s, they increasingly became technologic repositories and the lessons of 'watchful vigilance' from the 1950s were obscured by an enthusiasm for machines: "the care of the critically ill patient entered into a realm where data from machines supplanted the intense observation of nurses and their expertise" (Fairman, 1992, p. 58). This preference for the medico-technical, task-orientated aspects of care appear to dominate the work pattern of nurses in the ITU, particularly when time is short (Mason, 1985). In a study of nurse–patient interaction in a high dependency unit, Rundell (1991) found that most contact was task-orientated, and nurses were seldom found initiating contact or promoting communication.

Do you think that it is a fair and just criticism that the early ITUs were overly technical at the expense of human intervention?

These findings only serve to underline the earlier observations of Jourard (1966), that in both nurse–nurse and nurse–patient interaction little physical contact was in evidence. He was forced to conclude that we live in an age of disembodiment, and that the experience of being touched, which 'enlivens our bodies', was sadly lacking. Ashworth (1980), in a quantitative study of five ITUs, found that nurses only spent 14% of their time communicating with patients and 7% of that time involved giving long-term information, orientating the patient or teaching. Salyer and Stuart (1985) concluded that the clinical care environment was depriving patients of essential human interaction because carers were distracted by the technology. This preoccupation often means that in the wake of apparent technological success, intense human needs are underregarded:

> "The accurate and relatively easy monitoring of a patient's physical condition can be achieved by technology but this may increase the risk that psychological needs may not be identified and help given." (Ingham, 1989, p. 73).

The computer may offer a more refined means of monitoring patients without disturbing them, but it decreases physical and other interpersonal contact (Clifford, 1986).

The technological imperative: patient stressors

Rome (1969), in his paper on the irony of the ITU,

talks about patients having to endure emotional stress as a result of being exposed to the very environment that has the potential to save their lives. A number of reasons are given for these 'patient stressors'. Glen (1991) refers to the 'ICU syndrome' with 'anxiety, stress and despair' being associated with significant behavioural changes. The common clinical signs of the syndrome are confusion, disorientation, hallucinations, paranoia and aggression. She points to several significant causes, including sleep deprivation, sensory deprivation, sensory overload and social isolation. Ashworth (1990) talks about anxieties being raised by "bleeps, hisses, flashing lights and alarms at a time when a patient's human resources are largely immobilised." Bergbom-Engberg and Haljamae (1988) found that 28.5% of patients, in their study, expressed feelings of insecurity; the main reasons given were fear of equipment failure, a lack of trust in the nurse on duty, difficulties in communication, a conviction that they were dying, and being unable to distinguish between what was real and unreal. Clarke (1985), writing about her own experience, spoke of problems with insomnia, anxiety, the inability to communicate and feelings of total dependency. She described how she felt particularly sensitive to nurses' reactions, and her shame and humiliation at losing control of body functions. Similarly, Smith (1987), in her autobiographical account, highlights problems of communication; getting enough rest because of frequent observations, background noise and bright lights; feelings of total helplessness and dependency on machinery, especially in the event of a power cut, and feelings of a lack of privacy.

Certain common themes emerge from the research which indicate that patients experience intense feelings of fear, helplessness, hopelessness and uncertainty, and are struggling to make sense of what is happening to them. Everyday life, for most individuals, is largely routinized, and underlying the routine is the tacit assumption that "until further notice the world will go on substantially in the manner it has so far" (Schutz, 1970). It is our experience from yesterday that offers the framework and meaning for tomorrow. An admission to ITU is often made in cases of emergency, or after life-threatening surgery, and is certainly not part of the everyday world and experience of most individuals. Life has lost its meaning and they are unable, because of physical restrictions, to use the usual medium of communication to begin negotiating a new framework of understanding. Part of that 'making sense' of the new situation comes from knowing what has happened to them and why they are in an ITU. How long have they been there? How much time have they lost? What has been done to them? What are the physical implications of their new state? What equipment are they attached to? Who are the people around them? What lies ahead of them?

High levels of patient stressors are an inevitable part of an ITU experience.

Research indicates that patient stressors can be greatly reduced by effective, humanistic nursing interventions that increase patient's knowledge and sense of control. Tosch (1988), in a study of retrospective recollections, found patients recalled feelings of imprisonment and death, and found physical touch, hearing details of what was happening and reassuring voices to be helpful. Communication, according to Ingham (1989), is probably the most important aspect of nurses' work in reducing patients' anxieties. Ashworth (1980, 1990) argues that it is the 'nursing lens' that can transform patients' perceptions of technological equipment and procedures. It is the nurse, by using verbal and non-verbal communication, who can put treatment and care into a meaningful context and orientate patients to times, places, people and situations. Communication, for the critically ill patient, plays an important part in maintaining their identity, their psychological structure and their personal integrity. She concludes that there is a need for the human resources of the critically ill to be mobilized to prevent anxiety and stressors reducing patients' immunity. What is the significance of this argument that humanistic nursing interventions can play a vital role in the recovery and well being of a patient in terms of nursing practice?

Do you think that patient stressors can be reduced by nursing interventions?

The technological imperative: the nursing dilemma

Clifford (1986) argues that high technology is now part of everyday life, and in the face of even more complexity it is essential that nursing services regard humanistic caring skills as equally important as technical skills. Communication can make a major contribution to a patient's emotional stability, and the therapeutic relationship should be seen as a major constituent element in nursing practice being "entwined in all stages of the nursing process" (Albarran, 1992; Rundell, 1991). The qualities needed to be a nurse in a modern ITU are seen as having the capacity to be sensitive, caring, technologically competent with the ability to think analytically. They need to be psychologically fit and technologically competent.

The ITU nurse needs to be emotionally sensitive and capable of handling modern technical equipment.

There is a recognition that nursing in ITU is a very different psychological experience to nursing on other units, since the staff are dealing with situations that are highly emotionally charged. Ashworth (1980) recognizes that the nurse is constantly caught in conflict between the need to show warmth and compassion and the need to remain sufficiently objective to avoid inappropriate sympathy. Earlier, Rome (1969) argued that nurses need to 'dilute' the emotional impact of this "total immersion in critical sickness" by the tactic of avoidance and retaining emotional detachment. Coombs and Goldman (1973), in their qualitative study of 'detached concern', found that although staff recognized the need to resist emotional demands, they did still remain susceptible to the pathos occurring around them, and the experience did not destroy their capacity to feel. What are the implications of this demand for a nurse to integrate two very different models of nursing? Does this call for a dual role, whilst going some way to reduce patient stressors, increase nurse stressors? Do you think that a nurse can combine both the qualities demanded?

Clifford (1986) argues that the issue in ITU is one of role conflict, as a balance is sought between the 'art' of nursing and the scientific technology involved. It would seem that nurses are caught in a 'catch 22' situation: at a time when preserving life is becoming more and more about technological intervention there is a growing acknowledgement that health is about more than physical well-being. Can, in the words of Henderson (1980), the "essence of nursing" be preserved in a technological age? Does the demand for nurses to integrate both the technical and the emotional mean that the foundations laid by the feminists and those seeking greater professionalization have been compromised? It would seem that nurses are being asked to return to their so-called 'traditional' role as the 'empathetic', 'intuitive' nurse. But is it a return as such, or are new roles being constructed for the nurse? Do these new roles contain the seeds of post-modernism as nursing theory and research increasingly draws on disciplines outside medicine?

The nursing dilemma: potential solutions

Any account of a developing body of knowledge and its application tends to the linear and chronological, failing to capture the true complexities and interactive nature of the process. Street (1992) notes:

"Nursing actions are dialectically related to nursing knowledge. This dialectic relationship represents the continual interchange between the practices engaged in by nurses and the particular forms of knowledge in which these practices are embedded and by which they are informed and transformed." (Street, 1992, p. 89).

In this chapter it is only possible to give a brief overview of some trends in nursing theory and nursing practice and discuss their significance as potential solutions to the nursing dilemma.

There have been a number of responses to the tension between technology and humanism. These responses, it is claimed, achieve synthesis between the concept of nursing as an art and a science, confirm its academic and professional status, and offer nurses new roles that moderate the inhuman face of modern technology. What is equally significant is that they all have their roots in a growing body of academic theory and research that has developed within nursing.

Nurse education and a consequent change in the nurse/doctor relationship is seen as one solution. Briggs (1991) distinguishes between the 'extended' role of the nurse, which centres around learning new technical skills, and their 'expanded' role which focuses on the caring component of nursing. Synthesis is possible by educating nurses to be "professional practitioners who will challenge the dominance of the medical profession and fight for nursing autonomy and a professional status." The well-educated nurse will have the ability to plan caring around research-based decisions rather than intuition and opinion. They will be able to negotiate a new 'collegial' style relationship, especially in the ITU, where consultant anaesthestists, Briggs argues, have a degree of empathy with nurses. The goal is not the autonomous nurse practitioner but the nurse who can be respected and valued for their own specific knowledge and input into a multi-disciplinary team. Shuldham (1986) calls for "collaboration founded on mutal respect." A renegotiation of the nurse–doctor relationship is also seen to be the solution by Carnevale (1991), with high technology being balanced by humanity through 'open clinical conversations'.

This renegotiation in the power relationship between nurse and doctor, it is argued, makes the nurse able to act as an effective patient advocate. An important part of advocacy involves ensuring that all angles of the patient's care and treatment are taken into account in decision-making. The critical care nurse, many claim, is the ideal health care worker to act in this role because they combine clinical expertise, technical knowledge, a continuing relationship with the patient and the assertiveness that can directly challenge the doctor's role (Atkinson, 1987; Penticuff, 1989, Albarran, 1992). Barger-Lux and Heaney (1986) see the nurse advocate as the only solution to the "unrestrained thrust of the technological imperative." The patient, they argue, has become secondary to the technology, something that threatens their dignity and worth.

A second alternative offers integration by challenging the 'replaceable' perspective (the idea that the nurse is less important with increasing techno-

logical intervention) with an 'irreplaceable' perspective, which argues that in the face of technology the nurse plays a more important role. Technology, far from releasing the nurse from the bedside, has made their presence more important, since any machine is only as good as the person using it. In the modern ITU there are more invasive techniques than ever before, and each patient needs to be monitored by a nurse who can anticipate machine malfunction, observe intelligently, and critically reflect on those observations using pre-existing knowledge (Clifford, 1986). With experience, the ITU nurse learns to integrate and interpret sensory cues, and develop what is called 'clinical intuition'. Strauss *et al.* (1985) argue that the nurse is monitoring machine medical work by using sight, hearing and touch in a unique way so that a piece of inhuman technology becomes an extension of the nurse.

It is the moderation of inhuman technology and bureaucracy by a renegotiation in the nurse–patient relationship that is the focus of primary nursing with its claim that a one-to-one relationship is the cornerstone of nursing practice. The central feature is a recognition that healing is about an interactive, holistic therapeutic relationship between a nurse and their patient. Primary nursing, it is argued (Pearson, 1983), offers the nurse greater autonomy, the patient greater informed choice in their care, and the nursing profession a new ideology which draws on the traditional professional/client model and humanistic psychology. It is both an organizational approach and a philosophy which has been implemented into practice on a research basis in a number of ITUs. There are three core values in primary nursing:

1. The central focus for the nurse is the patient not the task. The nurse–patient relationship is seen to be paramount.
2. A commitment to decentralization of decision making to the bedside.
3. A belief that individual nurses grow and develop via peer review, the development of personal knowledge and a supportive, nurturing environment (Manley, 1990).

Research has shown this new model of nursing is beneficial, leading to a better quality of patient care, more patient satisfaction, more job satisfaction and greater cost-effectiveness (Manley, 1990). Research at the Oxford Nursing Development Unit has pointed to yet another potential gain: relationships between staff became more social and less functional when primary nursing was introduced. Authority was based on knowledge rather than position (Pearson, 1983). Could it be that primary nursing offers some compensation for the 'iron cage' of bureaucracy which Weber saw as a major threat to human relationships, individual creativity and autonomy?

Primary nursing, however, has not been without its critics. Constable (1991) argues that the responsibility for a single patient over a prolonged period can be very stressful. Salvage (1990) is cautious about describing it as the 'new nursing' because she sees it as a 'jumble of old and new ideas' that have not yet shown whether they contain the seeds of a more radical reorientation of nursing.

Whatever its critics may say, primary nursing offers a potential solution to the nursing dilemma whilst meeting current demands for change in four main areas:

1. That nursing be regarded as a self-accountable profession free of traditionally ascribed female roles.
2. That nursing be more firmly rooted in research and theory.
3. That nurses practise greater humanistic intervention and acknowledge holistic approaches to health.
4. That health professionals give more regard for patient's rights and autonomy.

Potential solutions to the conflicting expectations of the role of the nurse:

1. Change the power relationship between nurse and doctor through nurse education.
2. Encourage nurses to become patient advocates.
3. Change the perception of the nurse in ITU by highlighting their indispensibility even in the face of increasing technology.
4. Introduce the concept of primary nursing.

The academic solution: humanistic and holistic philosophies

This call within primary nursing for a holistic approach to health reflects a much broader change within nursing, both in terms of philosophy and practice. The development of nursing as an academically credible discipline with its own discrete, specialist body of knowledge has meant that terms such as 'nursing process', 'models of nursing' and 'nursing theory' are now part of the everyday language. Aggleton and Chalmers (1986) trace the development back to the 1960s, citing the American influence of Bonney and Rothberg and their call for a more systematic assessment of patients and their needs; Yura and Walsh's identification of discrete stages in nursing care, together with parallel developments in the field of psychology and sociology. The roots of nursing theory are eclectic, and reflect a growing desire to develop a body of knowledge which portrays nursing as both an art and a science.

Writers differ in the number and type of nursing models they choose to delineate. The majority, however, begin with a 'traditional', or 'biomedical' model, and then discuss others such as Henderson's Model, the Roper, Logan and Tierney's Activities of Living Model, Neuman's Health Care Systems Model, Johnson's Behavioural Model, Orem's Self-Care Model, Riehl's Interactionist Model, Roger's Unitary Field Model and the Paterson and Zdera Humanistic Model. The significant issue is the evident trend in nursing models away from those rooted in a physiological approach to those which incorporate some recognition of the social and/or psychological dimensions of health. For the purpose of this chapter, there are two specific models, or theoretical strands, that are important to highlight: first, the call for a humanistic approach in nursing, and second, the recognition of holism in nursing.

Humanistic nursing, as a theoretical concept, emerged for Paterson and Zderad (1988) in the 1960s, rooted in existentialism and phenomenology. It evolved as they, and other nurses, reflected and questioned their nursing experience. They describe it as "a heuristic culmination of their lived world of nursing" (p. 95). For them, nursing was a 'human transaction', a lived dialogue', 'an existential act' that was not a matter of 'doing' but of 'being': the nurse "available with her total being in the nurse–patient situation." Their aim was to "study, describe and develop an artistic science of nursing" which took account of the human context. Nursing, for Paterson and Zderad, is an art because it is the skilled application of scientific principles. It is possible, by a synthesis between the art and science of nursing to 'enrich' nursing practice and "offer a unique path to human knowledge."

Humanistic approach in nursing: central to this concept is the importance of human interaction between nurse and patient.

This perception that nursing should be about the quality of life, valuing human beings and freedom of choice has gained increasing credibility and links with a second significant development in nursing: the growing call for 'holism'.

Several of the nursing models, both traditional and interactive, reflect a fragmentary perspective about individuals which is uniquely Western. Any exploration of conceptions of health from other parts of the world reveals a very different holistic approach. There are four key beliefs in the concept of holism (Smuts, 1962). First, that an individual will always respond in situations as a unified whole. Second, that individuals are different from, and more than, the sum of their parts. Third, that there is an interactive relationship between the physical and psychological functioning of an individual and their environment. Fourth, that within people are vast untapped sources of energy which can be used for self-healing. The key to utilization is the active involvement of the individual in the healing process and a recognition that any treatment only complements the will of the individual to regain their health.

Holistic practice is based on the principle that individuals are multidimensional and closely linked to an equally complex universe. They are not just physical bodies, but people who have minds, spirits, life histories and pre-existing relationships with the world. Holism offers a radical challenge to the Descartian reductionist notion of the body as a machine that can be understood by breaking it down into its constituent parts. It involves a rejection of traditional medical paradigms and, in doing so, not only transforms the nature of the doctor–patient relationship, but challenges the narrow medical definition of legitimate modes of healing. It accepts the potential efficacy of alternative, or complementary, therapies with their stress on the importance of harmony between the biological, the psychological, the spiritual and the universe. Health, from a holistic perspective, requires an unimpeded flow of energy both within the body and between the body and the outside world.

Holistic approach in nursing: central to this concept is the wholeness of the individual and the need to see a person's illness in terms of their social, spiritual and psychological context.

This holistic approach to nursing is perhaps best reflected in the Martha Roger's unitary field model of nursing. Biley (1992) contends that, although other significant innovations have come from North America in terms of nursing process and nursing models, Martha Roger's science of unitary human beings has remained obscure. Her theory, which draws from anthropology, astronomy, mathematics, physics and philosophy, is rooted in three propositions:

1. Energy fields are the fundamental unit of the living and non-living.
2. There is constant interchange between the two energy fields and this mutuality of relationship between human and environmental fields means that changes in one field lead to inevitable changes in another.
3. Universal order is a force innate to all energy fields.

According to Rogers, the major concern of nursing is to promote 'symphonic' interaction between man and environment by directing and re-directing the patterning of energy fields so that individuals maximize their health potential. Roger's theory, Biley (1992) argues, offers the vital theoretical and philosophical framework, totally consistent with the "demands of a new age, ecologically concerned society" (p. 26).

What is the significance of humanistic nursing and holistic philosophies in terms of debates about post-modernism? They both offer an alternative to purely medical models of nursing, and challenge the traditional Cartesian division between the mind and the body. They develop pluralistic theories of nursing by drawing on academic disciplines other than science and medicine, and in doing so, achieve what the Frankfurt School called for: a combining of 'the fact' and 'the value', the incorporation of 'the social' into 'the scientific'. Nursing, from these perspectives, is both an art and a science.

Clearly, a recognition of holism in nursing, and in the ITU in particular, offers features that can be associated with post-modernism. In the next section, the impact of humanism and holism will be explored in terms of empirical research and nursing practice. Has the academic call for greater plurality been accepted both at an individual and an institutional level? Are complementary therapies gaining acceptance as legitimate modes of healing within the profession? One can only argue that there has been a significant move towards post-modernism in nursing if the principles are being implemented in practice.

Holism in practice

There are many complementary therapies available, the majority of which have their roots in ancient civilizations. Stevenson (1992) details a number which might be appropriate for nursing, including acupuncture, shiatsu, osteopathy, chiropractice, homeopathy, herbal medicine, kinesiology, iridology, hair analysis, pendulum diagnosis, divining, massage, therapeutic touch, reflexology, spiritual healing, Alexander technique, hydrotherapy, aromatherapy, meditation, visualization, chanting, the use of music, yoga and tai chi.

A number of these modes of healing have been used by Passant (1990) in the care of the elderly at Oxford. Trained in massage and healing techniques, together with a diploma in nutrition, her aim was to "work together to bring peace and harmony to body and mind" (p. 28). She found the use of herbal oils improved patients' skin textures, reduced pressure sores and induced sleep. She introduced a nutritional regime that eliminated the side effects of certain food additives. She taught patients "that the mind can move anywhere even though the body may be immobile", and this visualization technique was used, together with music and 'sounds of nature', to encourage relaxation and control pain. The overall finding was that fewer drugs were prescribed, especially laxatives and sedatives. On the basis of Passant's experience, Baldwin (1991) argues that there must be a place for complementary therapies in conventional medicine since they offer simplicity instead of complexity, the natural instead of the artificial.

The use of reflex zone therapy (RZT) in a maternity unit is reported by Evans (1990). The stimulation which RZT gives to the local blood supply is thought to improve the functioning of the organs which relate to the areas of the foot treated. It is argued that energy balances, between the different systems of the body, are brought back to a state of balance and the healing process enhanced. She quotes a number of examples where both mother and baby have benefited from this type of therapy. On the basis that alternative therapies include all the essential ingredients that should be part of nursing care, such as giving time to patients, making them feel comfortable and secure and touching them in a significant way, Smith (1990) argues that they should run parallel with the nursing process at its best. It is the concept of touch that will be explored in the next section.

Holism: the significance of touch

It has been seen earlier that nursing research supports the premise that humanistic nursing interventions can reduce patient stressors in the ITU. The importance of verbal and non-verbal interaction between nurse and patient, in particular the use of touch, has been recognized with an acceptance that each tactile act carries both physiological and psychosocial meaning. Weiss (1979) argued that a framework was needed so that the nature and meaning of touch could be better understood. What message does a nurse's pattern of touch give to a patient? As the focus on the concept of touch has intensified, so the nature of touch has become more closely defined, and today there is a ready acceptance of distinctions between so called 'procedural', 'casual', 'caring' and 'therapeutic' touch. Estabrooks and Morse (1992) found that touch was more than mere skin-to-skin contact, it was a multidimensional, social activity, the skills of which were learnt over a lifetime. They describe it as a "gestalt involving voice, posture, affect, intent and meaning within a context, as well as tactile contact" (p. 450). Three types of complementary therapies using touch will be explored: massage, aromatherapy and therapeutic touch. (See also Chapter 5.)

The instinctive use of touch to heal can be traced through history, and is well documented in early literature. Modern techniques of massage began at the end of last century, and were extensively used during the First World War for the treatment of nerve injuries, but subsequently replaced by electrical apparatus and modern drugs (Oldfield, 1992). It is claimed that massage improves circulation, aids digestion and stimulates the lymphatic system. It is thought to have a profound effect on the nervous system, relieving nervous tension and lowering heart rate and blood pressure. It is also believed to encourage the production of endorphins that can reduce pain and create a feeling of well-being (Oldfield, 1992). Fromant (1991) argues that the way nurses touch and handle patients says a great deal about the way they feel about them and their illness. Using an example from the intensive care unit at Addenbrooke's Hospital, Cambridge, she illustrates the value of massaging an intubated and ventilated patient with a mixture of essential oils. This alternative, prescribed by the consultant, brought the patient relaxation and meant she was able to fall into a natural sleep without the use of additional sedatives. She concludes that touch should be one of the therapeutic tools a nurse uses.

Aromatherapy involves the use of essential oils produced naturally in plants and flowers. The oils may be absorbed through the skin during massage or inhaled. Just two examples of its use in ITU settings will be mentioned here. Firstly, Dunn (1992) in her study in the ITU at Battle Hospital, Reading. Over a period of 14 months, 122 patients were randomly allocated into one of three groups to receive either aromatherapy using lavender oil, massage without an essential oil, or a period of rest. This happened on three separate occasions. The evaluation consisted of three elements: physiological assessments (blood pressure, heart rate, heart rhythm and respiratory rates); behavioural assessments (motor activity, somatic changes and facial expressions); and patient assessments (self-reported levels of anxiety, mood and ability to cope). Although the results were not conclusive in that no statistical difference was found between the groups on the physiological measures, the patients in the aromatherapy group reported much greater reductions in their levels of felt anxiety. This result raises a question that will be discussed later: can complementary therapies be evaluated using quantitative techniques when one is dealing with subjective states that are difficult to define and even harder to measure?

A smaller study, using the same research framework as Dunn (1992), was carried out by Hewitt (1992) in the ITU at the Royal Sussex County Hospital, Brighton. She found, 30 minutes after treatment, that patients in the aromatherapy group showed greater decreases in heart rate, blood pressure, respiratory rates, pain levels and wakefulness than patients in the other two groups. It should be noted, however, that these figures were not analysed for statistical significance. She concluded that patients did benefit from the caring touch, and that aromatherapy can help patients in intensive and coronary care units to relax.

A number of writers, whilst acknowledging the importance of touch, argue that it is the nature of that touch which is significant, and therapeutic touch is qualitatively different from other forms. The term was coined by Kreiger who, as Professor of Nursing at New York University, began its implementation in the early 1970s. It is rooted in the ancient practice of laying-on of hands, but does not carry any religious connotations and there is no need for the practitioner or patient to exercise any 'faith'. There are four essential steps Kreiger (1975) describes:

1. The process of centring where the nurse assumes the intention to help the patient.
2. The use of the hands as sensors to assess the patient's energy flow and needs.
3. The use of the hands to redirect areas of accumulated tension or energy.
4. The directing of energy to the patient.

It is a nursing intervention which involves the use of hands as the focus to facilitate healing during a period of consciously directed energy exchange. It is on this basis that Sayre-Adams (1992) argues that therapeutic touch can be put firmly into Martha Roger's nursing theory of unitary human beings. Therapeutic touch is an energy field interactions where the role of the nurse is to repattern, or rebalance, the energy field and promote relaxation and pain relief. As with all holistic approaches it is argued that self-healing can only take place in a state of relaxation, and that the therapy itself is merely facilitating natural, hither to latent human potentials.

The question that has preoccupied a number of researchers has been whether therapeutic touch can be shown to be more effective than procedural touch. Heidt (1981) found evidence to support its claims: patients who received therapeutic touch experienced significant reductions in post-test anxiety scores, differences that were statistically significant when compared with those who received casual touch or no touch at all. Quinn (1984) also tested the hypothesis by comparing the effect of 'real' and 'mimic' therapeutic touch. Mimic touch lacked practitioner centring, patient assessment and aims to repattern. The interaction was video recorded and post-test anxiety levels were more reduced in subjects who experienced real therapeutic touch. The conclusion was drawn that therapeutic touch is a healing mediation that can facilitate patient recovery. Glick's study (1986), however, using a distinction between 'caring' and 'procedural' touch, showed no statistically significant difference. She concluded that "although the study failed to show statistical significance, the results, which were in the direction of the hypothesis, are supportive of previous research on touch and anxiety" (p. 65).

The aim of all these studies was to measure the effectiveness of a holistic intervention in some quantitative way. A number of writers, whilst acknowledging the need for evaluation, would argue it is difficult to use traditional, scientifically proven research methods since one is dealing with the 'art' of nursing not the 'science' (Fromant, 1991; Stevenson, 1992). Benefits are seen to lie at a personal energy level, in the subjective and experiential realm. Subjective states are difficult to define: people have feelings about their existence but they are qualities that cannot be addressed by modern science and measurement. It is on this basis that Byrne (1992) calls for new and imaginative 'holistic' research methods, and for scientific medicine to broaden its view of health rather than reduce complementary therapies to mechanical techniques. She argues that quantitative techniques are blind to whatever cannot be measured, timed or weighed; they fail to take account of the importance of actors meanings and interpretations.

The study by Samarel (1992) is a good example of the use of an alternative research tool. Using qualitative research, and Martha Roger's conceptual framework, she explored patients' 'lived experience' of receiving therapeutic touch. She describes their experience as being dynamic, multidimensional, involving both developing awareness and personal growth. The positive feedback from her respondents included references to senses of physical, mental, emotional and spiritual well-being. She concludes that a nursing intervention that can achieve such a positive influence has potential for use in all areas of nursing care, and needs to be explored further. Rankin-Box (1991) also calls for competent research to measure the efficacy of alternative therapies because: "it is imperative that professional standards are maintained and therapies do not surreptitiously slide into nursing practice using a backdoor approach" (p. 14).

The process of legitimation

Holism, with its acceptance of complementary modes of legitimate healing, represents more than a collection of techniques; it reflects a different perspective and a significant change in concepts of health and illness, not just at an individual level but at a cultural level. It is possible to identify five stages in the progressive legitimation of a marginal activity. First, individuals recognize that other individuals are engaged in, and committed to, the same 'fringe' therapeutic practices, and that some form of association would be beneficial. This first stage represents the change from individual practice to counter-cultural practice. Second, this association of individuals gains increasing recognition as it exercises pressure on existing professional bodies and wider society. The third stage is difficult to locate chronologically, but is a gradual semantic change: what was once 'fringe' and 'alternative' becomes 'complementary'. This stage represents the transition from counter-cultural practice to sub-cultural practice. Fourth, there is a growing concern, often generated by the appropriate professional bodies, that any new practice needs to be legitimated by credible academic research and theory drawing on other academic disciplines. This concern leads to the fifth stage, a focus on educational standards and a call for greater control over who practises what holistic therapies and which qualifications are acceptable. This final stage in the process of legitimation contains its own irony: the once 'charletons' and 'quacks' begin to define other marginal practices in the way they themselves were once defined.

There is evidence that within nursing, professional bodies are facing a growing call to recognize complementary therapies and incorporate them into mainstream practice. In 1991, the Royal College of Nursing (RCN) Complementary Therapies in Nursing special interests group was established, with a reported membership of over 500 (Denton, 1992). One of the group's remits was to examine standards of education; there are an increasing number of courses being offered in complementary therapies, often specifically designed for health professionals. In addition, there has been a call to define standards of acceptable practice and a central register of all nurses who are qualified and willing to offer complementary healing. It is interesting to note that the RCN indemnity insurance scheme covers members who use 'non-invasive' complementary therapies and acupuncture in the care of their patients; this, it is argued, demonstrates that complementary therapies are recognized as part of nursing care. A further indicator of recognition is the convening in October 1992 of the first UK conference to explore the use of complementary therapies in nursing.

There is therefore considerable evidence to support the view that within nursing significant steps have been taken in the process of the legitimation of complementary therapies. There is also evidence that this is being reflected in society as a whole. Calnan and Williams (1992), in a study of the general population, found that individuals were ambivalent in their attitudes towards modern scientific medicine. This, they argue, is a result of a much wider demystification of science. They speculate that an increasing number of people turning to complementary medicine are doing so to symbolize an estrangement from contemporary forms of technological intervention which they increasingly define as 'unnatural'. What the Williams and Calnan study points to is a potential cultural shift as sections of the population appear to be disillusioned and moving away from a dominant, dichotomized Western view of health and illness.

In her study, Sharma (1990) found no evidence that it was 'marginal' people who were using so called 'marginal' medicine. People used alternatives because they experienced a chronic disorder that was not successfully treated under the National Health Service. Failures in conventional medicine led to a more experimental attitude, and this led to a more eclectic approach to health care. Users of complementary therapies commented on three contrasts with conventional medicine: a more equal relationship in the consultation; a feeling that they were able to exercise greater control; a recognition that they were seen as a whole person, their illness being put into its personal context. Could it be that, as anthropological studies have shown, the ritualistic and magical elements of the exchange between healer and sufferer are just as important as the actual content of the physical treatment offered (Evans-Pritchard, 1937)?

CONCLUSION

Modern technology, according to Antonovsky (1992), creates tensions and potential conflict because it increases complexity, offers new choices, generates more information and calls for greater adaptive change. Historically, responses to the challenge of technological change have ranged from the nihilism of the Luddites to the positive acceptance witnessed during the industrial revolution. Antonovsky (1992) argues that the problem lies not in the technology itself but in the human response it generates. Is it possible to manage the tensions by becoming the 'masters' of the technology rather than its 'slaves'?

There has been a recognition that 'high-tech' in the ITU is a double-edged sword; on the one hand, it offers the potential of extending life, whilst on the other, it is seen as dehumanizing and potentially depriving patients of dignity and worth. The question has been asked whether the price being asked is too great to pay (Pellegrino, 1979). Could it be that the way forward lies not in a Luddite revolution or an unquestioning acceptance of medical technology, but in what Antonovsky refers to as 'civility': a new order where the coercion to accept one dominant scientific, medical paradigm is replaced by an acceptance of plurality, heterogeneity and fragmentation? A position where the biomedical and the ethnomedical can complement one another, the fact and the value can be given equal recognition and the art of nursing be integrated into the science.

The utilization of complementary therapies by appropriately qualified nurses and the legitimation of those practices by both the relevant professional and academic bodies could be a sign that we are seeing the contours of a new era appearing on the horizon as society moves towards post-modernism.

KEY TERMS

Modernism

This refers to an age in history that is characterized by a secular value system rooted in science and technology. The organization in 'modern' society is highly sophisticated in terms of the division of labour and the differentiation of knowledge.

Post-modernism

This refers to an age beyond 'modernism' where the values of Western science, scientific medicine and technology no longer dominate society. 'Post-modernism' is characterized by a plurality of values drawn from a wide range of very different academic disciplines and cultural experiences.

The Enlightenment

or the 'Age of Enlightenment' refers to a period during the 18th century when it was believed that all human problems could be solved by the application of rational scientific methods of study. Human action would become predictable, and the state of mankind could only improve as scientific advances were made. Progress was inevitable and seen to be of positive benefit.

Cartesianism and Descartes

Rene Descartes is often referred to as the founder of modern philosophy who rejected traditional forms of knowledge arguing that it was possible to construct a complete, all-inclusive science of nature. This 'new' science, it was claimed, was certain and 'the truth', something that did not need verification from other academic disciplines.

Paradigm

Sometimes referred to as a 'perspective'. It is a recognized approach within sociology to understanding or interpreting the social world and social action.

Sociology

Is a social science which is concerned with the study of social interaction between individuals, between individuals and groups and between individuals and institutions in society.

ACKNOWLEDGEMENTS

I would like to thank a number of friends and colleagues for their support through discussion and critical review of this chapter, in particular Don Bradley, Brian Millar, Jim Richardson, Fran Biley and Julie Scholes. I would also like to thank Dawn Hewitt and Jimmy Cooper (ITU West Sussex Hospital, Brighton), Chrissie Dunn (ITU Battle Hospital, Reading) and Jean Sayre-Adams (Didsbury Trust) for the information they gave me on holism in practice.

REFERENCES

Aggleton, P., Chalmers, H. *Nursing Models and the Nursing Process*. Basingstoke: MacMillan, 1986.

Albarran, J. W. Advocacy in critical care – an evaluation of the implications for nurses and the future. *Intensive and Critical Care Nursing*. 1992; 8: 47–53.

Antonovsky, A. Modern technology. Plenary Address at the XIIth International Social Science and Medicine Conference. Peebles, Scotland, 1992.

Ashworth, P. *Care to Communicate*. London: Royal College of Nursing, 1980.

Ashworth, P. High technology and humanity for intensive care. *Intensive Care Nursing*. 1990; 6: 150–160.

Atkinson, B. Management of the intensive care unit. *Nursing*. 1987; 16: 584–589.

Baldwin, S. Complementary health. *Nursing*. 1991, November 21–December 4; 4(46): 15–17.

Barger-Lux, M. J., Heaney, R. P. For better and worse: the technological imperative in health care. *Social Science and Medicine*. 1986; 22(12): 1313–1320.

Bergbom-Engberg, I., Haljamae, H. A retrospective study of patients' recall of respirator treatment (2); Nursing care factors and feelings of security/insecurity. 1988.

Biley, F. The science of unitary human beings: a contemporary literature review. *Nursing Practice*. 1992; 5(4): 23–26.

Boyle, S. The nursing role in critical care. *Surgical Nurse*. 1992; 5(1): 17–19.

Briggs, D. Critical care nurses' roles – traditional or expanded/extended. *Intensive Care Nursing*. 1991; 7: 223–229.

Buckenham, J., McGrath, G. *The Social Reality of Nursing*. Australia: AIDS Health Science Press, 1983.

Byrne, C. Research methods in complementary therapies. *Nursing Standard*. 1992, 2 September; 6(50): 54–56.

Calnan, M., Williamson, S. Images of scientific medicine. *Sociology of Health and Illness*. 1992; 14(2): 233–253.

Carnevale, F. A. High technology and humanity in intensive care: finding a balance. *Intensive Care Nursing*. 1991; 7: 23–27.

Clarke, K. J. Coping with Guillain Barre syndrome (a personal experience). *Intensive Care Nursing*. 1985; 1(1): 13–18.

Clifford, C. Patients, relatives and nurses in a technological environment. *Intensive Care Nursing*. 1986; 2: 67–72.

Constable, B. Intensive disagreement. *Nursing Times*. 1991; 23 January; 87(4): 66–67.

Coombs, R. H., Goldman, L. J. Maintenance and discontinuity of coping mechanism in an intensive care unit. *Social Problems*. 1973; 20(3); 342–355.

Cooper, J. Personal communication. ITU, West Sussex Hospital, 1992.

Crawshaw, R. Technical zeal or therapeutic purpose – how to decide? *Journal of American Medical Association*. 1983; 250: 1857–1859.

Crook, S., Pakulski, J., Waters, M. *Postmodernism: Change in Advanced Society*. London: Sage, 1992.

Denton, P. Make your voice heard. *Nursing Standard*. 1992, 2 September; 6(50): 50.

Dunn, C. Staying in touch: A report on the randomised controlled trial to evaluate the use of massage and aromatherapy in an intensive care unit. Unpublished B.Sc. Dissertation, 1992.

Durkheim, E. *The Evolution of Educational Thought*. (Trans. P. Collins). London: Routledge and Kegan Paul, 1977.

Eagleton, T. Awakening from modernity. *Times Literary Supplement*. 20 February 1987.

Estabrooks, C. A., Morse, J. M. Towards a theory of touch: the touching process and acquiring a touching style. *Journal of Advanced Nursing*. 1992; 17: 448–456.

Evans, M. Reflex zone therapy for mothers. *Nursing Times*. 1990, 24 January; 86(4): 29–31.

Evans-Pritchard, E. *Witchcraft, Oracles and Magic Among The Azande*. Oxford: Clarendon Press, 1937.

Fagerhaugh, S., Strauss, A., Suczek, B., Wiener, C. The impact of technology on patients, providers and care patterns. *Nursing Outlook*. 1980, November: 666–672.

Fairman, J. Watchful vigilance: nursing care, technology and the development of intensive care units. *Nursing Research*. 1992; 41(1): 56–60.

Figlio, K. The historiography of scientific medicine – an invitation to the human sciences. *Comparative Studies in Society and History*. 1977; 19: 265–273.

Frankfurt Institute. *Aspects of Scoiology*. (Trans. J. Viertel). London: Heinemann, 1973.

Fromant, P. Let me rub it better. *Nursing*. 1991, November 21–December 4; 4(46): 18–19.

Fuchs, V. R. The growing demand for medical care. *New England Journal of Medicine*. 1968; 279: 192.

Giddens, A. *The Consequences of Modernity*. Cambridge: Polity Press, 1990.

Glen, A. Psychological Aspects of critical care. *Surgical Nurse*. 1991, June; 4(3): 15–17.

Glick, M. Caring touch and anxiety in myocardial infarction patients in the intermediate cardiac care unit. *Intensive Care Nursing*. 1986; 2: 61–66.

Heidt, P. Effect of therapeutic touch on anxiety of hospitalised patients. *Nursing Research*. 1981; 30: 32–37.

Henderson, V. Preserving the essence of nursing in a technological age. *Journal of Advanced Nursing*. 1980; 5: 245–260.

Hewitt, D. Massage with lavender oil lowered tension. *Nursing Times*. 1992, 17 June; 88(25): 8.

Hobsbawm, E. J. *The Age of Revolution, 1789–1848*. New York: Mentor, 1962.

Hofoss, D. Health professions: the origin of species. *Social Science and Medicine*. 1986; 22(2): 201–209.

Horkheimer, M. *Critical Theory: Selected Essays*. New York: Herder and Herder, 1972.

Illich, I. *Limits to Medicine. Medical Nemesis: The Exploration of Health*. London: Marion Boyars, 1976.

Ingham, A. A review of the literature relating to touch and its use in intensive care. *Intensive Care Nursing*. 1989; 5: 65–75.

Jourard, S. M. An exploratory study of body-accessibility. *British Journal of Clinical Psychology*. 1966; 5: 221–231.

Keat, R. *The Politics of Social Theory*. Oxford: Blackwell, 1981.

Kennedy, I. *The Unmasking of Medicine*. London: Paladin, 1983.

Kleinman, A. Culture, Illness and Care. *Annals of Internal Medicine*. 1978, February.

Kreiger, D. Therapeutic touch: the imprimatur of nursing. *The American Journal of Nursing*. 1975; 8: 152–155.

Lyotard, J. *The Post-Modern Condition*. Minneapolis: University of Minneapolis Press, 1985.

Manley, K. Intensive caring. *Nursing Times*, 1990, 9 May; 86(19): 67–69.

Mason, V. Nurses and doctors as healers. *Nursing Outlook*. 1985; 33(2): 70–73.

McKeown, T. *The Role of Medicine*. Oxford: Basil Blackwell, 1979.

Melia, K. *Learning and Working: The Occupational Socialisation of Nurses*. London: Tavistock, 1987.

Oldfield, V. A healing touch. *Nursing Standard*. 1992; 6(44): 21.

Passant, H. A holistic approach in the ward. *Nursing Times*. 1990, 24 January; 86(4): 26–28.

Paterson, J. G., Zderad, L. T. *Humanistic Nursing*. New York: National League for Nursing, 1988.

Pearson, A. (Ed.). *Primary Nursing: Nursing in the Burford and Oxford Nursing Development Units*. Beckenham: Croom Helm, 1983.

Pellegrino, E. D. *Humanism and the Physician*. Knoxville: University of Tenenesse Press, 1979.

Penticuff, J. K. Infant suffering and nurse advocacy in neonatal care. *Nursing Clinics of North America*. 1989; 24(4): 987–997.

Quinn, J. F. Therapeutic touch as energy exchange: testing the theory. *Advances in Nursing Science*. 1984; 6(1): 42–49.

Rankin-Box, D. Complementary therapies in nursing. *Nursing*. 1991, November 21–December 4; 4(46): 12–14.

Rome, H. P. The irony of the ICU. *Psychiatry Digest*. 1969, May: 10–14.

Royal Society of London. *Philosophical Transactions 1: 1665–1666*. New York: Johnson Reprint Company, 1963.

Rundell, S. A study of nurse–patient interaction in a high dependency unit. *Intensive Care Nursing*. 1991; 7: 171–178.

Salvage, J. The theory and practice of the new nursing. *Nursing Times*. 1990, 24 January; 86(4): 42–45.

Salyer, J., Stuart, B. Nurse–patient interaction in the ITU. *Heart & Lung*. 1985; 14(1): 20–24.

Samarel, N. The experience of receiving therapeutic touch. *Journal of Advanced Nursing*. 1992; 17: 651–657.

Sayre-Adams, J. Therapeutic touch – research and reality. *Nursing Standard*. 1992, 2 September; 6(50): 52–54.

Schutz, A. *On Phenomenology and Social Relations*. Chicago: University of Chicago Press, 1970.

Sharma, U. M. Using alternative therapies: marginal medicine and central concerns. In: P. Abbott, G. Payne. *New Directions in the Sociology of Health*. London: Falmer Press, 1990.

Shuldham, J. The nurse on the intensive care unit. *Intensive Care Nursing*. 1986; 1: 181–186.

Smith, C. In need of intensive care – a personal perspective. *Intensive Care Nursing*. 1987; 2: 116–122.

Smith, M. Healing through touch. *Nursing Times*. 1990, 24 January; 86(4): 31–32.

Smith, P. *The Emotional Labour of Nursing*. Oxford: Macmillan, 1992.

Smith, P., Redfern, S. The quality of care and student's educational experience in hospital wards. In: Eds. J. Wilson-Barnett, S. Robinson. *Directions in Nursing Research*. London: Scutari, 1989.

Smuts, J. *Holism and Evolution*. New York: Viking Press, 1962.

Stanton, D. J. The psychological impact of intensive therapy: the role of nurses. *Intensive Care Nursing*. 1991; 7: 230–235.

Strauss, A., Fagerhaugh, S., Suczek, B., Wiener, C. *Social Organisation of Medical Work*. Chicago: University of Chicago Press, 1985.

Stevenson, C. Appropriate therapies for nurses to practise. *Nursing Standard*. 1992, 2 September; 6(50): 51–52.

Street, A. F. *Inside Nursing: A Critical Ethnography of Clinical Nursing Practice*. Albany: State University of New York Press, 1992.

Toffler, A. *The Third Wave*. London: Pan Books, 1980.

Tonnies, F. *Community and Society*. New York: Harper & Row, 1957.

Tosch, P. Patients recollections of their post traumatic coma. *Journal of Neuroscience Nursing*. 1988; 20(4): 223–228.

Weber, M. *From Max Weber: Essays in Sociology*. (Trans. and Ed. by H. Gerth, C. W. Mills.) London: Routledge and Kegan Paul, 1970.

Weber, M. *Economy and Society*. (Trans. and Ed. by G. Roth, C. Wittick.) California: University of California Press, 1978.

Weiss, S. J. The language of touch. *Nursing Research*. 1979; 28(2): 76–80.

16
COMMUNICATION IN CRITICAL CARE NURSING

Julie Pearce

CHAPTER AIMS

This chapter aims at helping the reader to explore a range of issues related to communication in critical care nursing. Specifically, it looks at the *nature* of communication in critical care settings. It offers scenarios that highlight communication problems in the field, and it identifies and discusses some of the research related to communication.

INTRODUCTION

Many of the chapters in this book have dealt with technical, psychological and social issues related to critical care nursing. Perhaps the most vital issue in the field is that of communication. This takes many forms: communication between patient and nurse, between nurse and doctor, between patient and relative. Communication can also be verbal or non-verbal. This chapter explores aspects of a whole spectrum of issues related to communication in critical care nursing.

COMMUNICATION

"We speak with our vocal organs but converse with our whole body" (Argyle, 1978).

The development of technology in medicine and subsequent growth in invasive and non-invasive devices for measuring, monitoring and regulating body systems has meant that the role of the intensive care nurse has extended and expanded, and continues to expand, to incorporate technical aspects of care. This phenomenon has tended to focus skills on physiological problems, sometimes at the expense of meeting the psychosocial needs of the patient and their family. The feature of quality within an experienced intensive care nurse is someone who has developed the whole range of skills which enables them to achieve a balance in the care provided.

The person admitted to the intensive care unit will be experiencing a physiological crisis and a physical threat to his or her survival. On the other hand, the uncertainty and life-threatening nature of the situation will pose a series of real, imagined or potential threats to family members, whose main concern will be for the safety and survival of the patient. The anxiety and distress experienced under these circumstances will have an impact on the well-being of the family, and may make excessive demands upon their abilities to cope (Millar, 1989).

The impact of the intensive care environment on the patient and their family has been well documented. The abnormal patterns of sensory information are received from the patient's internal and external environments; the patient has to make sense, or to interpret these signals, when their cognitive abilities have been affected by the pathophysiology of the illness, the drug therapy, and the inability to communicate easily, either verbally or non-verbally (Ashworth, 1980; Hudak *et al.*, 1986). The patient has to cope with and deal with their thoughts, feelings, emotions, and experiences in relative isolation.

This situation may lead to feelings of dependency, isolation, loss of control over events, fear, anxiety, difficulty in sleeping, and perceptual distortions characterized by disorientation, restlessness, body image distortions, paranoia and depression. These experiences may reduce the patient's motivation and will to survive.

In an excellent two part article on body image, Helen Platzer (1987) writes about a patient's experience or memory of his stay in intensive care. The patient was ventilated for a period whilst suffering from a viral-bacterial auto-immune disease. He recalls:

"My mind had started playing tricks in the intensive care unit. The thought that I was abroad was confirmed by the foreign names and travel posters pinned on the walls. Another fascinating assumption was that I had a tube leading through my stomach to my backside, where it was attached to a toy model of an Austin A40. It was a counterweight for my intravenous tube! I would lie in bed wondering how they got it there in the first place. Medical science is an amazing thing!"

This description illustrates vividly the nature of the perceptual distortions that are experienced by patients. The patient was able to rationalize the experience later; however, at the time the experience was very real to him. There has been little research which focuses on the patient's recall of experiences following intensive care (Heath, 1989). We have little knowledge of how often patients have these experiences, and perhaps more importantly, the relative contribution that perceptual disturbances have on the outcome of illness and recovery.

Communication is fundamental to any human relationship and forms the basis of all human interaction. Communication is not optional; any encounter with another person, however brief, involves the exchange of information through verbal and non-verbal behaviour (Porritt, 1990). To patients and families within intensive care, the interpersonal skills of those caring for them will make a significant contribution to their overall experience of critical illness. They rely on those caring for them for information, support, reassurance, comfort, empathy, security. Behaviours which express this commitment are motivated by humanistic values which cannot be replaced by technology.

The nurse is involved in the total care of patients and their families. The dependency of the patient, the complexity of critical illness and strategies for supporting life add to the complexity of the assessment of need, information and data gathering, observation, decision making, and coordination of the skills and knowledge offered by each member of the multidisciplinary team towards providing continuous, high quality care. The nurse often plays a key role in coordinating care and communication on behalf of the team, and facilitates continuity of patient care and empowerment of family members.

The search for effective strategies which minimize distress and facilitate coping must be acknowledged as essential components in the process of caring for patients and their families. The person's perception of the experience may be modified through effective communication and the interpersonal skills and qualities of those caring for them. We should not underestimate the therapeutic contribution that effective communication makes to the well-being of the family, and possibly the outcome of critical illness for the patient. It presents a real challenge to the intensive care nurse.

The large amount of literature available on communication can be found within psychology, sociology, anthropology and nursing. Communication is a complex phenomenon in itself, and is therefore difficult to define. Nearly every communicative element, function or effect has been the focus for definition at some time. It has been described in relation to: its structure (sender-message-receiver); its function (encoding-decoding); and in terms of its intent (expressive-instrumental). It has been described as a process of transmitting stimuli, conveying meaning, and as a procedure by which one mind and behaviour affects the mind and behaviour of another (French, 1983; Pegano and Ragan, 1992; Wilmot, 1987). The person's ability to communicate effectively is based upon their awareness of how and what they are communicating, and how the interactive process influences the other person (Porritt, 1990).

What does it mean to be a competent communicator? Communication includes both cognitive and behavioural abilities; the person must have knowledge about the communication process, and also the skills to enact that knowledge. Competent communicators are able to use their knowledge and skills towards achieving desired goals (Pegano and Ragan, 1992). For example, during a pre-operative interview prior to cardiac surgery, the nurse may want to find out from the patient their current knowledge regarding their condition, the surgery, and their expectations of the outcome of surgery, so as to assess the patient's need for information. Competence is based upon the nurse's ability to define their communication goals for a particular situation, and to choose the communication behaviours which will give the best chance of meeting the desired goal. On the other hand, competence is also based on the perception of the other person with whom the nurse is communicating. Wiemann (1977) summarizes the process as: selecting interactional choices, accomplishing interpersonal goals, and recognizing the interpersonal and contextual constraints of communication situations.

Before examining the literature on interactional theories and the application of verbal and nonverbal communication skills within the context of critical care nursing, it may be useful to examine a number of typical situations or case scenarios. This may be a useful method of demonstrating what the interpersonal goals for the nurse may consist of, how these goals may be achieved, and the contextual constraints that are placed on the interactive process within each situation.

Case scenario I: admission of a patient to intensive care

Paul is a 25 year old man who was admitted to the accident and emergency department having been involved in a motor car accident. Paul had been a back seat passenger when they were involved in a head on collision with another vehicle. Paul had been trapped inside the car for 35 minutes before being cut free by the emergency services. He was intubated by the paramedics at the scene of the accident before being taken to hospital.

Paul was unconscious with a Glasgow coma score of 4. His pupils were equal, size 8 and reacting to light. He was in sinus tachycardia with a heart rate of 160 beats per minute, and blood pressure of 100/60 mm Hg. Multiple abrasions were noted on his face and chest. Blood was found in Paul's ears along with battle's signs. Fluid resuscitation was commenced.

Paul developed surgical emphysema; the chest x-Ray revealed a pneumomediastinum. A chest drain was inserted. Paul was taken to theatre via the CAT Scan for insertion of an intracranial monitoring system which gave an initial reading of 10 mm Hg. He was then transferred to the intensive care unit for further management and care. The initial diagnoses included a diffuse head injury with a base of skull fracture and a Le Forte type III facial fracture, cardiac contusion with pneumomediastinum.

Paul's mother and father had been contacted by the police and they have now arrived at the hospital with Sarah, Paul's sister. They are directed to the intensive care unit and wait anxiously for some news of his condition.

This scenario is a fairly typical situation that nurses within critical care face on a daily basis. The initial emphasis of nursing care must be to meet the patient's physical and physiological needs efficiently and effectively, working with the multidisciplinary team to achieve homeostasis. The nurses face the challenge of utilizing their skills in accurately assessing the patient's problems, through the continuous cycle of observation and data collection, planning, implementation and evaluation of the care provided.

Once this has been achieved, the nurse's attention turns to the family. The family is experiencing a major situational crisis caused by the unexpected, unpredictable events which have led to Paul's admission to the intensive care unit. Family members have not had the opportunity of planning and preparing for the situation which will interrupt the normal pattern of life for them. The challenge for the nurse is to enable the family members to find within themselves the resources to cope with the situation (Wright, 1986).

Personal experience and the literature demonstrates to us the importance of being able to meet needs for open and honest information which enables the patient and the family to make sense of the situation. The nurse must assess their ability to utilize the information and begin to interpret and accept what has happened. This will be an ongoing process through the patient's stay in intensive care and beyond. The family will also have a great desire to be near the patient (Molter, 1979; Coulter, 1989). The family must be prepared for their first and subsequent visits to the unit. This is a stressful time for the family; the nature of the distress is complex involving their concerns about:

☐ the outcome of the illness and the long-term effects of the patient's condition;

☐ the alteration in family roles and patterns of communication and support;

☐ the establishment of trust in hospital carers;

☐ their ability to cope with environmental stimuli;

☐ the comprehension of complex medical information; and

☐ their ability to cope with the patient's physical appearance, behaviour and emotions.

The interpersonal goals for the nurses involved in Paul's care will be to:

☐ begin to develop an open, trusting relationship with family members, which will enable them to feel able to ask questions, and to be with Paul whenever they wish and when it is practical;

☐ assess the family's ability to cope with information about Paul's condition and management;

☐ repeat and re-enforce information, interpret medical and technical language, and work towards an understanding of the situation and events;

☐ prepare the family for visiting Paul for the first and subsequent times within the intensive care unit;

☐ demonstrate their care and concern for Paul as a person and his family through verbal and non-verbal behaviours;

☐ assess family members' abilities to cope with the situation, identifying previous crisis events the family have experienced and the coping strategies they have utilized;

☐ begin to identify the individual needs of family members and to plan care appropriately.

The creation of a supportive atmosphere in which family and friends feel free and comfortable to be with the patient does not happen through chance. It is an outward manifestation of the philosophy upon which care is based and is, therefore, a complex phenomenon composed of the underlying beliefs and values, and the interpersonal skills held by the nursing team.

Case scenario II: preparation of a family for cardiac surgery

Katie is a six year old girl who is awaiting cardiac surgery for correction of a cardiac defect. Katie has been into hospital many times during her life, and has already undergone two palliative surgical procedures. Katie's mother and father are keen to have as much information about the operation as possible; however, they have found it difficult to talk to her sister Sophie, who is 8 years old, about the details of the operation and care that Katie will receive.

The nursing team work out a plan of pre-operative preparation for the family along with the play specialist who will be involved in preparing Katie and Sophie for Katie's operation.

The interpersonal goals for the nurses involved in the preparation of Katie's parents will be to:

☐ assess their understanding of Katie's condition, knowledge of the surgery and the events that will surround the operation;

☐ explore their previous experiences of hospital admission and their abilities to cope with the situation as a family;

☐ give information, building on previous knowledge, about the operation, stay in intensive care and rehabilitation and clarify medical information;

☐ begin to develop an open, trusting relationship with Katie's parents so that they will feel able to ask questions and continue to participate in Katie's care whilst in hospital;

☐ assess their understanding of information given and begin to identify their expectations of the hospital stay and Katie's operation;

☐ offer them the opportunity of visiting the intensive care unit before the operation.

Hospitalization is known to be a stressful experience for children and their parents. The first hospital admission makes a strong impression on parents, and any future hospitalizations will be interpreted in the light of previous experiences. The literature suggests that a child's vulnerability to hospitalization is influenced by the existing quality of relationships in their family life, and parental views and attitudes to hospitalization (Sargent, 1983). It appears that the distress experienced by children may be modified by parents (Hall, 1987).

Pre-surgical information and preparation is essential to parents as it facilitates cognitive appraisal and rehearsal of events and minimizes the dissonance between expectation and actual experience. A major source of parental stress relates to the changes that occur to their usual parental role. The role revision that takes place involves the transition from parents of a reasonably healthy child to that of a critically ill child (Carnevale, 1990; Jay, 1977).

Pre-operative preparation should include information about the child's defect and the events surrounding the surgical procedure; socialization to the unit and hospital systems; discussion of parental role alteration and potential changes in the child's behaviour and emotions; and identification of how the parental role may be re-established through involvement and participation in decision making and care of their child.

The interpersonal goals of the nurses involved in preparing Katie and her sister for Katie's operation will be to:

☐ begin to explore what Katie knows about her condition and what is going to happen whilst she is in hospital;

☐ find out what words Katie uses to express herself and the meanings she attaches to

those words when she is talking about her condition and stay in hospital;

☐ begin to develop a relationship of trust with Katie and Sophie;

☐ begin to prepare Katie and Sophie for the events surrounding the operation and the stay in the intensive care unit utilizing appropriate strategies, i.e. play situations, allegorical story of a child who has cardiac surgery, visual aids, e.g. pictures of other children in the intensive care unit and dolls;

☐ assess their level of understanding of the information they have gained.

Pre-operative preparation programmes for children are designed to reduce the emotional sequelae of hospitalization and surgery. Several techniques have been evaluated and found to be effective in reducing anxiety in children.

Allegorical stories enable children to cope with the worries and fears precipitated by illness, medical procedures and surgery (Fossen and Husband, 1984). Stories with appropriate symbolic themes not only supplement explicit discussions of experiences and sensations the child's care will generate, but also allow exploration of fears that may be of a particular concern for the individual child. These include fear of mutilation, separation anxiety, loss of control, and fear of death, issues that are not often addressed by explicit preparatory procedures.

Story books may be used by individuals without special training in counselling or emotional support of children. Parents can be especially effective readers, and because this role reinforces their natural supportive relationship with their child and facilitates open discussion of emotional issues within the family, this should be encouraged (Fossen and Husband, 1984).

Play is a voluntary, intensely personal experience; children act out their ideas, fears, feelings and fantasies, and in doing so, learn to cope with their experiences. Structured play and the utilization of 'dolls' enable the nurse or play therapist to explore with the child factual and sensory information concerning the surgery and intensive care environment. This is particularly useful in the younger child, where preparation must be gradual to allow the assimilation and integration of complex and potentially threatening information (Chan, 1980).

Bates and Broome (1986) discusses the benefits of using play therapy, dolls and stories with younger children, and verbal explanations, diagrams and films with older children.

Nursing staff have a continuous relationship with the family during the child's intensive care stay. Nurses share the responsibility of supporting the family through a major life event with the multidisciplinary team. However, nurses are seen by parents as being a key source for information, interpreters of medical information, and facilitators in helping parents to understand and find meaning in events as they occur. Nurses are also involved in supportive-educative activities which enable parents to participate in their child's care, and enable parents to communicate with other health care professionals about their child (Pearce, 1992).

Case scenario III: surviving the experience of critical illness

Mr Bill Thomas is a 65 year old gentleman who was transferred to the intensive care unit three weeks ago for management of his respiratory failure. Bill has chronic obstructive airways disease with corpulmonalae and a pneumonia which is resolving. He is currently on an SIMV with pressure support via a tracheostomy. Bill's main problems centre around the long process of weaning from mechanical ventilation. He finds it difficult to communicate his needs; he tires easily, has problems sleeping at night, has a poor appetite, and he feels depressed.

This third scenario is again fairly typical of the challenges faced by intensive care nurse. The main aim of care is to facilitate weaning from mechanical ventilation; this may be a long and difficult journey for Mr Thomas. The experienced nurse will move the emphasis of care to psychological support, using interpersonal skills to discover how to enable Mr Thomas to communicate his needs, feelings and emotions. The nurse will negotiate a weaning programme which will allow him to see that he does have some control over the situation and events.

Negotiation will no doubt take a great deal of time, patience, skill and creativity on both sides, but the end result will be a patient who feels valued, less dependent, able to contribute to his or her own plan of care, and this will probably improve the motivation to succeed and survive.

Communication aids may be helpful, such as picture cues, letter boards, non-verbal signs and signals. The nurse may use closed questions which enable the patient to nod or shake the head appropriately. This is a useful strategy for patients who have difficulty breathing and low energy levels.

The interpersonal goals for nurses caring for Mr Thomas will be to:

☐ achieve successful weaning from mechanical ventilation;

☐ assess Mr Thomas's communication difficulties and identify the most appropriate strategies which will optimize Mr Thomas's abilities to communicate his needs;

☐ explore with Mr Thomas his expectations regarding the weaning programme, and negotiate an achievable daily plan which allows rest and sleep at night;

☐ assess Mr Thomas's ability to cope with the weaning programme using non-verbal signals such as facial expression and body posture, clinical signs, and discussion of his progress;

☐ explore ways of improving Mr Thomas's sleep pattern and appetite, negotiate achievable daily plans to achieve this.

Once Mr Thomas is self-ventilating and maintaining good respiratory gases, it will be time to think about preparing Mr Thomas for his transfer to the medical unit. This may be a difficult transition for Mr Thomas, he may feel apprehensive about leaving the unit. The interpersonal goals for the nurses caring for him will be to prepare him for the environmental changes that will occur, as well as the psychosocial and emotional impact of the transfer. The nurse may want to explore his feelings and anxieties about the move, and to reassure him that these are normal feelings to have and that it will take him some time to adjust completely to his new surroundings. If time allows, the primary nurse or ward staff from the medical unit could be invited to visit Mr Thomas for brief periods before his transfer takes place. The important issue for Mr Thomas is that continuity of care is maintained between the ward areas, so that he feels confident and comfortable with his new carers.

THE FUNDAMENTALS OF COMMUNICATION THEORY

We have already begun to examine the complexities of communication through a number of typical practical scenarios in which the process of communication features as an important element in the care of the patient and their family. Communication is a social skill, and is learnt through the process of socialization from child to adult, and later through professional socialization. Nurses learn from the practical experience of communicating with patients and their families, through reflection and development of self-awareness, and through knowledge derived from communication theory.

The environment is where interaction occurs, for example, the health care setting, an organization, an institution. The social context is the part of the environment where interaction takes place. The status and power of the persons involved, and the roles and rules that apply will affect the dynamics of the interaction.

Exploration of the knowledge derived from both information and transactional theories offers a framework from which an understanding of the inter-relationship between the components of the communication process may be realized (French, 1983; Pegano and Ragan, 1992; Wilmot, 1987).

Information theory

In the past, communication has been seen simply as the process of transmitting information from one person to another. The four elements required are the sender, the message, the transmission channel and the receiver. These elements are linked and can be represented by the communication model outlined in Table 16.1.

Table 16.1. Communication model.

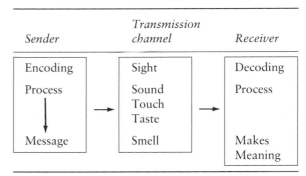

Sender	Transmission channel	Receiver
Encoding	Sight	Decoding
Process	Sound	Process
	Touch	
	Taste	
Message	Smell	Makes Meaning

The need to communicate something to the other person arises within the sender; it may be thoughts, feelings, ideas or information. The sender has a mental image of what he or she wants to communicate and these are translated or encoded into a set of symbols which are transferred or transmitted as a message to the receiver through an appropriate sensory channel. The coded messages may be verbal or non-verbal in nature, and are produced through motor functions which enable the sender to transmit the message using muscles to gesture, create posture and facial expression, and to write, draw, or produce sound (Porritt, 1990).

The receiver decodes or converts the coded message into meaning and therefore, requires knowledge of the symbols and signals being used and the sender and receiver must share the same encoding and decoding processes, for example, the same language. The meaning derived through the decoding process may or may not be an accurate interpretation of what the sending person intended to communicate.

The transactional nature of interpersonal communication

The model described above tends to stress the linear nature of the communication process where the message is passed from the sender to the receiver in a uni-directional fashion. Communication is an ongoing process in which the participants are simultaneously sending and receiving messages. It is more useful to see the communication process as a transactional process in which both participants play the roles of speaker, listener and observer, encoder and decoder, sender and receiver at the same time (Wilmot, 1987). The participants affect each other's behaviour, and both engage in a process of negotiating the meaning of messages.

The transactional model of communication enables us to focus on the important functions of listening, interpreting and giving feedback or checking out the accuracy of our interpretation of the messages received (Wilmot, 1987; Porritt, 1990).

Interpretation and feedback

The skilled communicator will check the interpretation of the messages given and received through a feedback mechanism. Ineffective or dysfunctional communication may result if the feedback mechanism is not employed.

The receiving person may take on the responsibility for checking that their interpretation of the message is correct, thus giving the sender an opportunity for adjusting the message to obtain a more accurate interpretation. This is particularly important for the nurse when communicating with a person (sender) who has difficulty encoding messages. This situation may be due to impairment of brain function and memory loss, which may diminish the sender's ability to select appropriate words or non-verbal cues. The anxious person or those in a highly emotional state may have difficulty in expressing exactly what they want to communicate.

Once the patient (sender) has decided upon a message, the next problem may be their inability to choose the correct transmission channel, or their choice of transmission channel may be limited by their inability to vocalize due to intubation, or severe dyspnoea. Alternatively, the patient may not be able to use appropriate non-verbal gestures, facial expressions and eye contact due to physical deficits as a result of the pathophysiology of the illness, mechanical constraints of the invasive monitoring, or the chemical constraints of sedation and muscle relaxants.

The nurse may use feedback techniques to check the interpretation of the messages she is receiving. This may be achieved through questioning, reflecting and summarizing. The nurse as the receiver needs to utilize the skills of the active listener:

1. Paying attention to what is being communicated using all senses.

2. Offering encouragement and rewarding the sender, particularly if communication is an effort for the sender.
3. Giving feedback.
4. Checking that the meaning of the message has been accurately interpreted.

When the nurse is the sending person, they may take the initiative in checking out the receiver's understanding of the information or message received.

Interference

Interference is any thing which will distort or prevent the message being sent or being received. These include: the degree of skill of the communicator, noise, the use of jargon, attitudes, values, socialization, other intrapersonal effects, e.g. physical, mental or psychological limitations, the degree of experience and knowledge relating to the message, and other environmental and sociocultural factors. It can be seen that distortion of the message being communicated may originate from factors within the individual person, both people, and the social context or the environment.

Barriers to effective communication

Encoding failure

A number of problems may arise in the thought processes which begin the sequence of communication events. These may range from impairment of brain functioning (e.g. altered level of consciousness), delirium, memory impairment (e.g. old age), brain damage through intracranial bleeding, or head injury which may diminish the ability to select appropriate words and non-verbal cues. Emotional factors (e.g. anxiety or anger) may result in the person having difficulty expressing themselves precisely (French, 1983).

Transmission failure

The person may be able to decide on the appropriate message to be sent; however, they may have difficulty in choosing and using the mode of transmission. The patient in intensive care may be intubated, and may be restricted in body movement by the number of invasive or non-invasive attachments, or may be experiencing paralysis of muscle groups either as a result of the pathophysiology of the illness, or through the use of sedation and muscle relaxants. These factors will impair the person's ability to speak and to communicate non-verbally through gestures and facial expression. Patients who are in respiratory failure and experiencing severe dyspnoea will have difficulty in expressing themselves verbally.

Channel interference

Once the message has been transmitted the symbols may be distorted in a number of ways. This may be due to transmission overload or attentional overload.

An example of channel overload is when two people are speaking at once, or if the person is speaking too rapidly. This often occurs when a patient who has a tracheostomy is communicating with the nurse. The nurse is dependent upon being able to lip read the patient and to interpret any non-verbal gestures which accompany the message. If the patient speaks too rapidly or is not able to emphasize the words sufficiently, then the nurse may have difficulty in grasping the whole message. The patient may also use gestures or hand signals which are too rapid which creates interpretation difficulties.

Examples of attentional overload involve competition for the receiver's attention. This can occur frequently within the critical care setting. The nurse may try to concentrate on receiving a message from the patient; however, an alarm sounds in the next bed area, the telephone rings and someone is asking for the keys to the drugs cupboard; this makes concentration and continuity difficult for both the patient and the nurse. There is evidence that we are able to close down various sensory inputs to pay attention to one in particular; however, we can still be distracted by stimuli impinging on other senses.

The patient may also experience attentional overload from the large number of abnormal sensory input that they receive from the environment, for example, noise of people and machines, artificial lighting, the number and intensity of interactions with members of the multidisciplinary team, and the pattern of nursing care.

The other important feature of channel interference relates to the relative permanence of the communication medium. The written word is a more permanent record of communication allowing the receiver to go back over the same cues. However, the spoken word relies on the memory of the receiver to keep track of the message. The receiver may ask the sender to repeat the message; however, it is unlikely that the verbal and non-verbal cues will be exactly the same each time.

Perceptual failure

This refers to an impairment in the person's ability to receive particular sensory stimuli. The position of the patient in bed may mean that they have a very limited visual field, therefore unless the nurse makes a point of coming close to the patient's face, they may miss eye contact and facial expression and other non-verbal cues.

The patient may have a functional loss of sight, or hearing through illness or advancing age, or a loss of touch sensations as a result of paraesthesia or anaesthesia. Certain drugs act on the central and peripheral nervous system which will lead to perceptual difficulties; for example, blurred vision, and an altered sense of smell and taste.

The extreme of sensory impairment is unconsciousness. Auditory sensation often returns before motor ability. This is why the critical care nurse communicates verbally and non-verbally with the unconscious person, even when the patient shows no signs of having received the message or generating a response.

Decoding failure

The receiver may have difficulty in making sense of the message received. This may be due to difficulty with language or dialect or the use of the non-verbal gestures within different contexts and cultures. Many decoding difficulties arise for patients and relatives when medical and technical language is used. Confusional states, pain, exhaustion, and some drug therapies may also interfere with a person's ability to derive meaning from the messages received.

Remedial action

The skill and ability of the nurse to identify and act on the causes of communication failure will enable communication problems to be minimized. The following strategies may be considered (French, 1983):

- [ ] simplify the message by cutting out irrelevant cues, e.g. words;

- [ ] strengthen the stimulus through mechanical means (e.g. hearing aids and spectacles) or reduce interference (e.g. noise and other stimuli, such as pain and tiredness);

- [ ] change the channel by using sign language, symbol cards, lip reading, written messages, and touch;

- [ ] give feedback and help the person to understand the cause of the communication failure. This may allow the sender or receiver to assist in taking action;

- [ ] give support, encouragement and reinforcement; this will help to minimize the frustration and loneliness felt by patients who have difficulty in understanding or being understood by other people.

VERBAL COMMUNICATION

Human communication is distinguished by the use of symbols which when they act together form language. Speech is a unique characteristic of human communication, people carry out the complex task of communicating verbally without any real awareness of what they are doing or how they are doing it. Words have recognized meanings; however, the meaning of a word may change depending on the context of communication or by the subtle way a word is used within a sentence.

Porritt (1990) uses the example of the word 'menopause' as in "Phyllis Smith has reached the menopause." If the statement is objective (the word is being used in its denotive sense) this means: Phyllis Smith is experiencing the hormonal changes that women undergo at the average age of 55 years. If, however, the term is being used in its emotional or connotative sense, this statement really means: Phyllis Smith is having all those ghastly symptoms of hot flushes, woolly head, fatigue, emotional distress and short temper.

A word does not always have the same meaning to everyone. Semantic differences can create many problems in communication. People carry the meaning of a word within their mental constructs having learned from their experience. The word itself is not the meaning. The use of medical and nursing jargon and abbreviations can confuse and obscure information which the person is trying to understand.

Speech allows us to ask questions, give information, orders and instructions, share intimate experiences or informal conversation. The meaning of any message is carried by both the deep and superficial structures of a sentence, and is normally accompanied by non-verbal signals.

Many authors have expounded on the importance of communication in relation to the critically ill. The most notable work is that of Pat Ashworth (1980). She has contributed enormously to our understanding of the nature of nurse-patient interaction and communication skills used by nurses within the context of intensive care nursing.

Ashworth (1980) suggested four aims for nurse-patient communication:

1. To establish a relationship in which the patient perceives the nurse as friendly, helpful, competent and reliable, and as recognizing the patient's worth and individuality.
2. To try to determine the patient's needs as perceived by him or her, and when necessary, to help the patient recognize his or her other needs as perceived by the nurse.
3. To provide factual information on which the patient can structure his or her expectations.
4. To assist the patient to use his or her own resources, and those offered by the ICU (e.g. information) to meet his or her own needs.

NON-VERBAL COMMUNICATION

Non-verbal communication is used subconsciously to express feelings, interpersonal beliefs and attitudes, and emotions, and has the potential of being five times more effective in conveying these sorts of message than verbal communication (Argyle, 1978). This is particulary the case when there is incongruence between what is being said and the unspoken behaviours of the person sending the message. For example, a nurse may ask the patient briefly, 'How are you?' whilst appearing to rush around looking at charts and monitors and fiddling with the arterial line or chest tubes, etc. The message the patient receives is 'Don't tell me how you are, I haven't got time'. When a person experiences this difference between the words and the actions, the words are ignored and the meaning of the message is taken from the actions (Porritt, 1990). There are a wide range of behaviours which come within the non-verbal category.

Facial movements

People distinguish one another by their faces. A person's face is their identity. People form and hold beliefs about a person's personality based on facial characteristics.

The face is one of the main expressers of emotion; it expresses happiness, surprise, fear, sadness, anger, interest, disgust, embarrassment etc. These emotions tend to show similar facial movements across cultures. However, different cultures may have rules about when it is appropriate to express emotion, and therefore differences occur in the frequency of usage and the situation in which it is expressed.

When two people meet, some evaluation will take place based on facial expression, and assumptions will be made about how that person is feeling before any exchange of verbal communication has taken place. This will probably lead to an accurate assessment unless the person is deliberately hiding their feelings.

Gaze and eye contact

When a person looks at another person, they are gazing; however, when both people look at each other, eye contact is occurring. There are three main purposes of eye contact:

- [ ] attracting the person's attention by sending information across a crowded room – we need to talk;
- [ ] it allows observation of all non-verbal messages being sent; and
- [ ] helps to synchronize the conversation, guiding who will talk and who will listen (Porritt, 1990).

The person who is listening tends to look at the person more frequently than the person who is doing the talking. There are certain cultural differences and even differences within a culture, e.g.

American and English women use more eye contact than men from those cultures (Henley, 1977).

Gestures and body movement

Gestures and body movements can add substantial emphasis to a message. The pattern of movements made are culturally determined, and serve to give the receiver/observer further clues about what a message means, e.g. a simple example is giving directions and pointing; or emphasizing how strongly one feels about a point – this may be a personal belief, attitude or emotion. Gestures and body movements include hand waving, beckoning, shrugging shoulders, thumbs up and head nodding (Morris, 1977).

Body posture

Social power relationships may be demonstrated by posture. Argyle (1972) described the dominant posture, which consists of standing erect, with head tilted back, and sometimes with hands placed on the hips. The submission posture involves a slight cower to look smaller, arching of the shoulders and bowing of the head.

In the sitting position, when someone is paying attention or showing active participation, they tend to sit forward. However, if the person sits crouched forward with their shoulders hunched, this possibly demonstrates that the person is tense and uncomfortable. Guarded and defensive behaviour may be indicated through a closed posture with the arms and legs folded.

Morris (1977) describes the phenomenon of the 'postural echo' which indicates friendship between two people. The two individuals act as mirrors to each other's posture; this demonstrates equality within a relationship.

Touch and body contact

There is much evidence to suggest that body contact is a basic animal need (Harlow, 1959). Touch and physical contact is a physical act, constrained and directed by cultural and behavioural rules, and the social and physical skills of the communicator. The context in which touch or bodily contact occurs is where it derives its meaning for the people involved. Touch is permitted in certain situations;

for example, by health care practitioners, hair-dressers, beauticians, etc.; bodily contact is interpreted here as being a necessary part of diagnosis, therapy or treatment and is not normally misconstrued as having any other meaning. There is also the bodily contact that occurs by accident, for example, the pushing of a crowd, the jostling of people on a bus or train. Touch in this context may cause embarrassment or annoyance.

This aspect of non-verbal communication will be explored more fully within the section focusing on touch within critical care nursing.

The use of space

The distance or proximity between people gives important signals about the desired degree of intimacy within a relationship. Hall (1966) discussed the cultural differences in the nature and extent of tactile communication permitted; he used the word 'proxemics' to refer to the distance maintained in encounters with others, describing four main areas of informal space:

☐ Intimate distance (<18 inches): used by those who have an intimate relationship with each other. It is interesting to note that a good proportion of the interpersonal communication which takes place between patients and nurses utilizes the intimate space; this is normally acceptable, although may create difficulties for both the nurse and the patient.

☐ Personal distance (18 inches–4 feet): used by those who have a close personal relationship with each other; for example, family and friends.

☐ Social distance (4–12 feet): this is normally an appropriate distance for professionals to interact with their clients and members of the public, often from behind a desk.

☐ Public distance (>12 feet): speakers on public occasions are usually placed at a distance of 12 feet or more from their audience.

In health care, practitioners invade both the intimate and personal distance which is normally reserved for special and significant people in our lives and caring, close, loving and sexual situations and relationships. Violation of the personal space may make the patient feel uncomfortable;

territoriality provides security, privacy, identity and autonomy for the owner of the space (Oland, 1978).

Appearance and dress

Information about the social status, occupation, financial state, person's attractiveness may all be inferred from the presentation of the person. This information will influence the assumptions made about the attitudes held by that person.

Patients within the critical care setting are normally nursed with the minimum of clothing and modesty is preserved using bed clothing. Clothes are also an extension of a person's body image, and therefore it is not difficult to understand that for the person who is recovering from critical illness, the type of clothing worn by patients will reinforce feelings of dependency and lack of perceived control over events.

The vocal aspects of speech

The non-verbal realm of speech is the vocal emphasis which accompanies speech. The tone of voice, level of pitch, patterns within the speech, pauses, volume, rate of speaking, positioning of emphasis and the use of silence all provide information about the message which is being sent.

Non-verbal communication in critical care nursing: the use of instrumental and expressive touch

Non-verbal communication is an important component of communication; however, there appears to be very little nursing research which focuses on this component of communication. This phenomenon may be due to the methodological difficulty of observing and recording non-verbal data, particularly within the complex environment of a critical care unit.

However, in the context of critical care nursing, non-verbal language is a powerful component of the patient-nurse relationship, particularly when the patient is unable to respond verbally. The unconscious or moderately sedated patient becomes a passive recipient of verbal communication, and the nurse has to find additional ways of communicating with the patient. To increase the effectiveness of communication, nurses need to develop their understanding of the symbolic and practical significance of non-verbal communication within the context of critical care nursing. This includes an awareness of the messages that are transmitted to the patient, and an awareness of its therapeutic value.

Touch is a major part of nursing care and also a powerful form of non-verbal communication. Touch conveys caring, a willingness to help and gives the patient a feeling of security and reassurance. This helps to reduce the patient's feelings of loneliness and isolation, and enhances their perception of comfort, identity and integrity, and facilitates the development of trust with the carer.

Touch is the earliest and most primitive form of communication – and a powerful source of social bonding. The unborn child has the capacity to perceive the sensation of touch. During birth, uterine contractions provide massive cutaneous stimuli which activate the physiological components of respiration and gastrointestinal function.

Tactile stimulation during infancy is essential for survival and the quality of subsequent development. Initially, the child is dependent upon its parents for the provision of touch experiences, communicating an assurance of love and security. The child then begins to carry objects to its mouth to experience their quality. This exploration of the world through touch enable the child to build an image of the world – and allows the child to distinguish itself from surrounding objects and beings. The child, in this way, begins to develop its own self-identity and body image.

As the child grows older, words replace touch and more emphasis is placed on symbolic communication; the use of touch becomes controlled by socially and culturally defined rules. However, these early tactile experiences influence the person's ability for learning in other areas of communication; and also the interpretation of touch in adulthood.

Touch can communicate a number of emotions. Laing (1959) suggested that people use touch to escape from a sense of aloneness. It provides a closeness with another person that cannot be replaced by verbal communication. Forer (1969) suggested that healthy forms of tactile contact

provide individuals with the means to maintain their separateness and individuality while still meeting their need for closeness and intimacy.

Bowlby (1958) suggested that an adult's need for tactile communication increases in situations of danger and illness. The ageing process may also increase a person's need for tactile contact as a means of gathering information about their environment, when visual, hearing and functional capacities are impaired.

Within the world of sophisticated technologies, the need for 'care' is essential for survival. Leininger (1977) emphasized the importance of including the concept of caring in our contemporary understanding of nursing; and awareness of the contribution of caring behaviours to the process of 'curing'.

The literature generally supports the relationship between the quality of non-verbal communication and the process of caring, and acknowledges the important role it plays in preventing the 'dehumanization' experienced by many patients.

An important area which can be affected in a positive way through expressive touch is the patients' perception of themselves; this includes their body image. Schilder (1970) conceptualizes body image as a dynamic concept which changes with alteration in position and movement of the body – sensory feedback from sight, touch, proprioception allows the person an awareness of his body size and position in space. Sudden environmental and social changes that occur as a result of critical illness – threatens the person's self-concept and distorts their mental picture of body image. Accompanying body image distortion there is also a loss of integrity; the person experiences difficulty in perceiving where their body boundaries are in relation to their external environment.

Zubeck's work in the 1960s allows us to see how quickly these perceptual distortions can occur. The researcher used voluntary subjects, and they were asked to experience various forms of sensory deprivation. Zubeck (1969) found that the subjects' tolerance of sensory deprivation was low; most experienced quite distressing sensations – altered body image, visual disturbances, hallucinations, and many displayed regressive behaviour.

The number of studies which have explored the patients' memory of their intensive care experience is small, again probably due to the methodological difficulties involved. Patients have reported quite bizarre experiences – however, we are not in a position to know how often they occur, and perhaps more importantly, the effects on patient outcome or recovery.

In a study published in *Intensive Care Nursing Journal* (Bergbom-Engberg *et al.*, 1988), a sample of 304 people who had been patients within an intensive care unit were asked to recall their experiences. More than 50% of patients were able to recall their experiences of being mechanically ventilated. The study concluded that the relationship and communication process between the ventilated patient and the nurse were the most important factors in inducing feelings of security for the patient. The quality of the interpersonal relationship appeared to make an important contribution to the patient's experience. Many patients felt that the development of trust and confidence in the nurse contributed more to the interpersonal relationship than purely the continuous presence of the nurse. In fact, if the patient felt that the nurse appeared to concentrate more on the technical equipment than on the patient, the nurse was considered to be less skilled, unpleasant, and less safe in their practice.

Touch as a mode of communication has been examined by a number of authors within a range of health care settings.

McCorkle (1974) investigated the effects of touch on patients with serious illness, and found that touch facilitated a closer relationship between the nurse and the patient, and this was associated with an increased verbalization of patient needs.

Barnett (1972) found that expressive touch appeared to be used more frequently in high stress areas, such as intensive care, labour ward, paediatrics and recovery areas.

Kubler-Ross (1969) observed that the acceptance of terminal illness by the dying person increases their need for non-verbal communication and tactile contact.

Ashworth (1980), in studying nurse-patient communication in the intensive care setting, found that 85% of nurses interviewed stated that they would use touch to convey reassurance, comfort and security to the patient.

The literature also recognizes that the person's need for privacy and personal space can be as important as providing human contact.

Weiss (1979) defined the act of touching using six tactile symbols: duration; location; action; intensity; frequency; and sensation. The author defined duration of touch as the total time over which the touch episode occurs. A longer duration of touch is essential for purposes of sensation and perception, and it allows more time for the recipient to become aware of the quality of the touch. It also allows the receiver a greater sense of body detail and perception of body boundaries. This may be of particular value to the patient in intensive care; whose awareness of body boundaries and body image may be distorted as a result of sensory disturbances.

The location of touch is related to the extent and number of areas of the body that are touched. Jourard (1966) demonstrated that a person's perception of how much their body is touched by others is related to a positive evaluation of self. Touches which are located towards the centre of the body, the trunk, convey messages of closeness, intimacy and feeling of well-being. The frequency of touch or the total amount of touching experienced by the recipient, contributes to personal perception of self worth; this is reflected within the person's self-esteem, body image, sexual identity and feelings of closeness with other people.

Nurses are socialized to view and react to touch and touching other people through cultural practices, family relationships, Professional Code of Conduct, and through nursing practice. Nurses are required to overcome the possible anxieties about touching other people whilst carrying out nursing care. The majority of touch is intrumental, that is task-related; however, less emphasis is placed on expressive touch and the psychosocial consequences of touching and being touched. It was on this basis that I decided to find out the answer to the question of whether intensive care nurses utilize expressive touch and to explore the nature of touch used in the care of the critically ill.

The title of the study was 'Nurse-patient communication in intensive care: a descriptive study exploring the nature and frequency of instrumental and expressive touch'. The aims of the study were to observe the frequency and type of touch used by nurses caring for patients in an intensive care unit, and to identify variables which affect the use and acceptance of instrumental and expressive touch.

Data was collected using non-participative observation of nurse patient interaction. Touch types and their components were recorded using an observation schedule which had been developed by Andree Le May and Sally Redfern (1986) at Chelsea College London. The instrument had originally been designed to observe nurse-patient touch and its relationship to the well-being of elderly patients. The data collection tool consisted of the following components:

Type of touch: Instrumental or expressive touch as defined by Watson (1975).

When touch occurs: The point during the interaction when touch occurs: approach; interface; separation.

Duration of interaction: The total length of time for each interaction.

Length of touch episode: Each episode was recorded as:

    F = Fleeting (corresponded to <2 seconds)
    S = Short (2–10 seconds)
    M = Medium (11–20 seconds)
    L = Long (>20 seconds).

Body area touched: Recorded on a manikin divided into body areas.

Response of the recipient to touch: The verbal response of the person being touched is recorded as silence; verbal; non-verbal.

Nature of verbal communication: By the toucher, e.g. treatment/care related; emotional/psychosocial support; social chit-chat; silence.

Nature of the interaction: What was happening at the time, e.g. basic care; technical care; observations; psychosocial support; teaching, etc.

Patient's position: During the interaction, e.g. lying or sitting in bed; sitting in a chair.

Nurse's position: During the interaction, e.g. standing, sitting, kneeling.

Biographical details included: age; sex; marital status; ethnic origin; and the socioeconomic status of both the nurse and the patient observed. In addition, the professional status and the intensive care experience of the nurse, and the diagnostic category, dependency category, and length of stay in ITU was recorded for the patient.

Training in the use of the observation schedule took approximately eight weeks. This included a period of time with Andree LeMay, and involved the use of the observation schedule in recording touch data from audio-visual tapes of nurse-patient interactions. The researcher spent two weeks using the observation schedule on the intensive care unit, where data collection was to take place. This was useful in three respects:

1. It allowed the researcher to develop an awareness of the potential distractions they were likely to encounter during the data collection period, e.g. noise and the activity levels of staff and relatives.
2. It allowed staff on the unit to become used to the researcher being there as a non-participant observer.
3. It enabled the researcher to decide on the use of a specified time interval for the recording of data. Each observation period was to be one hour in length – this was divided into five minute periods alternating between five minute period of data collection followed by a five minute period for checking the previous data.

The schedule had undergone four checks for inter-observer reliability in acute and long stay care of the elderly wards.

The sample included 15 adult patients who were selected randomly from a ten bedded intensive care unit over a two week period. This included both short- and long-stay patients, presenting a variety of acute medical and surgical conditions and nursing dependencies. Consent was obtained either from the patient or from a close relative on the day prior to data collection.

The unit was organized through patient allocation, therefore the nurse was assigned to the patient without prior knowledge of who was to be observed by the researcher. The nursing staff involved consisted of registered and enrolled nurses with a range of experiences in intensive care nursing. Consent was obtained from the nurse prior to data collection. Confidentiality and anonymity were preserved by coding data.

Each nurse-patient pair was observed for three, one hour observation periods – avoiding shift overlaps and meal times. In total, 45 hours of observation was completed over a two week period.

There are a number of limitations to the study due to the relatively small sample size and the lack of validity and reliability testing of the data collection tool within the context of critical care nursing. However, the study does provide a descriptive basis for further study and as with most research it creates more questions. The knowledge that is gained from this type of study will make a small contribution to the development of practice, education and theory.

The opportunity to observe nurse-patient interaction provides new insights into the communication skills and the quality of the nurse-patient relationships achieved by intensive care nurses. Subsequent development of practice occurs through synthesis of knowledge and dissemination of knowledge through education, and role modelling.

In the same way, nursing theory can be redefined and strengthened by discovering additional facets in relation to the nature of caring and the therapeutic potential surrounding the role of the nurse in critical care. Nurses are exploring the therapeutic potential of their role, and we are now beginning to see more formalized modes of expressive touch emerging – through massage, aromatherapy, shiatsu. The therapeutic potential is realized through the central concepts of caring, nurturing, holism, humanism, partnership, empowerment and autonomy. The challenge of providing holistic care necessitates review of the principles on which practice is based, and also confronts the individual nurse with their own strengths and weaknesses.

CONCLUSION

Nurses are the key providers of intimate physical care and psychological support. This creates opportunities for human closeness which should be used to therapeutic effect. Many complex and inter-related variables influence the use of expressive touch by intensive care nurses and these relate not only to the skills, knowledge and resources available, but also to the personal attitudes and beliefs held by nurses about patients and the nature of caring.

This chapter has explored a range of issues relating to communication in critical care nursing. The point, now, is to reflect on your *own* communication skills and see to what degree they do or do not match those described in this chapter.

FURTHER READING

Adler, R., Rodman, G. *Understanding Human Communication*. 3rd Ed. New York: Holt Rinehart & Winston, 1988.

Albarron, J. W. A review of communication with intubated patients and those with tracheostomies within an intensive care environment. *Intensive Care Nursing*. 1991; 7(3): 179–186.

Argyle, M. *Bodily Communication*. London: Methuen, 1984.

Benner, P. *From Novice To Expert*. Menlo Park, California: Addison-Wesley, 1984.

Crotty, M. Communication between nurses and their patients. *Nurse Education Today*. 1985; 5(3): 130–134.

Cunliffe, P. H. Communicating with children in the intensive care unit. *Intensive Care Nursing*. 1987; 3(2): 71–77.

Eagan, G. *The Skilled Helper*. 3rd Ed. California: Brooks Cole, 1985.

Easton, J. Alternative communication for patients in intensive care. *Intensive Care Nursing*. 1988; 4(2): 47–55.

Faulkner, A. *Nursing: A Creative Approach*. London: Baillière Tindall, 1985.

Hyland, M. E., Donaldson, M. L. *Psychological Care in Nursing Practice*. Oxford: Scutari Press, 1989.

Ingham, A. A review of the literature relating to touch and its uses in intensive care. *Intensive Care Nursing*. 1989; 5(2): 65–75.

Ley, P. *Communicating With Patients: Improving Communication, Satisfaction and Compliance*. London: Chapman and Hall, 1988.

Long, L. *Understanding and Responding: A Communication Manual For Nurses*. Jones and Barlett Pub. Inc., 1992.

MacKereth, P. A. Communicating in critical care areas: competing for attention. *Nursing (London)*, 1987; 3(15): 575–578.

McMahon, R., Pearson, A. *Nursing As Therapy*. London: Chapman and Hall, 1991.

Pratt, J. W., Mason, A. The meaning of touch in care practice. *Social Science and Medicine*. 1986; 18(12): 1081–1088.

Rundell, S. A study of nursing process interaction in a high dependancy unit. *Intensive Care Nursing*. 1991; 7(3): 171–178.

Wallace, L. Videotape modelling of communication skills in a coronary care unit. *Intensive Care Nursing*. 1987; 2(3): 107–111.

REFERENCES

Argyle, M. *The Psychology of Interpersonal Behaviour*. 2nd Ed. London: Penguin Books, 1972.

Argyle, M. *The Psychology of Interpersonal Behaviour*. 3rd Ed. Harmondsworth: Penguin, 1978.

Ashworth, P. *Care to Communicate*. Royal College of Nursing, London, 1980.

Barnett, K. A survey of the current utilisation of touch by health team personnel with hospitalised patients. *International Journal of Nursing Studies*. 1972; 9: 195–209.

Bates, T., Broome, H. Preparation of children for hospitalisation and surgery: a literature review. *Journal of Paediatric Nursing (US)*. 1986; 1: 10–15.

Bergbom-Engberg, I., Hallenburg, B., Wickström, I., Halijomäer, H. A retrospective study of patients' recall of respirator treatment (1): Study design and basic findings. *Intensive Care Nursing*. 1988; 4(2): 56–61.

Bowlby, J. The nature of the child's tie to his mother. *International Journal of Psychoanalysis*. 1958; 39: 350–373.

Carnevale, F. A description of stressors and coping strategies among parents of critically ill children. A preliminary study. *Intensive Care Nursing*. 1990; 6: 4–11.

Chan, J. M. Preparation for procedures and surgery through play. *Paediatrician*. 1980; 9: 210–219.

Coulter, M. The needs of family members of patients in intensive care units. *Intensive Care Nursing*. 1989; 5: 4–10.

Fossen, A. Husband, E. Bibliotherapy for hospitalised children. *Southern Medical Journal*. 1984; 77(3): 342–346.

Forer, B. The taboo against touching in psychotherapy. *Psychotherapy: Theory, Research, and Practice*. 1969; 6: 229–231.

French, P. *Social Skills For Nursing Practice*. London: Croom Helm, 1987.

Griffin, A. P. A philosophical analysis of caring in nursing. *Journal of Advanced Nursing*. 1983; 8: 289–295.

Hall, E. J. *The Hidden Dimension*. New York: Doubleday, 1966.

Hall, D. Social and psychological care before and during hospitalisation. *Social Science and Medicine*. 1987; 25(6): 721–732.

Harlow, H. F. Love in infant monkeys. In *Scientific American (1974) Papers on Socialisation and Attitudes*. San Francisco: WH Freeman, 1959.

Heath, J. What the patients say ... recollections of patients on intensive care units. *Intensive Care Nursing*. 1989; 5(3): 101–108.

Henley, N. M. *Body Politics: Power, Sex, and Nonverbal Communication*. Englewood Cliffs, New Jersey: Prentice-Hall, 1977.

Hudak, C. M., Gallo, B. M., Lohr, T. S. *Critical Care Nursing; A Holistic Approach*. Philadelphia: JB Lippincott Co., 1986.

Jay, S. Paediatric intensive care; involving parents in the care of their child. *Maternal Child Nursing Forum*. 1977; 6: 195–204.

Jourard, S. M. An exploration study of body accessibility. *British Journal of Social and Clinical Psychology*. 1966; 5: 221–231.

Kubler-Ross, E. *On Death and Dying*. New York: MacMillan, 1969.

Laing, R. D. *The Divided Self*. Harmondsworth: Penguin, 1959.

Leininger, M. The phenomenon of caring (part V): caring, the essence and central focus of nursing. *Nursing Research Report*. 1977; 12: 2, 14.

McCorkle, The effects of touch on seriously ill patients. *Nursing Research*. 1974; 23(2): 125–132.

Millar, B. Critical support in critical care. *Nursing Times*. 1989; 85(16): 31–32.

Molter, N. Needs of relatives of critically ill patients: a descriptive study. *Heart and Lung*. 1979; 8(2): 322–339.

Morris, D. *Manwatching: A Field Guide To Human Behaviour*. St Albans: Triad Panther, 1977.

Morrison, P., Burnard, P. *Caring and Communicating*. London: MacMillan Press, 1991.

Oland, L. *The Need for Territoriality*. In: A. Yura, M. B. Walsh (eds.). *Human Needs and the Nursing Process*. New York: Appleton-Century-Crofts, 1978, pp. 97–140.

Pearce, J. S. *Parental Satisfaction Survey Report: Cardiothoracic Intensive Care Unit*, Southampton General Hospital. Unpublished Report, 1992.

Pegano, M. P., Ragan, S. L. *Communication Skills for Professional Nurses*. Newbury Park: Sage Publications, 1992.

Platzer, H. Body image – a problem for intensive care patients (Part 1). *Intensive Care Nursing*. 1987; 3: 61–66.

Porritt, L. *Interaction Strategies: An Introduction for Health Professionals*. London: Churchill Livingstone, 1990.

Porter, L., Redfern, S., Le May, A. The development of an observation schedule for measuring nurse–patient touch using an ergonomic approach. *International Journal of Nursing Studies*. 1986; 23(1): 11–20.

Rogers, C. *On Becoming A Person*. London: Constable, 1967.

Sargent, A. L. The sick child and the family. *Journal of Paediatrics*. 1983; 102: 982–987.

Schilder, P. *The Image and Appearance of the Human Body. Studies in the Constructive Energies of the Human Psyche*. 2nd Ed. New York: International Universities Press Inc., 1970.

Watson, W. H. The meaning of touch. *Journal of Community*. 1975; 25: 104–111.

Weiss, S. J. The language of touch. *Nursing Research*. 1979; 28(2): 76–80.

Wiemann, J. M. Explication and test of a model of communication competence. *Human Communication Research*. 1977; 3: 195–213.

Wilmot, W. *Dyadic Communication*. 3rd Ed. New York: Random House, 1987.

Wright, B. *Caring In Crisis*. London: Churchill Livingstone, 1986.

Zubeck, J. P. *Sensory Deprivation: 15 years of Research*. New York: Appleton-Century-Croft, 1969.

17
COUNSELLING IN CRITICAL CARE NURSING
Philip Burnard

CHAPTER AIMS

The chapter is designed to identify those skills which can help the critical care nurse to function as an effective nurse counsellor. This is not to say that simply reading the chapter will enable a person to become a counsellor. Counselling skills are most readily learned in practice, or through the use of experiential learning methods (Burnard, 1989). On the other hand, a discussion of the skills can help the nurse to begin to identify the skills that he or she has and the skills that might be needed.

INTRODUCTION

Being a patient in a critical care setting is traumatic for many people. First, it can be traumatic, both physically and psychologically, for the patient. It can also be traumatic for the family and friends of the patient. Effective counselling skills are a vital prerequisite of skilled and compassionate care in this field. Also, such skills are useful in situations where staff care for staff. The business of being a nurse in this domain can also bring its problems. As we have seen in other chapters of this book, stress and burnout can face many nurses who constantly care for those in a crticial care environment.

Any discussion of counselling is likely to be a little one-sided. The approach discussed in this chapter is largely one concerned with the nurse being *client-centred*. This is in line with current nursing philosophies which stress patient autonomy and choice. It is, however, only *one* approach; others will be referred to, and the reader should become acquainted with a *range* of approaches and theories towards counselling if he or she is to become a counsellor in this field. The aim, in this chapter, is to offer practical *counselling skills* which can be used by any nurse working in the critical care field.

The chapter is aimed directly at the reader, and he or she is addressed as 'you'. Counselling is, after all, a personal activity. Thus the discussion in this chapter is written in a discursive and directly personal tone.

EXPLORING THE ISSUES

The key skills in counselling process are non-judgemental listening and the giving of full attention. The aim, as we have noted, is to emphasize and to enter the world of the other person: to attempt to see the world as they see it. The stage is more about standing back and taking the broader view of what the client is saying than about focusing and attempting detective work.

Carl Rogers (1983) uses the phrase 'an expanding frame of reference' to describe the slow but developing understanding of the other person. It is as though we begin with almost no understanding of the person in front of us, then we get to know them a little better and then the jigsaw begins to become more and more complete. It never *will* be complete, of course. We never can know someone completely and, anyway, they are continually changing. We can, though, get a much fuller picture than the one we start with.

The ability to suspend judgement comes into play in this stage. We are not there to criticize, moralize or judge. We are simply there to listen. This is not particularly easy. It is worth noting that we all seem to have an internal censor inside our heads when we listen to another person. As they talk, the censor tells us "yes: that's alright", or "no: that's wrong", and so on. Notice how that internal censor works even as you read. My guess is that you are constantly evaluating what you are reading. That evaluation often takes the shape of whether or not what is written is right or wrong. So it is when we listen to another person. In counselling, though – and particularly in this stage – we are required to put the censor out of action and merely to take in and listen. It is rather like visiting a large house and wandering from room to room and refraining from passing judgement as to whether or not we like or dislike what we see. We are there merely to *see* the rooms.

Listening and attending

Listening is the most important skill of all. The most skilled counsellors often operate almost silently: they listen far more than they talk. I read once of a woman in an Indian town who set up a stall with a big placard in front of it which read: I LISTEN. Apparently, she was never without someone in front of her stall. If we can learn to really listen to another person we are not only on the way to becoming good counsellors but also to becoming good friends and colleagues.

Before we start a discussion of the skills of listening and attending, consider the people you know that you would call 'good listeners'. What *tells* you that they are good? What do they *do*? 'Well', you might say, 'they listen!' The point is, though, that not only do they listen, they also SHOW that they listen. It is one thing to be a good listener. It is

another to demonstrate the skill. In order that listening is effective, it must be visible.

Initially, then, it helps to adopt behaviours that show that you are listening. These are not fool-proof. It is quite possible to adopt the behaviours and *still* not listen. The point is that if we can adopt the behaviours and add the necessary relationship skills, we are completing the circle – we listen and we are seen to be listening. The behaviours are suggested by Egan (1990) and are these:

☐ Sit squarely. Face the client rather than sit next to him or her. Sitting facing the client means that we are able to see his or her expressions, gestures and all of the non-verbal and para-linguistic aspects of speech. Most of all, we can see their eyes and they can see ours. It may be an exaggeration (and a cliche) to say that the eyes are the windows of the soul, but they do have a large part to play in communication.

☐ Sit in an open position. Do not fold your arms and cross your legs. On the other hand, be flexible about this. Egan was writing largely for an American audience. In the UK, it is common for most people to cross their legs when sitting down. However, the more open you can be in your posture, the more open you are likely to appear to the client.

☐ Lean slightly towards the other person. Do not overwhelm them, but leaning towards them shows that you are with them. If you find this unlikely, try sitting with someone and leaning *away* from them. You will soon see the effect.

☐ Maintain comfortable eye contact. Do not stare and do not 'follow the client's eyes'. No one likes to feel pursued. But do be ready to take up the eye contact of the client, when he or she looks up.

☐ Relax. You do not have to rehearse what YOU want to say. You do not have to think out why the person is talking the way that they are. All you have to do is sit and listen to their story. Initially, this is often difficult. As you develop counselling skills, though, you learn to trust yourself. You begin to know that you will be able to respond once the other person has finished speaking. You will know *when* to respond by their eye contact. Normally, when someone in a conversation wants the other person to say something, they look at that person. Do not be too ready to rush in and fill temporary silences. Just sit and listen and relax.

Egan suggests the acronym SOLER as an easy method of remembering these behaviours:

- ☐ S: sit squarely,
- ☐ O: open position,
- ☐ L: lean forward,
- ☐ E: eye contact,
- ☐ R: relax.

Remember, though, that cultural differences come into play when listening takes place. Those differences are particularly evident when it comes to eye contact. People from far eastern countries, for example, will tend not to make eye contact with people they consider to be occupying a superior role. West Indians often do not make eye contact when they are *talking* but only when they are *listening*. It is impossible in a book of this size to consider all the possible regional variations but do not assume that the SOLER behaviours will necessarily be appropriate in all situations. The key issue, when counselling people from another culture, is to take the lead from them. Notice how they respond to you and do your best to acknowledge and respect the differences. Also, if you are likely to counsel lots of people from different cultures, read as much as you can about those cultures and talk to other health care professionals who have had cross-cultural experience. The most important thing is to avoid *ethnocentricity*: the idea that the way that YOU do things in your culture is necessarily the RIGHT way.

Listening behaviours are linked to the internal state of the counsellor. The counsellor is not simply using a set of behaviours; he or she is also doing something inside the head. This is where the concept of awareness is useful. Figure 17.1 illustrates three zones of attention.

In zone one, the client's attention is focused directly on the client. The counsellor who's attention is in zone one is fully alert, noticing how the

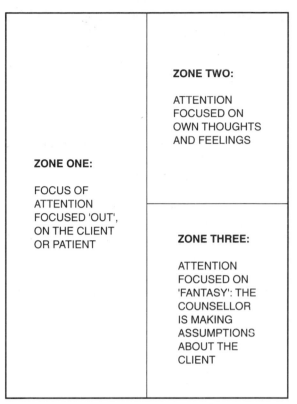

Figure 17.1. Three possible zones of attention.

client looks and fully taking in the words that the client is using.

As people talk, however, attention wanders into zone two. We think about what we are seeing and hearing. It is in this zone that the censor, described above, resides. Somehow, we have to learn to silence the censor and to return our attention to zone one. This can be a conscious effort. It is quite possible to NOTICE what is happening to your attention and to redirect it. Try it now. Stop reading this book and allow your attention to drift into zone two: become preoccupied with your own thoughts and feelings. Notice the degree to which your censor is at work and put it out of action. Then return to the book and concentrate fully on what you read. In doing this you are consciously moving from zone one to zone two and back again.

Zone three is more problematic. It is here that we 'make things up'. It is the zone of fantasy. When our thoughts and feelings are not satisfied by what we see or hear, we simply fill in the details and fantasize. Again, this can be demonstrtated fairly easily. Stop reading this book and move into zone two. Note what you are thinking and feeling. Now, do something else: think about the writer of this chapter. What do I look like?

Unless you have met me, you have just moved into the zone of fantasy! You have no means of knowing how I look, and yet you are able to offer some sort of answer to the question.

We often work in the domain of fantasy. When someone walks in the room we do not simply note what they look like. We go beyond that. We make a quick (and fallacious) assessment of them. We note whether or not we are likely to *like* them. We establish whether or not they are like us. We may put them into all sorts of other categories. And yet all of this categorization is built on almost no factual input!

The point of all this for the counsellor is simply this: as far as possible, when sitting with the client, stay out of the zone of fantasy. Stick to what the client is telling you. Listen to what they say. If something is not clear, ask for clarification. If you suspect something to be the case, ask the client. Do not jump to conclusions and try, as far as possible, to stay in zone one: stay with the client for as long as possible. For it is in zone one that you will really get to know the patient. All you will do in zone three is invent.

Listening to the client involves these two elements: external behaviours – showing that you are listening; and internal behaviours – purposely focusing your attention on the client. That combination is useful throughout the counselling relationship. If it can be sustained, it can lead to counselling becoming much more focused on the client's world than on the counsellor's belief system. In the end, what matters is what the client thinks, feels and does. The relationship, if you like, belongs to the client. The time spent counselling is time for the client to work through his or her own problems. It is not time for the counsellor to rehearse his or her own theories about human nature or about what is 'wrong' with the client.

Using open questions

Asking questions is a major part of the task of being a counsellor. There is a world of difference, though, between the questioning of an interrogator and the questioning of a counsellor. The interrogator or even the interviewer is there to get information. The counsellor uses questions in a different sort of way. The counsellor uses questions in order to help the client and the counsellor to illuminate the client's world. It is as though the counsellor is testing the ground by saying 'is it like this? . . . 'or like this?' . . . The counsellor does not so much seek out information for its own sake, but more to clarify. Skilful questioning is never obtrusive and certainly not intrusive.

Open and closed questions

It is usual to discriminate between two extremes in questioning: open and closed questions. The open question is the question to which the counsellor cannot guess the answer. Open questions are not usually answered with one word but by a series of sentences. Thus, the following are examples of open questions:

- ☐ How do you feel about that?
- ☐ What happened after that?
- ☐ What are your thoughts about it?

Open questions are particularly useful in helping the client to open up and to expand on what he or she is saying. They are useful 'memory joggers', and are frequently used in any stage of the counselling process, but are of particular value in exploring the client's problems and issues.

Closed questions, on the other hand, usually have a definite answer, and one that the counsellor can usually make a guess at. If this is not the case, the counsellor will usually have some idea of what *sort* of answer is likely to be forthcoming. Thus, these are examples of closed questions:

- ☐ How many children do you have?
- ☐ Has your wife visited you today?
- ☐ What is your GP's name?

Whilst closed questions are useful for gathering very particular pieces of information and are thus helpful in 'filling in the jigsaw', they can also often appear to be intrusive or just nosy. It is probably better to restrict the number of closed questions that you use. In a way, the process is self-limiting. If you *do* use too many closed questions, the conversation will tend to slow down or stop, anyway. Consider the following example:

> "When did you come into hospital for the first time?"
> "Earlier this year, I think . . ."
> "What, in January or February?"
> "February, I think it was."
> "Was it this hospital?"
> "Yes."
> "Did you have an operation?"
> "Yes."
> "What sort?"
> "I think it was called a laparotomy."

Too many closed questions soon lead to silence. Having made this distinction between open and closed questions, it is important to note that there are *degrees* of openness and closedness in questioning. Sometimes, what appears to be an open question, becomes a closed one. Consider this example:

> "How did you feel about having the operation?"
> "O.K. No problem."

Here, what seemed to the counsellor to be an open question was turned into a closed one by the client. It is worth considering why this happens. Quite often it happens because the counsellor has chosen the wrong *sort* of question to ask: that is, the wrong sort of question about the wrong sort of issue. In the example above, it seems likely that the counsellor thought that the issue of 'leaving your family' was an important one. It also seems that the issue was not a particularly burning one for the client. The counsellor had misjudged the sort of question to ask. If you find a lot of your open questions being turned into closed ones, ask yourself whether or not you are asking the *right* questions.

Questions to avoid

There are certain sorts of questions that are best not asked at all. These can be identified fairly easily in theory, but are sometimes difficult to avoid in practice. To avoid them it is necessary to remain clear about the *aims* of asking questions, and clear about avoiding judgement. Here are some of the sorts of questions to avoid.

Loaded questions

These are questions that reveal the counsellor's own particular beliefs and prejudices about the client. An example of a loaded question is: "Did you feel guilty about the way you treated your family?" The implication is that the client *should* have felt guilty. Also, whatever the answer the client puts him or himself in a difficult position. If the answer is 'yes', guilt is acknowledged. If 'no', it sounds as though the guilt that was appropriate was not felt! This sort of question is sometimes called a *leading* question. Perhaps the most famous leading question (which, again, would cause real difficulties, however it was answered) is: "Have you stopped beating your wife?"

Multiple questions

Sometimes, in the quest to get things right, it is possible to roll a number of questions into one: "How did you feel about being in hospital? Did you think that you were treated fairly well? Did you feel you could have managed better on your own . . . ? The obvious problem, here, is: which question is the client supposed to answer? Try to ask only one question at a time.

Unclear questions

This is a variant of the multiple question. When we are anxious or trying hard to be clear, it is possible to do exactly the opposite and to become very muddled. Then, sometimes, our questions become very unclear: "What did you do . . . I mean, what did you want to happen, sort of, before everything was sorted out at home and everything . . . ?" As a general rule, short questions are usually more effective than lengthy ones. If you find yourself getting into a mess, *acknowledge* that you have done so and start again. Remember, it is OK to make a mess of things sometimes: it lets the client know that you are human, too.

Intrusive questions

The aim of counselling is to help the client to problem solve. The aim is not to collect all sorts of very personal data about the other person. It is sometimes tempting to want to probe the other person's life a little. Sometimes, our nosiness gets the better of us. It is important that we do not ask questions that could embarass or offend the client, such as "Do you still feel sexually attracted to him?"

The issue of intrusiveness has to be put in context. Clearly, there are times, as the relationship develops, when such a question *might* be appropriate. However, in the early stage of the counselling process, it seems unlikely that it would be. If you feel tempted to ask very personal questions, ask *yourself* why you are asking it and what your motivation might be for asking it.

Empathy building

Empathy is the ability to enter into the other person's frame of reference: to feel as they feel. Empathy building is the process of *conveying* that shared experience with the client. Thus empathy building statements are always tentative, and also seek to try to ensure that the counsellor is 'matching' what the client is feeling. This is never easy, but it gets easier as the relationship deepens. Sometimes, the counselling relationship is a bit like a trance that you both slowly go into and both slowly emerge from at the end of your time together. It becomes as though only the two of you matter and that only the two of you exist for the time that you are talking. Any interruption, such as a 'phone ringing or someone else coming into the room, seems an intrusion.

Empathy building statements, then, are those that illustrate that you are matching the feelings and experience of the other person. Examples of empathy building statements are: "It feels as though . . .", "I get the impression that . . .", "Is it the case that . . . ?"

You always know if your empathy building is not going the way you would like it. The client lets you know fairly quickly. When this happens, it is probably best to stop attempting empathy building statements at all and to concentrate on listening with greater accuracy. Sometimes, empathy building statements do not 'work' because the counsellor is trying too hard. When this happens, again, it is best to relax a little and allow the client to talk more. Remember: the relationship belongs to the client. The time you are together is the client's time. There is absolutely no need to rush the process and,

anyway, most human relationships refuse to be rushed. You cannot force empathy: it has to be really there.

Reflection

Reflection (sometimes called 'echoing') is a familiar and well known counselling strategy. Two sorts can be described. First, there is straightforward reflection of the last thing that the client said. Thus, when the client begins to falter in what he or she is saying, the counsellor repeats back the last few words that were spoken: "When I first came into hospital . . . I thought that everything would be fairly simple . . . you know, a quick operation and then I would be able to go back home . . ."; "You thought you would be able to go back home . . ."; "Well, I never expected that all these complications would set in and that I would have to be in hospital for so long. It came as a dreadful shock to wake up and find myself in here!"

This type of reflection acts as a simple prompt. The client is momentarily lost in the conversation and the counsellor gently nudges him back on track. It is important to note that a reflected comment should not become a *question*. It is important that the comment is reflected back with much the same tone and volume that it was uttered by the client. If it *does* become a question, it will be *answered* as a question: "We all liked it, I think, because we knew what was happening . . ."; "You knew what was happening?"; "Yes"(!).

The second type of reflection is where something is reflected back from the *middle* of what the client has been saying: something that was emphasized by them or which appears to be an emotional issue. An example of this sort of reflection is as follows: "I was alright when I first came in. I knew why I was here and so did my wife. My children hated it. They hated coming to see me here. I don't know . . . I suppose its difficult for them to understand, really . . ."; "Your children really hated it . . ."; "They seemed frightened of the place. They used to go very quiet when they came to see me. Then they stopped coming all together. My wife helped them a lot and gradually they came round . . .".

Even people who have fairly monotonous voices emphasize certain things as they talk. To use this second, selective form of reflection, it is important to remain very attentive, and for that attention to remain 'free floating'. It is no good hanging onto a phrase to feed it back as a selective reflection! It is impossible to know, in advance, when the other person is likely to stop talking. Five minutes later, the selective reflection that you had planned may be 'out of date'. Thus, the need to maintain free floating attention: attention that takes everything in but which also gently shifts as the client shifts the focus of the conversation.

Reflection can be a useful way of gently encouraging the other person to continue his or her train of thought. It has to be used wisely, though. It can easily be misused and when it is, the conversation takes on a slightly odd character. it is likely, too, that the client will notice the oddness and comment on it, thus: "We were happier when we moved in Liverpool. It was bigger and we were used to life in the town, anyway . . ."; "You were used to the town . . ."; "Well, we had moved from London and we had always lived in a built up area. We never really got to grips with living in the country . . ."; "You didn't get to grips with living in the country . . ."; "No. That's what I just said!"

The great advantage of the use of reflection, though, is that it allows the client to remain in control of the conversation and allows him or her to take that conversation along the track that he or she chooses. Also, reflection makes sure that the client does not *add* any advice or suggestions to what is going on. Reflection remains one of the most effective aspects of client-centred counselling and is discussed, at length, by Rogers in his work on the topic (Rogers, 1967, 1983).

Checking for understanding

When we are counselling it is important that we understand what the other person is saying and what he or she is talking about. We all tend to invest some words with personal meanings; sometimes we use the wrong word for what we are trying to convey. At other times, we simply let everything pour out at once and it is not clear to the other person what we might mean. The intervention, known as checking for understanding, refers to the idea that we need to be able to stop occasionally and check what the other person is meaning. If we

do *not*, we run the risk of either getting confused or of missing the point.

Two sorts of checking for understanding can be described. First, there is the checking that can take place during a counselling session to check exactly what it is that the other person is saying. This is illustrated in the following example: "So I was very worried, really. I mean, I often used to think that I was the only one . . . I started having fits . . . People at work . . . I don't know, it was OK at home but sometimes people don't accept you, do they . . ."; "So you are saying that you were accepted at *home* but not so much at work . . . ?"; "Yes, everyone at home was fine. Some of the people at work, though . . . they made it clear that they didn't like me having fits."

When people are particularly wound up or excited, they often leave out important bits of information or they run together a range of ideas. In the example above, the nurse has temporarily stopped the person and asked him to clarify what he is saying. This not only makes sure that the nurse understands the conversation but it also encourages the speaker to become a little more focused.

The second sort of checking for understanding occurs when the counsellor sums up what has been talked about at the end of a session or whenever a natural break occurs. An example of this sort of checking is as follows: "Yes, everyone at home was fine. Some of the people at work, though . . . they made it clear that they didn't like me. Some were downright hostile to me. I don't want to talk about that at the moment. It still feels uncomfortable"; "So let me just sum up, if I can, what we've been talking about so far. First, you feel that you are 'different' to some of your family and to some of the people at work. You also feel that your family can accept you as you are but that the people at work can sometimes be hostile?"; "Yes. That and the problem of the job, itself. Yes. That just about sums things up for me at the moment."

This sort of checking for understanding can be used to close a counselling session. Some people like this approach as a means of rounding things off or of making sure that both parties really have understood each other. Some counsellors, though, find it a little contrived and choose *not* to sum up in this way. It is arguable that it is sometimes *better* not to summarize what has been talked about in that it can lead to an artificial feeling that everything is somehow rather 'neat' and well packaged. Life is rarely so straightforward, and sometimes it pays to leave things a little ragged round the edges. Also, the 'summing up' approach can sometimes also lead to the client packing away his or her problems at the end of the session. Whilst this may sometimes be an important thing to happen, some might argue that it is better for the client to leave the counselling session still thinking about the issues that have been discussed. This sort of counsellor may prefer a rather abrupt ending to the session and might avoid any sort of summary at the end, thus: "Yes, everyone at home was fine. Some of the people at work, though . . . they made it clear that they didn't like me. Some were downright hostile to me. I don't want to talk about that at the moment. It still feels uncomfortable"; "O.K. Let's leave it there. Its four o'clock and its time for us to stop. I'll see you again on Friday and we can discuss things further."

Think about which approach *you* prefer: the summing up or the abrupt ending. It is important to be clear about one thing here. We are not considering what you would prefer if you were a *client* but what you would prefer as an approach in counselling. As ever, it is important to try to be clear about *what* you do in counselling and *why* you do it.

Levels of disclosure

As the counselling relationship deepens and the counsellor and client get to know each other better, so the amount and depth that a client reveals will deepen. The depth of disclosure is a useful barometer of the relationship. If disclosure is not occurring, then the counselling relationship has probably not got very far. A useful device is to think of three levels of disclosure: first, second and third (Cox, 1978).

1st level of disclosure: safe disclosure

At this level, only safe issues are disclosed. Disclosures tend to be of the 'everyday' sort: e.g. "I got up a bit late this morning"; "I still find work a bit of a problem."

2nd level of disclosure: disclosure of feelings

Here, disclosure is about *feelings*: e.g. "I feel really angry about what is happening . . ."

3rd level of disclosure: deep disclosure

At this level, the client reveals hidden and very personal things: e.g. "I never really had a childhood"; "I think I'm homosexual."

Everyone discloses at the first level: it is the safe, 'everyday' level. Whenever we express something about ourselves to another person in the street or in a shop, we are disclosing at this level. Once we get to know someone a bit better, though, we tend to disclose at the second level more often: the 'feelings' level. Generally, we will only disclose our real feelings to another person if we feel a certain amount of trust with them. The third level is a different level altogether. It is the level of disclosure that we only reach with very close friends or with counsellors or therapists. Third level disclosures are disclosures of deep existential issues: things that really worry us and of which we rarely talk. If you think of three things that you would not like your colleagues to know about, you have identified three areas that would be the subject of third level disclosure.

Third level disclosures are not made easily. Often a person leads up slowly to making them. Sometimes, the person edges up and then backs away. Here is an example of a 'near' third level disclosure:

> "There is something else, of course, something I'm not really talking about . . ."
> "I thought there was . . ."
> "It's just that, well, you know . . . Oh! It doesn't matter. Lets talk about something else."

Here, the psychological moment has passed. The person tried to make a third level disclosure but found it impossible. What can you do in counselling when this point is reached? First, it is important not to rush things. The 'I thought there was', intervention may have made the other person feel under pressure. Often, the best intervention as someone heads, painfully, towards third level disclosing is for the counsellor to remain silent. Just sitting and listening is often the approach that helps the other person to disclose. If disclosure does not occur, then it is better if the client is allowed to move on: the disclosure will probably come at a later date. It is usually the case that once someone has made up his or her mind to disclose something important to someone else, then the disclosure *does* take place: the timing is not so important. Certainly it is impossible (and unproductive) to *push* someone towards a particular disclosure.

The level at which disclosure takes place depends on a number of things. It depends, at least on:

- [ ] how much the client trusts the counsellor;
- [ ] what the client judges the counsellor will 'make' of the disclosure;
- [ ] the urgency of the need to disclose;
- [ ] the atmosphere that exists in the room, and so on.

Counselling rarely stays for very long at the third level. Often, after a deep disclosure, the client returns to fairly light disclosure for the next two or three sessions. It is important that the client does not feel under any pressure, here, and that he or she chooses when and how he or she makes disclosures. The other thing to bear in mind is how the *counsellor* receives such disclosures. Sometimes, the most personal things about another person strike chords in us. We react to third level disclosures according to our own personal history and experience. It is important, after a third level disclosure, for the counsellor to think carefully about his or her own feelings. Finally, it is vital to remember that what is a third level disclosure for one person is not for another. The things that the client 'holds on to' might not seem worth holding on to from the counsellor's point of view. It is important not to trivialize or to glibly reassure over third level disclosures. Remember that we are all different. What bothers me may not bother you. Paradoxically, though, it is often true that we *do* share certain common fears and anxieties.

The other issue that arises out of disclosure is the degree to which the *counsellor* should disclose things about him or herself to the client (Burnard and Morrison, 1992). Jourard (1964) notes that "disclosure begets disclosure." If I tell you something personal about myself it is likely that you will tell me something about yourself. This can, of course, be overdone. First, it is possible to overwhelm the client by too much counsellor disclo-

sure. Consider, for example, the following:

Counsellor   "It may help if you know that I have been divorced, like you. At the time, I went through a very bad phase of depression. It was a very difficult time for me and for the family. Now, how are things for you . . . ?"

Arguably, the counsellor has told too much, too quickly. Second, it is possible to find yourself in a position of what Luft (1969) calls 'parralaction': holding a parallel conversation with the client in which you are both trading experiences but not really allowing each other to expand on what is being said. It would be hard to call this sort of conversation counselling: it is more an exchanging and comparing of experiences. Certainly, this sort of exchange is not usually a useful one in counselling where the emphasis should be on the *client's* experience. The counsellor may disclose things about him or herself, but these are usually kept short and sweet. Sometimes, for example, it is useful to share an experience with the client when you sense that the experience may parallel that of the client. The important thing, though, is to make the disclosure and then move quickly back to the client's world.

These, then, are issues of disclosure. Whilst disclosure *can* beget disclosure, it is important not to overwhelm or swamp the other person. It is also important not to turn the relationship into a therapeutic one for yourself. Sometimes, excessive disclosure on the part of the counsellor can lead to the client feeling sorry for the counsellor and to worrying about whether or not he or she really should be talking about his or her problems, given that the counsellor is so troubled! This is a less than ideal situation!

Finally, think about how you *handle* other people's disclosure. Some people are embarrassed by other people telling them personal details. Sometimes, too, it is possible to become something of a counsellor *voyeur*: the other person's disclosure becomes interesting and the counsellor wants to pursue what is being said more out of nosiness than out of therapeutic intention.

Train yourself to notice how much people tend to disclose to you as a matter of everyday course,

and what you do when people *do* disclose. In the counselling setting, it is important that third level disclosures are accepted and not met with moralization or disapproval. If they *are* then it is unlikely that the client will make further third level disclosures.

Moving on

Finally, the judgement has to be made about when to move on in the relationship. This initial period of exploration naturally leads on the to the next: the stage of identifying priorities. Perhaps the most important thing to bear in mind here is that *the priorities will emerge*. It is not, in the end, up to the counsellor to decide what those priorities are. As the relationship matures, it begins to become clear to both parties what the most important issues are.

Priorities emerge in many different ways. Sometimes, there are one or two particular issues to which the client keeps returning. Then, both parties begin to notice and begin to identify those issues as priorities.

Sometimes, the words that the client use indicate the sorts of things that may be priorities. We have noted above that many people live in a feeling, thinking or concrete domain. The person who constantly uses expressions such as 'I think' and 'I believe that what is going on here is . . .', may have problems in dealing with their feelings. On the other hand, the person who always uses 'feeling words' may have avoided any recourse to systematic problem solving. Alternatively, the 'concrete' person may avoid reflecting, at all, on his or her life situation and that fact becomes the priority. As we have seen, it often helps if people consider how they feel, how they think and also what *actually happens*.

Sometimes, the client will acknowledge particular issues as important ones. Then, he or she naturally leads the counselling relationship into the next phase. It is not a question of moving the relationship on, the relationship moves as a natural process.

Above all things, it is important not to risk this early phase. It is easy to search for 'green apples' — issues that *appear* to be major problems but which are not identified as such by the client. Mostly, this initial exploratory phase has its own life span. Mostly, the relationship steadily develops until it becomes clear exactly what issues need to be highlighted.

Coping with feelings

Whilst the issue of feelings is raised here, it is fully acknowledged that feelings can emerge at any stage in the counselling relationship. All of the things discussed in this chapter are applicable to other stages in counselling. The important thing, here, though is the working through of some of the bottled up feelings so as to move on to the next stage: that of exploring alternatives.

Counselling people often means coping with emotions. A considerable part of the process of helping people in counselling is concerned with the emotional or 'feelings' side of the person. In the UK and North American cultures, a great premium is placed on the individual's being able to 'control' feelings and thus overt expression of emotion is often frowned upon. As a result, we learn to bottle up feelings, sometimes from a very early age. Sometimes, just letting a person express his or her feelings can be therapeutic.

Before going further, a caution has to be noted. It is often noted that people are individual in their responses. It is difficult to make general statements about 'how human beings work'. If we *do* make generalizations, we are likely to find exceptions to them. It should be noted, then, that whilst the points made in this chapter are true of many people, they are not necessarily true of *all* people. Some people, for example, do not particularly like or want to express strong feelings. There is no need to have an elaborate theory of 'resistance' of denial here, but merely to note that different people do things differently. There should be no hint from the counsellor that people *should* release or face emotions. It is important to pay close attention to the individual's needs and wants.

Feelings

It is possible to distinguish between at least four types of emotion that are commonly suppressed or bottled up: anger, fear, grief and embarrassment. It is suggested that there is a relationship between these feelings and certain expressions of them. Thus, in counselling, anger may be expressed as loud sound, fear as trembling, grief through tears and embarrassment by laughter. It is suggested, too, that there is a relationship between those feelings and certain basic human needs.

We all have the need to understand and know what is happening to us. If that knowledge is not forthcoming, we may experience fear. We also need to make choices in our lives, and if that choice is restricted in certain ways we may feel anger. Thirdly, we need to experience the expression of love and of being loved. If that love is denied us or taken away from us, we may experience grief. To these basic human needs may be added the need for self-respect and dignity. If such dignity is denied us, we may feel self-conscious and embarrassed.

What is perhaps more important is that the expression of pent-up emotion is often helpful in that it seems to allow the person to be clearer in his thinking once he or she has expressed it. It is as though the blocked emotion 'gets in the way' and its release acts as a means of helping the person to clarify his thoughts and feelings. It is notable that the suppression of feelings can lead to certain problems in living that may be clearly identified.

Exploring possible alternatives

How, then, do you and the client decide on what is to be done? Sometimes, this stage is fairly simple – the question is asked 'What has to happen now?' and the client identifies a course of action. Sometimes, though, the client is still confused or uncertain about what needs to be done. Sometimes, too, the client is very reluctant to *do* anything. As we have noted earlier in this book, it is often easier to remain in the domain of thinking and feeling: doing is sometimes more difficult. For other people, the issue is that they want *things* to change but they do not want to change themselves. It is as though the client is saying "Show me how I can make my situation change but make it so that *I* do not change." The truth seems to be, though, that if we want change to occur in our lives then we must also change.

Problem solving

Formal problem solving is sometimes useful here. The stages of a problem solving cycle are these:

- [ ] identification of the problem;
- [ ] generation of all possible solutions;
- [ ] selection of a particular solution;
- [ ] institution of the particular solution;
- [ ] evaluating the effectiveness of the solution.

The process of *brainstorming* is the most useful way of generating a wide range of possible solutions. It is helpful if all sorts of solutions are generated: the more extreme, the better. For example, a client who discovers that she no longer wants to return to her husband might generate the following list of 'brainstormed' solutions. Some seem feasible but others, at first sight, seem highly unlikely:

- [ ] Never go home,
- [ ] Walk out, once I'm home,
- [ ] Disappear,
- [ ] Talk to husband,
- [ ] Talk to family as a group,
- [ ] Talk to the children on their own,
- [ ] Go and see a RELATE counsellor,
- [ ] Take a long holiday,
- [ ] Go to sea,
- [ ] Go to stay with my sister in Australia,
- [ ] Have an affair,
- [ ] Go home and argue,
- [ ] Go home and stay.

The list could no doubt be added to. In the end, certain options seem to rule themselves out, but the *process* of generating *unlikely* as well as *likely* solutions often opens up other possibilities. For example, the 'go to sea' option seems to be a reasonably unlikely option, but thinking about it may raise possibilities of moving, of a holiday, of working overseas, and so on. The brainstorming stage, then, should be a slow, open-ended one.

Recording counselling

At this point, it is important to consider whether or not you will *record* your counselling sessions. What is discussed in this section is of relevance to any part of the counselling relationship.

To record or not to record? Before we discuss a method of recording counselling, it is worth considering whether sessions should be recorded at all. First, the advantages of recording:

☐ a series of records allow you to check progress: yours as a counsellor and the client's in terms of the effectiveness of the relationship;

☐ records allow you to review what has happened between you and the client;

☐ records enable other people to see what you have been doing in your counselling sessions.

Now, the disadvantages:

☐ records can give a false sense of what is happening in a person's life. If you read a record card from last week, just before you counsel, the danger is that you will expect the client's life to pick up from that point when you meet him or her. In fact, though, the client has lived another week since you made your record. A lot can happen in a week;

☐ the real problem and potential disadvantage is the issue of confidentiality. If you make a record, you make a formal document which (presumably) is the property of the hospital or health district. This raises a number of subsequent questions. How *much* do you record of what someone has said? Who will see the records? Can you write *anonymous* records that do not name the client?

The question of whether or not you keep records of counselling is a far from simple one. You need to think long and hard about the issue, discuss it with your senior nurses and lecturers and then make a decision. It may, of course, be possible to write notes in other documents relating to the patient's care as a contrast to keeping separate 'counselling notes.'

Taking action

The final part of this penultimate stage of the counselling relationship belongs very much to the client. It is the stage in which the client *acts* as a result of counselling. Just as we noted that the 'talking has to stop' at some point, this becomes particularly important here. For effective counselling must always lead to *action* on the part of the client. The client has to change something about the way they do things or the way they live. Reflection on this idea will offer evidence of the truth of it. In the end, counselling can *never* just be about talking: action has to occur. And yet this is very often the most difficult part of the whole process. Freud noted about neurotic people that the last things they wanted to loose were their symptoms. Many people want *things* to change without changing themselves. Clearly, though, if 'life' is to change for the client, then the client must do some changing.

It is helpful if the counsellor talks through this 'action' phase of the relationship very carefully with the client and helps to *plan* the course of action. Like all change, it is usually best if life-change takes place slowly and gradually. However, it is important to make sure that it *does* take place! Often, we are quite good at persuading ourselves and other people that we have changed when, in fact, the changes have been so slight as to be unnoticeable and certainly ineffectual. During this phase of action, the counsellor will act as a supportive friend and be prepared to 'catch' the client if he or she fails. Often, too, the client will regress slightly during this change period. Regression refers to the idea that we slip back a little when we are threatened. Given that change is nearly always threatening, it seems reasonable to allow some slippage. In other words, the client may have come a long way in their thinking or feeling, only to slip back a little when they try to *change*. Again, support is required here, and the counsellor should allow the regression and not try too hard at making the client return to a more adult status.

This is not yet the time to terminate the counselling relationship, although the end is not far away. It is important that both parties allow the change element to take place successfully before termination is talked about. Anyway, neither client nor counsellor is likely to *want* to talk about ending the relationship at this point: it is far too traumatic for the client, and usually a phase in which the counsellor feels very much involved.

One thing often occurs as a result of the client instituting change: other people, around the client, change too. It is rather like a person becoming more assertive. As the assertive person is met by friends and family, they are perceived as 'different' and those friends and family begin to treat the assertive person differently. So it is with action following counselling. That action *must* occur after counselling seems inevitable. It is also inevitable that the client will be perceived differently as he or she changes. Again, it is part of the counsellor's role to support the client during this, often difficult, stage.

Something else happens, too. As the client changes, so does the client-counsellor relationship. After all, the counsellor is one of the important people in the client's life. So it happens that the client, as he or she tries action as a result of counselling, is likely to modify his or her view of the counsellor. Often, it is a case of the counsellor being seen as more 'human' and that often means 'more flawed'. As the client grows in confidence (and this is a gradual process) so too does he or she come to realize that the counsellor is quite an ordinary person after all. Once this happens, the client also comes to realize that he or she may be able to manage without the counsellor's help after all. Then it is apparent that the beginning of the end of the relationship is in sight.

This can be quite a painful process for the counsellor. The client is changing whilst the counsellor is not. For weeks the client has been fairly dependent upon the counsellor and now he or she is beginning to become much more independent. And yet the counsellor has remained fairly constant. As a result of this changing relationship, it is not uncommon for the *counsellor* to begin to review his or her life-position. There is nothing like another person's changing to cause us to question our own stasis! Handled well, this can be a taking off point for the counsellor as well as for the client. It can be a period in which the counsellor reflects both on his or her relationships and his or her skills. It can also do much to help the counsellor to face up to the fact of the inevitable partings in life.

CONCLUSIONS

This chapter has been concerned, mostly, with the *client-centred* approach to counselling. It must be acknowledged that this is only *one* approach to the topic. Other writers have discussed more *prescriptive* approaches to counselling and yet others have acknowledged that a *balanced* approach, in which neither party is wholly 'in charge' of the relationship may be appropriate (see, for example, Heron, 1990; Dryden, Charles-Edwards and Woolfe, 1989).

This chapter has illustrated a typical 'cycle' of counselling and has identified some of the skills that need to be practised in order to work round that cycle. Every critical care nurse is likely to need to demonstrate counselling skills at some point in his or her career – even if only to listen and to 'be with' the patient or client. The skills can be learned, and it is recommended that you consider your own skills and your own needs in this important domain of nursing.

STUDENT LEARNING QUESTIONS

1. To what degree is it reasonable to train critical care nurses as counsellors?

2. A distinction has been made between *being a counsellor* and *having counselling skills*. Which category do you feel is more appropriate for nurses?

3. What applications does counselling have outside of the critical care field?

4. Who should train nurses in counselling skills?

FURTHER READING

Baruth, L. G. *An Introduction to the Counselling Profession*. Englewood Cliffs, NJ: Prentice Hall, 1987.

Burnard, P. Existentialism as a theoretical basis for counselling in psychiatric nursing. *Archives of Psychiatric Nursing*. 1989; III(3): 142–147.

Dryden, W., Charles-Edwards, D., Woolfe, R. (Eds.). *Handbook of Counselling in Britain*. London: Routledge, 1989.

Ivey, A. E. *Counselling and Psychotherapy: Skills, theories and practice*. London: Prentice Hall, 1987.

Murgatroyd, S. *Counselling and Helping*. London: British Psychological Society and Methuen, 1986.

REFERENCES

Burnard, P. *Teaching Interpersonal Skills*. London: Chapman and Hall, 1989.

Burnard, P., Morrison, P. *Self Disclosure: A Contemporary Analysis*. Aldershot: Avebury, 1992.

Cox, M. *Structuring the Therapeutic Process*. London: Pergamon, 1978.

Dryden, W., Charles-Edwards, D., Woolf, R. (Eds.). *Handbook of Counselling in Britain*. London: Routledge, 1989.

Egan, G. *The Skilled Helper*. Pacific Grove, CA: Brooks/Cole, 1990.

Heron, J. *Helping the Client*. London: Sage, 1990.

Jourard, S. *The Transparent Self*. New York: Van Nostrand, 1964.

Luft, J. *Of Human Interaction: The Johari Model*. Palo Alto, CA: Mayfield, 1969.

Rogers, C. R. *On Becoming a Person*. London: Constable, 1967.

Rogers, C. R. *Freedom to Learn for the Eighties*. Columbus, Ohio: Merril, 1981.

18

CULTURAL ISSUES IN CRITICAL CARE NURSING

Jim Richardson

CHAPTER AIMS

This chapter will explore issues of culture as they may relate to the work of the critical care nurse. As a complex abstract idea, culture is not always easy to clarify, so the important ideas in this area will be introduced and illustrated by examples and case histories. Specifically, this chapter aims to:

☐ provide a definition of what is meant by culture;

☐ illustrate the relevance of cultural ideas in critical care;

☐ explore means of systematically assessing another's cultural ideas and needs;

☐ show the value to critical care nurses, and for those for whom they care, of nurses understanding their own cultural orientation;

☐ show how an understanding of cultural ideas can improve the collaboration between nurse and patient and thereby improve satisfaction with and effectiveness of care.

INTRODUCTION

The working environment of the critical care nurse is full of tensions and demands. The pace is rapid and decision making must be swift. The patient has, by virtue of his presence in the critical care area, immediate problems which may be life-threatening. The nurse's assessment of the patient's needs and his or her actions to satisfy these must keep pace with ever-changing situations. There is always the potential for sudden, catastrophic changes in the patient's condition. Modern technology provides more and more complex diagnostic, monitoring and therapeutic equipment, yet while this helps in the care of the acutely ill patient, it may add to the pressures by placing demands on the nurse for the safe and accurate use of this technology. The technical competence required of the nurse in using such technological assistance can easily become the most important demand on nurses, and blind them to the more human psychological and emotional components of the situation.

The fear and anxiety which always accompany serious illness or injury are enhanced in the high pressure critical care unit. Patients, when conscious, are fearful and utterly reliant on nurses and doctors for their continued survival. Relatives and friends of the patient may be powerless, vulnerable and petrified in the strange beeping, buzzing and hissing world of the modern critical care unit. This patient and family fear is transmissible to critical care unit personnel, adding to the pressures.

Nevertheless, amid this rather frightening scenario, critical care nurses have some advantages in their working environment. Each patient has his own nurse, perhaps even several nurses, and this allows the nurse the opportunity to get to know the patient and his or her family more closely. Concentrated contact between nurse and patient and family in the midst of a tense situation may allow the parties to come to know much about each other very rapidly as the social 'niceties' are bypassed.

In the care situation the most effective and satisfying results are achieved through the cooperation of the hospital staff, the patient and those important to him or her. This collaboration is dependent upon all concerned understanding what each person involved feels is important and achievable in the situation, and how it should be achieved. This shared understanding is dependent upon each considering the others' viewpoint. It is at this point that cultural factors emerge as being vitally important for the patient and his well-being. Disharmony between carer and cared for as regards cultural issues will lead to friction and even loss of collaboration, which can only hamper efforts to satisfy the patient's health needs.

WHAT IS CULTURE?

At first sight culture is an easy idea to define; everyone feels that they know what this means. Just a few moments spent on trying to explain this concept will, however, show how difficult it is to neatly define culture. Culture is a large and complex idea, and its definition is not helped by the range of ways in which we use the word in English. Culture might be used to describe a 'race' or 'nationality'. Equally, we tend to think of culture as those expressions of the intellectual development of a society such as art, literature, opera and ballet. Just think of what is implied when someone is described as a 'culture vulture'!

Anthropology and transcultural nursing have produced many definitions of culture. It will be useful at this point to consider some of these definitions to allow us to be clear just what we are talking about here.

Helman (1990) proposes that

". . . culture can be seen as the inherited 'lens' through which individuals perceive and understand the world that they inhabit, and learn how to live with it. Growing up within

any society is a form of enculturation, whereby the individual slowly acquires the cultural 'lens' of the society. Without such a shared perception of the world, both the cohesion and continuity of any human group would be impossible." (p. 3)

Murray and Zentner (1989) describe culture as

". . . the sum total of the learned ways of doing, feeling and thinking, past and present, of a social group within a given period of time. These ways are transmitted from one generation to the next or to immigrants who become members of the society. Culture is the group's design for living, a shared set of socially transmitted assumptions about the nature of the physical and social worlds, goals in life, attitudes, rôles and values." (p. 239)

From these two definitions we can begin to identify some of the important features of culture.

Culture is:

☐ learned as we grow up and live in our community;

☐ our beliefs – those things we feel are true about the world we live in and the people we live with, things we accept as real – this may include religious belief;

☐ our values – the things we think are important, our principles which guide our actions and form the basis of our opinions;

☐ our habits – the predictable ways in which we behave, our customs and rituals, the ways in which we behave in everyday life;

☐ passed from generation to generation, it is our heritage;

☐ the 'glue' which binds communities together, it forms a shared identity;

☐ dynamic, it changes according to the time and the place in which we live;

☐ important to us, it is the basis for many of the judgements and decisions we make;

☐ important to us to the point that we may be prepared to defend it;

□ so much part of us that we may not be aware of how it influences us;

□ influences how we see others who do not share our culture;

□ helps to determine our response to difficulties and crises.

For nurses, culture may only become an issue when faced with the situation in which the patient comes from a cultural background radically different from the nurse's own. It has become a truism that Britain is a multicultural society, and all critical care nurses will experience caring for people with a different cultural outlook to their own. In this case, culture will become a focus. This has led to a tendency to see culture as being important only when dealing with people with backgrounds which are seen as 'exotic' or 'unusual'. This is understandable – but is far from being the whole story.

If we examine again the features of culture outlined above, it will become clear that culture is a very subtle idea. Culture can be seen as a factor in regional and class differences within a society, and even in our professional rôles. Indeed, if we apply the definitions of culture we have outlined it can be seen that nursing itself forms a culture.

NURSING AS A CULTURE

Nursing beliefs

Nursing knowledge founded on the basis of the experience of practice and the results of nursing research shape the beliefs that nurses hold in common. Research evidence indicates how pressure sores can be avoided by turning the debilitated patient regularly to avoid sustained pressure on delicate and vulnerable tissues. Nurses generally believe this evidence and act on the basis of it. Not all nursing beliefs are so firmly based on fact: many nurses believe that when patients are given flowers, red and white blooms should not be displayed in the same vase. There is a vague belief that this is 'unlucky'.

Nursing values

Nursing values might include those ideas embodied in the UKCC Code of Professional Conduct (UKCC, 1992). These indicate the principles which nurses hold in common. Indeed, The Code of Professional Conduct includes the clause,

> "recognise and respect the uniqueness and dignity of each patient and client, and respond to their need for care irrespsoive of their ethnic origin, religious beliefs, personal attribute, the nature of their health problem or any other factor;" (UKCC, 1992, Clause 7.)

Other ideas might include tenets such as the view that nurses should not take industrial action by withdrawing their labour in any attempt to improve their pay and conditions. Such values may not be absolute – there may be degrees of acceptance of such ideas.

Nursing behaviour

Nursing behaviour is often shared and identifiable as being specifically nursing in such things as the wearing of uniforms, despite their impracticality, and registration and school of nursing badges. On occasion, nursing behaviour may be stable but have little in the way of logical underlying justification. Walsh and Ford (1989) has named such behaviour nursing rituals. These might include such behaviours as always transporting patients in beds or on trolleys head first, or the addition of a handful of salt to the post-operative patient's bath water!

Transmission of nursing culture through generations

Nursing beliefs, values and habits are transmitted by formal nurse education which must be successfully undertaken before we will admit the new nurse to the culture of qualified nurses (Bradby, 1990). Equally strongly influential in the formation of nursing culture are those informal education influences placed on the student nurse in clinical practice, when those valued behaviours necessary for acceptance in a close-knit and supportive nursing team are learned. As pointed out by Ashworth and Morrison (1989), there may be considerable differences between these formal and informal educational influences.

Nursing culture is dynamic

Nurses are now coming to accept nursing students as students rather than apprentices in a way which would have been unthinkable even a decade ago. Also, with changes in nursing philosophy, nurses are embracing their work as the holistic care of people rather than as a set of tasks to be done in a disjointed way.

SOME IMPORTANT CULTURAL IDEAS

When someone begins to accept the features of a culture through upbringing or education this process has been named *enculturation* or socialization. Nurses become encultured throughout their education and career.

When a new culture is encountered, and features of the culture are accepted, this process has been named *acculturation* or *assimilation*. It is important to realize that the original culture remains intact and only changes very slowly under the influence of the new. The student nurse may accept features of nursing culture, but retain all the features of that culture within which he or she was brought up. The new culture is superimposed on the old, and the resulting new mixture may be unique to that individual.

Professor R. who came to Britain 30 years ago to study and who is now an eminent university academic, would appear in his everyday life to have completely assimilated British culture. When he is admitted to the critical care unit with multiple injuries following a road traffic accident, however, he and his family request that amulets are brought to the unit to ensure his recovery. The use of such amulets belongs to Professor R.'s original culture, and he has only returned to their use in this time of danger and difficulty. His original culture is thus seen to be intact and of great comfort to him in a situation of adversity.

When people first encounter a new dominant culture they may experience considerable stress until they learn to accommodate and live within this new culture. Any nurses who have worked for any period of time abroad will recall how disorientating it can be when you are suddenly unsure of the basis of values and beliefs upon which those around you act. How to behave when customs and behaviour are very different can be highly stressful; the world becomes unpredictable and difficult to interpret. Brink (1979) has labelled this phenomenon *culture shock*, a term which neatly illustrates the profound effect this experience can have on the individual. Think of the poor terrified student nurse on the first day of a placement on the critical care unit!

A South East Asian refugee who fled from his home in a remote mountainous area of Laos as a result of the Vietnam war found his way to the United States. He found the experience of American culture quite unexpected. He described himself as "being like a goat in a herd of cows." (Rairdan and Higgs, 1992)

When considering any culture it will become obvious that there will be some smaller subgroups within this cultural group with slightly different aims and beliefs. This throws up the idea of the *subculture*. A subculture is a group within a group. To extend the nursing analogy, critical care nurses can be seen as a subculture. The subculture is embedded in the greater culture but is distinctive in sharing most beliefs, but also in possessing some particular identity of its own.

It is vitally important that critical care nurses do not make assumptions about a patient's beliefs, values and valued behaviours on the patient's *perceived* culture. It is, of course, particularly easy to do this when the patient is very ill, perhaps unconscious, and communication is limited. Such baseless assumption can be called *stereotyping*. **It should be clear that the only way to be sure of getting accurate cultural information about a person is to ask him or her!**

Mrs F., an Iranian lady, who has lived and worked

in the UK for the last 15 years, has spent some time on the coronary care unit following episodes of cardiac arrhythmias which have been hard to control. On discharge to the ward she commented that she found it strange that while she saw other patients being offered meals with meat she had been given no meat while on the CCU. The nurses, on learning that Mrs F. was an Iranian by origin, had ordered a vegetarian diet for her as they assumed her to be a Muslim. This was not, in fact, the case. In addition, Muslims do not tend to be vegetarian, but they do not, as a rule, eat pork.

Since everyone feels their own culture – beliefs, values and habits – to be especially correct, it is easy to slip into believing that everyone should share these same beliefs. By extension, anyone who deviates from these views might be seen as being wrong. This is the basis of *ethnocentrism* (Thiedermann, 1986). Ethnocentrism is simply a form of egocentrism, that is, not an intentionally selfish attitude but rather the inability to see another's point of view (Ruiz, 1981; Bonaparte, 1979).

Baby J. is admitted to the neonatal intensive care unit immediately after her birth. She has, among other medical problems, a severe degree of cleft lip and palate. Her father, who comes from a culture which values sons highly, is frank in his disappointment that his new baby is a daughter not a son. He expresses concern that it will be difficult to find a husband for his daughter in the future in the light of her lip deformity. The nurses are outraged and respond angrily. Relations between this new father and his daughter's nurses remain inflamed and unproductive for some time.

Prejudice is an unpleasant tendency to categorize people on the basis of their membership of a cultural group, and to treat them in a less favourable way as a result. Prejudice is characterized by not being related to any provable fact, and is often very difficult indeed to change or eradicate. It is frequently based in ignorance and 'fear' of the unknown.

Miss K. is being cared for on the surgical critical care unit as a result of complications following a

termination of pregnancy. This young woman has had three terminations before this operation. One of the nurses says "I can't stand these young people who think they can use abortion as a method of contraception. When she's awake she's going to get a piece of my mind. It's disgusting."

The critical care nurse's own culture as a factor in patient care

It should be clear that in all our interactions with other people we tend to use our cultural beliefs as a yardstick or even 'gold standard' in making our judgements. We are therefore **all** naturally egocentric. Our cultural orientation is so deeply part of ourselves that we use it as our 'lens' or the 'filter' through which we view others. This is such a familiar part of us that we employ these ways of thinking almost unconsciously. When asked to describe our own cultural beliefs, most of us would be initially stumped for a ready answer. To become clear about our own culture is an important aspect of self-awareness. We cannot objectively appraise another's cultural orientation and needs if we are not clear about the basis on which we are ourselves working in this area.

Readers may find it a useful exercise to complete a cultural assessment for themselves as outlined below. This will assist in reflecting on one's own cultural background.

Cultural assessment

Most of the assessment tools used by nurses such as Roper's Activities of Living (Roper *et al.*, 1983) will, when used sensitively, allow the nurse to gather adequate information about patients' cultural backgrounds. This will tend to be rather superficial in that it concentrates on behavioural features such as what and when people like to eat, how they like to wash and dress, and what their pastimes are. This sort of information is often sufficient when the nurse and patient share a cultural background in some measure and can feel confident about common understandings with regard to beliefs and values.

Difficulties can arise when the nurse and patient

have different beliefs and values and cannot be certain of this comfortable common understanding. In this case, a more thorough cultural assessment can be undertaken to clarify the issues and establish a frame of reference for all involved. As with all assessment procedures, cultural assessment need not be undertaken at one sitting and may be completed over a period of time as nurse and patient come to know each other. This is an important point, since many of the cultural tools available to us are American in origin and tend to be quite complicated and even cumbersome in use. Leininger (1985, 1988), a nurse and anthropologist, was one of the first to propose the use of cultural theory in nursing care planning and developed her 'Sunrise Model'. This is a comprehensive evaluation of cultural issues in care, but is complex and it may seem difficult to apply these ideas in practice. Giger and Davidhizar (1990, 1991) have further developed these ideas and simplified them although retaining comprehensiveness.

Giger and Davidhizar's model of cultural assessment

proposes that the nurse gather information about the patient in the following areas:

☐ *communication* – this in itself is such a large area that adequate assessment covering verbal and non-verbal aspects is a large task;

☐ *space* – this refers to the social space desired by an individual and preference for proximity with others;

☐ *social organization* – this refers to the form of family and community from which the individual comes;

☐ *time* – this category deals with finding out whether an individual is past, present and future orientated (this idea is explored in more depth later in the chapter);

☐ *environmental control* – this deals with the degree to which the individual feels in control of surroundings and events;

☐ *biological variations* – this explores racial factors such as skin and hair colour and texture and susceptibility to disease.

Rosenbaum (1991) proposes a fairly brief cultural assessment guide, but this runs into difficulties since it seems to assume that the patient is highly articulate in English. Questions such as "Can you teach me about how you see your life in relation to the world around you" would surely be rather difficult for anyone to respond to! This guide is, nevertheless, of interest to the nurse who seeks concise information about the range of issues on which information may be required when completing a cultural assessment.

Parfitt (1988) has succinctly described the value of cultural assessment in the critical care unit, and examines this topic from the specific point of view of the critical care nurse.

As has been pointed, out values are a core characteristic of cultural identity. Just a moment's thought about what values are and how information can be gathered about them will reveal what a mammoth task this could be when necessary as part of a cultural assessment. One interesting approach to this problem was introduced by Florence Kluckhohn, an American sociologist, in the 1950s. She proposed a system of classifying cultural value orientations (Kluckhohn, 1976) which, while complicated at first sight, with some practice can be quite easily used in practice to establish a patient's value orientation. This classification organizes value-related information into five categories.

Man's basic nature – in this area a culture/person may view mankind as:

☐ basically evil – may or may not be capable of improvement;
☐ neither good nor evil – variable and changeable, may not be predictable;
☐ basically good – may or may not be susceptible to being corrupted.

The patients' views in this area will influence how he sees those around him and interpret his intention towards them. If he sees man as basically bad it will be easy for him to be pessimistic about and distrustful of other people. In this situation he will need to be permanently on his guard, and may be reluctant to cooperate with others.

Mrs C. has been ill for some time with a rare neoplastic disease, and is presently suffering a relapse. One of the senior medical staff has been working very hard indeed on Mrs C.'s behalf. This doctor is often to be found visiting her in the evenings, closely monitoring her treatment, discussing alternative strategies with colleagues, searching the medical literature for new treatment possibilities for Mrs C. Rather puzzlingly, Mrs C. responds to this health worker's professional attention in a very sullen manner. She seems to actively resist his efforts. She has been heard to say, "What's she up to? What does she *really* want from me? What's in it for him? What *is* she after?" Mrs C. finds it hard to accept this doctor's good-will and altruism. She tends to view man as basically bad.

Man's relationship to nature – this category relates to how the patient sees her relationship with her environment:

- ☐ 'man-under-nature' – according to this belief nature is all-powerful and man cannot affect it or prevent its effect on him;
- ☐ 'man-in-nature' – here man is seen as living in harmony with nature, but the balance may be delicate and any disturbances in the balance may be held to explain illness (Durie, 1985);
- ☐ 'man-over-nature' – this viewpoint holds that nature can be subjugated and nothing should be impossible.

These factors may be very influential in how the patient and his family see the health crisis. In the first point he may feel hopeless and fatalistic, and be disinclined to comply with medical and nursing treatment. Those who hold the second view described may feel that only those treatments aimed at restoring a natural balance will be successful in dealing with their health problem. They may be prepared to comply only with strategies clearly aimed at achieving this. For those ascribing to the third viewpoint, anything is possible; modern medicine can provide the answer to all ills.

Mr Z., a 98 year old man, has suffered a catastrophic cerebrovascular accident. He has been deeply unconscious for some time, and has shown absolutely no signs of recovery. Mr Z.'s long-standing cardiac disease is deteriorating, and he is now in frank heart failure. His distraught family are convinced that not enough is being done for him. They are demanding that he be referred for neurosurgical treatment, and are convinced that this will be a helpful course of action. Holding a 'man-over-nature' philosophy, Mr Z.'s family are certain that if only the health care team will try hard enough, modern medicine holds the key to all problems. They cannot countenance the inevitability of Mr Z's death.

Staff Nurse Q. has been involved in some conflict with colleagues. He has on more than one occasion responded to situations of medical emergency such as cardiac arrest with what his co-workers see as a lack of urgency and speed. The conflict has reached crisis level, and the ward sister attempts to discuss the matter with Nurse Q. "Oh!" he exclaims, "but why should I rush and hurry? I will do everything I can for my patients but after all it is all in God's hand. What will be will be." Nurse Q.'s fatalistic attitude is clearly derived from a 'man-under-nature' orientation.

Time dimension – this factor determines how a person views his experience:

- ☐ past orientated – much store is placed on what has been learned by experience and on tradition. Elders are highly valued for their wisdom in this orientation – they have experienced much and learned from it;
- ☐ present orientated – only the here and now is important. The past is past and is now irrelevant and the future is too unpredictable to be taken into account in making decisions;
- ☐ future orientated – the past is gone and the present is only significant for how actions now can improve conditions in the future.

The past orientated person will want any health care to accord with what he has learned in the past. He may have strong beliefs about what causes illness and how that illness should be treated. In this case he will be reluctant to cooperate if treatment plans do not accord with his beliefs. Since the accrued wisdom of older people is much respected, he may wish to consult a senior member of the family about treatment options. For the present orientated person, this moment's comfort and sensations are what are important. For the future orientated person, the important thing is to look forward; he may be prepared to tolerate even very unpleasant procedures or treatment side-effects if this strategy can be expected to produce a future improvement in health.

X.J. is a three year old boy who has been treated for primary tuberculosis. He has come to hospital with tuberculosis meningitis, and his parents readily admit that they abandoned giving him his long-term tuberculosis drugs some time ago. On gentle questioning the nurse is able to find out that they stopped the drug because they saw their child as well and simply could not conceive the future consequences of their action. This family's orientation to the present was instrumental in their not complying with the drug regime.

The immunization programme offered to young children in our society, among other things, assumes a future orientation. No parent likes to expose a child to a painful injection and possibly a subsequent fever, but with a future orientation a short-term minor discomfort and small degree of risk from the vaccine can be tolerated in exchange for future protection from dangerous infectious diseases.

The purpose of existence – in some ways this might be seen as 'the meaning of life'!

☐ being – simply living and experiencing, pleasure is sought and no developmental changes are considered;

☐ being-in-becoming – the inner life is emphasized, life is to be experienced but experience brings reflection and greater understanding;

☐ doing – action is of paramount importance, achievement is highly valued.

It can be seen here how different degrees of motivation with regard to therapeutic methods and resulting collaboration between patient and health care personnel might be affected by value orientation in this area.

Mrs J. has come to hospital with severe abdominal pain, so severe in fact that she was shocked on admission. On being given an analgesic drug and obtaining complete pain relief as a result, Mrs J. expresses her complete satisfaction with the situation. The nurses find it very odd that Mrs J. does not seem at all concerned about the cause of the pain. Mrs J. simply wanted to be rid of the pain and when that has been achieved she is content. Her orientation is in being.

How people relate to each other – under this category consideration is given to how we form families and communities and the ways in which we derive social support:

☐ lineal – links between generations are maintained, the extended family is valued. The importance of heredity and traditions maintained over generations is emphasized;

☐ collateral – the value of one generation is predominant, the nuclear family is characteristic of this outlook. The goals of this small group are most significant;

☐ individual – the goals and interests of the individual are most highly valued, no group is identified though support may be derived from same-age peers.

This category describes the forms of community which mankind tends to form. This gives an indication of how interests might be defined and protected. Sources of help and succour available to the patient are defined by the sort of social organization he belongs to as outlined in this category. Some ideas of the influences on people, particularly in adversity, can be gained by an impression of the values held in this area.

Mrs S. has been diagnosed as having a rectal tumour. She has been advised that she should have surgical treatment as soon as possible. She has refused to consent to this treatment. In trying to establish why Mrs S. does not wish to undergo surgery, the hospital staff discover that Mrs S. has written to her family abroad about her condition.

She will not decide about treatment for now because her elderly grandmother will travel to Britain, and Mrs S. wishes to await her arrival so that she can consult her grandmother before taking this important decision. Coming from a lineal orientation, Mrs S. wishes to benefit from her grandmother's wisdom and experience at this crucial point in her life.

For the nurse working in a British critical care unit, some issues may be of particular importance for consideration with regard to their cultural components.

COMMUNICATING

Language is important in telling us many things about the person we are talking to. The particular language spoken, the regional dialect or accent or the slang used convey much information about the individual. This information may be used to form judgements about people almost as a reflex – without thought or analysis – this is an aspect of ethnocentrism. Care should be taken to be aware of these value judgements. In communicating with another we are able to give information and provide comfort and reassurance. Not to understand what is being communicated to one, whether the route is verbal or non-verbal, can be a very frightening experience (Haigh, 1988). Without a common language communication can be reduced to a very crude level raising considerable ethical problems, particularly in the following example. What does this tell us about 'informed consent' or patients' rights?

Mr T., an elderly man from the Indian Subcontinent who speaks no English, is being treated for acute septicaemia arising from a gangrenous leg. His leg should be amputated as a matter or urgency and the surgical team, none of whom speak Mr T.'s mother tongue, are attempting to communicate this fact. Voices are raised in frustration and embarrassment and attempts are being made to speak clearly and slowly. Mr T. is patently understanding none of this. Eventually communication is reduced to someone miming a leg being sawn off. All the health care personnel involved are left feeling ineffectual and brutal after this episode.

Critical care nurses are at an advantage concerning communication, since many of their patients may have difficulty in communicating perhaps because of disturbances in consciousness or if an endotracheal tube is in use to assist ventilation. With experience of care in such situations the critical care nurse can develop a high degree of expertise in communicating in adverse situations. Many means of alternative communication are available in the critical care environment, ranging from picture boards to flair and creativity in body and sign language – mime and dance! The example above, however, illustrates the limitations of this approach.

All this means that when faced with the patient who does not speak English, and a large group of relatives, in a tense situation the critical care unit nures will have the advantage of experience and insight.

Gestures should be used with care as their interpretation can vary from culture to culture, and innocent gestures familiar in British society may have the potential to cause offence for someone from another society.

The nurse who has been looking after Mrs P., a Greek lady, all morning waves goodbye as she goes off duty. She is amazed to see the look of horror which this friendly gesture has produced on Mrs P.'s face. The nurse had been unaware that in Greece to show someone the palm of your hand with your arm extended is a highly insulting gesture. Mrs P. is appalled as it does not occur to her that anyone could use such a gesture in a way different from that used by Greeks. Mrs P. feels deliberately insulted and very hurt, and communication has broken down.

This shows the potential for damaging misunderstandings to occur when nurse and patient do not share a common language – verbal or non-verbal. Awareness of this fact will go far in preventing its actually happening in practice.

The use of interpreters and link-workers has

lately become much more prominent in health care settings. Many minority communities will provide interpreters and are able to provide an appropriate interpreter on request. Hospitals will sometimes produce lists of people on the staff who speak another language and who can help out with interpreting in a case of urgency before formal interpreting services can be arranged. The value of these practices in assisting communication between nurse and patient cannot be overemphasized, but some care must be exercised here too. The use of interpreters needs careful thought and a good deal of sensitivity.

Mrs A., a 30 year old Pakistani lady, has been admitted following a very large vaginal haemorrhage. Finding that he cannot speak to Mrs A. because they do not have a common language, a junior doctor calls the 'informal' Urdu interpreter on the hospital list. This interpreter turns out to be a male kitchen porter. Mrs A. is reluctant to talk to this man because her culture discourages contact with a man other than her husband or a close relative. Also, the interpreter's different social status from her own causes her some social discomfort. The whole situation takes a distinct turn for the worse when the doctor, blissfully unaware, attempts to elicit information about Mrs A.'s obstetric and gynaecological history. This clumsy attempt at communication is made worse since the interpreter has no understanding of these 'women's things'. Everyone is mortified with embarrassment, no useful information has been gleaned, and Mrs A. is now very frightened and distressed.

From this some of the important principles which must be taken into account when using interpreter services can be seen. The interpreter should:

☐ have some understanding of the topics which will be under discussion; what is often involved is not simple translation but interpreting to ensure that the patient understands. Difficult and strange ideas may need much explanation;

☐ be bound by the same duty of confidentiality as other health care workers;

☐ be acceptable to the patient with regard to gender, marital status, age and the social class to which the interpreter belongs;

☐ be prepared to translate what the patient says exactly, and not edit what is said for re-translation.

Help may be available from members of the patient's own family who have a better command of English than the patient. In this context, the unfortunately widespread habit of using a child as interpreter should be avoided. Children learn English rapidly on attending school while maintaining their mother tongue as the home language. In this circumstance the child may be *capable* of interpreting, but there is a great risk of the child being frightened by some of the ideas being discussed, or by the responsibility of the task. This risk is naturally even greater in the critical care environment in the context of a relative being dangerously ill.

In cases where communication between nurse and patient is difficult, some very simple rules may prove helpful.

When talking to the patient who has difficulty understanding you should:

☐ take time in trying to communicate;

☐ try to avoid attempting to communicate in a noisy or distracting environment;

☐ try to ensure that the patient is comfortable before attempting to communicate;

☐ sit down and ensure that the patient can see your face clearly;

☐ speak slowly and clearly;

☐ avoid long complicated sentences containing more than one thought;

☐ be aware of your use of slang or jargon – using these will not help understanding;

☐ do not be tempted to raise your voice – this is guaranteed to be unhelpful;

- do not mouth words in an exaggerated fashion – you will only look foolish;

- be careful not to communicate a patronizing or condescending attitude – someone who does not understand English well does not have to be treated like a small child.

The will to communicate in an egalitarian fashion with the patient is communicable even in the absence of a shared language. With care you can communicate respect and concern even if nothing else is possible. This is a good deal better than nothing at all.

DIET

As an important contributory factor to good health, food is of significance to all cultures. Our tastes, choice and definition of what is important to eat, how we eat it and when we eat it are learned as part of growing up in our family and society. Food is essential to our survival and satisfies hunger – one of our most basic drives. Certain foods are reserved for ceremonial situations or special occasions and festivals such as Christmas, Easter and the Hindu festival Diwali.

Since food is generally recognized as being an important contributory factor to well-being and the establishment and maintenance of good health, it is natural that the importance of food is emphasized when someone is unwell. This is a common human belief, but each culture interprets and expresses this belief in its own distinctive way. Every critical care nurse will be aware of the importance sometimes attached to feeding by the family of a critically ill person. On occasion the patient's family may be quite simply desperate to see feeding started, and seem to place enormous faith in the beneficial effects of giving food.

In ill-health the food taken is sometimes seen as having a therapeutic effect. A well-known example of this is the use of chicken soup in some Jewish households as a food specifically to be taken when unwell.

Eating has an important social function; we enjoy eating *with* people and we offer food to those who are important to us. In this way food can be held to be a tangible expression of our affection and

regard for another person. The offering of food or drink can also be used to communicate concern. Consider how often, in the British hospital environment, people who are distressed are offered a cup of tea.

In many cultures food is seen as being 'hot' or 'cold'. This classification has nothing to do with the actual temperature of the food, but describes what is felt to be the effect the food has on the body (Karseras and Hopkins, 1978). An illustration of this can be seen in the Chinese concepts of *yin* and *yang*. Yin is the cold, wet, dark principle, while yang is hot, dry and light. All of life depends on these two principles existing in balance; any disturbance in the harmony between the two will result in a disruption of health. This is known as the *humoral theory of health* (Kleinman *et al.*, 1978). The body's organs are seen as either yin or yang in nature, so disturbances in an organ's function may be amenable to treatment using a diet composed of foods of the appropriate principle. A yin disorder may be treated with yang foods. Traces of this sort of belief may be seen in the idea of 'feed a cold and starve a fever', or in the custom of taking hot drinks to help a cold.

There is a very wide difference between communities as regards which foods or disorders are seen as 'hot' or 'cold'; the only way to be certain of a patient's beliefs in this area is to ask in detail. If a health care worker's advice runs contrary to a person's nutritional beliefs and customs, the patient may quite simply refuse to comply. In this area, therefore, it is important that dietary factors are discussed and negotiated to ensure their acceptability to both patient and nurse or dietitian. Clearly, the sick person and their family may be greatly alarmed if the dietary regime is felt to have a potentially negative effect.

Health care workers should be aware that families may attempt to use this form of dietary therapy in parallel with orthodox treatment.

Mr X. has undergone a very major surgical procedure. While still sedated and being artificially ventilated, enteral feeding using one of the commercial feeding formulas is started. Mr X.'s family is quite clearly alarmed and unhappy about this. They appear to understand explanations about the importance of giving Mr X. the nutrients he requires to recover, but are still anxious. When the nurse takes time to sit down and discuss the family's worries about the feeding regime with them, it transpires that they are worried that the enteral formula is milk. They can see it in the bottle and it looks like milk. They explain that they believe that Mr X.'s medical problem is a 'cold' disorder and their dietary belief is that cow's milk is a 'cold' food. That being so, as far as they are concerned, the feeding regime can only make Mr X.'s problem worse. When the nurse explains about the constitution of the formula the family are greatly relieved and much more inclined to co-operate with the health care team in Mr X.'s treatment.

In the light of this factor, it is important during dietary assessment not only to establish what a patient's normal dietary habits are, but also what foods he would like to be offered while he is unwell and recuperating. It is alarming, perhaps even offensive, for a patient to be offered food which he finds unpleasant or unsuitable.

Given the importance which most people attach to food, it is not surprising that many cultures define food which is unfit for consumption; this food may be seen as unclean or polluting. The rules governing this and the acceptable methods of handling and preparing food are complex.

Some examples of dietary restrictions

These notes on dietary laws are only guidelines; clearly, individualized care demands that every attempt is made to gather person-specific information, rather than relying on rote-learned guidelines. People vary enormously in the degree to which they adhere to the habits of the cultural group to which they belong.

Hindu
May be many restrictions, beef and beef products forbidden. Possibly strict vegetarian. Prohibition extends to *all* foods containing these products and also any foods which have been in contact with forbidden foods.

Muslim
All pork products prohibited. Other meats only acceptable if the animal has been slaughtered in the ritual *halal* fashion. Jewish *kosher* meat may be acceptable. The use of alcohol is forbidden.

Jewish
Complex system of dietary laws which may have originally had a partial explanation in early public health laws; many of the foods forbidden are those which spoil easily in a hot climate and could cause food poisoning. The Jewish religion has its origin in a hot climate in the Middle East. Other features are quite simply an everyday demonstration of faith. Pork products are prohibited. Meat acceptable only if it comes from an animal slaughtered in the ritual *kosher* way. Acceptable animals for consumption must have cloven hooves and chew the cud; fish can only be eaten if they have fins and scales. The eating of predatory animals is forbidden. Meat and milk or dairy products may not be combined in one meal.

Fasting is a feature of many cultural groups, but most of these groups are clear that the ill person is not expected to fast. Patients may feel, however, that they should make an attempt to fast on holy days. The nurse can help by discussing the advantages and disadvantages of such a course of action. The nurse should be aware of the possible effect of fasting on tired and anxious relatives, for example, during the Muslim Ramadam or the Jewish Days of Awe.

PAIN

Pain as a phenomenon is composed of many factors; the physiological which is universal and the psychological which is a learned, culture-dependent characteristic. The psychological aspect is influenced by what a person's culture tells him or her that pain means, by his group's accustomed response to pain, past experience of pain, the context in which the pain occurs, and what he or she understands the pain to indicate in that particular situation (Sofaer, 1992; Madjar, 1985). The topic of pain is one in which misunderstandings can easily arise if the patient and nurse belong to very different cultural traditions and respond differently to pain (Cavillo and Flaskerud, 1993).

The classical study of Zborowski (1952),

although written 40 years ago, is still interesting in throwing light on the cultural response to pain. In his work, Zborowski studied the pain responses of four cultural groups in a New York hospital. The groups studied were Italian, Jewish, Irish and 'Old American'. Startling differences were noted.

The Italian patients were very sensitive to pain and vocal in their response to it, but tended to forget the experience as soon as the pain was alleviated. Their concern was the immediacy of the pain.

The Jewish patients were also seen to be very sensitive to pain, and would complain loudly. They wanted the support of many people during the pain experience. In contrast to the Italians, however, the Jewish patients continued to suffer even after their pain had been alleviated with analgesic drugs. Once free of pain they tended to begin worrying about the implications of the pain and whether it might indicate a serious complication in their recovery.

The Irish patients were notable in their stoical response to pain, they did not complain and preferred to be left alone while in pain. They placed great stock in "bravery". When asked about their pain they found great difficulty in describing the pain or the emotion it caused them to experience. The researcher concluded that for the Irish patients pain was a lonely experience since they could not communicate how they felt about it to anyone.

The 'Old Americans' tended to respond to pain in a manner similar to the Irish but they, in contrast to the Irish, were able to give a lucid account of their experience of pain.

It is *always* unwise to place too much importance on generalizations about cultural groups; each individual can be assumed to be unique and will respond in his own individual fashion. These examples of responses to pain are useful, however, to the critical care nurse in demonstrating the range of possible responses to pain.

It should be noted that research has demonstrated that nurses tend to be poor at estimating the pain experienced by a patient regardless of the cultural background of either party (Davitz & Davitz, 1980). This provides a powerful argument for patients being encouraged to assess their own pain – only they can truly know the degree of their pain.

It is also interesting to look at Haywood's research (1975) in this light. If information is the prescription against pain, how much more important is communication with patients who may have difficulty understanding?

The axiom coined by McCaffery (1983) is especially relevant when cultural factors may seem to cloud the issue,

> "*Pain is whatever the experiencing patient says it is, existing whenever he says it does.* This definition involves a very important attitude towards the patient in pain – *the patient is believed.*"

Of course, the matter of the patient's pain may be very difficult to assess when there are linguistic barriers but sensitivity in closely observing patients for clues which might indicate that they are suffering pain will assist in this task.

DRESS AND HYGIENE

Many cultural groups maintain very distinctive styles of clothes. Often clothing styles will arise from the culture maintaining an enhanced sense of modesty. For some groups certain items of clothing have ritual significance.

Mr G., a young Sikh, has been involved in a motorcycle accident. He has a complicated fracture of his left femur which will be treated by open reduction and pinning when his condition has been stabilized. The nurses are attempting to splint his leg while he waits to go to theatre. A somewhat farcical situation has arisen as Mr G. refuses point blank to part with his underpants. Thinking that Mr G. is bashful the nurses arrange for two male colleagues to undertake the task. Mr G. still refuses to be divested of his underwear. None of the nurses appreciate that Mr G.'s underpants are a ritual garment, *kacha*, and it is their religious significance which makes Mr G. determined to keep his shorts on (Sampson, 1982).

Some items of jewellery and cosmetics may also have ritual importance for people from cultural minorities, much as a wedding ring is important. Such jewellery should not be removed unless absolutely necessary before consulting the patient or their family.

Hygiene needs are common to all people, but how these are satisfied varies from culture to culture. While the British patient may enjoy a soak in a hot bath, many Asian people much prefer to wash themselves under running water. Some cultures use only their left hands to cleanse themselves after elimination. The left hand is then seen as 'dirty' and its use is restricted in other activities such as the handling of food. Patients with such a belief will use their right hand for eating and may be shocked and repulsed if a nurse offers them a bread roll from the left hand.

Ritual ablutions may be necessary for people belonging to certain religious groups, such as Muslims, before they can pray. It is of great importance that the nurse facilitates this even when, in the critical care environment, this may pose a challenge to ingenuity to organize.

Most people are naturally modest; no-one would wish to lie around naked in the company of strangers. The value of modesty is, however, particularly emphasized in some Asian cultures, especially in the presence of the opposite sex. A feature of the critical care environment, when the patient is in need of intensive and continuing monitoring and interventions, is that to facilitate easy access to the patient the patient is often nursed naked, usually covered only by a single sheet. Occasionally, through need or staff inattention, even this is dispensed with.

Mrs J. underwent surgery this afternoon for a ruptured aortic aneurism. She is anaesthetized and on a ventilator. Her condition is still dangerously unstable. She is being intensively cared for by three nurses, and she is naked and exposed on her bed in the open critical care unit, although screens have been placed to shield her from the gaze of others. Mr J., who is mild-mannered and visibly very frightened and distressed, wishes to see his wife. The nurse in charge of the unit has spoken with him, explained the situation and outlined the kind of care his wife requires. The sister has taken care to explain about all the equipment being used in his wife's care so that he will not be frightened by it when he sees it. She then escorts Mr J. to his wife's bedside. As soon as he sees his wife Mr J. explodes with fury, shouts wildly and violently throws the flowers he has brought on the floor. He then dissolves into helpless tears. Only much later do the nurses find out that Mr J.'s first reaction was that the nurses were treating his wife disrespectfully by keeping her naked. This, in combination with his extreme tension and distress, made him react in this, for him, uncharacteristic way.

BIOLOGICAL DIFFERENCES

There are a number of biological differences between racial groups which may be important for the critical care nurse to note.

For people with dark or black skins the presence of cyanosis can be difficult to detect if the nurse is unused to caring for coloured people. This can be catastrophic. For someone with a black skin cyanosis, or for that matter jaundice, is most easily seen on tissue which is less pigmented such as the nail beds or the oral mucus membrane. The skin of the bridge of the nose can be blanched using light pressure; in the presence of cyanosis, tissue colour will return slowly from the edge of the pale area to the centre (Baxter, 1993). In the case of pallor, the person with a brown skin may appear sallow and yellowish while the black patient may look ashen grey as the natural underlying red tones are lost. Jaundice can be seen in the sclera.

Black people when ill and bed-ridden may easily suffer from dry skin and hair, and the nurse must take action to moisturize both. The patient's family can be of great assistance in deciding how best to accomplish this (Baxter, 1992, 1993).

Certain racial groups have a particular susceptibility to certain genetic disorders. Examples of these include sickle cell anaemia (Ferguson, 1991; Franklin, 1990) in the Afro-Caribbean community, and cystic fibrosis among Caucasians (Goodchild and Dodge, 1985).

VULNERABILITY

The powerlessness of the critically ill patient and his or her family will evoke many different responses. At this time the system of spiritual belief may become highly important as a support and solace. Most religious groups have spiritual leaders who can be called upon to visit the critical care unit to offer spiritual comfort and pastoral support to the patient and their family – and also the unit's staff. The nurse must make every effort to recognize spiritual distress (Burnard, 1987), and to make religious ceremonies and observances possible. A degree of privacy offered for this communicates respect. Items of religious significance such as religious medals, amulets and idols may be of utmost importance to the patient, and should be handled with reverence.

The spiritual needs of patients who are agnostic or atheist must not be ignored (Burnard, 1988). As with all individuals, atheists or agnostics will have their own unique spiritual needs. Only by talking to the person can nurses begin to gain some idea of how they might begin to meet these needs.

DEATH AND DYING

Death is the universal human experience, and one of nursing's primary functions is to ensure dignified death when this becomes inevitable. Every culture has specific ceremonies connected with dying. When considered carefully these, although widely variable in the form of their expression, are motivated by the same underlying human motivation. The desire is to take leave of the person, to communicate loss and the respect for the dying or dead person, and to secure a safe passage to the afterlife.

The complexity and variability of ceremonies, rituals and customs surrounding death can be bewildering, and though the nurse may gain some understanding of the needs of various cultural groups in this respect, he or she should always be guided by the bereaved family in this respect. There are several detailed books available to nurses with much information and guidance on the care required by patients and their families immediately before and following death (see Further Reading, Neuberger, 1987; Green and Green, 1992).

POST-MORTEM EXAMINATIONS

Following death an autopsy may be required in certain well-defined situations (Green and Green, 1992, Ch. 6). This is an unenviable prospect for families, but some communities particularly dislike the need for this procedure.

The Autopsy

Christians
No specific objection to the procedure, but the body must be treated with reverence.

Christian Scientists
Unlikely to agree to the procedure unless it is required by law.

Rastafarians
Unlikely to agree to the procedure unless it is required by law.

Buddhists
No specific objection to the procedure, but the body must be treated with reverence.

Baha'is
No specific objection to the procedure, but the body must be treated with reverence.

Jews
Jews prefer to bury the dead very quickly after death. The autopsy is prohibited under Jewish law, and will not be tolerated unless specifically required by law. The Jewish family may find the prospect of a post-mortem examination extremely upsetting. Very thorough explanation of the need for the procedure will be required (Berkovits, 1988).

Muslims
Muslims prefer to bury the dead very quickly after death. The autopsy is prohibited under Jewish law and will not be tolerated unless specifically required under law. The Jewish family may find the prospect of a post mortem examination extremely upsetting. Very thorough explanation of the need for the procedure will be required (Henley, 1982a).

Hindus
No specific objection to the procedure, but the body must be treated with reverence. The Hindu family may well be reluctant to agree to the procedure however (Henley, 1982b).

Sikhs

No specific objection to the procedure, but the body must be treated with reverence. The Sikh family may wish the funeral to take place quickly, and attempts should be made to avoid a post-mortem examination delaying this (McAvoy and Donaldson, 1990).

ORGAN DONATION

Cultural groups and individuals vary in their acceptance of organ donation following a sudden death. Since different views exist even within families, the following notes provide rough guidance only. Only by requesting organ donation can you be sure of the bereaved family's views.

Attitude towards posthumous organ donation

Buddhist
No religious objection to organ donation.

Christian
No religious objection to organ donation.

Jehovah's Witness
Decision a matter for the individual.

Hindu
No religious objection to organ donation.

Sikh
No religious objection to organ donation.

Jewish
No religious objection in principle, but the success of the procedure must be well established. No vital organ may be removed until death is definitely established by the lack of vital signs.

Muslim
Often refused, although recently there has been more willingness to consent.

(Source: Leaflet produced by the UK Transplant Co-ordinators Association (1989) *Organ Donation: religious and cultural issues*.)

RESPONSES TO PARTICULAR MODES OF TREATMENT

There are many cultural or religious groups who may have misgivings about specific modes of treatment. For the Jewish patient whose religion specifically forbids the use of pork products, the need for the use of porcine skin to cover a large skin defect can be difficult to bear. Judaism, like many religions, has a 'Law of Life' (Berkovits, 1988) which states that all laws apart from those related to serious crimes can be ignored if the patient's health or life is at stake. This would ostensibly allow the use of porcine skin without the infringement of Jewish religious law. The patient may, nonetheless, remain very uncertain and dubious, and may well find the opportunity to discuss the matter with his Rabbi helpful.

The Jehovah's Witness patient is prohibited from accepting a blood transfusion, while Muslim or Roman Catholic faiths forbid termination of pregnancy. Needless to say, this does not mean that women from Muslim and Roman Catholic backgrounds never have terminations.

Any misgivings would be revealed in the normal process of obtaining informed consent for the procedure. The current legal position is that when the patient in question is an adult and competent to make a decision then that decision should be respected by health care personnel. The situation is rather less certain when the patient is unconscious and health care workers are required to take what could be life-saving actions without the benefit of being able to discuss the matter with the patient (Dimond, 1985).

CONCLUSION

This chapter has attempted to paint a picture of the diversity of beliefs, values and customs held by humankind, and how these might have an impact on health care personnel, particularly those working in critical care areas. For such an extensive subject the ideas have, by necessity, been explored only superficially. The central message must be that even in our diversity we are similar; to promote common understanding all that is required is a little extra effort and investigation. Such shared understanding can only reduce for the patient and his or her family the terrors and tensions of the modern critical care area and severe life-threatening illness and injury. Thereby, too, critical care nurses can improve their job satisfaction and the quality of the professional service they offer to those in their care.

It should be clear that it is superficial and sometimes potentially dangerous to learn long 'shopping lists' of characteristics of each minority group. This is not to say that you should not read widely to broaden your understanding of people from the variety of cultural backgrounds which you are likely to encounter. To this end, a selection of further reading is provided.

Each patient cared for is an individual, and in order to provide the highest standards of individualized *holistic* care, it is a truism to state that the only way to be truly aware of another person's beliefs is to ask him or her.

STUDENT LEARNING QUESTIONS

After reading this chapter you will find it useful to return to the short case histories found in the boxes in the text, and spend some time considering the important issues in more depth. When doing this try to:

- [ ] think what patient *beliefs*, *values* and *habits* are involved in the patients' (or relatives') reactions;

- [ ] what information or resources the nurse needs to prevent such problems arising;

- [ ] what alternative strategies the nurses might have used had they been better informed.

For each of the case histories, consider if this situation could have happened in the area in which you work. If so, what can you do to prevent such a thing happening?

KEY TERMS

Acculturation

The process of learning one's culture through education and upbringing.

Culture shock

The uncomfortable sensation of being surrounded by a culture which is not one's own and which is difficult to understand.

Enculturation

The process of learning a cultural pattern which is *supplementary* to one's original cultural pattern.

Ethnocentrism

The inability to appreciate another's cultural viewpoint, unconscious use of one's own cultural viewpoint as a benchmark in judging others.

Prejudice

The willingness to treat someone less than fairly or think badly of them on the basis of the person's perceived cultural group membership, often not based on fact or amenable to reason.

Stereotyping

The assumption of cultural characteristics based on group membership, a fixed mental image, may not be based on fact.

Subculture

A group within a group which shares some of the cultural characteristics of the larger group but which also is distinguished by its own particular features.

FURTHER READING

Boyle, J. S., Andrews, M. M. *Transcultural Concepts in Nursing Care*. Scott, Glenview, Illinois: Foresman, 1989.

Brink, P. J. (ed.) *Transcultural Nursing: A book of readings*. Englewood Cliffs, NJ: Prentice-Hall, 1976.

Dobson, S. M. *Transcultural Nursing*. London: Scutari Press, 1991.

Donald, J., Rattansi, A. (eds.) *'Race', Culture and Difference*. London: Sage/Open University Press, 1992.

Giger, J. N., Davidhizar, R. (eds.) *Transcultural Nursing: Assessment and intervention*. St Louis, IL: Mosby-Year Book, 1991.

Green, J., Green, M. *Dealing with Death: Practices and Procedures*. London: Chapman & Hall, 1992.

Helman, G. J. *Culture, Health and Illness. Second edition*. London: Butterworth-Heinemann, 1990.

Mares, P., Henley, A., Baxter, C. *Health Care in Multiracial Britain*. London: Health Education Council/National Extension College, 1985.

(Note: This handbook is designed for health professionals. It is a useful reference and guide to other resources.)

Neuberger, J. *Caring for Dying People of Different Faiths*. London: Austen Cornish, 1987.

Quereshi, B. *Transcultural Medicine: Dealing with patients from different cultures*. Dordrecht: Kluwer Academic, 1989.

REFERENCES

Ashworth, P., Morrison, P. Some ambiguities of the student's rôle in undergraduate nurse training. *Journal of Advanced Nursing*. 1989; 14: 1009–1015.

Baxter, C. Caring for the patient's hair. *Community Outlook*. September 1992; 29–31.

Baxter, C. Observing skin. *Community Outlook*. January 1997; 21–22.

Berkovitz, B. *A Guide to Jewish Practice for Nurses and Medical Staff* (Beth Din Leaflet No. 9). London: Court of the Chief Rabbi, 1988.

Bonaparte, B. H. Ego Defensiveness, open-closed mindedness and nurses' attitude toward culturally different patients. *Nursing Research*. 1979; 28(3): 166–172.

Bradby, M. Status passage into nursing: another view of the socialisation into nursing. *Journal of Advanced Nursing*. 1990; 14: 1220–1225.

Brink, P. J., Saunders, J. M. Cultural shock: theoretical and applied. In Brink, P. J. (ed.). *Transcultural Nursing: A book of readings*. Englewood Cliffs, NJ: Prentice-Hall, 1976.

Burnard, P. Spiritual distress and the nursing response: theoretical considerations and counselling skills. *Journal of Advanced Nursing*. 1987; 12: 377–382.

Burnard, P. The spiritual needs of atheists and agnostics. *Professional Nurse*. 1988; 4(3): 130–132.

Cavillo, E. R., Flaskerud, J. H. Evaluation of the pain response by Mexican American and Anglo American women and their nurses. *Journal of Advanced Nursing*. 1993; 18: 451–459.

Davitz, L. L., Davitz, J. R. *Nurses' Responses to Patients' Suffering*. New York: Springer Verlag, 1980.

Dimond, B. *Legal Aspects of Nursing*. London: Prentice-Hall, 1985.

Durie, M. H. A Maori perspective of health. *Social Science and Medicine*. 1985; 20(5): 483–486.

Ferguson, M. Sickle cell anaemia and its effect on the new parent. *Health Visitor*. 1991; 64(3): 73–76.

Franklin, I. *Sickle Cell Disease: A guide for patients, carers and health workers*. London: Faber & Faber, 1990.

Giger, J. N., Davidhizar, R. (eds.) Transcultural assessment: a method for advanced nursing practice. *International Nursing Review*. 1990; 37(1): 199–201.

Giger, J. N., Davidhizar, R. (eds.) *Transcultural Nursing: Assessment and intervention*. St Louis, IL: Mosby-Year Book, 1991.

Goodchild, M. C., Dodge, J. A. *Cystic Fibrosis: Manual of diagnosis and management. Second edition*. London: Balliere Tindall, 1985.

Green, J., Green, M. *Dealing with Death: Practices and procedures*. London: Chapman & Hall, 1992.

Haigh, H. 'OK?' – Communication across the language barrier. *NATN News*. April/May 1988; 11–15.

Hayward, J. *Information: A prescription against pain.* London: Royal College of Nursing, 1975.

Helman, G. J. *Culture, Health and Illness. Second edition.* London: Butterworth-Heinemann; 1990.

Henley, A. *Caring for Muslims and Their Families: Religious Aspects of Care.* Cambridge: National Extension College/DHSS, 1982a.

Henley, A. *Caring for Hindus and Their Families: Religious Aspects of Care.* Cambridge: National Extension College/DHSS, 1982b.

Karseras, P., Hopkins, E. *British Asians – Health in the community.* London: Wiley; 1977.

Kleinman, A., Eisenberg, L., Good, B. Culture, illness and care: clinical lessons from anthropologic and cross-cultural research. *Annals of Internal Medicine.* 1978; 88: 251–258.

Kluckhohn, F. R. Dominant and variant value orientation. In Brink, P. J. (ed.), *Transcultural Nursing: A book of readings.* Englewood Cliffs: Prentice Hall; NJ: 1976.

Leininger, M. M. Transcultural care. Diversity and universality: a theory for nursing. *Nursing and Health Care.* 1985; 6(4): 209–212.

Leininger, M. M. Leininger's theory of nursing: cultural care, diversity and universality. *Nursing Science Quarterly.* 1988; 1(4): 152–160.

Madjar, I. Pain and the surgical patient: a cross-cultural perspective. *The Australian Journal of Advanced Nursing.* 1985; 2(2): 29–33.

McAvoy, B. R., Donaldson, L. J. *Health Care for Asians.* Oxford: Oxford University Press, 1990.

McCaffery, M. *Nursing the Patient in Pain.* London: Harper & Row, 1983.

Murray, R. B., Zentner, J. D. *Nursing Concepts for Health Promotion.* London: Prentice-Hall, 1989.

Neuberger, J. *Caring for Dying People of Different Faiths.* London: Austen Cornish, 1987.

Parfitt, B. A. Cultural assessment in the intensive care unit. *Intensive Care Nursing.* 1988; 4: 124–127.

Rairdan, B., Higgs, Z. R. When your patient is a Hmong refugee. *American Journal of Nursing.* March 1992; 52–55.

Roper, N., Logan, W., Tierney, A. (eds.) *Using a Model for Nursing.* Edinburgh: Churchill Livingstone 1983.

Rosenbaum, J. N. A cultural assessment guide: learning cultural sensitivity. *Canadian Nurse.* 1991; 87(4): 32–33.

Ruiz, M. C. J. Open-closed mindedness, intolerance of ambiguity and nursing faculty attitudes toward culturally different patients. *Nursing Research.* 1981; 30(3): 177–181.

Sampson, S. *The Neglected Ethic: Religious and cultural factors in the care of patients.* Maidenhead: McGraw-Hill, 1982.

Sofaer. B. *Pain: A handbook for nurses. Second edition.* London: Chapman & Hall, 1992.

Thiedermann, S. B. Ethnocentrism: a barrier to effective health care. *Nurse Practitioner.* 1986; 11(8): 52–59.

United Kingdom Central Council for Nursing, Midwifery and Health Visiting. *Code of Professional Conduct.* London: UKCC, 1992.

Walsh, M., Ford, P. *Nursing Rituals: Research and Rational Actions.* London: Butterworth-Heinemann, 1989.

Zborowski, M. Cultural components in response to pain. *Journal of Social Issues.* 1952; 8: 16–30.

Section 5
CRITICAL CARE AND THE FUTURE

A key challenge of the future will be harnessing the explosion in information technology, which has an increasing impact on our personal and professional lives. This section offers an insightful and stimulating vision of these developments.

19
INFORMATION TECHNOLOGY AND CRITICAL CARE

A view from USA

Nancy Rollins Gantz

"What works for us, intellectually speaking, in one time and circumstance may not for anyone else or at another time. In today's world, and most certainly in tomorrow's, every situation calls for completely novel solutions."

Developing A 21st Century Mind (Sinetar)

CHAPTER AIMS

This chapter will focus on the first line nurse manager who is unfamiliar with computers and desires the basic education and the starting point for computerizing a critical care unit. Throughout the chapter you will see a very strong theme; that hospitals should be actively and thoughtfully moving in this direction to become thoroughly computerized – most especially high acuity, multi-system failure patients in critical care units where information is enormous and time is critical. With the data and sophistication, and the patient outcomes and the shortened length of stays that are upon us, nurses cannot function productively, efficiently or with job satisfaction without having some kind of computerized system that complements their practice and productivity.

The key terms in this chapter are:

- [ ] patient focused;
- [ ] outcome driven;
- [ ] user friendly;
- [ ] constant change;
- [ ] efficiency;
- [ ] health care user involvement;
- [ ] nursing process; and
- [ ] innovation.

INTRODUCTION

As the health care climate continues to be in a constant state of change, so does technology and acute care hospitals within the health care giver environments. In fact, change is happening more quickly in critical care increasing more ethical, legal, outcome-driven, patient-focused and technology-steered decisions having to be made, because of cost containment, government influences, rules and regulations, community involvement with a direction towards patient care satisfaction. The progress that has been demonstrated over the past 25 years at the hospital bedside with computers and advanced technologies has not only advanced the professional practice of nursing, but has put all hospitals, physicians and ancillary staff in a disputable position. This awkwardness has gone beyond what institutions can financially support in advanced technology and critical care procedures.

As a nurse manager, several ramifications become of primary importance and, usually, the least of importance is computerization. As a new manager you must learn the budget, you must learn operations, you must learn personnel, you must learn to mould into the culture of the hospital as well as collaborate with the people that are a part of the hospital. So technology gets pushed back into a corner. This is unfortunate. As a general aim of this chapter, I wish to show that technology needs to be pushed to the front and made a high priority for institutions, after one has their feet on the ground and feels comfortable in the new critical care setting they are in. I also want to show that this chapter is geared at getting physicians involved in computers as well as other ancillary departments. It would be worthless to have a decentralized unit that was computerized if it was not networked into the entire health care system. The hospital as it is would defeat the advantages and capabilities of computerization, i.e. efficiency, productivity and system-wide networking. Physicians are key players in technology and critical care, and they continue to be key players as well, as will administration. As a nurse manager, one of the primary responsibilities in the 21st century is not only to convince but to prove and demonstrate the essential need for computerization in critical care units.

HISTORICAL ISSUES

"Today, the opportunity to affect one of health care's boundary conditions – the information management capabilities in health care – is within our grasp. And it is believed that if enough individuals become embued with this sense of the possible, the reality will emerge." (Dick and Steen, 1991).

Understanding and using computers in critical care is not always a simple task. One must do their homework and become educated to the vast vocabulary, usage and capabilities in the area before they can methodically and with a sense of education implement as well as maintain a computerized system. This chapter is a reflection of the past, and current literature and research that has been contributed to by numerous nursing leaders. This shows the new nurse manager what is essential to the current day and what must be looked at, and their efforts should be concentrated on this rather than on operational duties that one can delegate or leave for later attention. One of the main issues is the nursing process: assessment, planning, implementation and evaluation of a clinical information system in a critical care unit for the new nurse manager who does not have the tools with which to accomplish this task. Through the years we have learned a great deal about selecting different computerized systems, and illustrated in this chapter will be the key points that one must look for when evaluating different systems for your individual hospital.

Tomasik (1988) estimates that more than 15,000 medical devices marketed under about 50,000 different brand names are available for use – nurses are introduced to a new piece of equipment almost every week.

If all nurse managers knew, and those who are very seasoned believed in, computers and pushed to computerize not only critical care units but the entire hospital, they would hurtle a milestone in health care delivery. Our health care delivery system is in great need of change in all countries. But I believe it is essential that the nurse manager be part of this plan and a part of this process, as well as a strong proponent and advocate of computerization. If we do not find ways to streamline our care and make nursing practice more efficient for our clinicians, health care will only continue to get more costly, less efficient and more difficult to provide. Reimbursement can get to the point where we are giving care with practically no resources. If it is done the right way, the nurse manager has a great impact on changing this through computerization.

Historically, physiological monitors in coronary care units and in anaesthesia for operating rooms were the first computerized instruments that we saw in a hospital setting. But over the last 25 years, those very simple, one-channel monitors have become multi-channelled, multi-functioned computerized technology that will essentially give us all the data needed on a critically ill patient who is near the end stage of life.

LITERATURE AND RESEARCH

The literature shows us that computerization has been around for many years. It started as a medical search. It started more so in the operating room where patients could be monitored during surgery for heart rate and respirations. This was done by anaesthesiologists, and then went into coronary care units where they monitored heart rates. The very first critical care units in the world were coronary care units. The computer was a powerful tool. It definitely began to modernize the nursing profession. Computers (bedside monitors) became essential equipment in many hospitals and community health agencies, academic and research centres, and other nursing environments around the world. Thus, computers became a part of a professional nurse's everyday life; and nursing, long recognized as a caring profession, was now digging into the technological areas. They became so engrained that as far as being a part of everyday life, nurses in the critical care environment could not give quality care to their patients. This bedside monitor needed to monitor not only their heart

rate, respirations, oxygen saturations, cardiac output, and pulse rate, but also the many other parameters that would otherwise have to be done manually. Research shows that we have come a long way in the past 25 years, and definitely to nursing's advantage. But, nursing still has a way to go. We have found ways to enable nurses with computers to document and store large volumes of data, to conduct and publish research so as to advance their professional practice, to educate and instruct students about nursing knowledge and skills in the critical care unit, as well as other areas of nursing, and to communicate information throughout the hospital/institution via the computer network.

Computers have also shown us through the literature that we do not look at a computer system as a 'cost savings' per se; rather, we look at it as increasing productivity and efficiency. And when you measure out productivity, productivity is cost, so indirectly, it is a cost saving, but a difficult process to prove to administrators. One must document, through time studies and other methods, that you are actually saving money by having a computerized system. That is why nursing managers and nursing informatic leaders must have a very methodical, well-documented, strategic plan to illustrate the need and the value of a computerized system.

In the past, nursing has focused on designing scientific staffing programmes to produce improvements in productivity in critical care. However, the 20th century gains in that direction will be insignificant to meet the needs faced by hospitals in critical care in the 21st century. Nurse managers must evaluate the quality of critical care in the 21st century, as it is our responsibility to push this forward, as indicated through the literature. There have been many great leaders in the computer field of nursing that have moved nursing to the point we have now reached, which is a sophisticated level. They recognize, also, that we have a great deal further to progress; computer systems need to be implemented rather than 'just talked about'. But it takes more than just one person or more than just one dollar or more than just one action. Through collaborating and educating ourselves as managers, staff, educators and professionals, we can be part of that movement.

PRACTICAL NURSING IMPLICATIONS

Assessment and planning

Strategic planning involves initiative and risk-taking. It is pro-active and directed. Strategic planning includes identifying, formalizing, implementing and evaluating unit plans on an ongoing basis (Gantz-Rollins, 1991).

Nurses spend at least 40–60% of their time charting at the bedside in critical care units, because of the high acuity and intensity of their patients. All that information must be recorded timely and accurately to get to the final outcome – that of giving the patient the quality of care needed and the ability to return to the community. Without monitors linked with a clinical information system, all this vital information has to be documented on paper, which becomes extremely time consuming and costly. In some neo-natal units, nurses spend up to 70% of their time charting, because of the vast measurement details that are needed for the doctors and clinicians to adequately care for critically ill infants. With the nurse shortage still a concern, it will become even more essential that systems in critical care units help make the job easier for fewer people. Nurses hold that key as hospital costs continue to escalate and patients continue to be more critically ill with more multi-faceted and multi-system failure involvement. We must remain aware of the cost of health care and the implications of these for consumers. Bedside computers that monitor physiological data have been around for 25 years. However, computers to generate the information from other technical equipment as well as bedside monitors for critical care are still fairly new. In the early 1980s, people started focusing on this because the acuity of the patients became higher. There were more interventions, more treatments, more procedures on which nurses were required to intervene; and they had less time in which to do those interventions. Coupled with that was a staffing shortage, the shortage of funds within the hospital, and pressure from administration to perform at a highly productive level with limited resources.

Literature still indicates that there is no complete or perfect system which meets the whole clinical technological needs of critical care units. This is in terms of productivity, computer response and flexibility. Different hospitals have their specific wish list, but no one company or conglomerate of organizations has yet developed it. This is an opportunity for managers to collaborate together from all over the world to determine what the specific 'wish list' should be, and then to make that system a reality that also adheres to financial restraints and which demonstrates improved patient outcomes. And then, ideally, this treatment could be modified for each specific hospital with their individual, specific needs.

Research has shown that nurses are taking control and managing computer systems more aggressively than they have in the past. It is the responsibility of the nurse manager to implement a computerized clinical information system in a critical care unit in a methodical, step-by-step process. There are many steps that one must take before implementing such a system. The first step is a commitment to the system and process. This commitment must also be secured from administration as well as the Vice President of Patient Care, the nursing staff and physicians. Without this commitment, figuration will not occur persuasively, and the unit will not achieve its potential in computerization. Therefore, one must present a well-organized, strategically-planned and methodically-driven proposal on how you want to assess, plan for, implement and evaluate a clinical information system, and the elements that are specifically required in the hospital unit. Bring it to administration after it has been presented and approved by the unit and physicians, and demonstrate its number one advantage and quality of increased productivity. The first step, besides your commitment, is involving the entire staff; the medical staff and other ancillary areas that will be using the system, such as respiratory, dietary, social service, pharmacy, billing and admissions. Commitment from these areas is essential, as without that commitment no computerized system will be maximized to its fullest potential.

A task force is then formed. It meets on a regular basis with a specific agenda that relates to the documented strategic plan. The first meeting should be the formation of goals, the mission and the vision, what it is you are out to accomplish by computerizing and bringing a clinical information system into your critical care unit.

Assessment: (Management Focus Group, 1989)

Present demand	Future demand
Define and evaluate present service.	Identify relevant factors.
Identify changes required.	Identify changes in service management.
Plan, implement and monitor change.	Identify changes in service delivery.

Sub-groups can be formed from this main committee to make things flow in a manageable manner and to accomplish the task swiftly. When evaluating a clinical information system, one needs to look at the hospital's culture, philosophy of nursing in critical care and the medical-surgical units, and where the computer would be positioned when interfacing with other departments. This is a critical component for success.

The original computer task force should also be the computer implementation committee, i.e. they should be the ones involved from start to finish in the implementation of the system, to install, orient personnel, and periodically evaluate it to make sure that it is meeting the needs of all the clinical practitioners.

Thomas and colleagues (Donovan and Lewis, 1987) stated, "The concept of culture is an important tool for understanding and changing the behavior of individuals in organizations . . . To relate the two concepts [of culture and climate], when an employee's personal beliefs and values are consistent with the prevailing culture, he tends to perceive the climate as 'good'. However, a perception of a 'poor' climate results when the beliefs and values are in conflict."

The very first event that needs to occur is to bring in the vendors of all the various clinical information systems you have identified that meet the requirements of what kind of system is needed in the specific critical care unit. When identifying those needs, one cannot only identify for today. One must look into the future; and the future cannot be just one or two years from now. The future is five, ten, twenty years down the road. It is estimated that the life of the computer system is seven years. However, the generation of a clinical information system is much longer because of the sophisticated technological support and ongoing, upgraded software. Some of the elements that need to be identified when looking at clinical information systems are:

1. Nursing and physician application.
2. Display performance.
3. Network capability.
4. Mainframe structure (small/large).
5. Software languages.
6. Customization – appreciation for each institution.
7. Implementation process.
8. User friendly.
9. Archiving abilities.
10. Confidentiality/legal issues.
11. Ergonomics.
12. Reliability of system during busy hours as well as slow periods.
13. Responsiveness/speed.
14. Availability of data.
15. Biomedical/institutional support.
16. Vendor support; software upgrades.
17. Researchability and its applications.
18. Cost (as compared to other systems).
19. Interfacing to peripheral devices/HIS systems and other ancillary departments.
20. Development of systemized nursing databases.
21. Potential problems, concerns or 'down' time.
22. Health care applications.
23. Total system analysis. Does it meet requirements?
24. Future capabilities and extension of system.

Traditional Mind

☐ Egocentric frame of reference.

☐ Split-perception; sees the part; confused by paradox; centres on the detail.

☐ Dualistic.

☐ Polarizes and separates; feels disconnected, cut off from, alienated.

☐ Fear motivated.

21st Century – Unitive Mind (Sinetar, 1991)

☐ Synergistic frame of reference.

☐ Whole – seeing: first sees whole (contextually), then understands part; resolves paradox, dichotomies.

☐ Non-dual.

☐ Integrates, unifies (feels itself part of the whole).

☐ Love (people) motivated – agape.

We will now work through the steps that are important and essential in bringing up a clinical information system in the critical care unit so that positive acceptance and usage is obtained by all health care users.

Implementation

The unit's physical structure must be considered to allow adequate space for clinical information systems to interface with computers. You need to look at how they will be mounted; whether you will have your computer system at the end of the bed or at the head of the bed, whether your computer system will be mobile or whether you will use a central station. There are many options available when one evaluates the unit for implementation, and it must be carefully analysed. Along with that analysis, biomedical engineers need to be consulted as they are typically the ones who assist in installation, troubleshoot problems, and repair technological equipment in the critical care setting.

Staff

It is critical that the staff is involved with the implementation of the bedside monitor and clinical information systems. Without this involvement, commitment and ownership will not occur. There are many ways one can go about doing this. One way is through creativity with posters, memos, availability of committee minutes and communicating continually at each staff meeting as to what is happening with the computer implementation committee. One must permit people who are inter-

ested to get involved. Encourage those people who are hesitant to become involved. It is surprising that a lot of nurses are shy about computers. However, once you get them involved they become interested and excited. Often, the people who are most antagonistic toward computerization and bedside monitoring become the advocates once the system is installed and usable. This is true with physicians as well. Ownership of computerization is a key factor. Without this one element that comes through involvement from initial onset of the decision to computerize the unit, the success of the unit's computerization will not be there.

Administration

The support of the administration is essential. Without the financial support there will be no system. Besides financial support, there must be interface between different departments and different ancillary areas. So this support and involvement must also be considered.

Administration is the key to the hospital and the operations of the hospital. They should be dealt with in a very logical and sophisticated manner. A nurse manager should look at them as their support system, and as somewhere they can go for assistance through difficult times, as well as to sort out problems that may occur. If this is not the case in such a hospital, it is the nurse manager's responsibility to attempt to build that trust and relationship between administration and his or her critical care environment.

Biomedical physics

One of the most important departments to a critical care unit is the biomedical physics department and their support. They are a clinically strong support system, knowledgeable and always there when one needs them. When the bedside monitors or the clinical information system has a problem or 'goes down', biomedical engineers come in to correct the problem in an expedient manner. Nurses cannot be expected to know all the various ways to disassemble the monitor or troubleshoot equipment. Therefore, biomedical engineers must be incorporated into critical care units and supported to an extreme manner. So use them to one's best advantage, and involve them in the computer implementation committee, the selection process, and in the demonstration projects of all the various vendors that are available. Value their input, as it is a backbone for clinical technology.

SUMMARY AND CONCLUSIONS

One must find a way to harness computers to help manage the mass of detail and information required to operate a sophisticated critical care unit. One must find a way to use the computer effectively and efficiently as a tool. A tool that will assist us in integrating, evaluating and simplifying care in a cost-effective way, and in assimilating the necessary data while continually using our human skills to make care humanistic.

Society has become very educated to the health care system and their needs and wants when they enter a hospital. And as a professional, one must be able to deliver that quality, outcomes and satisfactions in a cost-driven and 'high touch' manner. Through computerization and the new era of the 21st century, we must demonstrate that this is the most effective and efficient way to provide the quality of patient care that the community is looking for, as well as meet the hospital's mission.

New technology has reduced the cost for treatment for many procedures; however, the overall cost has increased because the total number of treatments has grown dramatically, offsetting any savings. However, this is changing, and it is changing rapidly as the government has actively become involved in health care, and has made a commitment to ensure that costs are reduced. Cost and technology have accelerated the growth in the outpatient market. The hospitals still dominate the outpatient market for many procedures, controlling over 60% of the market, and technology will assist this. The hospital inpatient market, while maintaining stable demand, has lost most of the overall market share due to the high demand of outpatient services. However, nearly half of that lost is offset by a shift to hospital outpatient services. The sickest patients will be in the hospital beds, and thus technology and computerization becomes essential.

By almost any estimation, computerized patient clinical records will be an important feature of all reformed health care delivery systems, drawing patient data currently scattered among various providers into an integrated format that is concentrated into useful information (see Figure 19.1).

The concept of community care networks or accountable health plans means we need to start working with our collaborative partners to better share information. "You can't transport a hard copy patient record from a clinic to a hospital, especially when the two organizations may be different entities," says William Reed, Vice President of Operations and Chief Information Officer at Geisinger System Services, Danville, Pennsylvania, USA.

Despite the increased optimism over computerized records, survey respondents show some lingering concerns: technology issues, financing, hospital strategy issues, and government policies and laws. Many observers say that scanning the current paper record is not a viable option, and would only slow down storage capabilities and automate currently inefficient processes. Advocation for the use of information technology to help change the process of manual patient care charting practices is extremely strong and valid.

What we can do in the meantime is start to integrate some of the clinical information that is floating around all our isolated systems. In fact, 40% of hospitals plan to follow that strategy over the next two years, saying their top priority is to enable information sharing across departmental lines. More generally, eight out of ten hospitals agree that President Clinton's reform plan will accelerate the advancement of information technology, and half of them say expand greatly. What will happen is that we will see a completely different focus on what kind of information is needed in an acute care hospital, and what we will be using.

In the past, hospitals have been revenue, procedure and visit driven; and in future, it will be outcome driven, clinical protocol driven, and patient satisfaction driven. Like many of our colleagues, we are concerned about whether federal fiscal policies will recognize the substantial information technology investments that assist and complement health care. Over the coming fiscal year, hospitals should expect to roughly double

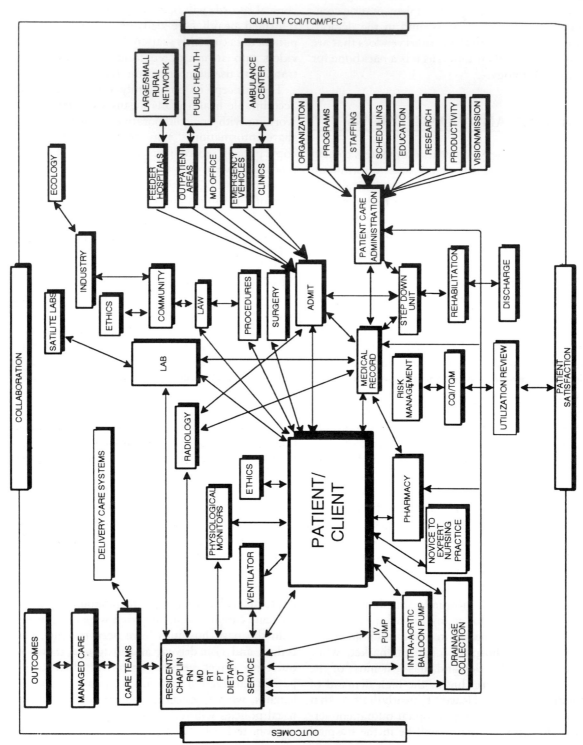

Figure 19.1.   Health care information flow (in reality).

their capital information technology budgets – a figure that will approach $4 million – although the budgeting process is not completed at the time of writing. About half that amount is slated for fibre optic infrastructure improvements, which will carry computerized records between entities. Although most hospitals feel information technology budgets for clinical information systems will increase somewhat or substantially over the next two years, that is not felt by all. This is where one as a nursing practitioner can have great influence and impact.

STUDENT LEARNING QUESTIONS

1. What *components* are critical and which are not when selecting a clinical information system or computer system?

2. *Who* should be involved in the selection process of a computerized system, and *why* should these people be involved?

3. Is cost the driving force behind implementing a computerized clinical information system in an acute care hospital?

4. Why have computers taken so long to get to the point they are today?

5. What responsibility do we as professionals, whether our role is in a management, staff or education role, have when it comes to clinical information systems?

KEY TERMS

Artificial intelligence

A term used to describe the use of computers in such a way that they perform operations analogous to the human abilities of learning and decision taking. Often used to embrace expert systems, knowledge-based systems and decision support systems, although strictly speaking, neither of these requires a learning ability.

Audit trail

A record of processes and events relating to a specific record, transaction or file. In a computer system, the trail will be stored as a file and is created during the routine processing of data as a separate activity, thus allowing the system to be audited, or subsequent reconstitution of files.

CD ROM

A compact disk read-only memory: a storage device using optical laser storage techniques.

Customizing

The modification of a standard hardware or software product to meet the needs of a specific user.

Data

A general expression used to describe any group of operands or factors consisting of numbers, alphabetic characters or symbols which denote any condition, value or state, e.g. all values and descriptive data operated on by a computer program, but not the program itself. The word data is used as a collective noun, and is usually accompanied by a singular verb: 'data are' may be pedantically correct but is awkward to say and therefore awkward to understand. Data is sometimes contrasted with information, which is said to result from the processing of data, so that information derives from the assembly, analysis or summarizing of data into a meaningful form.

Expert system

A means of making available to non-experts a data base of expert knowledge as, for example, in initial diagnosis of medical ailments or comparison of legal precedent. Expert systems differ from decision support systems (pre-defined rules), knowledge-based systems (knowledge but no expertise), and artificial intelligence systems (using methods of reasoning similar to human thought).

Informatics

The science or art of processing data to provide information.

Information technology

A portmanteau phrase to cover all aspects of the art of science of processing data to produce information.

Interface

This term is used to refer to the channels and associated control circuitry providing the connection between a central processor and its peripheral units. It may be used more generally to refer to the connection between any two units.

Local area network

A network designed to provide facilities for inter-user communication within a single geographical location. It does not use public facilities or standards. Contrasted with wide area network.

Management information system

A system which may perform routine commercial processing functions, but which is designed so that such processing will also produce information that will be presented to management, including top management, to assist in decision making. The implication is that the results will be produced speedily, perhaps requiring real-time processing to enable management to ascertain the progress of the organization in terms of satisfying its major objectives.

Network

A series of interconnected elements which form an overall system or structure. Examples of the use of this term include: (i) Network database: a database structure in which elements are not organized in set records on files, but one in which related data elements are linked by pointers. Thus, any desired record or file can be created by following pointers and assembling records to contain relevant data elements. (ii) Communications network: a system of computer devices (nodes) interconnected by communications circuits to permit files, transactions and data to be interchanged to fulfil the information and data processing needs of a community or business organization. (iii) Event network: in critical path analysis, a computer model or diagram which represents the relationship between various activities which must be completed to fulfill a given task.

Update

To apply transactions to a data file in order to amend, add, or delete records and thus ensure that the file reflects the latest situation.

User

1. A general term for any individual or group ultimately making use of the output from a computer system. 2. In an operating system, an invididual exercising control over, or using, a particular resource.

FURTHER READING

Ball, M. J., Douglas, J. V., O'Desky, R. I., Albright, J. W. *Health Care Information Management Systems*. New York: Springer-Verlag, 1991.

Ball, M. J., Hannah, K. J., Gerdin Jelger, V., Peterson, H. *Nursing Informatics – Where Caring and Technology Meet*. New York: Springer-Verlag, 1988.

Birdsal, C. *Management Issues in Critical Care*. St. Louis: Mosby Year Book, 1991.

Bleich, M. R., Bratton, J. M. *Information Management and Computers*. Baltimore: Williams & Wilkins, 1990.

Boyer, A. W. *Computer Information Systems: An Introduction*. Cincinati: South-Western Publishing Co., 1983.

Brimm, J. E. Computers in critical care. *Critical Care Nursing Quarterly*. 1987; 9(4): 53.

Coile Russell, C. *The New Hospital*. Maryland: Aspen Publishers, 1986.

Dick, R. S., Steen, E. B. *The Computer-Based Patient Record*. Washington, DC: National Academy Press, 1991.

Drucker, P. F. *Managing for the Future*. New York: Truman Talley Books, 1992.

Duff, I. Street Smarts in Hospital Purchasing. *Journal of Cardiovascular Nursing*. 1989; 2(2): 4.

Groom, S. Automation of the Medical Chart. *Computers in Health Care*. 1987; 8(14): 22.

Hammer, M., Champy, J. *Re-engineering The Corporation*. New York: Harper Business, 1993.

Hayne, A. N., Bailey, Z. W. *Nursing Administration of Critical Care*. Maryland: Aspen Publication, 1982.

Herzlinger, R. E. *Creating New Health Care Ventures – The Role of Management*. Maryland: Aspen Publication, 1992.

Inlander, C. B., Morales, K. *Getting the Most For Your Medical Dollar*. New York: Wings Book, 1991.

Inlander, C. B., Weiner, E. *Take This Book to The Hospital With You*. New York: Wings Books, 1993.

Kennedy, P. *Preparing For The Twenty-First Century*. New York: Random House, 1993.

Malia, F. M. Caring in a technologic age: Education for adaptation. *Focus on Critical Care*. 1987; 14(3): 21.

Miller, J. B. *The Corporate Coach*. New York: St. Martin's Press, 1993.

Saba, V. K., McCormick, K. A. *Essentials of Computers for Nurses*. Philadelphia: J. B. Lippincott, 1986.

Saba, V. K., Rieder, K. A., Pocklington, D. B. *Nursing and Computers: An Anthology*. New York: Springer-Verlag, 1989.

Seuss. *Oh, The Places You'll Go!* New York: Random House, 1990.

Simms, L. M., Price, S. A., Ervin, N. E. *The Professional Practice of Nursing Administration*. New York: Wiley, 1985.

Snook, I. S. *Hospitals – What They Are and How They Work*. Maryland: Aspen Publication, 1992.

Staggers, N. Using computers in nursing. *Computers in Nursing*. 1988; 6(4): 164.

Stefan Chik, M. F. Point-of-care information systems: Prioritizing bedside applications. *Computers in Health Care*. 1987; 8(4): 42.

Taylor, P. L. (Ed.). How computers are improving patient care. *Health Technology*. 1988; 2(6): 224.

Templeton, J. M. *Looking Forward – The Next Forty Years*. New York: Harper Business, 1993.

REFERENCES

Dick, R. S., Steen, E. G. (Eds.). *The Computer-Based Patient Record*. Washington, DC: National Academy Press, 1991. (Committee on Improving the Patient Record Division of Health Care Services, Institute of Medicine.)

Donovan, M., Lewis, G. Increasing productivity and decreasing costs: The value of RN's. *Journal of Nursing Administration*. 1987; 17(9).

Gantz-Rollins, N. J. In Ed. C. Birdsall. *Management Issues in Critical Care*. St. Louis: Mosby, 1991, p. 268.

Management Focus Group. *Key Managing Issues for Health Care – A Monograph*. Birmingham: Management Focus Group, 1989.

Sinetar, M. *Developing a 21st Century Mind*. New York: Ballantine Books, 1991.

Tomasik, K. QA update: Nursing and technology. *Quarterly Review Bulletin*. 1988; 14(8): 254.

Index